Better Patient Care
Through
Nursing Research

Better Patient Care
Through
Nursing Research

Second Edition

FAYE G. ABDELLAH,
R.N., Ed.D., Sc.D., LL.D., F.A.A.N.

Assistant Surgeon General
Chief Nurse Officer, U.S. Public Health Service
Department of Health, Education, and Welfare
Washington, D.C.

EUGENE LEVINE, Ph.D.

Deputy Director, Division of Manpower Analysis
Public Health Service, Department of Health, Education.
and Welfare, Washington, D.C.

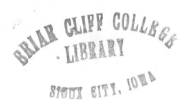
Macmillan Publishing Co., Inc.
NEW YORK

Collier Macmillan Publishers
LONDON

Macmillan Publishing Co., Inc.
866 Third Avenue, New York, New York 10022

Collier Macmillan Canada, Ltd.

Library of Congress Cataloging in Publication Data

Abdellah, Faye G.
    Better patient care through nursing research.

    Bibliography: p.
    Includes indexes.
    1. Nursing—Research.   I.   Levine, Eugene, joint author.   II.   Title.
RT81.5.A25   1979   610.73'07'2   78–15701
ISBN 0–02–300110–0

    Printing: 2 3 4 5 6 7 8   Year: 9 0 1 2 3 4 5

PREFACE

THIS BOOK is the product of our twenty-five years of experience in nursing research. As we have struggled to develop tools for research and to describe how to use them in manuals, articles in professional journals, and workshop reports, we have had to deal with the many conceptual and analytical principles of research presented in this book. In executing a large variety of studies in the nursing field we have had to put these principles into practice. Whatever values this book may have for the reader have resulted from these years of experience and the stimulation we have received from research workshops, seminars, university teaching, and from our colleagues in both federal and nonfederal agencies.

This book appears at a time when research in nursing is emerging as a defined area of research. Research undertaken in the next decade can shape the direction of nursing for many years to come. For this reason we feel it important to present in one volume the basic concepts of research in nursing, particularly those concerned with health care. No attempt is made to present an all-inclusive work on research but rather to provide the reader with an overview of what is involved in the research process.

Although literature on the methodology and content of research is available, we believe that this book will fill the need for a presentation of how some of the important methodological tools can be applied to problems that are uniquely those of nursing. Throughout the book, many examples of the application of the methods of research to nursing and health care situations are presented. Focus is placed upon the discipline of nursing because of its generic base. Hundreds of actual studies undertaken in the nursing area and related health fields are cited as illustrative material throughout the book.

The orientation of the book is predominantly practical. Although theoretical concepts are introduced from time to time, the attempt is to explain these in down-to-earth language and to show their application to actual research situations. The book is liberally sprinkled with such "how-to-do-it" aids to the understanding of the research process as:

> Selecting a topic for research
> Determining when to carry out a research project
> Searching the literature for pertinent material

v

Writing the protocols for a research project
Selecting the appropriate research design
Deciding when to use an experimental design
Controlling the effects of extraneous factors in the study
Defining and scaling the variables to be studied
Collecting needed data
Computing the major summary measures and calculating
    tests of significance
Interpreting the findings of the research

This book is divided into four parts. Part I serves as a general introduction to research in nursing. The history of nursing research is traced, the influences of the physical and social sciences on research in nursing are discussed, an analysis of the question—what is research—is presented, and the role of theories and models in research is examined.

Part II presents a thorough description of research methodology, beginning with the way in which research problems are formulated, moving through all the major steps in the research process, and concluding with how to interpret and communicate the findings of a study.

Part III contains a discussion of the methodology and findings of numerous research projects in nursing, many unpublished and never before available in the literature. These are systematically grouped according to their major purpose and method.

Part IV reviews the present status of nursing research and suggests areas and specific projects for further research. The role of the federal government and the foundations in stimulating and supporting research is also discussed.

This book has been developed in such a way as to meet the needs of the users of research—administrators, teachers, practitioners—as well as the doers of research and students who are preparing themselves to undertake research. Research users might find particularly helpful the material dealing with what is research, the past, present, and future course of nursing research, and the case studies of completed research in nursing. Researchers might find useful the systematic review of research tools, the presentation of some of the newer research concepts and tools, and the discussion in Chapters 10 and 15 of what we have called "research tactics" —the administrative and financial matters that have to be considered in undertaking research. For the student, all chapters in the book should contain something of value. Particularly geared to the student are such features as the problems for further study at the end of each chapter in the first three parts of the book, an extensive glossary of important terms at the end of the book, and a bibliography of relevant research literature that has been indexed to provide easy reference to research topics.

In undertaking this book and at various stages in its preparation, we have asked ourselves what value we think it will have for its readers. We feel we can summarize our answer as follows:

First is its comprehensiveness. We have attempted to put together into one volume all of the basic material that can be of use to those interested in nursing research. Thus, we have included such topics as conceptualization in research, quantification of variables, and interpretation of data, which are either omitted or treated very lightly in other works. In attempting to achieve comprehensiveness, we have risked the possibility of treating some subjects superficially. We hope the many references to the literature on topics deserving further study will alleviate this.

Second is its uniqueness. We have included a considerable amount of material not available elsewhere. This includes a typology for nursing research, analyses of many unpublished studies, a presentation of theories and models of use in nursing, and the bringing together in one place of the major efforts that have been undertaken to develop new methodologies for nursing such as measures of patients' needs for care, criteria of patient welfare, and administrative measures of the effectiveness of nursing service. Another unique feature is the presentation of nearly 200 problems that we hope will be of special help to teachers and students in provoking thoughtful discussion and stimulating further study.

Third, we have attempted to incorporate all of the latest approaches and ideas in research methodology, including the use of models and theories, controls in experimental design, methods of scaling quantitative and qualitative variables, complex types of sampling plans such as cluster and sequential sampling, and Bayesian inference.

Fourth, we have attempted to come to grips with some of the thorny questions that have frequently troubled researchers in developing and conducting a study. We are hopeful that this book will shed some light on the following questions:

How can I decide if I should undertake a research project?
How can a theory be helpful to research?
How can I find out what other researchers in the field have done?
How can I make my research problem more specific?
What kind of research design shall I use?
How many subjects do I need to include in my study?
What does a test of statistical significance really do?
Should I use a parametric or nonparametric test of significance?
How can I control bias and error in my research?
What does a random sample really mean?
What are the best ways of collecting and tabulating the data?
How can I interpret the findings of my study to maximize their practical significance?
How can I determine the budget and personnel needed for my research?
What are some sources of financial support for nursing research?

The authors are aware that a work of this magnitude contains limitations. We take complete responsibility for any errors of commission or omission this book may possess.

We would be quite remiss if we did not acknowledge the many individuals who over the past years have influenced our thinking in this area. It is impossible to acknowledge all those individuals by name and to them individually and collectively we wish to express our gratitude.

FAYE G. ABDELLAH
EUGENE LEVINE

ACKNOWLEDGMENTS

Grateful acknowledgment is made to the following for the use of copyrighted materials:

Addison-Wesley Publishing Company for permission to quote from *Probability with Statistical Applications*, by Frederick Mosteller, 1961, p. 146.

American Journal of Public Health for the quotations from "Patient Care Research: Report of a Symposium," by Ruth Freeman *et al.*, **56**:965–969, June 1963; and from "Matching in Analytical Studies," by William G. Cochran, **43**:684–691, June 1953.

American Sociological Review and the authors for the quotations from "Models and Theory Construction," by James M. Beshers, **22**:32–38, February 1957; "Randomization and Inference in Sociological Research," by Robert McGinnis, **23**:42, August 1958; "Confidence Intervals for Clustered Samples," by Leslie Kish, **22**:154–165, April 1957; and "A Critique of Tests of Significance in Survey Research," by Hanan C. Selvin, **22**:519–527, October 1957.

American Journal of Nursing for quotation from "Reflections on Nursing Research," by Rozella M. Schlotfeldt, **60**:494, April 1960.

American Nurses' Foundation, Inc., for permission to quote from *Content and Dynamics of Home Visits of Public Health Nurses, Part I*, by Walter L. Johnson and Clara A. Hardin, 1962 and to reprint the "Classification System of Topics," p. 51.

Appleton-Century-Crofts (Meredith Publishing Company) for permission to quote from *Nursing Research: A Survey and Assessment*, by Leo W. Simmons and Virginia Henderson, 1964, pp. 71 and 72.

Florida State Board of Health and the author for permission to reprint tables from *Epidemiology of Polio Vaccine Acceptance*, by A. J. Johnson *et al.*, Monograph No. 3, 1962, p. 35.

G. P. Putnam's Sons for permission to quote from *Interpersonal Relations in Nursing*, by Hildegard E. Peplau, 1952, p. 132.

Harcourt, Brace and World, Inc., for permission to reprint quotations from *An Introduction to Logic and Scientific Method*, by Morris R. Cohen and Ernest Nagel, copyright 1934, by Harcourt, Brace and World, Inc., © 1962, by Ernest Nagel and Lenora Cohen Rosenfield, pp. 199, 200, 248, 263, and 289.

Holt, Rinehart and Winston, Inc., for permission to quote from *Research Methods in Social Relations*, by Claire Selltiz *et al.*, 1962, pp. 435, 481, and 196–197; and from *Research Methods in the Behavioral Sciences* by Leon Festinger and David Katz, eds., 1953: "Experiments in Field Settings," by J. R.

P. French, Jr., p. 101 and "Problems of Objective Observation," by Helen Peak, p. 256.

Hospitals, J.A.H.A. for permission to quote from "A Critical Incident Study of Hospital Medication Errors," by Miriam A. Safren, **34**:62, 64, May 1, 1960; and to print Figure 1, "Patient Condition Questionnaire to Be Completed by Head Nurse," from "Effective Use of Nursing Resources: A Research Report," by Robert J. Connor *et al.*, **35**:34, May 1, 1961.

Institute of Industrial Relations, University of California, Los Angeles, for a selection from *Tenderness and Techniques: Nursing Values in Transition* by Genevieve R. Meyer, 1960, p. 13.

Journal of the American Statistical Association and the author for permission to quote from "Sampling in a Nut-Shell," by Morris J. Slonim, **52**:143–161, June 1957; and "Statistics and Science," by E. J. G. Pitman, **52**:323, September 1957.

McGraw-Hill Book Company for permission to print material from *From Dream to Discovery: On Being a Scientist,* by Hans Selye, 1964, pp. 40 and 280.

Milbank Memorial Fund Quarterly for permission to quote from "Research Techniques in the Study of Human Beings," by William G. Cochran, **3**:125, April 1955.

National League for Nursing for permission to reprint Exhibits 5 and 6 from *A Study of Pediatric Nursing,* by the National League of Nursing Education, 1947, p. 98.

Nursing Outlook, for permission to quote from "The Nature of a Science of Nursing," by Dorothy E. Johnson, **7**:292, May 1959.

Nursing Research for permission to reprint or cite several studies reported in the journal from 1957 to 1964.

Psychological Bulletin for permission to quote from "Factors Relevant to the Validity of Experiments in Social Settings," by Donald T. Campbell, **54**:297–312, 1957.

Science for permission to quote from "Statistics—Servant of All Sciences," by J. Neyman, **122**:401, September 2, 1955.

The American Nurses' Association for permission to cite and excerpt the clinical papers originally presented at the Clinical Sessions, 1962, A.N.A. Convention monographs 1, 2, 3, 5, 9, 10, 11, 14, 17, 19, 20, 21; Clinical Sessions, 1964, A.N.A. Convention monograph 3.

The American Psychologist for permission to quote from the article "Gradualness, Gradualness, Gradualness," by Robert S. Morison, **15**:193, March 1960.

Queens College, of the City of New York for permission to reproduce excerpts of some of the instruments from "Employer Expectations vs. Staff Nurse Performance," by Emma Spaney and Ruth V. Matheney, 1962.

The Journal of the Kentucky Medical Association and the author for permission to quote from "An Approach to Health Problems in Kentucky," by R. K. Noback, **56**:33–37, January 1958.

The Journal of Nursing Education and the author for permission to reprint an excerpt of the "Luther Hospital Sentence Completions Form," from the article "A Method for Evaluating the Attitudes of Prospective Nursing Students," **2**:2, May–June 1963.

The New Yorker Magazine for permission to quote from the article, "Center of a New World," by Christopher Rand, pp. 58, 60, April 18, 1964.

The Saturday Evening Post for permission to quote from the article "Why Philosophy?" by Susanne K. Langer, **234**:19–35, May 13, 1961.

The Saturday Review for permission to quote from "Through Happiness with Slide Rule and Calipers," by Joseph Wood Krutch, p. 14, Nov. 2, 1963.

W. B. Saunders Company for permission to use material from *Elementary Medical Statistics* by Donald Mainland, 1963, pp. 17 and 95.

The authors also are indebted to the many principal investigators who gave us permission to cite their materials. These are: Rena E. Boyle, Martha Brown, Dr. W. D. Bryant, Mildred A. Disbrow, Dr. Amasa B. Ford, Professor Gerald J. Griffin, Dr. Ann M. Hart, Dr. Donald P. Hayes, Dr. Marjorie J. Hook, Professor Dorothy E. Johnson, Dr. Marguerite E. Kakosh, Dr. Lawrence C. Meltzer, S. J. Miller, Dr. Mary K. Mullane, Ester C. Pfab, Frances Reiter, Dr. Frieda I. Shirk, Professor Howard E. Wooden.

CONTENTS

1

INTRODUCTION TO NURSING RESEARCH

This part of the book is intended to provide an introduction to research in nursing, particularly an understanding of the setting in which research in nursing is developing.

Chapter 1 explores the many factors that have contributed to the present stage of development of nursing research. Some of these factors have had a major influence on the direction that nursing research is taking. Also included is a historical resumé of milestones in nursing research.

Chapter 2 focuses upon a discussion of the need for research and the role of the nurse as a researcher, particularly as a member of an inter-disciplinary team.

Much, if not all, of nursing research is dependent upon the contributions of the life sciences and the social sciences. Examples of how some of these concepts have relevancy for nursing are discussed.

Chapter 3 clarifies some of the basic concepts about research. Before one can undertake research it is important to understand the concepts. What is research is discussed in detail. What research can and cannot do is explored.

Chapter 4 presents various approaches to placing nursing research within a framework of theory. Examples of theoretical approaches used by other disciplines are considered.

Chapter One

EVOLVEMENT OF NURSING RESEARCH

NURSING RESEARCH may be thought to be a systematic, detailed attempt to discover or confirm the facts that relate to a specific problem or problems. It has as its goal the provision of scientific knowledge. The use of the scientific method and a scientific attitude is indicative of progress in research.

NURSING RESEARCH—ITS ROOTS

The tremendous growth and interest in nursing research during the past decade are remarkable when one considers that the first organized and continuing effort to do studies of nursing problems on a national basis was in 1949 when the Division of Nursing Resources of the U.S. Public Health Service was established to carry out research and consultation in nursing.[1]* In spite of Florence Nightingale's pioneering efforts to do research in the health field, professional nurses did not pursue research of nursing practice to any great extent during the quarter century after her death (1910–1935). Nurses have been preoccupied with pressures of hospital expansion, development of health agencies, and increasing demands for nursing services. The nursing profession's organized efforts were toward the improvement of the nurse practitioner and nurse educator and not in the preparation of the nurse scholar nor the nurse investigator in research. The study of nursing practice itself and the study of the art and science underlying the practice of nursing are only beginning to be recognized as "musts" for the profession.

The lack of a formal mechanism by the professional organizations for carrying out research during this period, such as the American Nurses' Foundation, later established in 1955,[2] did not deter individual nurses

---

* The Division of Nursing was organized in 1960 and combined the Division of Nursing Resources and the Division of Public Health Nursing. The Division encompasses both intramural and extramural research programs.

from carrying out projects of their own in which they sought to find new knowledge about nursing.

The National League for Nursing has had a notable history in pioneering in initiating and conducting studies in nursing since 1952. The former National League for Nursing Education through its study unit established in 1930 ". . . developed record forms for basic schools of nursing, a comprehensive record system, a national testing service, a method for collecting and dissemination of basic school data, and established criteria for both a hospital nursing service and schools of nursing."[3]

Since 1912, the then National Organization for Public Health Nursing kept census data about the distribution and preparation of public health nurses by official and nonofficial public health agencies. This was later continued by the United States Public Health Service. Analyzing cost of service and education in public health nursing agencies was one of the first methodological studies to be developed in nursing.

To seek out the roots of nursing research one would need to study the time period spanning the years 1900–1964. That great nurse scholar and historian Mary M. Roberts in her major contribution to the profession, *American Nursing, History and Interpretation,* has unfolded a dramatic period in nursing, particularly in nursing research.[4] It is not the purpose of the authors to make an assessment of nursing research during this period, but one cannot discuss current research without looking at some of the major milestones and pioneering efforts in nursing research. Only a few of these major contributions have been highlighted in the following paragraphs:

1920   A comprehensive hospital and health survey was carried out by Josephine Goldmark under the direction of Dr. Haven Emerson.[5] This study identified the many inadequacies of housing for student nurses and the paucity of instructional facilities.

1922   The first recorded time study of institutional nursing was released by the New York Academy of Medicine.[6] This was a report of the nursing section's survey of New York hospitals. Significant findings of the survey indicated wide discrepancies in practice such as physicians writing multiple orders for patients beyond a point that they could be carried out effectively by adequate nursing personnel. Likewise, at the time of the study there were 52 schools of nursing in the New York area for which no evidence could be shown regarding the cost of nursing education and nursing service. During this same year, at an annual meeting of the National League of Nursing Education an initial effort was made to look at the cost of nursing education.[7]

1923   A milestone in nursing education was reached by a comprehensive study of nursing education made by the Committee for the Study of Nursing Education.[8] This was a classic study in nursing research in that it was the first representative study of schools of nursing and public health agencies with firsthand observation of nurses at work as public health nurses, as teachers, and as administrators. Many of the recommendations of this committee are still to be achieved. A major recommendation was that the hospital should be so supported that it is independent of the school for its permanent nursing staff, and the school in turn must be able to maintain an independent education program. This study provided a method for carrying out large-scale representative studies which was subsequently used in carrying out national nursing surveys. The final report, entitled *Nursing and Nursing Education in the United States,* was published in 1923.

1923   The Yale University School of Nursing, established in 1923, was to grant its first bachelor's degrees to two graduates of the school three years later.[9] University education was thus forging the way to prepare nursing leaders who were scientifically and culturally prepared. Vanderbilt University School of Nursing (1925) and the Western Reserve University School of Nursing (1923), also endowed institutions, were to pioneer in many experiments in nursing education. These three programs carried on the pioneering efforts initiated in 1899 when the first step toward university recognition of the nurse's need for higher education was undertaken by Teachers College, Columbia University, and later in 1910 when the University of Minnesota established the first basic school of nursing to become a part of a university system.

1926   The Committee on the Grading of Nursing Schools appointed May Ayres Burgess to direct a monumental study extending over an eight-year period.[10, 11] The broad function of the committee was to study ways and means for insuring an ample supply of nursing service at a level essential for the adequate care of the patient. The study encompassed three major projects. The first was directed at the supply and demand for nursing service; the second a job analysis; and the third the grading of nursing schools. The first project was reported in the now classic publication *Nurses, Patients, and Pocketbooks.*[12] The findings are still meaningful today in that in spite of more nurses in practice there are still too few qualified to meet the many demands.

1934   The second project of the Committee on the Grading of Nursing Schools was reported in the publication *An Activity Analysis of Nursing.*[13]

The third project, the grading of nursing schools, utilized a survey approach in which each participating school was graded on each item, in relation to all other schools in 1929 and in 1932.[14] Statistically this project was sound, but the interpretation of the data required a great deal of additional review and study. Consequently, the schools were not classified. This was not to become a realization until 1950 with the establishment of the National Nursing Accrediting Service.

1935   ANA first published *Some Facts About Nursing: A Handbook for Speakers and Others,* which published yearly compilations of statistical data about registered nurses.

1938   Economic security was under scrutiny by the American Nurses' Association, which conducted a study of incomes, salaries, and employment conditions of nurses (exclusive of public health nurses).

1940   A major breakthrough in providing basic information about the cost of nursing service and nursing education was made by Pfefferkorn and

Rovetta.[15] An earlier study by the Committee on the Costs of Medical Care provided a series of factual reports on the overall costs of medical care, including nursing service.[16]

1941 The United States Public Health Service conducted a national census of nursing resources in cooperation with state nurses' associations.

1943 The National Organization of Public Health Nursing made a survey of needs and resources for home care in 16 communities. This was reported in *Public Health Nursing Care of the Sick*.

1948 The Brown report, scholarly and objective, brought to a focal point many of the issues facing nursing education and nursing services for the past half century.[17] The recommendations put forth in this report spearheaded many of the research studies that were to be carried out in the next ten years. Studies of in-service education, nursing functions, nursing teams, practical nurses, role and attitude studies, the nurse technician, nurse-patient relationships, hospital environment, economic security, are examples of the studies that were to find their roots in the recommendations of the Brown report.

Nursing Schools at the Mid-Century, a report of the National Committee for the Improvement of Nursing Services, was a direct effort on the part of the committee to implement some of the recommendations of the Brown report.[18] An Interim Classification of Schools of Nursing Offering Basic Programs (1949) was prepared, which classified the schools in Class I, II, III, according to criteria for judging a good school. *Nursing Schools at the Mid-Century* provided a factual report of the basic nursing schools. The National Nursing Accrediting Service (1950) under Dr. Helen Nahm's able direction was to take on the major task of establishing a sound system for accrediting schools of nursing.

1948 The Division of Nursing Resources (now the Division of Nursing), U.S. Public Health Service, pioneered in carrying out statewide surveys and developing manuals and tools for nursing research.[19]

1949 ANA conducted its first national inventory of Professional Registered Nurses in the United States and the territories of Alaska, Hawaii, and Puerto Rico. The seventh inventory will be published in 1979. Inventory data are also reported in *Facts About Nursing*.

1952 The professional organization's first official journal for the reporting of studies related to nursing and health research was published in June 1952. The journal was named *Nursing Research* and pioneered in reporting studies significant to furthering nursing research. One of its main functions was to provide a means for the investigator to communicate ongoing research.

1953 Under the leadership of a social anthropologist, Dr. Leo Simmons, and a renowned expert nurse teacher and practitioner, Virginia Henderson, a survey and assessment of nursing research was initiated by the National Committee for the Improvement of Nursing Services, under the auspices of Yale University. A major purpose of the Yale survey was to find, classify, and evaluate the research in nursing during the past decade.[20]

The establishment of the Institute of Research and Service in Nursing Education, Teachers College, Columbia University, under the able leadership of its first director, Dr. Helen Bunge, marked another major milestone for nursing research. This was the first formalized mechanism within a university to carry out nursing research. The institute had three main purposes, aimed at strengthening and improving education for nursing through research by: (1) conducting research on selected problems in nursing and nursing education; (2) disseminating the results of the research undertaken by the institute; and (3) assisting in the preparation of nurses for the conduct of research in nursing.

1954   ANA Committee on Research and Studies established to plan, promote, and guide research and studies relating to the functions of the Association. It existed for 16 years and published the *ANA Blueprint for Research in Nursing* (1962), and *The Nurse in Research: ANA Guidelines in Ethical Values* (1968).

1955   The American Nurses' Foundation, a center for research, supported mainly by the American Nurses' Association was established. It serves as a receiver and administrator of funds and as a donor of grants for research in nursing. The foundation also conducts its own programs of research in nursing and provides its own consultation services to nursing students, research facilities, and others engaged in nursing research.[21]

Studies sponsored by the American Nurses' Foundation and the American Nurses' Association (1950–1957) appeared in *Twenty Thousand Nurses Tell Their Story*.[22] This, too, was a milestone for nursing research and marked a major achievement in reporting 34 studies dealing with such areas as nursing functions, job satisfaction, role, and attitude. Several of the recommendations of the Brown report (1948) were achieved by the completion and reporting of these studies.

In 1961 ANF assumed the responsibility for an Abstracting Service, and from 1962 to 1974 the service was a part of the Foundation's programs. Susan D. Taylor developed the system and made use of volunteer abstractors. The abstracts were designed to make information about the results of research readily available.

1955   The Nursing Research Grants and Fellowship Programs of the Division of Nursing of the U.S. Public Health Service were established to stimulate and provide financial support for research investigators and research training in nursing. The P.H.S. act authorizing the extramural grant and award programs provides that the Surgeon General of the P.H.S. shall encourage and render assistance to appropriate public authorities, scientific institutions, and scientists in the conduct and coordination of research related to the cause, diagnosis, treatment, control, and prevention of physical and mental diseases.[23]

1957   Nursing research gained still greater impetus by the establishment of the Department of Nursing in the Walter Reed Army Institute of Research. The institute has two main objectives—namely, to evolve a program of military nursing research projects that are patient care oriented, and to evolve and implement a program to develop a small core of competent nurse practitioner-researchers.[24]

1957   The Western Interstate Commission for Higher Education (WICHE) sponsored the Western Council on Higher Education for Nursing with Faye G. Abdellah as the first consulting director and Jo Eleanor Elliott who became its permanent director in July 1957. The Council was established to improve the quality of higher education for nursing in the West with an early focus placed on the preparation of nurses for research, the development of new scientific knowledge, and the communication of research findings. Since 1968 WCHEN sponsored several research conferences. The Southern Regional Education Board (SREB) and the New England Board of Higher Education (NEBHE) were regional counterparts to WICHE.[25]

1959   NLN Research and Studies Department created (name changed to Division of Research). Examples of functions include conducting research studies, providing consultation to NLN staff, and maintaining information about NLN research projects. Publications include *NLN Nurse Career Pattern Study* (1975), and *The Open Curriculum Study* (1974, 1975, 1976).

1959   Abstracts of Studies in Public Health Nursing, 1924–57 by Hortense Hilbert published in *Nursing Research,* 1959.

1963   The Surgeon General's Consultant Group on Nursing issued a report on its study of the nursing situation in the United States. Among its many findings and recommendations the group found that "the potential contributions of nursing research to better patient care are so impressive that universities, hospitals, and other health agencies should receive all possible encouragement to conduct appropriate studies." (p. 53).[26] The group recommended a substantial increase in federal government support for research in nursing and for the training of researchers.

   Nursing Studies Index, Volume IV, 1957–1959, by Virginia Henderson, completed. The remaining three volumes have been published. The Index provides a valuable guide to the analytical and historical aspects of the literature on nursing published in English from 1900 to 1959.[27] Volume I, 1900–1929 (published 1972); Volume II, 1930–1949 (published 1970); Volume III, 1950–1956 (published 1966).

1964   *Nursing Research, A Survey and Assessment,* was completed by Leo W. Simmons and Virginia Henderson. It provides a review and assessment of research in the areas of occupational orientation, or career dynamics, and nursing care.[28]

1965   ANA Nursing Research Conferences (1965–1973) were sponsored by the U.S. Public Health Service. The first of nine conferences was held in New York. These conferences provided a forum for critiquing nursing research and for providing opportunities for nurse researchers to examine critical issues.

1966   *International Nursing Index* established. Lucille E. Notter was its first editor.

1970   ANA Commission on Nursing Research officially formed. The Commission was the first to prepare position papers on human rights in research and participated in the dissemination of research. Papers of the Commission included *Human Rights Guidelines for Nurses in Clinical and Other Research* (1974), *Research in Nursing: Toward A Science of Health Care* (1976), *Preparation of Nurses for Participation in Research* (1976), and *Priorities for Nursing Research* (1976).

1970   *An Abstract for Action* by Jerome P. Lysaught. The purpose of this report was to identify recommendations for change in nursing in terms of increased research into practice, improved educational systems, clarification of roles and practice, and increased financial support for nurses and nursing.[29]

1970 *Overview of Nursing Research 1955–1968* by Faye G. Abdellah. A comprehensive overview of nursing research projects supported in part by the Department of Health, Education, and Welfare to provide a "state of the art" assessment of nursing research, the knowledge available, and the gaps and needed research.[30]

1971 ANA Council of Nurse Researchers established by the ANA Commission on Nursing Research. The Council was formed to advance research activities, provide for the exchange of ideas, and recognize excellence in research. The Council published *Issues in Research: Social, Professional, and Methodological* (1973).

1971 *Extending the Scope of Nursing Practice.* A report of the Secretary's Committee to Study Extended Roles for Nurses. A position paper of the health professions supporting the expansion of the functions and responsibilities of the nurse practitioner.[31]

1973 The American Academy of Nursing established under the aegis of the American Nurses' Association with 36 charter fellows. The purposes of the Academy are to advance new concepts in nursing and health care; to identify and explore issues in health, in the profession, and in society as they affect and are affected by nurses and nursing; examine the dynamics within nursing; and identify and propose resolutions to issues and problems confronting nursing and health, including alternative plans for implementation.

1977 *Nursing Research* celebrates twenty-fifth anniversary year. Dr. Helen L. Bunge, first volunteer editor, helped *Nursing Research* grow as a scientific periodical. Hortense Hilbert and Barbara Tate served as part-time editors until Lucille E. Notter became the first full-time editor in 1961. *Nursing Research* became the first nursing journal to be included in MEDLINE, the computerized information retrieval service.

1977 *An Overview of Nursing Research in the United States* by Susan R. Gortner and Helen Nahm. Provides a historical perspective of the development of nursing research in education, practice, and traced research resources.[32]

1977 *U.S. Public Health Service's Contribution to Nursing Research—Past, Present, Future* by Faye G. Abdellah traces the role of the PHS in the development of nursing research.[33]

NURSING RESEARCH—ITS FUTURE

We believe that nursing is a service to individuals and to families, therefore to society. It is based upon an art and science that mold the attitudes, intellectual competencies, and technical skills of the individual nurse into the desire and ability to help people, sick or well, cope with their health needs.

The primary task of nursing research is the development and refinement of nursing theories which serve as guides to nursing practice and which can be organized into a body of scientific nursing knowledge. A concomitant task of nursing research is the discovery and development of valid means of measuring the extent to which nursing action attains its goal—these to be stated in terms of patient behavior.[34]

The purpose of this book is to provide a framework from which nursing research can develop, one which places the ultimate test of the significance of the research upon the patient.

References

1. E. M. Vreeland, "The Nursing Research Grant and Fellowship Program in the Public Health Service." *Am. J. Nursing,* **58:**1700–1702 December 1958. See also "Nursing Research Programs of the Public Health Service." *Nursing Res.,* **13:**148–158, spring 1964.
2. The American Nurses' Foundation, "Research—Pathway to Future Progress in Nursing Care." *Nursing Res.,* **9:**4–7, winter 1960.
3. National League for Nursing, Research and Studies Service, "The National League for Nursing—Its Role in Nursing Research." *Nursing Res.,* **9:**190–195, fall 1960.
4. Mary M. Roberts, *American Nursing, History and Interpretation.* New York, Macmillan Publishing Co., Inc., 1954.
5. Haven Emerson and Josephine Goldmark, *Cleveland Hospital and Health Survey,* "Nursing," Part IX. Cleveland, Cleveland Hospital Council, 1920.
6. E. H. Lewinski-Corwin, "The Hospital Nursing Situation." *Am. J. Nursing,* **22:**603, 1922.
7. "Sub-Committee Report on the Cost of Nursing Education." Twenty-Eighth Annual Report of the National League of Nursing Education, 1922, p. 93.
8. *Nursing and Nursing Education in the United States.* Report of the Committee for the Study of Nursing Education and a Report of a Survey, by Josephine Goldmark. New York, Macmillan Publishing Co., Inc., 1923.
9. Annie W. Goodrich, *The Social and Ethical Significance of Nursing.* "A Description of the Yale University School of Nursing." New York, Macmillan Publishing Co., Inc., 1923.
10. May Ayres Burgess, *A Five-Year Program for the Committee on the Grading of Nursing Schools.* Committee on the Grading of Nursing Schools, New York, 1926.
11. *Nursing Schools Today and Tomorrow.* Final Report of the Committee on Grading of Nursing Schools, New York, 1934.
12. May Ayres Burgess, *Nurses, Patients, and Pocketbooks.* Report of a Study of the Economics of Nursing conducted by the Committee on the Grading of Nursing Schools, New York. 1928.
13. Ethel Johns and Blanche Pfefferkorn, *An Activity Analysis of Nursing.* Committee on the Grading of Nursing Schools, New York, 1934.

14. S. P. Capen, "A Member of the Grading Committee Speaks." *Am. J. Nursing,* **32:**307–311, 1932.

15. Blanche Pfefferkorn and Charles A. Rovetta, *Administrative Cost Analysis for Nursing Service and Nursing Education.* New York, National League for Nursing Education, 1940.

16. *Medical Care for the American People.* Final Report, No. 28 of the Publications of the Committee on the Costs of Medical Care. Chicago, University of Chicago Press, 1932.

17. Esther Lucile Brown, *Nursing for the Future.* A report prepared for the National Nursing Council. New York, Russell Sage Foundation, 1948.

18. Margaret West and Christy Hawkins, *Nursing Schools at Mid-Century.* A report of the Subcommittee on School Data Analysis for National Committee for the Improvement of Nursing Services. New York, National League for Nursing, 1950.

19. Faye G. Abdellah, "State Nursing Surveys and Community Action." *Pub. Health Rep.,* **67:**554–560, 1952.

20. Virginia Henderson (editorial), "Research in Nursing Practice—When?" *Nursing Res.,* **4:**99, February 1956.

21. American Nurses' Foundation, Inc., *The First Three Years.* New York, American Nurses' Foundation, Inc., 1958.

22. Everett C. Hughes, Helen Hughes, and Irwin Deutscher, *Twenty-Thousand Nurses Tell Their Story.* Philadelphia, J. B. Lippincott Co., 1958.

23. E. M. Vreeland, *op. cit.*

24. Harriet Werley, "Promoting the Research Dimension in the Practice of Nursing Through the Establishment and Development of a Department of Nursing in an Institute of Research." *Military Med.,* **127:**219–231, March 1962.

25. J. E. Elliott, *Communicating Nursing Research 1967–1974.* (Final Report, USPHS Research Grant No. NU-00289.) Boulder, Colo., Western Interstate Commission for Higher Education, 1974.

26. *Toward Quality in Nursing: Needs and Goals.* Report of the Surgeon General's Consultant Group on Nursing. U.S. Public Health Service Publication No. 992, Washington, Government Printing Office, February 1963.

27. Virginia Henderson, *Nursing Studies Index,* Vol. IV, 1957–1959. Philadelphia, J. B. Lippincott Co., 1963.

28. Leo W. Simmons and Virginia Henderson, *Nursing Research: A Survey and Assessment.* New York, Appleton-Century-Crofts, 1964.

29. Jerome P. Lysaught, *An Abstract for Action.* New York, McGraw-Hill Book Co., 1970; *An Abstract for Action: Appendices,* 1971.

30. Faye G. Abdellah, "Overview of Nursing Research." *Nursing Res.,* Part I, **19:**6–17, January–February 1970; Part II, **19:**151–162, March–April 1970; Part III, **19:**239–252, May–June 1970.

31. Department of Health, Education, and Welfare, *Extending the Scope of Nursing Practice.* A Report of the Secretary's Committee to Study Extended Roles for Nurses. Washington, D.C., Government Printing Office, November 1971.

32. Susan R. Gortner and Helen Nahm, "An Overview of Nursing Research in the United States." *Nursing Res.,* **26:**1:10–33, January–February 1977.

33. Faye G. Abdellah, "U.S. Public Health Service's Contribution to Nursing Research—Past, Present, Future." *Nursing Res., 26:244–249, July–August 1977.

34. Rozella M. Schlotfeldt, Reflections on Nursing Research." *Am. J. Nursing,* **60:**492–494, April 1960, p. 494.

Problems and Suggestions for Further Study

1. Review the life of Florence Nightingale, and cite specific incidents in which she undertook pioneering efforts to do research in the health field.

2. What were some of the studies developed by the former National League for Nursing Education? Select one of these studies, and show what influence it had in our present-day approach to problems.

3. Describe the first recorded time study of institutional nursing conducted in 1922. What methods used in this study would be useful in present-day studies of what nurses do with their time?

4. Compare the organizational structure of the following and describe the goals of each:

   Division of Nursing, U.S. Public Health Service
   Institute of Research and Service in Nursing Education,
       Teachers College, Columbia University
   The American Nurses' Foundation
   The Walter Reed Army Institute of Research
   Division of Research, National League for Nursing

5. Evaluate the comment that prior to 1950 most of the research studies in nursing were directed toward nursing education rather than nursing service.

6. Discuss the various ways in which nurses have participated in research activities other than conducting nursing studies.

7. Read Ellwynne M. Vreeland's article, "Nursing Research Programs of the Public Health Service" (*Nursing Res.,* **13:**148–158, spring 1964), and parallel significant developments in nursing with those events important to the development of nursing research.

8. Considering the concern with the rising costs of health care, discuss the ways in which nursing research could be helpful in containing these costs.

9. Read Rozella M. Schlotfeldt's article "Nursing Research: Reflection of Values" (*Nursing Res.,* **26:**4–9, January–February 1977). Discuss the author's conclusion that commitment to research is a key prediction of nursing's fulfillment of its potential.

Chapter Two

RESEARCH IN NURSING

NEED FOR RESEARCH IN NURSING

THE TURBULENT ATMOSPHERE that surrounds nursing research today has been brought about by the many medical and technical advances in recent years. But, there are certain other significant factors that are having their impact upon the nursing profession and, perhaps more than anything else, upon focusing the need for research upon nursing practice.

Many medical and nursing leaders believe that there is a thirty-year gap between existing knowledge directly affecting nursing and its application. This gap exists in both nursing education and nursing service. Much research is needed to test this knowledge to see if it is still valid in light of emerging concepts affecting patient care. Let us examine these concepts and view them in terms of needed research that should be undertaken or subjected further to scientific inquiry. Attention should be given to these emerging concepts lest nursing fail to find a justifiable role among the health professions.

The Patient as a Person

No single concept has greater significance for nursing research than that of viewing the patient as a person. The contributions of the social sciences challenge our ritualistic preoccupation with the prescribed physical care of the patient. If the latter focused upon the basic health needs of patients such as hygienic care, maintaining nutritional needs of patients, elimination, this form of preoccupation might be viewed as essential nursing care. But as we are well aware, meeting the basic health needs of patients has long since been delegated to the nonprofessional worker. Today, nursing's preoccupation is with the technical aspects of nursing care, the highest status symbols being attributed to those tasks formerly carried out by the physician such as administering intravenous solutions. What then is the nurse's role?

As the professional student nurse becomes more proficient in the technical skills, she builds an ever increasing gap between herself and her patient. As a result, she is less able to identify the patient's total needs as a senior as compared to her ability to do this as a freshman.[1] Research is needed to find the facts as to why this change occurs.

Some medical personnel predict that eventually nursing personnel will be largely replaced by electronic computers. Precise measurement of patient care is certainly a goal toward which to strive. The addition of electronic equipment in operating rooms, recovery rooms, and intensive care units should free the nurse of routine observations, but her skill and judgment will still be required to interpret these observations. Automation can help to save the nurse's time, but to what avail if she does not spend this time constructively with her patients?

Many activities at the patient's side, such as taking and recording temperature, pulse, respirations, blood pressure, making and adjusting beds, checking intravenous infusions, suction, and traction, have been mechanized or automated.[2]

At present covert nursing problems cannot be detected by electronic equipment. It is also quite probable that only 10 per cent of patients will spend part of their hospitalization in areas equipped with electronic equipment. Can one say that since the remaining 90 per cent of patients have no need for such equipment, these units will therefore become minimal care units? Is the concept of the "patient as a person" to remain a myth? Research is needed to spell out the nurse's role in the electronic age and to protect the patient from becoming a part of the automation.

The Clinical Nurse Specialist Making the Nursing Diagnosis

The concept of a nursing diagnosis is now an acceptable function for nurse practitioners. Making a nursing diagnosis has become an independent function of the professional nurse.[3, 4] Nursing diagnosis is defined as the determination of the nature and extent of nursing problems presented by individual patients receiving nursing care and their families. The unique function of the professional nurse is conceived to be the identification or diagnosis of the nursing problem and deciding upon a course of nursing action to be followed for the solution of the problem.

The clinical nurse specialist is a professional nurse on a unit similar to the team leader who assumes the responsibility for identifying or diagnosing the problems presented by patients and assumes the responsibility for patient care over a 24-hour period and is not confined to an 8-hour shift. The clinical nurse specialist shares with the physician the responsibility for patient care; identifies systematically and accurately the nursing needs of patients; devises and implements patients'/clients' care plans; organizes subteams of nurses to carry out the care plans; carries one's own case load; makes observational studies of patients' needs and evaluates their requirements; translates research findings into practice; and institutes improvements for patient care.

The responsibilities of the nurse practitioner are similar to those of the clinical nurse specialist and differ only in degree and depth. In general, nurse practitioners assess patients'/clients' needs; carry out patient care, including the use of specialized equipment for monitoring or therapeutic purposes; make decisions for carrying out appropriate nurse actions; assist in the development of patient care plans; and initiate preventive measures to protect the patient from complications.

Patients' Common Medical and Nursing Needs

The concept of common medical and nursing needs as related to patient care challenges several ritualistic patterns in nursing service and nursing education. If patients have recognizable common medical and nursing needs, segregation by diagnosis, sex, and age becomes unrealistic.

It has been demonstrated that it costs a hospital $300 more a year to staff each bed by the traditional pattern than by grouping patients by their common medical and nursing needs.[5] The saving is based upon better utilization of medical and nursing personnel. This is a significant factor in a period in which many feel we are faced with nurse shortages, which would seem to be the result of poor utilization of available skills rather than a numerical shortage.

Identification of patients' needs and then grouping these patients by their common medical and nursing needs is the heart of the now widely accepted Progressive Patient Care program.[6] If one accepts this concept as it is related to nursing education and nursing service, ritualistic systems in both education and service need to be studied to determine which are useful and which are not.

Liberalization of Nursing Education

This concept has received increasing scrutiny since the work of Russell.[7] He has pointed out that ". . . professional practice today calls for individuals who have a wide range of knowledge, keen intellect, and clarity of vision concerning human values." This demands that the nursing curriculum include a major portion, possibly two years, of study in the humanities: history, philosophy, and political science. The objective is to help the student develop an attitude toward continual self-education long after she has graduated. Much study and research need to be undertaken to develop a common core curriculum that provides a generic base for all the health professions.

Nursing as a Science

This is one of the most controversial concepts today. The controversy centers around the interpretation of the profession of nursing as a practice and/or a science. In its development thus far as a profession, nursing is more easily defined as a practice rather than as a science. However, the fact that the latter is unclear does not mean that a nursing science does not exist. Many nursing leaders feel that a nursing science will emerge.[8] This can be furthered by a series of studies that can test the physiological and anatomical basis of nursing practices.

Self-Care as a Form of Extending the Patient's Therapy

A broader concept of patient care is emerging:

> The nurse today must teach patients to care for themselves. She must assume greater responsibility in the whole process of therapy. She must divide her responsibilities with other hospital workers and cooperate with other specialties in the health field. These changed responsibilities require the nurse practitioner to have a deep knowledge of people and to possess keen judgment, in addition to having a grasp of the basic sciences that underlie health.[9]

The self-care unit is a part of a "P.P.C." program and provides an opportunity for the professional nurse to teach patients to care for themselves by learning to take their own medications, simple treatments, and when indicated to prepare a special diet. Self-care thus provides a way of extending the physician's therapy for the patient while he is still under hospital supervision.

Research needs to be undertaken to find out how this concept can be applied and how nursing personnel and professional nursing students can make full utilization of this area.

The Hospital as a Community Health Center

This concept is placed last as it represents a long-range goal to be achieved. If the professional nurse is to function within a community health center, all of her professional skills will come into demand. In such an environment, the hospital is one element. Official and nonofficial health agencies, nursing homes, and other long-term facilities are additional elements of the health center.

The nurse's competencies must extend beyond the hospital walls. She must be equally concerned about the tubercular, mentally ill, and chronically ill patient in the community as she is about the acutely ill in the hospital. To function in a community health center environment demands full knowledge of total health needs of patients as well as the resources within the community. Identification or diagnosis of the patients' total needs whether in the hospital or community becomes paramount.

These seven concepts have been presented to point up much needed research to be undertaken to help the professional nurse better understand her changing role as a member of the health team and the changing environment in which she must function.

CONTRIBUTIONS OF THE SCIENCES TO NURSING RESEARCH

The very roots of nursing practice stem from the biological and physical as well as the social sciences. Interpreted in its broadest sense, science is a systematic method of describing and controlling the material world.

Science had its beginnings before 600 B.C. when recordings of scientific fact related to medicine and surgery, astronomy, and mathematics were made.[10]

The early beginnings of basic science as we now know it were attributed to the Greeks who desired knowledge of "things" as a means of understanding and realizing the harmony and order of the world. They preferred to discuss abstract principles, and few accurately recorded observations and experiments were made.[11]

Action research as we know it today is attributed to the Egyptians and earlier Babylonians who recorded and studied mainly those facts in the material world that had practical application.

We have learned today, particularly in nursing research, that science begins with small phenomena (observable facts and events) that tend to have probable solutions. The Greeks preferred to look at broad philosophical questions and were not concerned if their answers had any practical application. A significant part of the scientific method involves reasoning. Perhaps Plato's and Aristotle's greatest contribution during the fourth century B.C. was that they taught man how to reason.

Aristotle (384 B.C.), noted for his collection and systematization of knowledge, was first to conceive the idea of organized research.[12] Copernicus, Kepler, and Galileo were masters in basing scientific concepts in observed data. The scientific method as we know it today was first employed by Galileo Galilei (1564–1643). His research endeavors were in the areas of physics and astronomy.

It was not until the seventeenth century that Francis Bacon (1561–1626) was able to demonstrate the value of inductive reasoning and of experimentation in testing basic concepts. Francis Bacon differed in the use of the scientific method in that he preferred to collect every fact that might clarify the subject rather than to use his judgment in selecting the questions that needed to be studied.

René Descartes approached scientific inquiry in a way opposite to Bacon's in that as a mathematician he believed in deductive reasoning. Boyle and Newton were later to arrive at a happy medium in utilizing a scientific method that included both the collection of evidence and deductive reasoning in selecting the research question and interpreting the findings of the inquiry.

As science developed it became more concerned with relationships. We first observe and then extract assertions which are the raw materials.

Science organizes these assertions into intelligible systems showing their relationships.

The technique of scientific inquiry was advanced greatly by the discovery of numerous ways of recording the behavior of "things" in quantitative terms. The Vernier scale (1631) and the micrometer (1638) were early techniques of measurement.[13]

The historical development of science places much emphasis upon fact. Events that have been given a specific kind of description can become fact. "A fact is an event so described that any observer will agree to the description."[14] Likewise, if a fact is not well established or erroneous, everything will crumble or be falsified, and errors in scientific theory will arise.

Science does not stop with the provision of facts. The goals of science are to collect truths based on facts and from these to establish laws, theories, and explanations. Thus, science begins with observations and leads to theories, laws, and finally the prediction of new knowledge. Making observations is the basic technique of the scientist, which places nursing in a strategic position to do research, as this is the research skill that the nurse develops more than any other. The decision-making process, also a skill of the nurse researcher, helps her to make use of her observations.

The mind of man must always be the most important instrument in research. Training in research must be largely self-training. Those attracted into nursing research may not necessarily be those with the highest intellectual competence, but rather those with creative ideas. Hebb[15] points out that the great scientist is not always one who thinks at a more complex level. His greatness is often attributed to his ability to avoid the complexities in which others become intellectually bogged down. The scientist ". . . sees the relevant issues, and often enough with no logical justification except that in the end it works because he has pushed apparently contradictory data to one side, leaving them to be explained later."[16]

This does not imply that the scientist does not discipline himself for rigorous intellectual thought. It is well known that the great discoveries such as Pasteur's would not have occurred if the scientist had not been intellectually prepared to perceive certain relations which he bases upon his knowledge accumulated in the past. Patrick[17] summarizes this intellectual process which makes up creative thought as preparation, incubation, illumination, and finally verification. Curiosity, an important element of creativity, atrophies after childhood unless transferred to an intellectual level.

It has been mentioned previously that the observational skills of the nurse play an important part in her development as a nurse researcher. Observations have meaning for the mind that is prepared to grasp their significance. Observers frequently miss what appear to be obvious facts. Knowledge acquired from the past and continued intellectual growth help the nurse to evaluate her observations objectively. Effective observation is noticing something and giving it significance by relating it to something else already observed or known. "Regard for learning of the past, tolerance and free discussion of novel suggestions and readiness for cautious experimenting when opportunity offers—these features are typical of the prepared mind."[18]

The Role of Chance in Discovery

New knowledge frequently results from an unexpected observation or chance occurrence arising during an investigation. The scientist must be prepared to interpret the clue and make the most of its possible significance. This requires a unique type of discipline on the part of the researcher. He must utilize his knowledge without preconceived ideas and consider all unexplained observations as sources of new knowledge.

Beveridge[19] stresses the importance of certain conditions being conducive to intuition: the unexplained hunch that may result in new knowledge. First, the mind must be prepared for prolonged conscious thinking about the problem. Competing interests or worries are distractions that take the mind away from this deep thought. Freedom from such interference is essential if intuition is to reach the conscious level. Second, intuitions often emerge when the problem is not being worked on at the conscious level. Third, discussing the problem with others often gives rise to positive stimuli. Fourth, and most important, intuitions must be written down.

The scientist.does not make his discoveries by happenstance. Cannon points out that serendipity occurs not because something new has been observed, but because some new relevance has been attributed to the observation.[20] Investigations begin with an operational hypothesis (a hunch) and continue with the formulation of deductions which are still tentative but sharpen up the original hypothesis.

The hypothesis is the most important mental tool the researcher has. He can make use of the hypothesis to suggest new explorations and observations. Most important of all he can use the hypothesis to help interpret the significance of an obscure event. Hypotheses can be used as tools to uncover new facts rather than as ends in themselves.

One might cite many examples to illustrate the importance of the role of chance in discovering new knowledge. The fruits of one's labors may not appear in his lifetime or even for many centuries. Continued research work and seeking the truth basic to intuition must often precede the realization of a hunch or idea upon which success depends.

A classic example of the role of chance in the uncovering of new knowledge is the discovery of radioactivity.[21] In 1896, Henri Becquerel investigated crystals of the double sulfate of potassium and uranium. These were exposed to sunlight for four hours. He then placed a grain of the uranium salt which had been exposed to the sunlight on thick, black sheets of paper which he used to shield photographic plates from light. When the plates were developed Becquerel discovered an outline of the grains of the phosphorescent salt that he described as a dark smudge. A significant consequence of this discovery was that it supported a hypothesis previously identified by Poincaré. The grain of salt had emitted a radiation like x-rays that affected the photographic plate across a screen that was opaque to light.

The untiring efforts of the English physicist Ernest Rutherford (1871–1937), Becquerel, and Pierre and Marie Curie identified these radiations in growing order of magnitude by three Greek letters, alpha, beta, and gamma. This was climaxed by Marie Curie's discovery of radium and polonium that led to radioactivity.

Taton[22] describes the invention of the ophthalmoscope (1851) as an example of the part intuition played in its development. The German physiologist and physicist Hermann von Helmholtz (1821–1894) is credited with this invention. Helmholtz was thoroughly cognizant of Brucke's theory of the illuminations of the eye. Brucke was within close reach of the invention of the ophthalmoscope. Helmholtz was able to achieve what Brucke did not because he asked himself what optical images are produced by the rays that emerge from an eye into which a light is thrown. Thus, previous knowledge, hard work, intuition, and motivation led Helmholtz to find out what happens behind the back of the eye and how one would go about illuminating the retina of the living eye.

Within our lifetime we have been able to experience and benefit from a well-known and significant achievement that resulted from the chance observation of the renowned English biologist Sir Alexander Fleming. The familiar story about his significant discovery of penicillin begins in September 1928. Whle studying mutation in some colonies of staphylococci, he noticed during a microscopic examination that plates of one of his cultures had been contaminated by a microorganism from the air outside.[23] Most investigators would have been infuriated by the contamination and started all over again. Fleming, on the other hand, studied the contamination in great detail. He observed that colonies of staphylococci that had been destroyed by microscopic fungi had been transparent in a large area surrounding the zone of contamination. Fleming surmised that this was due to some antibacterial substance secreted by the contaminating organism. He then proceeded to study the properties of the newly discovered antibacterial substance.

Extending over more than half a century similar observations had been made by Tyndall, Pasteur, and Joubert, but it was Fleming who was successfully able to demonstrate the antibiotic effect of the secretion of microscopic fungus (penicillium) upon staphylococci. What motivated Fleming to persist in making his great discovery? Man's ability to reason is the force that guides the actions of most investigators. One purpose to formulate hypotheses is to judge the validity of ideas resulting from intuition. Other reasons include deciding what observations should be followed in greater detail in weighing the evidence to support or not support new findings, making inferences from the findings, and finally making application of this new knowledge.

Discovery follows a similar pattern in the physical as well as the biological sciences. The latter pose many more problems because of the complexity involved in dealing with living organisms whether they be man, animals, or microbes.

Illustrative of research in the biological sciences, Watt[24] describes the history of serotonin, a clinical substance found in the blood platelets, in the gastrointestinal tract, and in the brain. It was discovered by an investigator looking for the cause of hypertension. This is an example of serendipity in that a secondary discovery was more significant than the original objective of the research. The important role of serotonin, particularly its effects upon heart disease, cancer, and mental illness, is beginning to be explored.

This is the century of biochemistry and biophysics. In our own time, we have found not only the antibiotics but also the atom and the electron. It seems safe to say that the bulk of medical research today is concerned with molecules and their particles—with the fine structure of protoplasm, of proteins, the chemical mechanics of cellular activities. These are the materials with which modern medicine must deal when it seeks to expand its power of service to man.[25]

As new chemical substances are discovered and new surgical and medical techniques devised, the nurse's role in clinical investigations—because she is with the patient for 24 hours—becomes even more important in making the necessary observations to provide data upon which the scientist and physician can make intelligent decisions about the course of therapy. All of this will require that the nurse have greater depth in training in the sciences.

One of the problems facing nursing today is the need for studies that test the anatomical, physiological, and biological bases of nursing practices. These practices derive from the concepts of both the physical as well as the social sciences.

Biochemistry is still another field in which new horizons of medical progress are evident. This science contributes to a better understanding of all diseases because man can be understood more clearly.

There have been many major contributions of experimental biochemistry to clinical medicine.[26] To cite only a few, many major nutritional disorders have been eradicated; there is better diagnosis and therapy of sprue, pernicious anemia, pellagra, beriberi. We know more about planning intelligent dietary regimens for obesity, pregnancy, diabetes, hypertensive cardiovascular disease, atherosclerosis, peptic ulcer.

Biochemistry has also contributed to a better understanding of disorders of specific tissues such as hepatic, biliary, gastric, and renal dysfunctions.

Understanding of the synthesis of an abnormal protein or complete failure of synthesis of a specific protein, as this relates to the diagnoses of hereditary disorders, has been increased because of the contributions of biochemistry.

One must also mention the contributions of biochemistry to increased knowledge of quantitative diagnosis of disturbances of composition and volume of extracellular fluid and endocrine disorders.

Use of Concepts from the Physical Sciences*

Circulating blood serves as a means of transporting substances to and from the cells, and the volume and pressure must be maintained within certain limits to meet changing demands of various organs.[27] The basic principles related to this concept become important in caring for patients where there is apt to be postsurgical hemorrhage or where hemorrhage is imminent, such as in a patient with a bleeding gastric or duodenal ulcer.

The application of dressings, bandages, casts, or traction may be constricting, and close observation is essential to avoid any interference with circulation. Knowledge of the circulatory system provides the nurse with basic principles that she can apply in emergency situations. For example, when bleeding occurs in an extremity, the affected part should be elevated above the heart.

Instruments, such as a sphygmomanometer, provide useful diagnostic data about the patient's changing condition which help both the physician and nurse make valid decisions regarding the patient's care. It is not sufficient that the nurse be able to take an accurate blood pressure reading; she must also be able to interpret this reading and make judgments about the systolic and diastolic readings.

The concepts of physics applied to nursing have wide application. For example, the principle that fluids flow from an area of higher pressure to one of lower pressure comes into play in the withdrawal and administering of fluids whether by means of an irrigating tube, an intravenous infusion, or a suction machine.

Maintaining a constant supply of oxygen to all body cells is a physio-

* See also: Dolores Krieger, "About the Life Process." *Nurs. Sc.,* **1:**105–115, June–July 1963.

logical concept upon which the survival of the organism depends. The nurse must have knowledge of the factors influencing the maintenance of this supply:[28]

1. An adequate supply of oxygen
2. A clear airway
3. An intact thoracic cage
4. An adequate diffusing surface in the lung
5. An adequate system of transportation

In order to make an intelligent decision about the appropriate nursing practices to use, the nurse must recognize which factor is interfering with providing a constant supply of oxygen. For example, the lack of oxygen in the environment is the interfering factor in patients undergoing an anesthetic. The same difficulties would be experienced by those individuals at high altitudes.

Maintaining a clear airway is vital for postoperative patients in chest surgery, for the asthmatic, and for the unconscious patient. The lack of an intact thoracic cage may be the interfering factor in chest injuries such as stab wounds or crushing injuries. The patient with pneumonia, pulmonary edema, or congestive heart failure does not receive sufficient oxygen because of an inadequate diffusing surface. The circulatory system of an anemic patient, or the patient with carbon monoxide poisoning, is unable to transport oxygen because of insufficient red blood cells.

Use of Social Science Concepts

The application of social science concepts to nursing practices is as important as applying the physical and biological concepts. However, because there is no immediate association of these concepts with survival there are less urgency and commitment on the part of nurses to utilize them. Lately there has been a greater understanding on the part of many nursing leaders of the importance of giving increased attention to these principles.[29]

The general issues studied by the behavioral scientist are critically important to medical and health research. The scientific study of behavior is just beginning to be developed and dates back less than one century. The physical sciences claim matter and energy whereas the behavioral sciences (psychology, anthropology, sociology, economics, political science) claim human behavior and human culture and, like the physical sciences, demand all the processes of symbolization and disciplined thinking.

The research methods used by the behavioral scientist are no different from those used by other scientists—namely observation, instrumentation, field and laboratory experiments, construction of models and theories, and application of statistical processes to analyze data.

Increased support for research in the behavioral sciences has been given by the Public Health Service's National Institutes of Health, which already support major basic research in neurophysiology and psychology. The National Science Foundation has also given increased recognition to the behavioral sciences by the establishment of a Division of Social Science.

Examples of large-scale studies in the behavioral sciences include studies of mass communications, personality deveolpment, effects of sensory deprivation, and how injury to the brain affects speech, memory, and problem solving. The anthropologist is concerned with changes in primitive societies, sociological research with communication, and psychological research with perception and problem solving.[30]

Significant to nursing research is that all the fundamental research tools used by the physical scientist are also used by the behavioral scientist. Observation, experimentation, and the development of working hypotheses are crucial tools for both, although the observations of the physical scientist are often more readily accessible than those made by the behavioral scientist.

The concept, "to identify and accept positive and negative expressions, feelings, and reactions," is particularly important in dealing with patients with psychoneuroses, psychoses, geriatric patients, and physical diseases that threaten physical appearance and/or vital functions.[31] Recognition of the importance of this concept helps the nurse to create an atmosphere in which the patient can express his positive and negative feelings and emotions.

Another social science concept vital to nursing care is, "to facilitate awareness of self as an individual with varying physical, emotional, and developmental needs."[32] This concept is applicable to all patients in varying degrees. The nurse is challenged to plan a program of care directed at the relief of the problems and needs of the whole individual. It means making provision for the combination of allied health services that can be directed toward helping the patient to a full and meaningful life. Thus, human life during the last 150 years has changed because of science and the techniques to which it has given rise.

THE IMPACT OF THE SOCIAL SCIENCES ON NURSING RESEARCH

The social sciences have had a twofold impact on nursing research. The first has been in the formulation of research problems. A review of completed research in nursing will quickly reveal the extent to which so many studies are formulated in terms of theories, models, and concepts that are derived from the field of social sciences. Second, the social sciences have had an important impact on the methods used in the design of nursing research. Many nursing studies have depended heavily on the logical approaches for conducting research, the instruments for data collection, and the techniques of data analyses, which have been developed in the social sciences.

The importance of the social sciences is underscored by the high proportion of social scientists who have been involved in nursing studies. In a review of 460 studies in nursing, Hilbert and Hildebrand have pointed out that about 22 per cent of all the investigators have been social scientists.[33] Only two groups—nurses (31 per cent) and physicians (30 per cent)—had a higher percentage of investigators. Moreover, these data show that social scientists rank next to nurses in the number of times they appear as authors or co-authors of research articles reported in the journal *Nursing Research*.[34]

In addition to the fact that social scientists compose a high proportion of the investigators on nursing research projects, many studies directed by nurse researchers employ social scientists as consultants in the design and execution of the studies.

In order to analyze the impact of the social sciences on nursing research it is necessary to delineate what these sciences include. In her work *Social Science in Nursing,* Macgregor has pointed out the difficulties in arriving at a definition of the social sciences.[35] Recognizing that disciplines such as political science, economics, and law can be classified as social sciences, Macgregor limits her discussion to those social sciences she terms the behavioral sciences: "All those intellectual activities that contribute more or less directly to the scientific understanding of problems of individual behavior and human relations."[36] In the behavioral sciences she includes sociology, social psychology, and cultural anthropology. For the purpose of the discussion that follows, the social sciences will be defined as including the basic disciplines of sociology, psychology, and anthropology, and all mixtures of these disciplines, such as social psychology.

Formulation of Research Problems

It should come as no surprise to find that a large share of nursing research that has been undertaken is dependent to some extent on the social sciences. Nursing is essentially a social activity in the sense that much of what a nurse does takes place within a framework of interpersonal relationships. From the basic relationship between a nurse and a patient to the complex system of relationships present in the organized structure of a total nursing service department, it is possible to identify a multitude of social activities in which the nurse takes part. We find studies in nursing at all levels of these social activities. At the nurse-patient level Whiting studied the perception of nursing personnel and patients of the relative importance of various facets of the nurse-patient relationship.[37] At another level of interpersonal relationships, Bennis and others investigated the organizational loyalty of groups of nursing personnel in outpatient departments.[38] At the highest level of complexity of interpersonal relationships, Burling and others studied the total social system of six hospitals.[39]

These studies, as well as many others that could be cited, applied many theories and concepts from the social science to the study of nursing problems. Role theory, small group theory, leadership, informal organization, status, communication, and job satisfaction are among the many social science ideas that have been used to investigate such problems as:

1. The sociopsychological causes of turnover of nursing personnel
2. Barriers to communication among nurses and patients
3. Causes of attrition among student nurses
4. Authoritarian versus democratic leadership in nursing
5. The consequences of the formation of informal groups in nursing service organizations
6. Definition and delineation of the role of the professional nurse

In addition to studies concerned with the interpersonal relations in nursing, some research, using theories and techniques from the field of psychology, has dealt with the psychological aspects of nurses and nursing. This has been concerned with such factors as personality, abilities, needs, perceptions, and attitudes of nursing personnel and students. For example, Navran and Stauffacher studied the comparative personality structure of psychiatric and nonpsychiatric nurses,[40] and Lentz and Michaels compared the personality of medical and surgical nurses.[41] Boyle investigated the ability of student nurses to perceive patient needs.[42]

Research Methodology

The use of methods developed in the social sciences has been widespread in nursing research. Examples are plentiful of nursing studies that have used such techniques for collecting and analyzing data as psychological tests, sociometric measurements, scaling techniques, and quantitative analysis of data such as factor analysis and the correlation of attributes. The following are brief descriptions of four of these techniques and of their actual use in nursing studies:

1. In sociometric measurements, using a device called a sociogram, members of a group may be asked to identify a small number of people who occupy extreme positions on certain characteristics such as the most liked, most disliked, most respected, least respected, and so on.[43] Sociograms are also used to identify groupings of individuals according to such factors as whom they find most congenial or with whom they would like most to engage in a particular activity. With the sociometric technique, a study was made of 40 patients in a Montreal hospital in which the patients

drew sociograms twice each day for a one month period.[44] It was found that such factors as age, sex, and language similarities had important influences on congenial groupings.

2. The Q-sort is a device for sorting into a few categories a large number of statements concerning the topic being studied (e.g., satisfaction with nursing care).[45] The sorter is instructed to place each statement into one of the categories according to some evaluative criterion. The number of statements that can be placed in each category is established in advance. An example of the use of the Q-sort technique is found in a study of attitudes toward psychiatric nursing care. In this study, hospital personnel and patients sorted 50 statements describing activities concerning psychiatric nursing care according to a scale of importance.[46]

3. Role analysis—a sociological technique—is based on the concept of a role as a patterned sequence of learned actions or deeds performed by a person in an interaction situation.[47] In nursing research a role analysis led to the classification of the roles of nurses as professionalizer, traditionalizer, and utilizer.[48]

4. A Guttman-type scale is one in which the different items composing the scale have a cumulative property so that a person who responds a certain way to, say, the third item on the scale is almost certain to have responded the same way to the preceding two items.[49] In a study of nursing in Israel, a Guttman-type scale was developed to measure interest in nursing as a career among high school girls.[50]

In a later chapter of this book, discussing measurement in research, other research methods from the social sciences having applicability in nursing studies will be described.

EVOLVEMENT OF NURSING AS A SCIENCE

Nursing will emerge as a science when a highly organized and specialized field of knowledge in nursing is based upon a self-consistent system of concepts that organize logically a given area of phenomena.[51] Nursing science is thus a degree of systematic logical organization of phenomena. Some forward steps have been made in organizing a substantive body of knowledge that can serve as an initial basis for such a science.[52]

The professional disciplines in general represent applied rather than basic sciences. They are committed to the task of utilizing knowledge to achieve some well-defined social goal. They draw heavily upon the basic sciences to derive their bodies of knowledge. They are sciences, however, and are concerned with the systematization of knowledge and with its expansion. These characteristics have very direct implications for the development of a science of nursing.[53]

Crucial to the development of a nursing science is the nurse's ability to make a nursing diagnosis and prescribe nursing actions that will result in specific responses in the patient. Nursing diagnosis is a determination of the nature and extent of nursing problems presented by individual patients or families receiving nursing care. The position is taken that it is an independent function of the professional nurse to make a nursing diagnosis and to decide upon a course of action to be followed for the solution of the problem.

Research can help to clarify underlying theories and concepts related to nursing, each step leading toward an identification of a nursing science.

Summary

The turbulent atmosphere that surrounds nursing research today has brought about many medical and technical advances. Specific concepts such as viewing the patient as a person, the clinical nurse specialist and nursing diagnosis, and grouping patients by their common medical and nursing needs must be given consideration if nursing is to find a justifiable role among the health professions.

The contributions of the sciences to nursing research have become increasingly important. In nursing research, scientific inquiry begins with observations of seemingly unrelated phenomena. These observations are then organized into intelligible systems that show the relationships among the phenomena. This is the approach used by scientists throughout the centuries. The research methodologies of the physical, biological, and social scientist are basically very similar. Observation, experimentation, and working hypotheses are crucial tools of all researchers.

Since many nursing studies have been conducted by the social scientist, the methodologies of this discipline are familiar to nurse researchers. Hopefully, as more nursing studies in the physical and biological sciences are initiated, the methodologies of these disciplines will become equally familiar.

References

1. Rena Boyle, *A Study of Student Nurse Perception of Patient Attitudes.* U.S. Public Health Service Publication No. 769. Washington, D.C., Government Printing Office, 1960.
2. Mark S. Blumberg, "Automation Offers Savings Opportunities." *Mod. Hosp.,* **91:**59–61, August 1958.
3. Department of Health, Education, and Welfare, *Extending the Scope of Nursing Practice.* A Report of the Secretary's committee to study Extended Roles for Nurses. Washington, D.C., Government Printing Office, November 1971.

4. Faye G. Abdellah *et al., Patient-Centered Approaches to Nursing.* New York, Macmillan Publishing Co., Inc., 1960, p. 9.

5. Charles D. Flagle, "The Problem of Organization for Hospital Inpatient Care." New York, Pergamon Press, Reprint No. 55, 1959.

6. Jack C. Haldeman and Faye G. Abdellah, "Concepts of Progressive Patient Care." *Hospitals, J.A.H.A.,* **33:**38–42, 142, 144, and 41–46, May 16 and June 1, 1959.

7. Charles H. Russell, ". . . on a Liberal Education." *Am. J. Nursing,* **60:** 1485–1487, October 1960.

8. Dorothy E. Johnson, "The Nature of a Science of Nursing." *Nursing Outlook,* **7:**291–294, May 1959.

9. Russell, *op. cit.,* p. 1486.

10. Sherwood F. Taylor, *A Short History of Science and Scientific Thought.* New York, W. W. Norton and Co., Inc., 1949, p. 20.

11. James R. Newman, *What Is Science?* New York, Washington Square Press, 1961.

12. Sir William C. Dampier, *A History of Science.* New York, Macmillan Publishing Co., Inc., 1949, p. 30.

13. Taylor, *op. cit.,* p. 145.

14. Edwin R. Guthrie, "Psychological Facts and Psychological Theory." *Psychol. Bull.,* **43:**1, January 1946.

15. D. O. Hebb, *A Textbook of Psychology.* New York, W. B. Saunders, 1958, pp. 200–219.

16. Hebb, *ibid.*

17. Catherine Patrick, "Scientific Thought." *J. Psychol.,* **5:**55–83, 1938.

18. W. B. Cannon, "The Role of Chance in Discovery." *Scient. Month.,* **51:** 204–209, 1940.

19. W. I. B. Beveridge, *The Art of Scientific Investigation,* rev. ed. New York, W. W. Norton and Co., 1957, p. 80.

20. Cannon, *op. cit.,* p. 204–209.

21. R. Taton (translated by A. J. Pomerans), *Reason and Chance in Scientific Discovery.* London, Hutchinson Co., Ltd., 1957.

22. Taton, *ibid.,* p. 84.

23. Alexander Fleming, "On the Bacterial Actions of Cultures of Penicillin with Special Reference to their use in the Isolation of B Influenza." *Brit. J. Exper. Path.,* Vol. X, 1929.

24. James Watt, "Nursing and Research in the Biological Sciences." *Nursing Res.,* **6:**57–60, October 1957.

25. Watt, *ibid.,* p. 57.

26. Philip Handler, "Contributions of Biochemical Research to Progress in Medicine." *J.A.M.A.,* **177:**840–853, September 23, 1961.

27. Madelyn Titus Nordmark and Anne W. Rohroeder, *Science Principles Applied to Nursing.* Philadelphia, J. B. Lippincott Co., 1959.

28. Faye G. Abdellah *et al., Patient-Centered Approaches to Nursing, op. cit.,* pp. 168–170.

29. Frances Cooke Macgregor, *Social Science in Nursing.* New York, Russell Sage Foundation, 1960.

30. "Strengthening the Behavioral Sciences." *Science,* **136:**233–241, April 20, 1962.

31. Faye G. Abdellah *et al., Patient-Centered Approaches to Nursing, op. cit.,* p. 195.

32. *Ibid.,* p. 199.

33. Hortense Hilbert and Edna M. Hildebrand, "Studies in Nursing—Notes and Observations." *Nursing Outlook,* **10:**44–46, January 1962.

34. *Ibid.,* p. 46.

35. Frances Cooke Macgregor, *op. cit.,* p. 36.

36. The Ford Foundation, Behavioral Sciences Division, *Report,* 1953, p. 13.

37. Frank J. Whiting, *The Nurse-Patient Relationship and the Healing Process.* Pittsburgh, Pennsylvania, Pittsburgh Veterans Administration Hospital, 1958.

38. W. G. Bennis, N. Berkowitz, M. Affinito, and M. Malone, "Reference Group and Loyalties in the Outpatient Department." *Admin. Sc. Quar.,* **2:**481–500, March 1958.

39. Temple Burling, Edith M. Lentz and Robert N. Wilson, *The Give and Take in Hospitals.* New York, G. P. Putnam's Sons, 1956.

40. Leslie Navran and James C. Stauffacher, "A Comparative Analysis of the Personality Structure of Psychiatric and Nonpsychiatric Nurses." *Nursing Res.,* **7:**64–67, June 1958.

41. Edith M. Lentz and Robert W. Michaels, "Comparisons Between Medical and Surgical Nurses." *Nursing Res.,* **8:**192–197, fall 1959.

42. Rena E. Boyle, *op. cit.*

43. Benjamin Wright and Mary Sue Evitts, "Direct Factor Analysis in Sociometry." *Sociometry,* **24:**82–98, March 1961.

44. B. Harvey and R. Mark, "Sociogramatic Study of Spontaneous Patient Groupings." *Canad. Nurse,* **54:**924–928. October 1958.

45. W. Stephenson, *The Study of Behavior: Q-Technique and Its Methodology,* Chicago, University of Chicago Press, 1953.

46. Donald R. Gorham, "An Evaluation of Attitudes Toward Psychiatric Nursing Care." *Nursing Res.,* **7:**71–76, June 1958.

47. Theodore R. Sarben, "Role Theory," in G. Lindzey, ed., *Handbook of Social Psychology.* Reading, Massachusetts, Addison-Wesley Publishing Co., 1954, vol. 1, pp. 223–258.

48. Robert A. Habenstein and Edwin A. Christ, *Professionalizer, Traditionalizer, and Utilizer.* Columbia, Missouri, University of Missouri Press, 1965.

49. Louis Guttman, "Measurement and Prediction," *Am. Sociol. Rev.* **9:**139–150, 1944.

50. Judith T. Shuval, "Perceived Role Components of Nursing in Israel." *Am. Social. Rev.,* **28:**37–46, February 1963.

51. Faye G. Abdellah *et al., Patient-Centered Approaches to Nursing, op. cit.,* p. 21.

52. *Ibid.*

53. Dorothy E. Johnson, "The Nature of a Science of Nursing." *Nursing Outlook,* **7:**292, May 1959.

Suggestions for Further Reading

1. Plato. "The Dialogues of Plato. The Republic Bk VII," *Great Books of the Western World*. Chicago, Encyclopaedia Britannica, Inc., 1952, Vol. 7, pp. 391–398.

2. Galilei, Galileo. "Dialogues Concerning the Two New Sciences," *Great Books of the Western World*. Chicago, Encyclopaedia Britannica, Inc., 1952, Vol. 28, pp. 131–260.

3. Harvey, William. "An Anatomical Disquisition on the Motion of the Heart and Blood in Animals," *Great Books of the Western World*. Chicago, Encyclopaedia Britannica, Inc., 1952, Vol. 28, pp. 267–496.

4. Aristotle. "The Works of Aristotle," *Great Books of the Western World*. Chicago, Encyclopaedia Britannica, Inc., 1952, Vol. 8, pp. 119–137.

5. Bacon, Francis. "Advancement of Learning," *Great Books of the Western World*. Chicago, Encyclopaedia Britannica, Inc., 1952, pp. 43–48.

6. Kant, Immanuel. "The Critique of Pure Reason," *Great Books of the Western World*. Chicago, Encyclopaedia Britannica, Inc., 1952, Vol. 42, pp. 93–115.

7. Einstein, Albert. *Relativity: The Special and the General Theory*. New York, Holt, 1920.

8. Huxley, J. S. *Science and Social Needs*. New York, Harper and Row, 1935.

9. Newman, James R. (ed.). *What Is Science?* New York, Washington Square Press, Inc., 1955.

10. Conant, James B. *On Understanding Science*. New York, Mentor Book, The New American Library of World Literature, Inc., 1951.

11. Sheldon, Eleanor B. "The Use of Behavioral Sciences in Nursing: An Opinion." *Nursing Res., 12:*150–152, summer 1963.

12. Berthold, Jeanne T. "Nurses and Behavioral Scientists: An Alternate Assessment." *Nursing Res., 12:*153–156, summer 1963.

13. "Nurse Practitioner Research and Evaluation," *Nursing Outlook* (entire issue), **23:**147–177, March 1975.

14. Bates, Barbara, "Doctor and Nurse: Changing Roles and Relations." *N. Eng. J. Med.,* **283:**129–134, July 6, 1970.

15. Bates, Barbara, *A Guide to Physical Examination*. Philadelphia, J. B. Lippincott Co., 1974.

16. Bloch, Doris, "Some Crucial Terms in Nursing. What Do They Really Mean?" *Nursing Outlook,* **22:**689–694, November 1974.

Problems and Suggestions for Further Study

1. How did Kepler (1571–1630) go about refuting the principles of traditional astronomy? If there was a nursing revolution as there was a "Copernican revolution" and later a "Keplerian revolution," what approaches might you use in challenging the principles of traditional nursing?

2. The ancient scientists were aware that practical applications could be made from their discoveries. Bacon (1561–1626) was a pioneer in furthering this new scientific attitude. If you were chosen to debate basic research in nursing versus applied research, what arguments would you put forth?

3. Which of your points would have been similar to those given by Bacon in support of applied research?

4. Distinguish between Newton's experimental and mathematical physics, and Aristotle's philosophical physics. Show how this distinction would relate to research in nursing. Discuss the difference between experimental and philosophical science, spelling out the nursing components.

5. Review some recent issues of the journal *Nursing Research*. In the reports of research that you find can you identify examples of the use of methodology from the social sciences? The life sciences? The physical sciences?

6. Comment on the proposition that nursing research can be more effectively pursued by persons who devote full time to the job rather than by part-time researchers.

Chapter Three

WHAT IS RESEARCH?

RESEARCH PROVIDES ANSWERS TO QUESTIONS

IN THE BROADEST SENSE, research can be considered as an activity whose purpose is to find a valid answer to some question that has been raised. That this is a broad definition is readily apparent, since it encompasses such activities not ordinarily thought of as research as a student answering the question, "What is democracy?" posed on an examination paper, or a mother replying to her child's query, "Mommy, why is the sky blue?"

Giving immediate answers to questions from information stored in one's brain is not generally classified as research because it is commonly held that research is directed toward questions whose answers are not immediately known. However, suppose our student is given the question, "Is the United States a democracy?" as a topic for a term paper and is allowed several weeks to gather his facts from appropriate source documents. Would this activity be considered research? Or, suppose the mother did not know why the sky is blue and deferred an answer to the question until she consulted an encyclopedia. Would this be research?

It would generally be held that these activities do not represent research, because of the further qualification placed on the definition: research is directed to questions that have not been previously answered. In other words, research is an activity directed to questions whose answers provide new knowledge to the world at large. Thus, consulting an encyclopedia to find out why the sky is blue may provide new knowledge to the mother as well as the child to whom she imparts the information. But this activity does not add to the storehouse of information in the world at large, since a valid answer to this question was formulated many years ago.

This does not mean that in order to qualify as research a study must be directed to a brand new, never-before-studied question. First of all, there are questions that are by nature so broad that many separate research studies are required before a valid answer is obtained. Take the question: What causes cancer? Thousands of independent research investigators are presently working on studies directed toward this question. Thousands of other researchers have sought answers to this question in the past. Most of these investigators, in order to make their research projects manageable, have narrowed the question down to one with much greater concreteness. Often the specific study seems to have little relation to the broad underlying question. Thus, what causes cancer has been the underlying question of recent research projects bearing the following titles:[1]

Character of the etiological agents of mouse leukemia
Acid extractable proteins of cancer cells
Inductive agents in normal and malignant tissues
Heredity in certain types of cancer
Relationship of virus infection to tumor growth

Furthermore, an enormous number of distinct research projects can be developed on various levels of specificity of the question itself—e.g., What causes *lung* cancer? What causes *lung* cancer in men? What causes *lung* cancer in American men? What causes *lung* cancer in American men in urban areas?

Similarly the question of how nursing care influences patient welfare has given rise to a large variety of studies using different methods of approach and concerned with different definitions of the question. Thus, some studies have defined nursing care as size of nursing staff available to give nursing care (average hours of care available per patient), while others have defined it as the method of organizing the nursing staff. Patient welfare can be defined as physiological phenomena such as blood pressure, psychological factors such as satisfaction with care, or in terms of the occurrence of certain events such as request for sedatives which are manifestations of both physiological and psychological phenomena.

Second, there are questions that are so difficult to answer that many different research studies, each building on the findings of previous studies, are required before a satisfactory answer is formulated. Remillard provides an interesting illustration of this in a discussion of the history of research into the question of where the noise from thunder originates.[2] This question has been subjected to study ever since Aristotle, over two thousand years ago, recognized that thunder derived from lightning. But this was not a satisfactory answer, since it does not tell us how thunder is actually produced, or why some types of lightning produce thunder while others do not. Nor does it answer a host of other subsidiary questions that are relevant to an understanding of the phenomenon. It was only in 1957 that a study built on the foundation of other research finally provided a comprehensive answer to the question.

Third, an investigator might direct his research to exactly the same question previously studied by another investigator because he has doubts about the validity of the earlier findings. His doubts may arise as a result of some imperfection he notes in the research design. Thus, in essence he repeats the earlier study but with a new or corrected design. Many examples are available of faulty research designs leading to spurious findings, which were later set straight in more properly conducted studies. The classic example is the research done at the Hawthorne Works of the Western Electric Company in the 1920's on the relationship between physical environment and worker productivity.[3] Because of improper research design (to be discussed in a later chapter)—which has become known as the Hawthorne effect—sociopsychological responses in the subjects under study were created that were primarily due to their participation in the study itself and not to the factors (e.g., physical environment) being studied.

Fourth, many studies are repetitions of previous studies and not only are directed toward the same question but also use the same method of procedure in seeking the answer. This process is called *replication*. Here the researcher is actually trying to confirm (or deny) the findings of the earlier research. In a sense these earlier findings may be considered as tentative. Only after the study has been repeated a number of times and similar findings have been obtained do we consider that a valid answer has been reached. In fact, few individual studies, and these primarily for a very limited population and concerned with a very narrow question, can be expected to produce final answers to a research question. What is usually required, particularly when the research is directed toward questions affecting human health and well-being, is a whole series of studies, a research program to provide definitive findings. To illustrate: in clinical trials of drugs, in which the effect of the drug on patients is evaluated, similar studies are independently carried out at the same time by different researchers among different groups of patients in different hospitals. These are known as multiclinic trials.[4] Each trial is attempting to answer the same question: Is the drug any good? Each trial would be considered as a research study even though in the strictest sense its aim is not to supply new knowledge.

QUESTIONS UNANSWERABLE BY RESEARCH

Not all questions are researchable. Research questions essentially deal with tangible, observable phenomena and require answers whose truth and meaning can be validated by others. In other words, research questions seek answers concerning facts: concrete things that exist in time or space together with the relationships between them.[5]

"Is there life on other planets?" is an example of a factual question. "Life" (or lack of life) is a phenomenon that can be objectively defined and observed. The existence of life on other planets is, therefore, a proposition whose truth is capable of being supported by tangible evidence. On the other hand, some questions do not seek factual replies but instead require answers that reflect judgments, preferences, or values.

The question, "Is Earth a more desirable place to live than Mars?" is not, as stated, a factual one. The characteristic "desirable" cannot be objectively observed, since its definition would vary according to the personal preferences of the observer. What is desirable for one observer may be totally undesirable for another. To some people desirability may be defined in terms of physical environment, such as climate, topography, soil fertility; and by this kind of definition the Earth could well be held in higher esteem. To others, desirability could be defined in terms of population density, so that for persons with preferences for a low population density Mars could be the more desirable place to live.

Now, if agreement can be reached as to the definition of the value term, if this definition is kept intact throughout the study, and if it involves phenomena that can be observed, the question thereby becomes researchable. In essence the value term is transformed to a factual one. Thus, if *desirable* is defined as the ability to support life productively, we have moved closer to a proposition on which factual evidence can be brought to bear.

There are other kinds of questions that in their literal form are not researchable. Questions concerning courses of action to follow often have to be reformulated because they involve value judgments. For example, consider the question, "Should our community build a new hospital?" It is not directly researchable because not all of the premises upon which the question will be decided can be based on factual evidence. Some of the case for or against the new hospital will rest on value judgments concerning the need for the hospital: a hospital is a good thing for a community to have, a community should see to it that its residents are provided with adequate health facilities, people should not have to travel too far to a hospital, health care is the most important thing on which a community spends money. The importance of these evaluations could far outweigh the factual evidence that could be brought to bear in seeking an answer to the question. This evidence could include projections of future bed needs based on population growth, hospital utilization trends, health status of the population, assessments of personnel resources available in the community to staff the hospital, appraisal of the economic ability of the community to support the hospital.

There is a third kind of question that is not researchable. There are questions for which no methodology is available at present to provide proper answers. In the health field, as well as in many other areas, vitally important questions have remained unanswered because appropriate methodology is lacking. For example, the question of how nursing care can maximize patient welfare cannot be pursued with reasonable chances of success until valid, objective measures of this phenomenon become available. At the present time only crude, indirect indicators of patient welfare exist. Definitive research in this area must await the development of appropriate research tools.

REASONS FOR DOING RESEARCH

Basic Research

Although all research can be said to stem from the desire to answer a question, research can serve various purposes. First, research may arise purely to satisfy a desire to increase the state of knowledge in a certain area. Here the end product of the research is an accretion of knowledge through the findings of the study. The findings may simply be a collection of numerical data as in a biological study of the weights of protein molecules, or a lengthy narrative document as in an anthropological study of some primitive society, or statements of propositions demonstrated to be true by the study as in a psychological study of the effects of food deprivation on the behavior of rats. Studies like these are sometimes called *basic* or *pure* research. The implication of this designation is that such research establishes fundamental facts, theories, or even laws in an area of knowledge that is essential to the undertaking of further research in this area. Findings from basic research can be considered to be building blocks upon which further research and increments in knowledge are based. As defined in a governmental report, basic research is "that type of research which is directed toward increase of knowledge in science. It is research where the primary aim of the investigator is a fuller knowledge or understanding of the subject under study."[6]

Another way to grasp the meaning of the term "basic research" is to consider Alexander Pope's famous quotation: "Not to go back is somewhat to advance and men must walk, at least, before they dance."[7]

All fields of endeavor advance in stages, each stage building on the knowledge gained in previous stages. Thus, before television became commonplace in everyone's living room, extensive research was necessary in many areas of electronics, including cathode rays, vacuum tubes, and amplifiers. And before a cure for cancer is found it will be necessary to obtain the answers to a host of important questions, including the very fundamental question of what is life itself. The stages that contribute to the advance in knowledge make up the process known as basic research. The research carried out at each of the stages does not necessarily have to be directed toward some immediate or even long-range practical purpose, such as the development of a new product or the finding of a cure for a disease. The purpose is primarily knowledge for knowledge's sake.

Although their results have not led to immediate action, the majority of research studies conducted in nursing can be classified as applied research, as many of these projects have been directed toward specific real-life goals. These goals have included:

Improvement of patient care
Alleviation of the nursing shortage
Enrichment of the curriculum in nursing education
Increasing recruitment into nursing
Optimizing the organization of nursing service

It has been said that individual studies in the field of nursing have not achieved these goals, but by providing new knowledge they are serving as steppingstones to their attainment at some time in the future. No single study can be expected to yield final answers to these major nursing problems because they are so global, so multifaceted and complex. Only a battery of studies, each building on the findings of previous research, can eventually provide definitive answers to these problems.

Applied Research

A sharp dividing line is often drawn between research whose end product is purely knowledge and research that is directed toward so-called practical purposes. The former is generally classified as basic research and the latter as applied research.

There are many purposes for conducting applied research. Briefly, these can be grouped into the following categories:

1. To solve a problem
2. To make a decision
3. To develop a new program, product, method, or procedure
4. To evaluate a program, product, method, or procedure

Problem Solving   Most research studies are initiated to find solutions to existing problems. In nursing, as in many other areas, there is no end to the number and variety of problems for which solutions need to be found. For example:

What is the most effective way to educate a professional nurse?
How much nursing care does a patient need?
How can recruitment into nursing be increased?
What can be done to reduce the drop-out rates in schools of nursing?
How should a nursing unit be designed to make the most efficient use of personnel time?
What is the maximum case load that could be managed in one day by a public health nurse?
How often is it necessary to take T.P.R.'s?

In problem solving the assumption usually exists that there is some deficiency or shortcoming in present ways of doing things and that improvement can be achieved through research. Improvement, then, is the key objective in problem solving. Improvement, it is hoped, will be accomplished by making changes as a result of the research. The aim of the research is to provide the appropriate facts on which to base the change.

Decision Making The process of decision making involves the selection of a course of action from alternative courses of action that could be taken. "Shall we establish a new three-year diploma school of nursing in our community?" is an example of a question that involves the making of a decision. The action that is contemplated by the decision is the establishment of a diploma nursing school, and the alternative is not to establish the school. Additional alternatives that could be posed are the establishment of other types of educational programs such as a two-year associate degree, a four-year baccalaureate degree, or a practical nurse program. Other examples of decision-making questions in nursing that could serve as bases for research are:

Does greater use of practical nurses rather than nursing aides improve the quality of patient care?
Should admissions to schools of nursing be restricted to high school students in the upper third of their class?
Should automatic data-processing equipment be used to assist in the provision of nursing care?
Is the team leader method of organization effective in nursing?
Should salaries paid to nurses be increased?
Is the nursing supervisor needed?

The function of research in decision making is to yield the facts upon which the selection of the course of action can be made most appropriately. However, facts are not the only elements considered in decision making. Other elements like value judgments also can influence the decision that is taken. But to the extent that the decision question involves matters that are essentially factual in nature, research can play an important role in decision making.

Developmental Studies Research can be a valuable aid in the development of methods, procedures, and programs in nursing. For example, if it is desired to devise a new training program for nursing aides, factual data, which can be systematically gathered through research, will be needed in designing the format, content, and scope of the program. If it is desired to create a new system of delivering medications to patients, a research approach can assist in developing a system that would be efficient and practical.

The number of programs, methods, procedures, and products that can be developed in the field of nursing is vast. The following is a listing of just a few of these:

A method for rating nursing performance
Programmed instruction methods (teaching machines) for nursing education
Measuring instruments for assessing adequacy of patient care
Procedure for forecasting patients' needs for nursing service
Devices for electronic patient monitoring
Procedures for effective matching of work load with staffing
A method of assessing job satisfaction of nursing personnel

Evaluative Research   To many people, applied research is synonymous with evaluative research. In evaluative research a program, method, procedure, or product is being tested to answer such questions as:

Has a desirable change occurred?
Is the product any good?
Has the patient been helped?
Has efficiency been increased?
Have costs been reduced?
Has service been improved?
Have the students learned well?
Can the patient take better care of himself?

Evaluative research essentially looks backward to assess what has been done, whereas decision-making research looks to the future and suggests what should be done. Evaluative research is very pragmatic. The underlying question is, "Has it made any difference to do something one way as contrasted with another way?" This difference must be real, meaningful, and practically significant.[8]

There are many examples of evaluative research. In the health field the testing of drugs, known as clinical trials, is a very important activity and one that has received much public attention in recent years. In the field of education evaluative studies are continuously being made of curriculum, selection procedures, and teaching methods. In manufacturing a procedure known as quality control is constantly applied to see whether the finished product meets desired specifications. And in the field of market research much effort is devoted to consumer evaluation of a company's goods and services.

It is obvious that many research studies classified as applied research cannot be fitted into one of the four categories just enumerated. Many studies are multipurposed and may even possess features of all four categories. For example, in the clinical trials of drugs the essential purpose is to evaluate the effectiveness of the drug under study. However, as a result of the evaluation a decision will be taken as to whether the drug will be marketed. In studies of the relationship between smoking and lung cancer the essential purpose is to solve the problem of what causes lung cancer.

If the cause is isolated these studies may well shed light on what kinds of programs should be developed to combat the disease.

Moreover, when studies are conducted for the purpose of developing a new product, method, or program, they are usually combined with an evaluative phase to test what has been developed after it has been put into practice. To illustrate this point:

In 1955 the Board of Directors of the Rochester Methodist Hospital (Rochester, Minnesota) asked the Building Committee to develop a design for a new building. As part of the developmental research the committee reviewed the existing literature, visited other hospitals, and studied available plans for the construction of new hospitals. As a first step it was decided to build an intensive care nursing unit. A Development Committee was appointed to gather data concerning the significant factors in providing care to acutely ill patients. As a result of the analysis of these data it was decided to construct the unit in the shape of a circle. The circular unit was selected because this design appeared to offer the greatest opportunity for most adequately providing patient-centered care. The Board of Directors decided to build an experimental circular unit of 12 private rooms and to evaluate the effectiveness of the unit as a facility for the provision of intensive nursing care by comparing it with a conventional rectangular unit. Among the criteria used in evaluating the units were patient satisfaction with care received, attitudes of surgeons and nurses, promptness in answering patients' calls, distances traveled and frequency of travel, and utilization of nursing time. The results of the evaluation appeared to indicate that the circular unit was superior to the conventional rectangular unit.[9]

Demonstrations

In the health field, particularly in the field of public health, the term "demonstration" is often used in connection with the process of research. Actually, demonstrations fall within the same area as developmental research but possess one feature that distinguishes them from true research. In developmental studies the aim is to develop a new procedure, program, or product, often without a specific application in mind but rather to be generally applicable to a variety of situations. By contrast, a demonstration takes a program, procedure, or product that has already been developed and shows how it can be applied to a specific situation. A demonstration, then, can be considered as the application phase of applied research and the research itself as the fact-finding and analysis stage.

A research project should uncover some new facts that can be applied to more than one isolated, specific situation. A demonstration takes facts that have been obtained by others and applies them to a specific situation. Most important, research is conducted on the basis of strict principles of research design, whereas a demonstration project does not have to concern itself with these principles.

Examples of demonstration projects are numerous in the field of public health. These have been concerned with such subjects as:

A referral system for patients discharged from hospitals
A procedure for evaluating the performance of nursing aides
Organization of a nursing care of the sick at home program
A method of analyzing the activities of nursing personnel
A system of forecasting patients' needs for nursing services
The use of disposable supplies on the hospital nursing unit

Why is it important to bear in mind the distinction between a demonstration and research? Often the two processes are confused, particularly the occasional mislabeling of a demonstration project as research. Often a demonstration project has many elements of a research study. A special group of persons may be chosen to participate in the demonstration similar to the study group in a research project. Also, statistical data may be kept as part of the demonstration, and the data may even be analyzed.

What is really a demonstration, which is actually a convincing argument for a certain way of doing something, may erroneously be labeled as research, which is a systematic, objective search for facts free of any special pleading. If someone is interested in promoting something, he has already made up his mind as to its virtues, and there is no need to engage in either developmental or evaluative research. However, if one is not sure about the proper way to do something, he can probably benefit from a research study which can at a later time lead to a demonstration project based on the findings of the study.

RESEARCH AIMS

Research studies can be broadly divided into two categories according to whether they are primarily concerned with discovering new facts or with assessing the relationship among facts. The former is sometimes called descriptive research, whereas the latter is termed explanatory research. In descriptive studies the research is primarily concerned with obtaining accurate and meaningful descriptions of the phenomena under study. In explanatory studies the primary interest is in investigating the *relationships* among the phenomena being studied.

Other terminology is often used to distinguish descriptive from explanatory research. Wold,[10] for example, uses the term "absolute" research as a designation for descriptive studies. The implication is that absolute research is directed toward phenomena as distinct and pure entities which are not dependent on or relative to other phenomena.

Kempthorne[11] suggests the use of the term "comparative" research as a synonym for explanatory studies. In explanatory research one phenomenon is frequently being compared with another phenomenon in terms of their effects on the subjects (people, animals, inanimate objects) being studied. For example, medical research is often concerned with investigating the effects of different modes of treatment on patients. Explanation of how to treat diseases can result from comparing or contrasting these effects.

Descriptive Research

Descriptive studies are concerned with an extremely broad range of phenomena. The following brief abstracts of actual studies reported in the literature of various disciplines indicate the great variety of subject matter of such studies:

Field	*Description of Study*
Meteorology	Using the Explorer VII satellite, a study was made of the amount of heat energy reaching various parts of the earth from the sun and to what extent invisible heat rays were radiating back into space from the earth. This "heat budget" study will provide valuable data for weather forecasting.
Physiology	Recent studies of sleep, using human subjects and highly sophisticated instrumentation, have indicated that during an eight-hour period the subjects were most deeply asleep in the first hour or so. They then gradually moved into progressively lighter stages of sleep until they finally awoke.
Zoology	The phenomenon of hibernation—of particular interest because of implications for space flight—has been intensively studied among animal populations. Among the many findings is that a mammal's body temperature during hibernation drops radically and its respiration rate slows down to a very small fraction of the rate when awake.
Astronomy	Among the many facts brought to light by the space probe of the planet Venus is the very high temperature of its surface—too high to support life as we know it.
Sociology	A study was made of the rate of suicide in different countries. Scandinavian countries ranked among the highest, followed closely by Japan.
Economics	Although median family income has risen to an all-time high in the United States, the number of people who are still living at substandard levels is very large according to a recent survey. Approximately 40–50 million persons, or one-fourth of the total population, were found to be living in poverty.
Medicine	A study of cardiovascular disease among African pygmies showed that in general the health of the pygmies was very poor. A very high rate of heart murmurs was found among the pygmies. But blood analysis showed very low levels of serum cholesterol.
Nursing	In a study of the image that families have of the services of found that 80 per cent of all the hospitals employed at least one part-time nurse and that the average part-time nurse worked about half as many hours per year as did nurses employed full time.

Field	*Description of Study*
Public health	In a study of the image that families have of the services of their health department, a number of distortions were found. For example, the health department was looked upon as a dispenser of medical care rather than of preventive services. Many families incorrectly thought the health department was responsible for the collection of garbage and refuse.
Administration	A study of the educational backgrounds of lay hospital administrators has shown that only a small percentage received formal training in a school of hospital adminstration. Training in schools of business administration was the most frequently reported type of educational preparation.

In descriptive research the end product can take many forms. This can be a lengthy narrative statement, sometimes called a case study, as for example the anthropological studies of primitive societies illustrated by Margaret Mead's *The Coming of Age in Samoa* and the sociological studies of whole communities as the Lynds' *Middletown*. Or, the end result could be a collection of detailed statistical tabulations, exemplified by the reports of the U.S. Census Bureau in its descriptive surveys of the population of the United States and the monographs of the National Center for Health Statistics concerning the health of the American people. Another type of descriptive research is historical research, which will be discussed in Chapter 6.

Explanatory Research

In explanatory research the aim is to go further than pure description. The aim is to discover why a phenomenon occurred. In explanatory research it is not enough to say that something happens. The ultimate aim is to find out why it happens.

To illustrate these distinctions, in descriptive studies the researcher observes certain phenomena, which can be labeled A and B. For his purposes, these phenomena are independent, discrete entities having no important relationship to each other. For example, assume that A represents the number of home visits to patients made by the staff of a public health agency during a certain period of time, and B represents the diagnoses of the patients who are visited. These facts are of interest by themselves as providing a description of the work of the agency. In other words, A can be examined independently of B and still provide meaningful facts.

In an explanatory study A would be studied in relation to B—that is, the number of visits would be related to the diagnoses of the patients. What is important in this type of study is not a description of A and B as isolated entities but, rather, the relationship between A and B. If we look at A and B separately we answer the questions: "How many visits are made by the staff of the agency?" "What kinds of patients compose the case load of the agency?" If we study the relationship between A and B we can answer the question: "How many home visits are made to patients in different diagnostic categories?" Expressed in the form of a *rate* of visits, the data might show that certain diagnostic categories receive considerably more visits than patients in other categories. Such a relationship goes much further in explaining the work load of the agency than does a study that regards visits and diagnoses as unrelated entities.

Explanatory studies are concerned with discovering how the phenomena under study are related to each other. Does A influence B, or vice versa? Or are A and B affected by a third factor, C? In essence then, explanatory studies are predictive studies in which the behavior of one phenomenon is investigated in relation to the behavior of another phenomenon. Since if we are able to predict we can also control, explanatory research offers a powerful tool in harnessing the forces of nature and making technological advances. This kind of research is in fact the essence of the scientific method.

Most studies classified as applied research are predictive or explanatory. In a problem-solving study, for example, we seek to isolate all the relevant factors associated with the problem under study, so that by explaining these relationships we can predict how these factors will behave in the future. Thus, in investigating the problem of why hospital costs are rising, such factors as poor administrative organization and inefficient physical layout might be isolated as important contributors to costs. By controlling these factors we can influence hospital costs, thereby exerting beneficial control over this important problem.

Evaluative studies are for the most part explanatory rather than descriptive. In these studies we are essentially trying to determine whether certain procedures, methods, products, or processes achieve better results than other ones. Thus, a study of whether thoroughly informing a patient about the nature of his illness favorably affects his rate of recovery can supply valuable facts for improving patient care. And a study of consumer preferences for the same product wrapped in different packages can result in increased sales for the manufacturer.

The examples of explanatory research are plentiful in all fields of knowledge. The following listing cites a few of these:

Field	*Description of Study*
Public health	A study was made of the extent to which an educational campaign influences the degree to which people will obtain vaccinations against poliomyelitis. It was found that the campaign was most effective among persons in the higher educational brackets and least effective among those with less education.

Field	Description of Study
Psychology	Two groups of rats were studied using the maze test. One group was placed in a cold room, having a mean temperature of about 55° Fahrenheit. The other group was placed in a room that was about 20° warmer. The rats in the cold room appeared to learn how to navigate the maze faster than those in the warm room.
Agriculture	The effect of several insecticides on ridding plants of Japanese beetles was studied. The most effective chemical was unfortunately also found to be destructive of the plants themselves.
Nursing	It was found that patients who received lesser amounts of nursing care made more requests for sedatives. This relationship was observed with particular clarity on weekends when staffing dropped to very low levels.
Education	When the students were encouraged to participate freely in the classroom discussion they appeared to learn more than when the instructor lectured during the entire class period.
Medicine	Numerous drugs were investigated as to their ability to depress the clot-forming mechanism and decrease the tendency toward thromboses. Promising as a therapeutic agent is streptokinase, a protein isolated from the culture broth of streptococcal bacteria.
Social psychology	It was found that the groups most successful in infantry combat were those in which leadership was democratic and permissive. Combat groups characterized by rigid, autocratic leadership had higher rates of casualties, surrenders to the enemy, and failures of mission.
Biology	In studies of the aging process it has been shown that the life span of an animal is proportional to the time taken by an animal to reach maturity. Thus, if the attainment of maturity is slowed up by artificial means the life span of the animal is thereby increased.
Sociology	Since it has often been claimed that good housing will diminish juvenile delinquency among children of slum families, a study was made of the rates of delinquency among children in several hundred families before and after their move to a new housing development. The data revealed that the delinquency rate dropped significantly after the move to the new housing development.
Administration	A study showed that it is possible for administration to greatly modify or to completely remove group resistance to change in methods of work. This is done by using group meetings to communicate need for change and obtain group participation in planning change.

As in the use of most classification systems, many studies cannot be rigidly classified as either descriptive or explanatory but have attributes of both categories. The well-known Kinsey studies are a good example of this dualism. Much of the data in these studies deal with detailed descriptions of the phenomenon, sex behavior. In addition, the reports also contain numerous analyses of relationships between sex behavior and other phenomena. Thus, in the report on males, Chapter 10 deals with the relationship between social level and sexual outlet, Chapter 12 is concerned with rural-urban background and sexual outlet, and Chapter 13 discusses relationship between religious background and sexual behavior.[12]

Another example of the mixture of description and explanation in research is the studies of Lazarsfeld and others of voting behavior in the United States.[13] Much of this report is concerned with a description of how a carefully selected sample of the population of Erie County, Ohio, voted during the elections of 1940. However, the main contribution of this study is the explanation it provides of voting and, in a broader sense, of political behavior. Among the significant explanations of this research are:

1. People tend to vote as they always do, in fact as their families always did.
2. Attitude stability is important in preserving feelings of individual security.
3. Individual tendencies to vote are reinforced by group processes.
4. The side that has the more enthusiastic support and that can mobilize grass-root support in an expert way has great chances of success in an election.

Frequently, descriptive research precedes explanatory studies in the same way as basic research precedes applied research. The history of science is full of examples of how descriptive research is followed by explanatory studies. Perhaps the best-known example is the work of Galileo, particularly his development of the law of falling bodies. Galileo is considered by many to be the father of modern experimental science, although this title is subject to some controversy among recent historians. However, there is no controversy about the superb skill he possessed as an observer of nature. Galileo's early descriptive research in the area of falling bodies consisted of accurate descriptions of the motion of a ball when it is dropped from the mast of a ship. More well known is his supposed dropping of two cannon balls of unequal size and weight from the Leaning Tower of Pisa, although whether this incident actually occurred is questionable. However, there is agreement about the fact that Galileo proceeded from descriptions of falling objects to the development of a theory in which he refuted Aristotle's notion that one of the factors that determines the speed with which an object falls is its weight. He argued that bodies falling freely in a vacuum have the same rate of speed regardless of size or weight. To check his theory he conducted a controlled study in which a brass ball was made to roll down a grooved board at various angles of inclination of the board. This was an example of explanatory research on the same phenomena, falling bodies, previously studied descriptively. From this research came confirmation of Galileo's theory known today as the law of falling bodies.

One conclusion from this Illustration is that descriptive research, in these situations, serves to generate hunches about the relationship among the various phenomena studied. These hunches are later tested in an explanatory study which confirms or rejects the hunches.

Of greater interest to the field of health research are the observations made by Galileo of a swinging chandelier in the Cathedral of Pisa. By his observations that each swing took the same amount of time he derived the law of the pendulum, which made possible the development of clocks. Being a physician, Galileo suggested that the swinging pendulum be used to time the pulse rate of patients. This illustration clearly shows the evolution from a basic descriptive study to an explanatory study to the actual development of a product (clock) and a procedure (taking of pulse rates).

METHODS FOR CONDUCTING RESEARCH

In the broadest sense there are two methods for conducting research: the experimental and the nonexperimental methods. Either of these methods can be used in conducting applied or basic research. Both can serve the purposes of either descriptive or explanatory research.

The simplest and perhaps the most useful distinction between experimental and nonexperimental research has been provided by Stuart Chapin in his very valuable little book *Experimental Designs in Sociological Research*. Chapin says that "an experiment is simply observation under controlled conditions."[14]

It follows then that nonexperimental research is observation without controlled conditions. Now what does this rather stark definition mean? The key words are "controlled conditions" because the critical distinction between experimental and nonexperimental research is the fact that in experiments the researcher consciously manipulates (controls) the conditions for the study—he actually interferes with "nature." In nonexperimental research "nature" is let alone—it is uncontrolled.

To illustrate, let us say we are interested in the problem of job turnover of nursing personnel in hospitals. From descriptive studies we see that this turnover is very high. It is so high that it undoubtedly adversely affects patient care. How can this high turnover be reduced? If we raise the salaries of nursing personnel, will it be reduced? This latter question undoubtedly possesses the ingredients for a research study. It is an important question whose solution could add valuable knowledge to the world at large. Moreover, it could feasibly serve as the basis for a study, since it poses a situation that is researchable. Methodologically, the basic question is, shall we conduct this research experimentally or nonexperimentally?

At the risk of oversimplification, but to illustrate the distinction between the two major methods of research, this study could be conducted experimentally as follows. In one type of design (not by any means the best design, as will be made clear in a later chapter), nursing personnel working in two hospitals that have identical rates of personnel turnover could be selected as the study population. Then, the salaries of the personnel in one hospital would be raised a substantial amount, say 20 per cent, while the salaries of the personnel in the other hospital would be kept at the same level they were before the study began. After a period of time the rates of job turnover would be measured in the two hospitals and a comparison made of any differences. If the turnover rate in the higher-paying hospital is considerably lower than in the hospital in which salaries are not changed, we would have some evidence that a solution to the problem of high personnel turnover has been found—the solution being the payment of higher salaries.

In the nonexperimental approach two similar hospitals, with differences in their salary levels, could be chosen as the study population. The turnover rates in the two hospitals would be compared. If the hospital with the higher salaries had significantly lower turnover rates we might infer that turnover could be reduced by increasing salaries.

It is obvious that the main difference between these two study designs is that in the experimental approach "nature" is consciously interfered with—the salaries of the personnel in one hospital are raised as part of the study. In the nonexperimental approach the salary levels are not interfered with, but are taken into the study in their natural state—that is, as they have been established prior to the study. In this approach the salary difference is only indirectly controlled. This is done by *selection* of hospitals that have different salaries to begin with.

The *time, order* and *manner* in which the study conditions are created —in the example given, the difference in salary levels between the two hospitals—are the characteristics that really distinguish experimental from nonexperimental research. In the former these conditions are created by the researchers themselves after the study has begun. In the latter the conditions are in effect *prior* to the beginning of the study. They have been created outside of the study, and only by the process of selection of study subjects do the researchers exert "control" over them.

Because of the time order of the establishment of the conditions for the study, experimental studies are sometimes called prospective or "carry-forward" studies, whereas nonexperimental studies are called retrospective, "carry-back," or ex post facto studies. The main attributes of the experimental approach, because it is prospective in nature, are these: In explanatory experimental studies it is possible to come closer to establishing cause and effect relationships among the phenomena studied than in nonexperimental explanatory studies. In experimental descriptive studies it is possible to achieve greater purity of description than in nonexperimental descriptive studies because of the stronger control exerted over the study conditions.

In explanatory experimental research, which is the kind of research that is fundamental to the advancement of scientific knowledge, the time sequence of the occurrence of the phenomena under study is controlled by the researcher during the course of the study. In the example cited the salary differential between the two agencies, which can be called A, is established by the researcher. After a period of time elapses he observes the turnover differential, if any, which can be called B. If B is significantly large, then the researcher can say—subject to the limitations imposed by study design and probabilistic inferences, discussed in later chapters—that A caused B.

In nonexperimental research the time sequence of the occurrence of the phenomena under study is *not* controlled by the researcher during the course of the study. The researcher attempts to trace a causal connection between B and A, but there is danger in studies like these that another factor, called C, not even considered by the researcher, may actually be responsible for B instead of the factor, A, he was supposed to be controlling by selecting study subjects who differed in the amount of A they possessed. For example, let us say that in the nonexperimental study of the relationship between salaries and turnover it was found that the agency with higher salaries had much less turnover than the agency with low salaries. We might then infer that low salaries cause high turnover. However, we could be quite wrong in this inference. We must consider the fact that the salary differential between the agencies existed prior to the initiation of the study. This differential might even have been a long-standing phenomenon. Thus, salary difference is not a stimulus in this study design in the same way it is in the experimental approach, where the salary is dramatically changed in one hospital just as Pavlov rang a bell to make a dog salivate.

Not being subjected to the stimulus of a sudden change in salary, as are the personnel in the experimental study, the reactions of the nursing personnel in the nonexperimental study to salary differentials are not at all comparable to those in the experimental group. For one thing, some personnel in the nonexperimental study may have taken the job in the hospital with lower salary with full knowledge and acceptance they were being underpaid because other features of the job were desirable—its convenient location to home. For these personnel the lower salary paid by the hospital would have no effect at all on turnover behavior. Conversely, some personnel in the agency paying higher salaries might be predisposed to leave for factors totally unrelated to salary. In other words, a multitude of uncontrolled factors besides salaries can influence turnover. Besides the personal factors there are numerous social factors that can affect turnover behavior. Perhaps the administrative climate in the lower-paying agency is friendlier, more permissive, more productive in fostering altruistic motives, than the agency that pays more. The presence of these characteristics can promote greater job stability even in the face of lower salaries.

It must be borne in mind that unlike the rather simple, mechanistic means-ends situation illustrated by Pavlov's animal experiments on conditioned reflexes, every social situation involving human beings has interwoven and interacting with the phenomena isolated for study many other individual and social factors that can influence the results of the study. This is as true for experimental as it is for nonexperimental research. The problem for research design, therefore, is to sort out and control the effects of these extraneous factors that we are not interested in so that we can draw valid and accurate inferences from the study. It is this problem to which the next part of this book is addressed.

Barriers to Experimentation

As has been indicated, the major advantage of experimental research is that it permits greater control over the phenomena under study, thus enabling the drawing of more valid inferences of causal relationships among the phenomena studied. However, because nature is interfered with in experiments, we often run into more practical difficulties in conducting these studies than in nonexperimental studies. This is particularly so in studies involving human beings. Some of the changes that might have to be made in conducting certain experiments could interfere so radically with the natural course of events as to be impossible to do. Other changes could offer hazards to health or even life. Still others might be so costly to undertake as to be prohibitive.

In the illustration provided of the study of the relationship between salaries and turnover, in the experimental design we are faced with the administrative problem of actually changing the salary level. In the "natural setting" of the nonexperimental design we do not change salaries but take them as they have been established outside the study by "natural" forces. In other experiments we may have to introduce rather drastic changes into the existing situation, as seen by the following examples:

1. In a study of the effects of different kinds of leadership on employee productivity, some employees may react negatively to the introduction of certain types of leadership, and may even quit the organization.

2. An experiment concerned with testing the impact of the structure of physical facilities on patient care might involve expensive renovations in the existing plant which may have to be scrapped at a later date.
3. A study of the effects of different amounts of nursing care on patient satisfaction with care might require some patients to receive such inadequate nursing care as to endanger their health and well-being.
4. Experimentation with various methods of organizing nursing homes could drastically disrupt the ongoing services provided to patients.
5. A study of lengthening the course of training for practical nurses from one year to two years may result in a drastic rise in the drop-out rates from these schools during the course of the experiment.
6. Experimentation with different methods of recording home visits made by public health nurses might result in a loss of valuable information that would normally have been kept.

Of course, if we develop a new system, method, or product, one whose use cannot be found in existing situations, there is no alternative to experimentation if we want to conduct an evaluation. The nonexperimental approach can be applied only where the phenomenon we are interested in studying already exists and is available for study. Thus, the evaluation of new drugs is generally conducted as an experimental study, because before the drug is released for general usage it is usually given a thorough clinical trial under rigid research conditions. If a drug is released to the general public without rigid experimental study, as in the case of the drug thalidomide, the consequences as discovered in a retrospective evaluation could be very unfortunate.

On the other hand, there are many questions that do not lend themselves to experimentation but can only be investigated through a nonexperimental case study approach. These are questions, generally in the area of descriptive research, that because of the uniqueness of the phenomena under study would make experimentation not only impractical but foolish. Moreover, it is this uniqueness that is the reason for the study, and therefore it should be described as naturally as possible. Particularly in such fields as anthropology, geology, astronomy, archeology, and sociology, the purpose of the study is often to describe the existing situation in its natural state as accurately as possible. Any kind of control over the research conditions, other than over the accuracy of the observations, could actually destroy the purpose of the study.

In certain kinds of comparative studies experimentation is out of the question, too. Consider a study directed to the question: "Does the system of nursing in Great Britain provide better patient care than the system of nursing in the United States?" Essentially this is a descriptive study in which observations would be made of actual nursing care provided in the two countries in their natural settings. However, on closer inspection the question actually goes beyond pure description and moves into the realm of explanatory research directed toward the relationship between two different systems of nursing and the quality of care. If the descriptions of these unique systems can be generalized to broader concepts that provide higher-level abstractions of the concrete empirical facts of nursing in Great Britain and the United States, it is even possible to conceive of an experimental approach to this study. That is, if nursing in Great Britain can be characterized as, say, authoritarian, stable, personalized, while that in the United States as permissive, mobile, depersonalized, it may well be possible to create these conditions in an experimental setting. Many areas of research exhibit just such an evolutionary development, progressing from a descriptive, nonexperimental study of a specific situation to a testing of general constructs through an experimental design.

Another disadvantage of the experimental method is the length of time it can take to successfully carry out such a study. Nowadays, answers to research questions are wanted in a hurry. It is sometimes impractical to consider conducting an experiment if another research approach could get an answer much more quickly even though the answer might not be as definitive. The following example illustrates this difference in time requirements:

Suppose someone wanted to answer the question: Is a graduate of a degree program more proficient as a bedside nurse in a general hospital than a graduate of a basic diploma program? If the study were conducted experimentally, a group of high school graduates could be selected and assigned to either a diploma program or a degree program, and followed up after they had graduated from nursing school and been employed as graduate nurses in hospitals. Then, their proficiency as nurses would be measured to see whether there were a difference in proficiency between the graduates of the two types of programs. If the study were conducted nonexperimentally a sample of graduate nurses in hospitals would be selected, their proficiency as bedside nurses would be measured, a determination made of whether they had attended a degree program or a diploma program, and an analysis performed to evaluate the difference in proficiency scores between graduates of the two types of programs. The study, if carried out experimentally, might take a minimum of five years and require much money and effort. If carried out nonexperimentally, it could possibly be done in about a year and with considerably less expense.[15]

Still another deficiency of experiments is their artificiality. Many experiments are constructed of such unnatural elements that they have little real-life applicability. One such unnatural element is the setting in which they are conducted. Special facilities are sometimes set up for the conduct of the study which are so unique as to permit little applicability of findings beyond the study setting. In addition, the subjects of the study are often atypical. Because they are a captive audience, students are frequently used in experimental work. But the reaction of students to the phenomena under study can be quite different from that of other persons. Also, animal studies are sometimes pursued, particularly in such fields as psychology and medicine, as analogues of human studies. Such subjects as animals are, of course, even further removed from the everyday world of humans than are students. Finally, even the phenomena under study in experiments are sometimes too artificial to have any practical meaning.

Because of these various difficulties in conducting experimental research in fields of study dealing with human populations—the time, the cost, the administrative difficulties, the possible artificiality—it often becomes necessary to severely restrict the scope of an experiment. The problem is narrowed down. The number of study subjects is reduced to a bare minimum. The period of study is stringently budgeted. These limitations, of course, restrict the value of the study. The problem often becomes so narrow and so specific that it can make only a minor, sometimes trivial contribution to advancing the state of knowledge. Great care should be taken not to reduce the scope of experiments to the point where they become mere sterile academic exercises. Experiments do offer the surest way of explaining causality and as such can make a valuable contribution to the advancement of scientific knowledge in nursing.

RESEARCH SETTINGS

Highly Controlled Settings

There are a variety of settings in which research can be performed. At one end of this spectrum is the highly controlled, specially devised setting called a laboratory, experimental center, research center, or test unit. These specialized research settings are set up outside of the actual life situation for the sole purpose of conducting research. Usually the kind of research carried out in these specialized settings would be experimental in methodology and for the most part explanatory in purpose. However, descriptive research could also be conducted in these highly controlled settings. In fact, the popular image of the research process is one in which the scientist, peering in a microscope in the dimly lit laboratory, is describing the behavior of the bacteria he observes in his slides.

Although specialized, highly controlled settings do enhance the purity of research observations, they suffer from the previously mentioned drawback of artificiality. This can be particularly bothersome in studies involving human beings. When a study proposes to put human beings in a special test unit, several things can happen. First, it may be difficult to obtain cooperation from people to enter these highly controlled settings because they may react negatively to being placed in a strange environment. Second, if people do agree to enter a strange environment they may then behave in completely unpredictable and unnatural ways. The famous "Hawthorne effect" is used to describe the way people who are put in a specialized research setting tend to respond to the conditions of the study just because they know they are participating in something special and therefore feel they have to behave in a special way. In show business terminology this is called "hamming it up." This behavior biases the study findings and leads to spurious conclusions. In research this behavior consists, for example, in exaggerating and distorting the facts in responding to research questions, in reacting favorably to a "treatment" even though no treatment was actually given, and in behaving much more productively and energetically in the experimental situation than normally would be the case.

Another aspect of artificiality in the use of highly controlled research settings is the fact that these settings may have such remote resemblance to the real-life situation they are supposed to represent that it becomes difficult to apply the findings of the study to the real world. In social psychology, for example, among the studies that have been done in rigidly controlled settings are those concerned with how people behave in small groups. Many of these studies attempt to create in a laboratory setting an analogue of the real-life situation. Thus, in studies of responses to different styles of leadership behavior a group of individuals may be subjected to a variety of artificially created administrative situations. A big leap has to be taken to translate the findings of these studies to the flesh-and-bone situations of actual day-to-day working conditions. Another example: in medical research on cancer various carcinogenic substances are rubbed on the backs of mice to see if cancerous growths are produced. But producing cancers on the backs of mice may have only a remote connection to the way cancers are actually produced on the skin and lungs of human beings.

With all the limitations of the use of specialized, highly controlled settings in research, there is much to be said in their favor. By being removed from the flow of normal day-to-day activities the study situation can be purified. Moreover, specialized settings enable the researcher to remove himself from the pressures and problems of the workaday world in order to concentrate on research matters in an undisturbed, unhurried way. And last, but by no means least, in specialized research settings it is possible to make real modifications in the environment, to manipulate the study conditions, in short, to conduct a true experiment with all the virtues that this method possesses.

Natural Settings

At the other extreme of research settings are natural settings. These are also called uncontrolled settings, field settings, or real-life situations. These settings are characterized by an absence of control over the environment. The setting is studied just as it is without any modifications. The only direct "controls" exerted by the researcher are mainly in relation to such matters as the selection of study subjects and the ways in which the data are analyzed.

By definition, only nonexperimental studies can be conducted in natural settings. However, both descriptive and explanatory purposes can be served by studies in completely uncontrolled settings, although explanatory research is less likely to be found in such settings than is descriptive research.

The terms "field surveys" and "case studies" describe particular types of natural setting research. A field survey usually gathers statistical data on a particular subject through questions asked of a group of persons in their natural habitat, either directly by interview or indirectly in a mailed questionnaire. The decennial census is one example of a field survey that uses interviews. The American Nurses' Association Inventory of Registered Nurses, based on questions asked of each nurse at the time she renews her license, is an example of a mailed questionnaire survey.

A case study is a detailed, intensive, factual description of individuals, groups of individuals, institutions, communities, whole societies, or even incidents, situations, inanimate objects, or animals. Such studies are characterized by lengthy narrative statements which describe in depth the subjects under study in their natural settings. The studies may delve into past history as well as report on the current situation. They may include statistical data as well as verbal description. They may contain explanatory and evaluative statements as well as descriptive data. Particularly good examples of case studies are anthropological investigations of primitive societies. In the field of patient care, illustrations of case studies abound. A study of the sociology of a hospital, entitled *The Give and Take in Hospitals,* is one example of the case study approach.[16]

Just as experimental research can be done best in highly controlled settings, other kinds of research can be conducted most advantageously in natural settings. By definition certain types of studies, such as anthropological and sociological case studies, have to be conducted in uncontrolled settings. In other studies the advantages of the use of natural settings include the following: they are generally less expensive than using specialized research settings, they are more factually descriptive of the existing situation, the problems of obtaining cooperation of study subjects is less formidable than in highly controlled studies, the artificiality of the controlled situation is eliminated, permitting more direct applicability of findings.

However, natural settings offer certain disadvantages to the researcher. For one, the questions for which answers are being sought by the research may not be easily approached, if at all, through a study conducted in a setting that is completely uncontrolled by the researcher. If, for example, we are interested in finding out whether certain types of patients receive better care in an intensive nursing unit than in a conventional unit, we will probably have to interfere with the natural situation to some extent, such as moving some patients into the intensive care unit who ordinarily would not be placed there. Moreover, in the evaluation of a new method, procedure, or product, it will be necessary to change existing conditions by introducing it into the natural setting. In addition, uncontrolled settings often pose formidable problems in delimiting the scope of the study.

But the major disadvantage of research in natural settings has already been suggested. This is the great difficulty in establishing causal relationships in such studies because of the presence of many intervening and disturbing factors.

Partially Controlled Settings

It is probably correct to say that the majority of studies involving human beings as subjects are conducted in settings that are not totally controlled. In explanatory studies conducted outside of a laboratory or test unit the researcher manipulates the environment only partially. Studies that fall into this category are labeled experimental field studies. Thus, in studies of the reactions of people to health education programs the researcher introduces the educational material into the community and observes the effect in terms of the behavior that results—say, the rate at which people go for health examinations. The "unnatural" element is the introduction of the educational program into the community. However, no other aspects of the settings are tampered with; they are kept the way they would have been had the study not been done it is hoped.

If this same study were conducted in a highly controlled setting, a group of subjects would be placed in a laboratory or a test room. They would then be exposed to the educational material, and their responses could be measured in terms of a written evaluation on a questionnaire.

Finally, if the study were done in a completely uncontrolled setting, it would be necessary to locate an existing community in which the educational program to be studied was already in operation—if such a community could be found. Another community, similar in composition but without the health education program, would be used to serve as a basis for comparison of the rates at which the members of the two communities took health exams.

Of the three approaches the last would be most subject to spurious relationships. In this uncontrolled situation differences in rates of seeking physical exams could well be due to factors other than the presence or absence of the health education program. The second approach, that of a completely controlled setting, could yield meaningful causal relationships. However, these relationships may be valid only within the study setting itself and not be applicable to the population at large.

The partially controlled setting is undoubtedly the most satisfactory compromise. This type of setting can probably yield results that would give a more valid evaluation of the health education program than can the totally uncontrolled approach. Moreover, findings from the partially controlled study would be applicable to a much wider population than the laboratory experiment. Thus, for many research questions a field experiment can offer the best of two worlds. It can yield data for predictive purposes, and it can apply to large populations. For these reasons field experiments have proven to be a popular approach to the conduct of research.

As a summary of the varieties of settings in which research can be done the following listing provides illustrations of actual studies in patient care conducted in different settings:

Highly Controlled Settings
1. In an experimental unit a study was made of the response to group psychotherapy of psychiatric patients.
2. Observations were made in a special nursery of the gain in weight of infants who were fed different formulas.
3. Detailed records were kept in the laboratory of the life span of the various strains of mice that were bred. These data will be useful in studies concerned with the control of cancer.
4. Several hospitals in this country are devoted completely to research. One of these, the Public Health Service's Clinical Center in Bethesda, Maryland, has over 400 research inpatients.

Partially Controlled Settings
1. One group of nurses making home visits interviewed the patients using tape recorders. The other group made notes after the visit was over. The effectiveness of the two systems was later evaluated.
2. The disposable syringes were introduced in two of the clinics. The attitudes of the physicians and nurses toward the syringes were recorded on a questionnaire.
3. The nursing school curriculum was altered to include a course in interpersonal relations that was given to the junior class. After completing the course the students' ability to talk to patients was evaluated when they took their clinical practice to see if they scored higher than students from schools that did not offer such a course.
4. One unit of the hospital was converted to an "experimental" unit. This unit was staffed completely by registered nurses. Two weeks after the patients who had been on these units were discharged from the hospital they were asked to rate the adequacy of the care they received. Their ratings were compared with ratings by patients who had been assigned to units that were normally staffed—with practical nurses and nursing aides as well as registered nurses.

5. In one group, every patient visiting the maternity clinic was told about the desirability of practicing weight control. In another group, literature on weight control was provided, without any oral communication. The third group received the information both orally and through the written material. At time of delivery the weights of the patients in the three groups were recorded and a comparison made of the differences among the groups.

Uncontrolled Settings

1. A study was made of the number of times the patients rang the call bell. It was found that female patients called the nurses 50 per cent more often than did male patients.
2. The National Health Survey found that chronic and disabling conditions were prevalent among a high proportion of persons aged 65 years or over.
3. The study showed that during the first year after graduation from a diploma school of nursing 20 per cent of the nurses had married. During the same period of time 35 per cent of the graduates of a collegiate school had married.
4. The curriculum of the school of nursing for the past 75 years was intensively analyzed. It was found that less than a fifth of the course content had not changed over the years.
5. The death records of nearly 10,000 men were reviewed. The occupations of those dying from coronary artery disease were compared with the occupations of those dying from other causes.

RESEARCH SUBJECTS

Just as research settings can vary, so can research subjects. In fact, the variety of possible research subjects is staggering in number. Research can focus on, for example, humans, animals, plants, or inanimate objects. Research can also be concerned with parts of people, such as a study of the effect of fluoridation on teeth or a study of the condition of feet among older persons. Or research can be concerned with human traits, attributes, or functions, and these may be physiological, psychological, sociological, political, economic, and so on.

Some research can have as its study population, not a concrete physical object, human or otherwise, but abstract ideas, theories, or formulations. Mathematical research is an example of such studies.

In the health field the primary subjects of most research studies are human beings. However, only a few studies are concerned with the whole person. Many studies are directed toward some selected aspect (or aspects) of human beings. The selection of specific traits as subjects for research is made clear from the following brief list of study subjects.

A study of private duty nurses who left the profession
A comparison of the personalities of medical and surgical nurses

The relationship between myocardial infarctions among older men and the
   amount of physical exercise they pursue
Absenteeism among nursing aides in general hospitals
Educational goals of staff-level public health nurses in state health depart-
   ments
Nursing care of mentally retarded children

The delimitation and definition of study subjects are, of course, dictated
by the purpose and problem of the study. The methods for actually selecting the individual members to participate in a research study involve such
concepts as the universe, sample, randomization, and allocation. These
concepts will be discussed in later chapters of the book.

WHO DOES RESEARCH?

Another way in which research can be classified is in terms of who
actually conducts the research. The doers of research can be classified
into several broad categories. At one end are the people who work full
time on research in organizations that are devoted almost entirely to research activities. Lazarsfeld calls these organizations research institutes.[17]
Several schools of nursing have established their own research institutes
such as at Wayne University and the University of Illinois.

At the other extreme is the person working in an operating organization
such as a hospital or public health agency who may occasionally engage
in research in order to satisfy a specific objective connected with his
operating responsibilities. Usually such research is conducted to solve
some current problem or to make a decision or to evaluate a procedure
or program. Thus, a director of nursing in a hospital may undertake a
study of the utilization of personnel because she is faced with a heavy
work load and does not have sufficient staff to meet it.

Between these extremes are a great variety of research doers. Thus, in
an operating organization such as a hospital, a special research office may
be set up that is staffed full time with people whose job it is to conduct
research. An example of this was the Operations Research Division of Johns
Hopkins Hospital, which was established to carry out hospital research.[18]
And in the Division of Nursing, U.S. Public Health Service, which has a
number of responsibilities besides research, several branches are devoted
exclusively to research activities.[19] In addition, professional organizations,
like the National League for Nursing, American Nurses' Association, and
American Hospital Association, have components that are concerned with
research.

Another type of research is that found in educational institutions. Faculty members often engage in research on a part-time basis while they
also maintain teaching responsibilities. Some faculty members even pursue

research on a full-time basis and are relieved of all teaching responsibilities. Students frequently engage in research as part of their academic requirements. In nursing many excellent studies have been conducted as master's theses and doctoral dissertations.

It can be said that the closer the researcher is related to an ongoing operating situation, the more likely the research will be applied rather than basic. Conversely, when research is conducted by personnel who are not administratively connected with an operating organization, the research is more likely to be of the basic variety. Moreover, the more detached the researcher is from the ongoing work situation, the greater is the possibility that the research he does can yield findings that have applicability beyond the immediate research setting. The less detached the researcher is from the operating situation, the more difficult it becomes to classify his activity as research rather than demonstration, management improvement, methods analysis, or just plain troubleshooting. One of the values in creating specialized settings in which to conduct research, such as experimental units, is the freedom these settings provide from the pressures of the day-to-day flow of work. Consequently, objectivity is enhanced and creativity is stimulated.

SUBSTITUTES FOR RESEARCH

The variety of purposes, methods, settings, subjects, and doers of research studies has been discussed. Among the purposes of research the following were indicated:

1. To obtain new knowledge
2. To solve a stated problem
3. To make a decision
4. To develop a program, procedure, or product
5. To evaluate a program, procedure, or product

Research can achieve these purposes with accuracy and validity by pursuing them in a systematic, planned approach according to an established set of principles of research design. Discussion of these principles forms the basis for much of the later material in this book. As will be seen, research is not a simple, easily accomplished activity but requires great effort, mental as well as physical, and demands considerable time, money, and patience. In view of these difficulties the question can be raised as to whether there are substitutes for the undertaking of formal research in order to achieve the purposes listed above that make fewer demands on human and economic resources. It is obvious there are. Every day, millions of decisions are made—in personal affairs, in business activities, in government. Yet, few of these, very few, are based on formalized research. Moreover, in all walks of life, problems are constantly being solved, most without recourse to formalized research.

There are numerous substitutes to research that can yield new knowledge, solve problems, and assist in decision making. Briefly, these substitutes are:

1. Trial and error
2. Experience
3. Empirical evidence
4. Common sense
5. Faith, custom, precedent, habit

Trial and Error

History reveals that much knowledge has been gained through the ages by the simple technique of trial and error. Try something, and if it does not work, try something else. Keep trying until the problem is solved. The history of medicine is full of many examples of the trial and error approach. Different treatments are used on patients until one is found that seems to work.

In a sense the method of trial and error is analogous to a poorly controlled experiment that lacks a theoretical underpinning. To illustrate this, suppose an administrator is concerned with the rising costs of operating his hospital. He decides to take some steps to reduce them. He makes a change in the situation, perhaps not filling vacant positions. This does not have an appreciable effect on costs, so he makes another change: he replaces some of his R.N. positions with aides. This does not appear to reduce costs much either, so he cuts down on the amount of annual leave granted to new personnel, and so on. Finally, the financial statement shows a reduction in the operating costs of the hospital. At this point he stops making changes and is convinced that he has found a solution to his problem.

There are several things wrong with this approach. First of all, he cannot be sure which of his changes, if any, was responsible for the reduction in costs. It probably was not the last change he made, because the effect of all the changes may be cumulative and interactive, and only the jumbled combination of changes may have produced the lowered costs. On the other hand, he cannot be sure that some factor he himself did not control and which he was unaware of was operating while he was making his changes. And it could well have been this factor that was actually responsible for lowering the costs. This outside factor could have been greater bed utilization during the period of trial and error, which could have resulted in an increase in the hospital's income.

Trial and error often produces an unstable solution which may have only a short-run effect on the problem it is supposed to solve. Moreover, a solution based on a trial and error approach usually has only local applicability, thus lacking one of the major virtues of a well-designed research study—the generalization of findings beyond the boundaries of the research setting. Finally, trial and error suffers from being conducted outside of the framework of theory. Without a theoretical framework as a guide, which can point out some of the negative consequences that could result from certain courses of action, solutions to problems that are obtained by trial and error may not be real solutions at all. Thus, in the example just cited, by reducing professional nursing care the administrator may reduce some salary costs, but this saving could be more than offset by a drop in the quality of nursing care provided to patients.

Experience

One of the definitions of a good, experienced administrator is that he can solve problems, make decisions, and evaluate programs off the top of his head, so to speak. This may well be true for the majority of situations he is confronted with, which are uncomplicated and straightforward. However, complex problems and decisions may demand considerably more data for their solution than the experiential background of the administrator can provide. As society advances, as knowledge in all fields multiplies, as problems become thornier, the need for research conducted outside of the rough and tumble atmosphere of the ongoing administrative process becomes greater.

Empirical Evidence

Many problems, many decisions, many needs to develop new programs or procedures, can be met by recourse to existing facts. There is a wealth of factual knowledge available to meet these needs in many areas of activity. "How many nurses do I need to staff my obstetrics unit?" is an example of a specific problem question. Study of available empirical data on existing patterns in large numbers of hospitals can serve as a guideline, rough as it is, for the staffing of a specific nursing unit. Research may not be needed for a whole class of problems like these which can be served adequately by existing data. On the other hand, there is danger in overreliance on using such data in solving specific problems. Data representing the average situation in a large population may hide important differences that exist among the individual members of the population. Moreover, data describing an existing situation tell only what is and not what should be. They are not norms or standards and should not be regarded as such.

Common Sense

One of the attributes of a "common-sense" approach to problem solving, decision making, or evaluating is that it operates from a heterogeneous and rather superficial collection of facts rather than an orderly and systematic arrangement of knowledge and theories. The common-sense approach may be quite workable in many situations and could serve as a practical substitute for formal research. In other situations—generally those that are complex and many-faceted—common sense has the same deficiencies as do trial and error and reliance on existing empirical data. Foremost among the deficiencies of these methods is their superficiality, which can result in "solutions" that are transitory and insubstantial. Moreover, common-sense knowledge, like that acquired by trial and error, may even turn out to be dangerous. For example, the common-sense "solutions" to the treatment of certain illnesses that medical historians so often describe have sometimes had undesirable consequences in terms of the health of human beings.

Faith, Tradition, Habit

Many decisions are made, many programs are launched, many procedures and methods are carried out, that primarily depend on what can be called faith, or reliance on custom, habit, or ritualism. To illustrate: for the past fifty years hundreds of hospitals have been built, each following the design of previously built hospitals with the rigid compartmentalization of patients according to such factors as major category of illness (medical, surgical, etc.) and sex. Recent studies, like those concerned with the system of hospital organization known as Progressive Patient Care, have shown that other ways of organizing patients, such as according to their nursing care needs, could well prove to be more efficient and economical.[20] Or, take the many nursing procedures that are performed. How many of these, like routine T.P.R.'s, are ritualistic and serve little useful purpose?

Reliance on faith, tradition, routine can sometimes perpetuate inefficient performance. An important attribute of research is that it often raises pertinent questions about the value of certain customary ways of doing things. In research the saying:

> Hath not old custom made this life more sweet
> Than that of painted pomp?[21]

is superseded by:

> These times do shift—each thing his turn does hold
> New things succeed, as former things grow old.[22]

WHEN IS RESEARCH NEEDED?

We have seen that there are many substitutes to the carrying out of formal research and that these can often serve as useful guides to the making of decisions, the solving of problems, or the development or evaluation of programs, procedures, and methods. However, when the situation becomes too complex the homely devices of trial and error, common sense, empirical evidence, and reliance on past behavior can prove to be inadequate. It is at this point that the need for formal research may become apparent.

But the decision to actually engage in research probably depends on one critical factor—the importance of the problem to be studied. Because research usually requires a large expenditure of human and economic resources, the decision to pursue a research study cannot be taken lightly. The importance of the problem must be demonstrated. In many cases, the importance of a problem can be evaluated in terms of three criteria: the frequency with which the problem arises; the amount of money that is affected by the existence of problem; and the degree to which human health and safety are influenced by the problem.

In addition, it is almost self-evident that two other criteria are important in deciding to undertake research. These are a genuine interest in a researcher to conduct the research, and the capability of expressing the problem in terms that can be researched.

These criteria can vividly be demonstrated by the problem of the shortage of nurses. This problem meets all the criteria just mentioned. The shortage of nurses is not localized to one institution or one field of nursing or one area of the country, but is spread throughout the country. Moreover, it can easily be demonstrated that large sums of money are affected by this shortage. But even more important is the possible harm to human health and safety by not having enough nurses to give adequate nursing care. Finally, many researchers can be found who have strong interests in solving the problem, and it has been adequately demonstrated that the problem is researchable.

The significant extent to which the problem of the shortage of nurses meets all the criteria for deciding when to undertake research helps to explain why so many studies have been focused on this problem in recent years. But a problem need meet only some of these criteria to show a need for research. Automobile manufacturers, for example, spend enormous sums each year on research concerning consumer preferences for automobile design. It is hard to justify this expenditure on the basis of frequency of the problem, because it certainly has been demonstrated by certain manufacturers of foreign cars that it is not necessary to change an automobile's styling each year. Nor can it be argued that car design (at least from the aesthetic standpoint) has a significant effect on the health and well-being of many people—other than the car manufacturers themselves, perhaps. However, it can be argued that enormous sums of money are affected by this problem. Automobile manufacturing is a multibillion-dollar industry, and mistakes in design, as demonstrated by the ill-fated Edsel automobile, can have serious monetary consequences.

Summary

The purpose of this chapter was to provide some notions of what research is—the various purposes of research, the methods for conducting research, the types of research settings, the kinds of subjects upon whom research is done, and finally some criteria for determining when research is needed. In this chapter, research has been shown to be an activity directed toward finding answers to questions that provide new knowledge to the world at large. More definitively, research can be defined as a planned and systematic activity directed at the discovery of new facts and/or the identification of relationships among facts.

The following is a typology of research studies that summarizes the various topics that were discussed in this chapter:

A Typology of Research

I. Reasons for doing research

    A. Basic or pure research: to establish fundamental theories, facts, and/or statements of relationships among facts in some area of knowledge that are *not* intended for immediate use in some real-life situation. Basic research is useful in advancing scientific knowledge and in furthering research

    B. Applied research: to obtain new facts and/or identify relationships among facts which are intended to be used in a real-life situation, specifically, to:
      1. Solve a problem
      2. Make a decision
      3. Develop a program, procedure, process, or product
      4. Evaluate a program, procedure, process, or product

II. Purposes of research

    A. Descriptive research: to discover new facts
    B. Explanatory research: to discover relationships among facts

III. Methods of research

    A. Experimental method: observation under controlled conditions
    B. Nonexperimental method: observation without controlled conditions

IV. Settings for research

    A. Highly controlled settings: research centers, laboratories, experimental units, test units
    B. Partially controlled settings: experiments in field settings
    C. Uncontrolled settings: field surveys, case studies, natural setting studies

V. Subjects of research

    A. Human beings
    B. Animals, plants, etc.
    C. Inanimate objects

VI. Doers of research

   A. Specialized research institutes devoted entirely to research
   B. Research branches of operating organizations such as hospitals, governmental agencies, and professional organizations
   C. Faculty members and students engaged full or part time in research studies
   D. Personnel in operating organizations with full-time operating responsibilities, with occasional need to conduct a formal study

VII. Substitutes for research

   A. Trial and error
   B. Experience
   C. Empirical evidence
   D. Common sense
   E. Faith, custom, precedent, habit

VIII. Criteria for determining when research is needed and should be undertaken

   A. Frequency of occurrence of problem
   B. Amount of money affected by problem
   C. Degree to which health and welfare of humans affected by the problem
   D. Genuine interest of researcher in doing the study
   E. Researchability of the problem

References

1. U.S. Department of Health, Education, and Welfare, Public Health Service, National Institutes of Health, *Public Health Service Grants and Awards, Fiscal 1961 Funds.* U.S. Public Health Service Publication No. 883, Part 1. Washington, D.C., Government Printing Office, 1961.

2. Wilfred J. Remillard, "The Ancient Mystery of Thunder." *Saturday Review,* **44:**31–34, July 1, 1961.

3. Fritz J. Roethlisberger and William J. Dickson, *Management and the Worker.* Cambridge, Harvard University Press, 1939.

4. Bernard G. Greenberg, "Conduct of Cooperative Field and Clinical Trials." *American Statistician,* **13:**13–17, 28, June 1959.

5. Morris R. Cohen and Ernest Nagel, *An Introduction to Logic and Scientific Method.* New York, Harcourt, Brace and Co., 1934, pp. 217–218.

6. Naval Research Advisory Committee, *Basic Research in the Navy* (Volume 1 of a Report to the Secretary of the Navy on Basic Research in the Navy, June 1, 1959), p. 2.

7. Alexander Pope, *Epistle 1.* Book 1.

8. Elizabeth Herzog, *Some Guidelines for Evaluative Research.* Childrens Bureau Publication No. 375, 1959. Washington, D.C., U.S. Department of Health, Education, and Welfare, 1959, pp. 15–26.

9. Madelyne Sturdavant, *Comparisons of Intensive Nursing Service in a Circular and a Rectangular Unit.* Hospital Monograph Series No. 8. Chicago, The American Hospital Association, 1960.

10. Herman Wold, "Causal Inference from Observational Data." *J. Royal Statistical Soc.* (Series A, Part 1), **119:**28–61, January 1956.

11. Oscar Kempthorne, *The Design and Analysis of Experiments*. New York, Robert E. Krieger Publishing Co., Inc., 1973.
12. Alfred C. Kinsey, Wardell B. Pomeroy, and Clyde E. Martin, *Sexual Behavior in the Human Male*. Philadelphia, W. B. Saunders Co., 1948.
13. Paul F. Lazarsfeld, Bernard Berelson, and Hazel Gaudet, *The People's Choice*. New York, Columbia University Press, 1948.
14. F. Stuart Chapin, *Experimental Designs in Sociological Research*, Westport, Conn., Greenwood Press, Inc., 1974, p. 1.
15. Eugene Levine, "Experimental Design in Nursing Research." *Nursing Res.*, **9:**203–212, fall 1960.
16. Temple Burling, Edith M. Lentz, and Robert N. Wilson, *The Give and Take in Hospitals*. New York, G. P. Putnam's Sons, 1956.
17. Paul F. Lazarsfeld, "The Sociology of Empirical Social Research." *Am. Sociol. Rev.*, **27:**757–767, December 1962.
18. Charles D. Flagle, "Operational Research in the Health Sciences," in L. M. Schuman (ed.), "Research Methodology and Potential in Community Health and Preventive Medicine." *Ann. New York Acad. Sci.*, **107:** Art. 2:748–759, May 22, 1963.
19. Dorothy G. Sutherland, "Nursing's New Look in the Public Health Service." *Nursing Outlook,* **8:**571–572, October 1962.
20. Jack C. Haldeman and Faye G. Abdellah, "Concepts of Progressive Patient Care." *Hospitals, J.A.H.A.,* **33:**38–42, 142–144, May 16, 1959.
21. William Shakespeare, *As You Like It,* Act II, Scene 1, Line 2.
22. Robert Herrick, *Hesperides: Ceremonies for Candelmas Eve.*

Suggestions for Further Reading

A good, brief discussion of the various kinds of research can be found in:
Bernard G. Greenberg, "Introduction to Research," in *International Conference on the Planning of Nursing Studies,* edited by Margaret G. Arnstein and Ellen Broe. London, International Council of Nurses, Florence Nightingale Foundation, 1956, pp. 51–65.

Discussion of the various kinds of research settings is found in:
Leon Festinger and Daniel Katz, *Research Methods in the Behavioral Sciences.* New York, The Dryden Press, 1953. Part 1, "Research Settings," pp. 15–172.

Good brief descriptions of the research conducted by famous scientists, including Galileo, Darwin, and Pavlov, are found in the paperback:
Lives in Science. New York, Simon and Schuster, 1957 (A Scientific American Book).

For a discussion of the term "demonstration," see:
Elizabeth Herzog, "Research, Demonstrations and Common-Sense." *Child Welfare, The Journal of the Child Welfare League of America,* pp. 243–248, June 1962.

For an extended discussion of natural setting research see:
Robert W. Habenstein (ed.), *Pathways to Data.* Chicago, Aldine Publishing Co., 1970.

A good description of the case-study method is found in:

Pauline V. Young, *Scientific Social Surveys and Research.* Englewood Cliffs, N.J., Prentice-Hall, 1949, Chap. XII, pp. 265–285.

A clearly written little book on the experimental method, written for high school students, is:

Philip Goldstein, *How to Do an Experiment.* New York, Harcourt, Brace and Co., 1957.

An excellent distinction between explanatory and descriptive research is contained in:

Herbert Hyman, *Survey Design and Analysis.* New York, The Free Press of Glencoe, 1955.

For a critique of experimental studies involving human subjects see:

Theodore X. Barber, *Pitfalls in Human Research: Ten Pivotal Points.* New York, Pergamon Press, 1976.

Problems and Suggestions for Further Study

1. Various definitions of research given in this chapter have used the term "facts." What are facts? In Cohen and Nagel's *An Introduction to Logic and Scientific Method* (pp. 217–219) there is an excellent discussion of what is meant by facts. The authors show that there are at least four kinds of facts. What are these? List some facts that you are familiar with that fall into these different categories.

2. List ten questions that could serve as the starting point for a research study. Briefly indicate whether each question would initiate basic or applied research. Are the questions as you have stated them researchable?

3. List some of the pros and cons of experimental versus nonexperimental research. Why can nonexperimental studies usually have greater breadth in terms of range of problems studied, number of study subjects included, and so on, than can experimental studies?

4. Can you think of any new procedures or products that should be developed in your area of work? List some of these and indicate briefly how you think a research study could help in the development of these procedures or products.

5. How does trial and error really differ from a research approach? What are some of the dangers in using a trial and error approach in patient care? Can you think of some examples of the use of trial and error in your personal life, your work?

6. Review some recent issues of the nursing and hospital journals (e.g., *Nursing Research*) to see if you can find any examples of reports of research studies. Select three of these, and using the typology of research given in the summary of this chapter, indicate into which categories under each major heading the research study you have selected would fall. Did you find any reports of experimental studies conducted in highly controlled settings?

7. Describe the kinds of problems, administrative and otherwise, you might run into if you wanted to undertake the following research studies:

    a. Testing a new way of giving a back rub to a patient
    b. Designing a new layout for the central supply room
    c. Investigating the question: Is private duty nursing obsolete?
    d. A study of the quality of nursing care provided in nursing homes
    e. A study of physicians' attitudes toward higher education among nurses
    f. Investigating the causes of drop-outs from a baccalaureate program of
       nursing education

8. Read the article by Miriam A. Safren and Alphonse Chapanis, "A Critical
Incident Study of Hospital Medication Errors" (*Hospitals, J.A.H.A.*, **31:**
32–34, 57–66, May 1, 1960). How would you classify this study according to the typology given in the summary? What, if any, were the study
conditions that were controlled by the researchers? To what extent could
the findings be applied beyond the study setting? Can you suggest other
ways such a study could be done?

9. Discuss what is meant by explanation in the use of the term "explanatory"
research. What is meant by the statement, if we can explain we can also
predict? Is this always true?

10. Give some examples of "common-sense" knowledge in nursing. How does
common-sense knowledge differ from scientific knowledge? What are the
limitations of common-sense knowledge, and what are its advantages?

11. Why is the second example 4 on page 58 of this chapter of the study of
the relationship between nurse staffing and adequacy of patient care classified as a partially controlled setting rather than a highly controlled setting? How could this study be more highly controlled than it is?

12. Can you conceive of studies involving animals in nursing research? How
could the findings of such studies be applied to human beings? What are
the advantages of using animals as subjects in research studies?

13. What are the disadvantages of conducting explanatory surveys in completely uncontrolled settings? Can cause and effect relationships be isolated
in natural settings or can they be studied only in a laboratory?

14. Give three examples of existing data (e.g., such as the data in *Facts about
Nursing* published by the American Nurses' Association), that could be
used in solving problems or making decisions in specific nursing situations.
A hint: how could the data on nursing salaries in *Facts* be used in a specific situation?

15. Do the criteria for determining when research is needed, given in this
chapter, apply to basic research as well as to applied research? Can you
think of other criteria that could be used to determine when research is
needed?

16. Discuss the kinds of basic research that could be done in your field of interest. In what sense would these projects be considered as basic research?

17. Can you think of examples of research that is being done that could have
been stimulated by the frequency with which the problem being studied
occurred? Can you think of examples where the research was probably
stimulated by the amount of money involved in the problem? By the
health and welfare of human beings?

18. Which of the following activities can be defined as research and which
cannot? If you do not feel they are research, what kind of activity or
process are they (e.g., demonstration, common sense, etc.)?

    a. Analyzing results of public opinion polls
    b. Writing a history of nursing
    c. Conducting a cost analysis of a school of nursing
    d. Developing the architectural plans for a new health center
    e. Administering intelligence tests to a group of applicants for a job
    f. Conducting a census of unemployment in a large city

19. There is a current trend toward the use of the term "evaluation research." What does this term mean? How does it differ from other kinds of research? Examples of evaluation research can be found in Gene V. Glass (ed.), *Evaluation Studies Review Annual*, Vol. I. Beverly Hills, Sage Publications, 1976.

Chapter Four

CONCEPTUALIZATION IN NURSING RESEARCH

IN NURSING RESEARCH, much emphasis has been placed upon finding solutions to operational problems rather than upon using scientific inquiry to get at the fundamental cause(s) of the problem. It is often more difficult to find and to formulate a problem than to find its solution. One prevalent difficulty in setting up nursing research on a scientific basis lies in posing the appropriate questions that need to be answered rather than in finding the answers.

In science, the questions that matter are of a particular kind. They are so formulated that the answers to them will confirm, amplify, or variously revise some part of what is currently taken as knowledge in the field.[1]

Every problem in science involves a question(s), but not every question qualifies as a scientific problem. Much emphasis in the literature has been placed upon the John Dewey process of problem solving but little can be found about the process of "problem finding."

What is the process of "problem finding"? Where does it begin? Unfortunately, there is no set formula that one can follow. One approach is to begin by challenging existing facts and questioning the evidence at hand. In research, facts are often included in generalizations that relate one fact to another. Thus, the facts can be correct but the deductions about the relationships among the facts may be false.

One might also begin by examining the facts to see if their application in present-day situations is still relevant. Examples of this can be found by examining some current nursing practices that have been or have become ritualistic rather than being based upon sound physiological principles. Such practices originally served very useful purposes in past situations. But situations change, and facts related to current practices must be examined in light of these changing situations.

Merton summarizes the process of "problem finding" in the three following steps:[2]

First: originate the question. State what it is you want to know.

Second: specify the rationale or conceptual framework (to be described later). State why you want to have this particular question answered.

Third: state the questions that point toward the possible answers to the originating questions in terms that satisfy the rationale for having raised the question.

One significant limitation in carrying out research in nursing is the lack of a conceptual framework for the proposed research. This lack becomes particularly acute when one is trying to identify specific criterion measures of the phenomena being studied.

In nursing, a conceptual framework is a theoretical approach to the study of problems that are scientifically based that emphasizes the selection, arrangement, and clarification of its concepts. The rationale, or conceptual framework, is a predictive tool that can tell us what will happen to other parts of knowledge or practice as a result of answering the research question. This helps to differentiate between the scientifically consequential and scientifically trivial question. In a sense, the conceptual framework provides the investigator with the evidence he needs to justify why he selected a particular question for study. Nursing is changing so rapidly that even its conceptual framework is unsteady, and doubts arise about the meaning of traditionally accepted words, such as "nurse," "nursing," "patient," "staffing pattern," "team nursing," "nursing function," "nursing skill." Can we continue to use such vague concepts if we are not quite sure what we are saying when we use them.

So long as we doubt what our general terms really mean, we cannot even think clear thoughts, for all thinking on a theoretical level is implemented wholly by words, and if the implements are faulty, thinking peters out in words.[3]

A conceptual framework in research can provide ways of looking at data and grouping facts into a rationale. It makes explicit what is implicit in our beliefs or denials. The conceptual or theoretical framework in nursing research can help to provide a clear and concise statement of knowledge in the area. Theory gives direction to the investigator as he seeks to uncover the truth based upon facts. Those researchers who purport to be disdainful of theory are proceeding with a blindfold over their eyes, for without it progress is not possible.

THE ROLE OF THEORY IN RESEARCH

A review of current studies completed in nursing research points to a major limitation of these studies—namely, the need for systematic knowledge founded on a broader base. The lack of this knowledge necessitates that any inferences drawn from the findings would usually have to be limited to the specific situations in which the research has been conducted.

The development of a theory for the research is the most direct way of systematizing knowledge founded on a broader base. A theory or conceptual framework for the research is the source of the rationale for the research.

Theory in research summarizes existing knowledge, provides an explanation for observed facts and relationships, and predicts the occurrence of as yet unobserved events and relationships on the basis of explanatory principles embodied in the theory.[4] Braithwaite[5] defines a theory as a set of hypotheses that form a deductive system. The latter is arranged in such a logical pattern that some of the hypotheses become premises of other hypotheses, which in turn become premises of still other hypotheses, thus forming a system of scientifically derived knowledge.

A scientific theory is composed of three parts. These are:

1. Definitions: These are operationally defined terms of words or phrases used in the statement of the problem. Whenever possible they should be expressed in observable and quantifiable terms.

2. Postulates: These are concepts or abstract ideas of universal significance which later may be translated into principles and laws. Each postulate must be documented from the literature or from previous research as yet not published.

   It is necessary to distinguish laws from postulates. Laws originate as postulates that eventually may become laws when the hypotheses tested are proven to be true. Peirce[6] refers to laws as generalizations from observation of facts that are representative of outward conditions. A law must not be based upon a chance coincidence among the observations from which it is derived.

   The validity of postulates is determined by testing deductions that derive from them. Deductions thus comprise the third part of a scientific theory.[7]

3. Deductions: These are commonly referred to as hypotheses. Deductions are conclusions reached by logically proceeding from a clarification of definitions to acceptable postulates (concepts) and then to hypotheses that can be tested in research.

   The testing of the hypothesis either serves to confirm the validity of the theory or leads to a modification of the postulates upon which the theory was based. The usefulness of a theory is dependent upon the deductions that can be made from it.

The degree to which the nursing profession progresses in defining a scientific body of knowledge that is uniquely nursing will be dependent upon research that will provide a body of facts from which generalizations and laws can be applied to the solution of a wide range of nursing problems. The development of scientific theories for application to nursing research can help to achieve this goal.

Theories are not "ivory-tower" phenomena but have great importance in developing research.[8] A good theory can serve as the basis for the successful exploration of phenomena and testing of hypotheses.[9] Theories can serve as important guides for the direction of the research by pointing to areas that are likely to be productive of meaningful relationships among the phenomena studied. The more research is directed by scientific theory, the more likely are its results to contribute directly to the development and further organization of a scientific body of knowledge in nursing.

Conceptualization—A Hallmark of Nursing Research

Methods of inquiry belong to all fields not just nursing. Who does research in nursing? The broad conceptualization of nursing research does not limit nor require that the researcher be a nurse. Likewise, nursing research has no distinctive setting. It can take place in a hospital, community, home, school. Those criteria that distinguish nursing research are those associated with identifying nursing phenomena—the actions and the theories that make up nursing practice. Phenomena in nursing are man made—artificial rather than natural phenomena. They are shaped and determined by normative judgments (rules, ideas that govern the profession).

There is an increased need for emphasis on studies that provide a conceptual basis for nursing and shaping the theory of nursing. It is here that the case study is so important. By examining the total one can see the normative judgments taken and avoid repetitive errors. One needs to discover the sets of values operating. Values cannot be separated from research.

A few direct attempts have been made to develop conceptual models for nursing research. A conceptual model can be defined as a diagrammatic representation of a postulate or concept.[10] A brief description of some of these models follows.

Development of a Methodology to Evaluate Patient Care

Howland[11] recognized the need for system models designed to provide organized information to assist in the management decision-making process related to patient care. Descriptions of man-machine systems in terms of task performance and resource utilization variables have been developed.

Howland and his research team specified certain characteristics of a systems research model. These are:[12]

1. It is designed to provide descriptive rather than prescriptive models of man-machine systems.

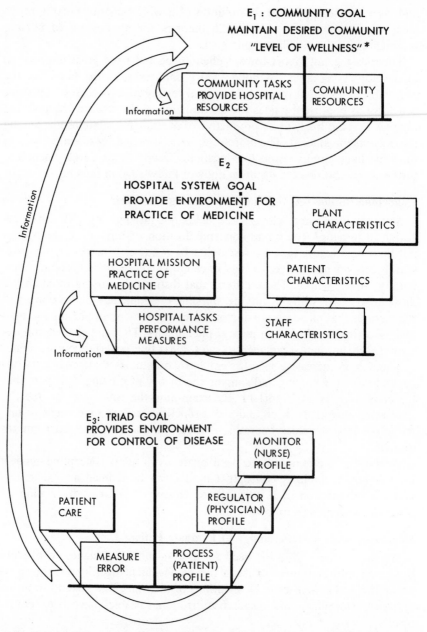

Fig. 4-1. Missions, tasks, and resources of the hospital system. (* Dunn, Halbert L., "Points of Attack for Raising the Levels of Wellness." *J. Natl. Med. Assoc.,* **49:** 225–55, 1957. *Courtesy* Howland, Daniel, *The Development of a Methodology for the Evaluation of Patient Care.* Systems Research Group of the Engineering Experiment Station, the Ohio State University and the OSU Research Foundation, June 1961, GN-W-4785; RF-940, p. 29, and "A Hospital Systems Model." *Nursing Res.,* **12:**235, fall 1963.)

2. It specifies relationships between levels of task performance and resource utilization.
3. It is based on empirical methods rather than upon formal mathematical systems.
4. It is problem-oriented rather than technique-oriented.

Figure 4-1 shows an overall hospital system broken down into community, hospital, and triad levels.

The nurse-patient-physician triad was developed by Howland[13] and McDowell[14] (see Figure 4-2). The investigators conceptualized the triad as a servo system in which the patient generates signals to the monitor. The monitor may respond to the patient signals at one of three levels. The first provides information about patient condition; at the second level the monitor determines the difference between actual and desired patient performance, and the difference information is made available to the regulator; at the third level the nurse serves as a monitor and takes necessary action for the regulation of the patient's condition.

The forward thinking of the Howland research team has brought together the concepts of homeostasis first envisioned by Cannon[15] and later developed by Wiener[16] and Ashby.[17]

The rationale basic to the "nurse-patient-physician triad" is that it is viewed as a self-regulating mechanism that constantly compares actual and desired patient condition and takes action to minimize the difference between the two. This action (which might be nurse action or physician action) is taken to reestablish and maintain the state of the patient within specified limits, or error bandwidth.[18]

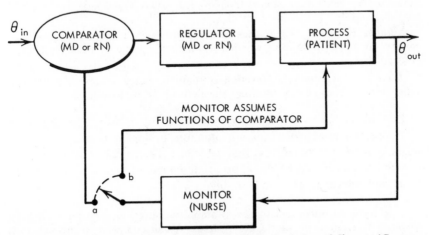

Fig. 4-2. Man—machine system for the control and regulation of disease. (*Courtesy* Howland, Daniel, and McDowell, Wanda E., "The Measurement of Patient Care: A Conceptual Framework." *Nursing Res.*, **13:**5, winter 1964.)

A Reaction Model

Hayes and Leik[19] envisioned developing a reaction model that might be used to predict behaviors related to interpersonal relationships. The investigators raised the question: Why are there such differences in reaction to essentially the same situations among several persons or in the same person over time? Basic to a model is the theory upon which it is built. The dimensions of the reaction model are "relevance" and "value," which affect all situations such as interpersonal relationships, nurse-patient interactions, nurse actions taken that affect the patient (e.g., nurse action and pain).

Following is an interpretation of the way in which Hayes and Leik[20] conceived the theoretical structure basic to their model.

Relevance

Operational Definition: Relevance is considered an omnipresent dimension of all situations to which one is exposed. The dimension or degree of relevance may range from low to high.

Postulates (concepts):
1. Experience and imagination help to establish the relevance of a situation.
2. High levels of satisfaction or deprivation substantially modify one's reaction to many situations.
3. What we believe to be the relevance of essentially the same situation may undergo substantial change as a product of our experiences with it.

Deduction (hypothesis): The more relevant we perceive a situation to be for us, the stronger will our reaction be.

Value

Operational Definition: Value refers to the individual's evaluation of the positive, neutral, or negative character of an object, someone's behavior, or a situation. The value dimension is bipolar—it has two high points, positive and negative, and one low point, neutral.

Postulate (concept): Experience contributes heavily to producing the standards of judgment in deciding whether a situation is primarily positive, neutral, or negative.

Deduction (hypothesis): Reaction strength increases as our judgment of values moves from neutral to either the positive or negative pole.

To illustrate, a situation test may be used to measure the degree of relevance and value placed upon a situation. Following is such a test that might be used. The situation is first described. The person must then select *one* choice that would be the appropriate course of action to take where value and relevance may both be high.

A professional nurse is assigned to ambulance duty in a hospital situation where there is an acute shortage of interns. A call comes in to proceed to a nearby lake where a child has been rescued. She arrives on the scene ten minutes after the child has been taken from the water. The parents are with the child. No one has attempted to resuscitate the child. The nurse knows that if she should be successful in resuscitating the child, the child would more than likely suffer considerable brain damage due to the lack of oxygen. If you were in this situation which one of the following courses of action would you follow?

1. Attempt to resuscitate the child and hope that brain damage would be minimal.
2. Explain the alternatives to the parents and let them decide.
3. Do not attempt to resuscitate the child, knowing that brain damage might be extensive.
4. Place the child in the ambulance and take her to the hospital.

The situation is then repeated. Everything is exactly the same with one exception—the child is the niece of the nurse on ambulance duty. You are asked to choose once again from the above choices.

Since all choices are possible there is no right or wrong answer. However, the choice the respondent makes does provide information as to the dimensions of relevance and value. The choice of these dimensions in repeated situation tests can help to predict types of behavior and provide clues to possible answers to the original question posed by Hayes and Leik—namely, why are there such differences in reactions to the same situation among several persons?

A Nursing Care Model

From the beginning of organized nursing practice in the battlefield, in the home, and in the hospital there has been a need for a way to predict nurse staffing patterns. Several attempts[21] have been made to study the nurse at work and then to plan staffing patterns based on empirical knowledge. This tends to perpetuate ritualistic nursing practices that no longer serve useful purposes; it also fosters the development of staffing patterns organized to meet the needs of the health agency or hospital rather than the needs of the patient.

In an attempt to derive nurse staffing patterns based on patient needs, the following nursing care model was developed.

In developing a conceptual framework from which a nursing care model[22] might evolve, the first step was to define operationally the terms from which the derivation of nurse staffing patterns might be traced.

Term	*Definition*
Nursing care	1. Assistance is provided a patient when, for some reason, he cannot provide for the satisfaction of his own needs.
	2. It is commensurate with the abilities and skills of the person providing the assistance.
	3. It is derived from a study of the patient's requirements for nursing care.
	4. It is directed toward making the patient better able to help himself.

Term	Definition
Personal need	A considerable variety of optimal conditions such as air, water, food, temperature, and intactness of body tissue is required for survival. When, for some reason, any of these necessities departs from the optimum, *a state of need* can be said to exist.
Self-help ability (S.H.A.)	An ability of the person to provide for the satisfaction of his own needs.
Impaired state	An impairment to the body or person that limits the individual's ability to satisfy his needs and results from injury, disease, malformation, or maldevelopment.

Once these definitions were spelled out the next step was to spell out the postulates and deductions related to nursing care requirements (see Figure 4-3 for an application of the model to a coronary patient).

Nursing Care Requirements

Postulate   As long as self-help ability is developed and maintained at a level in which need satisfaction can take place without assistance, nursing care will not be required. Need satisfaction will then be a function of S.H.A., etc.

Deduction   Need satisfaction will then be a function of self-help ability and nursing care.

Need for Impairment Care

Postulate   When, as a result of an impaired state, self-help ability is reduced to a minus state and certain personal needs cannot be satisfied, a need for impairment care will arise.

Deduction   Impairment care is a function of the need for sustenal care, for remedial care, and for restorative care.

Need for Sustenal Care

Postulate   When self-help ability is diminished as a result of an impaired state and the patient cannot of his own accord provide for the satisfaction of his personal needs, care must be administered to augment self-help ability to the extent that the personal needs can be satisfied.

Deduction   The need for sustenal care will be a function of the reduced state of self-help ability and unsatisfied personal needs.

$$N\ CaSus = f\ [(SHA\ -) \times (Np)]$$

(The need for care, sustenal, is a function of self-help ability minus, multiplied by the patient's personal needs.)

The development of the postulates (concepts) necessary to explain the effect(s) of the application of the stimulus and a rational presentation of what is taking place are often designated as theoretical research.

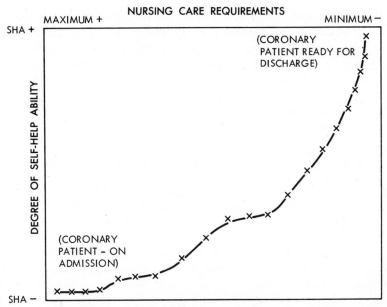

Fig. 4-3. Progression of coronary patient during three weeks of hospitalization according to self-help ability and nursing care requirements.

If an investigator does not provide a conceptual framework for his research, he is in danger of basing his research on an isolated postulate or hypothesis that really does not tie in with other acquired knowledge. A postulate is significant only if it occurs together with others in statements of lawfulness that we have reason to believe are true. A conceptual framework can state functional relationships between qualitative phenomena and is not limited to statistical relationships.[23]

A concept that is frightening to some is patient-centered care. One hears, "Isn't this what we have always been doing?" Is this just another cliché for "total patient care," "comprehensive care," "nursing the whole patient?" It has been pointed out that all concepts basically theoretical must be implemented by words. If the words selected to implement the theoretical framework are ambiguous, interpretation of the concept itself can only lead to confusion and frightened thinking.

If we fail to admit our natural fears we shy away from the concept and state that it is esoteric and beyond us. The concept of patient-centered care can be clarified only by presenting the facts about the concept. What words can be selected to translate it into meaningful terms? Operationally one might agree that patient-centered care is assistance provided a patient in meeting his individual requirements for nursing care when for some reason he cannot provide for the satisfaction of his own needs.

The concept can be clarified further if criteria are spelled out that can be used to identify its implementation—that is, if patient-centered care were being provided in a patient care situation, one might use the following criteria to determine if the objectives were being met:

1. The patient is able to provide for the satisfaction of his own needs.
2. The nursing care plan makes provision to meet four needs—sustenal care, remedial care, restorative care, and preventive care.
3. The care plan extends beyond the patient's hospitalization and makes provision for continuation of the care at home.
4. The levels of nursing skills provided vary with the individual patient care requirements.
5. The entire care plan is directed at having the patient help himself.
6. The care plan makes provision for involvement of members of the family throughout the hospitalization and after discharge.

Any concept not defined clearly in terms that are universally acceptable will create confusion and withdrawal from its use. One must continue to question each concept to determine how it fits into a theoretical framework. The danger is in withdrawing from the concept and saying, "That's beyond me." One must never give up a continuing search for the truth based upon facts. An investigator who takes time to spell out a sound conceptual framework is more likely to base his research upon facts rather than upon conjecture. The following might serve as a conceptual framework from which a nursing care model might evolve.

List of 21 Specific Needs Presented by Patients at Different Stages of Illness[24]

Basic to all patients

1. To maintain good hygiene and physical comfort
2. To promote optimal activity: exercise, rest, and sleep
3. To promote safety through prevention of accident, injury, or other trauma and through the prevention of the spread of infection
4. To maintain good body mechanics and prevent and correct deformities

Sustenal care needs

5. To facilitate the maintenance of a supply of oxygen to all body cells
6. To facilitate the maintenance of nutrition to all body cells
7. To facilitate the maintenance of elimination
8. To facilitate the maintenance of fluid and electrolyte balance
9. To recognize the physiological responses of the body to disease conditions—pathological, physiological, and compensatory

10. To facilitate the maintenance of regulatory mechanisms and functions‘

11. To facilitate the maintenance of sensory function

12. To identify and accept positive and negative expressions, feelings, and reactions

13. To identify and accept the interrelatedness of emotions and organic illness

Remedial care needs   14. To facilitate the maintenance of effective verbal and nonverbal communication

15. To promote the development of productive interpersonal relationships

16. To facilitate progress toward achievement of personal and spiritual goals

17. To create and/or maintain a therapeutic environment

18. To facilitate awareness of self as an individual with varying physical, emotional, and developmental needs

Restorative care needs   19. To accept the optimum possible goals in the light of limitations, physical and emotional

20. To use community resources as an aid in resolving problems arising from illness

21. To understand the role of social problems as influencing factors in the cause of illness

Model for the Study of Pain

The physical sciences are particularly important in determining the physiological basis of nursing practices. Following is a theoretical framework developed by two nurse research students in studying the problem of the frequency with which pain accompanies intramuscular injections administered in two selected sites.[25] The two sites selected for study were the gluteus maximus muscle and the vastus lateralis muscle.

Definition:

Pain is seen as a specific sensation with a special and separate mechanism for the detection and transmission of pain impulses. A distinct feeling state accompanies the sensation. The sensation and the feeling state together constitute the pain experience.

The investigators made an intensive review of the literature and were able to identify the following postulates (concepts) that had bearing on their research.

Postulates:

1. Each structure such as skin, subcutaneous tissue, fascia, muscle, periosteum, bone, and blood vessels has a characteristic pain sensation.

2. Each structural category demonstrates specific variations within its group which are consistent from individual to individual.

3. Pain threshold does not vary markedly from person to person, but there are certain localized conditions that will modify it in the individual.

4. Diseases of the nervous system modify the cutaneous sensitivity.
5. Muscles differ in their relative sensitiveness in the same individual. Deep muscle pain can modify the cutaneous pain threshold purely by reason of the fact that in certain instances both may be served by the same set of nerves.

A patient's previous experience with pain will have a decided effect upon the patient's response.

The investigators hypothesized the following deductions:

Deductions:[26]
There is no difference in the frequency with which pain occurs concomitant to an initial injection of a given medication into the inner aspect of the upper outer quadrant of the gluteus maximus muscle as compared with the frequency with which it occurs during a similar injection into the longitudinal midpoint of the vastus lateralis muscle as reported by the patient.

There is no difference in the frequency with which pain occurs concomitant to an initial injection of a given medication into the inner aspects of the upper outer quadrant of the gluteus maximus muscle at 6:00 A.M. as compared with the frequency with which it occurs during a similar injection given at 6:00 P.M. in the same site as reported by patients.

There is no difference in the frequency with which pain occurs concomitant to an initial injection of a given medication into the longitudinal midpoint of the vastus lateralis muscle at 6:00 A.M. as compared with the frequency with which is occurs during a similar injection given at 6:00 P.M. in the same site as reported by patients.

Model for Study of Aggression

As in the physical sciences, questions essential for formulating the problem for which the social sciences can help can have greater relevancy if they stem from a sound theoretical framework. A nurse investigator majoring in anthropology was interested in the problem of aggression, specifically the way in which it is controlled in primitive societies.[27] Understanding this would hopefully give her a better understanding of the ways in which patients suppress and repress drives and needs. Following an intensive review of the literature she was able to find evidence to show that although aggression is rigidly controlled in interpersonal relations, the drive or need remains. Since aggression cannot be expressed freely in interpersonal relations, it must be expressed more indirectly, symbolically, and in disguised forms. She further rationalized that religious systems provide for such expressions by the mechanisms of projection, displacement, and rationalization.

A further spelling out of the rationale or theoretical framework led the investigator to formulate the following hypothesis: The greater the control over the expression of aggression in interpersonal relations by the members in societies, the greater the expression of aggression in religious practices and beliefs.

Religion was defined as a set of beliefs and practices with respect to supernaturals that the members of a society report and/or that the investigator observes.

Model for Study of Emotional Stress

Another example of formulating a theoretical framework for a problem utilizing social science concepts was a study of patients undergoing major surgery in a general hospital to determine the level of emotional tension preoperatively and postoperatively.[28] This investigator hoped to differentiate levels of emotional tension in patients undergoing major surgery.

Examples of definitions spelled out as part of the investigator's framework were:

Anxiety: an apprehension of threat or danger
Emotional tension: behavioral and physiological reaction to a stress situation
Stress: type of stimuli most likely to arouse anxiety in most individuals
Stress situation: a circumstance in which adjustment is difficult or impossible, but in which motivation is very strong

Postulates were also spelled out that helped to show the derivation of such concepts as: Surgery is almost uniformly a source of stress depending on how the patient perceives it.

Individuals react differently to stress. Most patients are fearful of surgery although they may not express this fear.

All human behavior is purposeful and goal seeking; it is energized by tension and anxiety; it is designed wittingly or unwittingly in terms of how an individual perceives himself in relation to others and in terms of skills and abilities that he brings into play when his personality is threatened and requires that he defend himself. These behaviors require transformation of energy derived from tension and/or anxiety.[29]

This next led to the deduction that "it is possible to differentiate levels of emotional tension in preoperative and postoperative patients."

Conceptual Framework for Study of the
Role of the Public Health Nurse

Faced with the problem of evaluating the readiness of a student to assume the role of a practicing public health nurse the investigators first analyzed the role into some of its components and then developed a means of assessing these components.[30] To develop a framework for the study of the role of the public health nurse required a specification of this role.

An expectations file was developed to provide a picture of the complexity of the role of the public health nurse. A coding system was developed to use the information in the expectations file to describe this role. The approach used by the investigators in searching for criteria for evaluation could form the basis for a theoretical orientation to research in public health nursing.

Framework for the Study of the Role of the Public Health Nurse

A. Counter Position Holding Expectation
1. Staff public health nurse.
2. Public health nurse director, consultant, or supervisor.
3. Nurse educator.
4. Professional nursing organizations (when the organization, rather than an identifiable counter position within the organization, expresses an expectation) and nurses other than public health nurses.
5. Community service agencies—including Department of Welfare, Tuberculosis Association, Cancer Society, Family Service Society, Mental Health Association, Crippled Children's Society, Urban League, and Health Department personnel exclusive of nurses and health officers.
6. Health officers.
7. Physicians, other than health officers.
8. Principals or teachers (public schools).
9. Patients.
10. Families of patients and other members of household.
11. Other consumers, including community groups and community leaders.
12. Members of allied professions not mentioned above, such as psychologists, sociologists, and anthropologists.
13. Miscellaneous, including USPHS and State Boards of Health when the specific counter position cannot be identified.

B. Statement of Expectation or Behavior
1. The *types* of expectation or behavior are:
   a. Nursing service for particular patients or family. (Examples: Talk to patients about low calorie diet. Give skilled nursing care to arthritic patients.)
   b. Nursing service or general nursing procedures transcending individual cases. (Examples: Interpret local health regulations. Take an active part in classroom teaching.)
   c. Policies relating the public health nurse to other professionals and community workers in ways neither directly concerned with patient or family care nor to general nursing procedures. Anything concerned with smooth, organized functioning of interdisciplinary and interprofessional groups. (Examples: Interpret to appropriate groups the health and welfare needs of the community. Hold meetings to discuss work of teachers and nurses in order to obtain closer working relationship.)
   d. Activities of public health nurses not directly related to patient or family care, and not primarily concerned with interprofessional relationships. Activities that are related to intraprofessional affairs, civic affairs, research or professional development of individual nurse. (Examples: Work through professional organizations for the advancement and improvement of public health nursing. Study and evaluate own job performance.)
   e. Knowledge and attributes assumed to be necessary for action in above categories and miscellaneous expectations. (Examples: Should be able to recognize deviations from normal growth and development. Should have the ability to help others help themselves.)
2. The *sorts of skills* primarily involved are:
   a. Technical nursing skills. (Examples: Visit tuberculosis patients in the home to demonstrate and supervise care. Visit the chronically ill at home to give injections.)
   b. Skill in motivating an individual or face-to-face group to adopt a course of action.

(Examples: Encourage arthritic to do as much for himself as possible. Plan, with patient, ways of meeting long-term medical needs.)

c. Skill in convincing a large group to adopt a course of action, by such means as lectures, written communiques, etc. (Examples: Make a talk to the whole school on accident prevention. Take every opportunity to influence public opinion against taking mental patients to jail pending hospitalization.)

d. Skill in applying medical or other scientific knowledge in a situation that is primarily noninstructional, such as ability to discuss patient's health problems with M.D. or others, or ability to refer patient to M.D. or others, when basic aim is not to motivate a course of action. (Examples: Work with teachers on psychological problems of pupils. Observe, evaluate, and report to the physician patient's reaction to drugs and treatment.)

e. Skill in giving instruction when the primary purpose is to increase knowledge or understanding rather than to motivate a course of action. (Examples: Explain hospital admission procedures, rules, and regulations to family of hospitalized mental patient. Interpret public health nursing to the community.)

f. Skill in gathering information—active or passive—regardless of its purpose. (Examples: Take histories on psychiatric patients. Find out why patient is reluctant to attend clinic.)

g. Other skills whose nature cannot be determined from the statement. (Examples: Establish rapport with the patient. Work with the patient, not for him.)

h. Any combination of the above when one skill does not seem predominant.

3. The *values* that underlie the expectations and behaviors are:

a. Direct service to particular patients or families. (Examples: Explain dietary regulations to diabetic patient. Give family health counseling.)

b. Deemphasis of individual health problems or emphasis on community health. (Examples: Apply measures for prevention and control of communicable diseases. Cooperate with professional groups in analyzing community health needs.)

c. Service to the nursing profession, and professional development of the individual nurse. (Examples: Work through professional organizations for advancement and improvement of nursing. Keep in touch with the newest developments in medicine and nursing.)

d. Advancement of the healing arts and improvement of health and welfare services. (Examples: Participate in developing methods for coordinating nursing service. Plan with other health personnel in order to secure completeness and continuity of service to families and individuals.)

e. Other, including any combination of the above.

4. The expectation or behavior refers to patients of the age group:

a. Premature.
b. Infant.
c. Preschool.
d. School.
e. Adult.
f. Old age.
g. All ages.

5. The expectation or behavior refers to the patient's condition or situation of:

a. Venereal disease.
b. Tuberculosis.
c. Communicable disease (other than above).
d. AP and PP.
e. Chronic disease, including cancer.
f. Orthopedics.
g. Mental health.
h. Disaster.
i. Accident prevention and safety education.
j. General health.
k. Vision, speech, and hearing.
l. Dental health.

C. Counter Position with which Nurse Interacts in Fulfilling Expectation
   Same counter positions as listed under A.

D. How Expectations are Transmitted to Nurse
   1. By face-to-face interaction between nurse and counter position holding expectation. (Example: A teacher tells the public health nurse of some expectation she—the teacher—holds.)
   2. Directly from the counter position holding the expectation via literature or lecture. (Example: A nurse educator writes of her expectations for public health nurses.)
   3. Indirectly, via another counter position in face-to-face interaction. (Example: The supervisor tells a staff nurse of some expectation of the health officer.)
   4. Indirectly, via another counter position, through literature or lecture. (Example: An article by a sociologist regarding the expectations social workers hold for the public health nurse.)
   5. Self-expectation of the nurse.

A MODEL OF NURSING SUPPLY, REQUIREMENTS, AND DISTRIBUTION

In an ambitious attempt to construct a comprehensive model of nursing supply and requirements, the technique of "system dynamics" was applied to the important variables currently impacting on nursing manpower and likely to impact in the future.[31] A major use of such a model is to analyze the effect of changes in these variables on the supply, demand, and distribution of nursing personnel and services. With the current emphasis on health planning, such analysis can help in the formulation of policy decisions concerning nursing manpower.

The model's relationships are grouped into four main sectors:

- *Nursing education*—representing the factors affecting the number of students in each major type of educational program and the graduation rates from these programs.
- *Nursing employment*—representing the factors affecting the number of nurses employed in each setting and various characteristics of employment in each setting, such as nurses' wages and nurses' roles.
- *Demand*—representing the health care provided in each sector of the health-care-delivery system, nursing needs, and nursing jobs available in each employment setting.
- *Demographic*—representing key demographic characteristics of the total population that impact on other sectors of the model, principally the demand sector.

The model is operational for the United States as a whole, although it could, with further development, be made applicable for smaller geographic areas. Such a model as this, dependent on a vast data base and a complex computing program can only be made operational with sophisticated computer resources. In fact, this model is an excellent example of a family of models (this one based on a technique known as simulation)

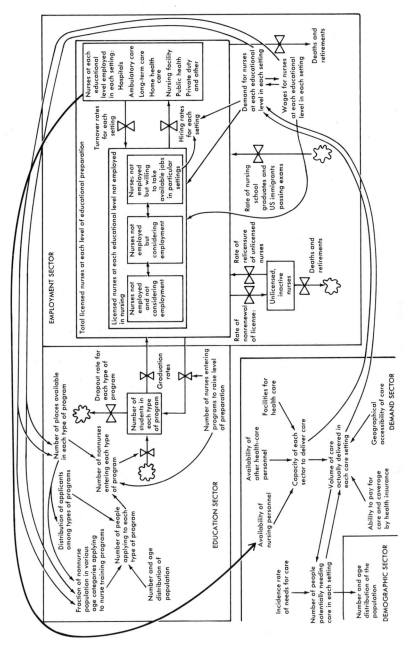

Fig. 4-4. Overview of the national model of nursing supply, requirements, and distribution.

89

that has been made possible by the development of high-speed electronic computers.

Summary

A major deterrent to nursing research is the lack of a conceptual framework for the proposed research. The development of a theory for nursing research is the most direct way of systematizing knowledge founded on a broader base.

A scientific theory is composed of operational definitions, postulates, and deductions. A few direct attempts have been made to develop theoretical models in the health field. However, much still needs to be done.

The building of a scientific theory for nursing research will directly affect the degree to which the nursing profession progresses in defining a scientific body of knowledge that is uniquely nursing.

References

1. Robert K. Merton, Leonard Broom, and Leonard S. Cottrell, Jr. (eds.), *Sociology Today*. New York, Basic Books, Inc., 1959, p. ix.
2. *Ibid.*, p. xiii.
3. Susanne K. Langer, "Why Philosophy?" *The Saturday Evening Post,* **234:** 35, May 13, 1961.
4. Claire, Selltiz, Marie Jahoda, Morton Deutsch, and Stuart W. Cook, *Research Methods in Social Relations*. New York, Holt, Rinehart and Winston, Inc., 1962, p. 481.
5. R. B. Braithwaite, *Scientific Explanation: A Study of the Functions of Theory, Probability and Law in Science*. Cambridge, England, Cambridge University, 1955.
6. C. S. Peirce, *Selected Writings of Charles S. Peirce,* "Values in a Universe of Chance," edited by Philip Wiener. New York, Doubleday and Co., Inc., 1958.
7. Robert M. W. Travers, *An Introduction to Educational Research*. New York, Macmillan Publishing Co., Inc., 1958.
8. *Ibid.*, p. 22.
9. Florence S. Wald and Robert C. Leonard, "Towards Development of Nursing Practice Theory." *Nursing Res.* **13:**309–313, fall, 1964.
10. Horace B. English and Ava Champney English, *A Comprehensive Dictionary of Psychological and Psychoanalytical Terms*. New York, Longmans, Green and Co., 1958, p. 326.
11. Daniel Howland, *The Development of a Methodology for the Evaluation of Patient Care*. Systems Research Group of the Engineering Experiment Station, Ohio State University and O.S.U. Research Foundation, June 1961, GN-W-9784; RF-940.

12. *Ibid.*

13. *Ibid.,* pp. 33–43.

14. Wanda E. McDowell, "Nurse-Patient-Physician Behavior: Nursing Care and the Regulation of Patient Condition." Paper presented at the American Nurses' Association 1962 Clinical Sessions, Detroit, Michigan.

15. Walter B. Cannon, *The Wisdom of the Body,* 2nd ed. rev. New York, W. W. Norton and Co., 1939.

16. Norbet Wiener, *Cybernetics.* New York, John Wiley and Sons, 1958.

17. William R. Ashby, *An Introduction to Cybernetics.* New York, Wiley and Sons, 1958.

18. Wanda McDowell, *op. cit.*

19. Donald P. Hayes and Robert K. Leik, "A Reaction Model." University of Washington (unpublished paper), 1962.

20. *Ibid.*

21. Everett C. Hughes, Helen Hughes, and Irwin Deutscher, *Twenty-Thousand Nurses Tell Their Story.* Philadelphia, J. B. Lippincott Co., 1958.

22. Faye G. Abdellah, "Criterion Measures in Nursing." *Nursing Res.,* **10:**21–26, winter 1961.

23. Robert M. W. Travers, *op. cit.,* p. 27.

24. Faye G. Abdellah *et. al., Patient-Centered Approaches to Nursing,* New York, Macmillan Publishing Co., Inc., 1960.

25. Marie Haddad and Vivian Holdsworth, "A Proposed Research Design." A project submitted in partial fulfillment of the course requirements of *Nursing 570a,* University of Washington, 1960.

26. *Ibid.,* pp. 1–2.

27. Lorraine Phillips, "Aggression and Religious Beliefs and Practices—A Proposed Research Design." A project submitted in partial fulfillment of the course requirements of *Nursing 570a,* University of Washington, 1960.

28. Marie L. Sadlick, "A Study of Patients Undergoing Major Surgery in a General Hospital to Determine the Level of Emotional Tension Pre- and Post-Operatively." A proposed research design. A project submitted in partial fulfillment of the course requirements of *Nursing 570a,* University of Washington, 1960.

29. Hildegard E. Peplau, *Interpersonal Relations in Nursing.* New York, G. P. Putnam's Sons, 1952, p. 132.

30. Ann C. Hansen and Harry S. Upshaw. "Evaluation Within the Context of Role Analysis." *Nursing Res.,* **11:**144–150, summer 1962.

31. Tom Bergan and Gary Hirsch, "A National Model of Supply, Demand, and Distribution." Summary Report. Boulder, The Western Interstate Commission on Higher Education, 1976.

Suggestions for Further Reading

1. Myrtle Irene Brown, "Research in the Development of Nursing Theory." *Nursing Res.,* **13:**109–112, spring 1964.

2. John Dewey, *How We Think.* New York, D. C. Heath Co., 1910.

3. Jean Baptiste Joseph Fourier, "Analytical Theory of Heat," *Great Books of the Western World,* Vol. 45. Chicago, Encyclopaedia Britannica, Inc., 1952, pp. 169–172.

4. David J. Fox, "A Proposed Model for Identifying Research Areas in Nursing." *Nursing Res.,* **13:**29–36, winter 1964.

5. C. G. Hempel, "Fundamentals of Concept Formation in Empirical Science." *International Encyclopedia of the Unified Science,* Vol. 2, No. 7. Chicago, University of Chicago Press, 1952.

6. Ada Jacox, "Theory Construction in Nursing: An Overview." *Nursing Res.,* **23:**4–13, *January–February,* 1974.

7. Dorothy E. Johnson, "Development of Theory: A Requisite for Nursing as a Primary Health Profession." *Nursing Res.,* **23:**372–377, *September–October,* 1974.

8. Immanuel Kant, "The Critique of Pure Reason," *Great Books of the Western World,* Vol. 42. Chicago, Encyclopaedia Britannica, Inc., 1952, pp. 68–69, 179–182.

9. Sir Isaac Newton, "Mathematical Principles of Natural Philosophy," *Great Books of the Western World,* Vol. 34. Chicago, Encyclopaedia Britannica, Inc., 1952, pp. 5–24.

10. Ida Jean Orlando, *The Dynamic Nurse-Patient Relationship. Function, Process and Principles.* New York, G. P. Putnam's Sons, 1961.

11. Hildegard E. Peplau, *Basic Principles of Patient Counseling.* Philadelphia, Smith, Kline and French Laboratories, 1964.

12. Walter R. Reitman, "Information-Processing Models in Psychology." *Science,* **144:**1192–1198, 1963.

13. P. D. Reynolds, *A Primer in Theory Construction.* Indianapolis, Bobbs-Merrill, 1971.

14. Joan P. Riehl and Sister Callista Roy, *Conceptual Models for Nursing Practice.* New York, Appleton-Century-Crofts, 1974.

Problems and Suggestions for Further Study

1. Trace the development of Newton's universal law of gravitation and show how a similar approach can be used to develop a theory of nursing.

2. Develop a patient care model spelling out the nursing components.

3. What is a good definition of the term "theory"? Can you cite some theories that have been established in your area of study or work? Is a theory the same thing as a hypothesis? A law? An axiom? What are the differences, if any? (See W. M. O'Neil, *Fact and Theory.* Sydney, Sydney University Press, 1969.)

4. What is the definition of scientific knowledge? How can research aid in the furthering of scientific knowledge? Give some examples of scientific knowledge in nursing.

5. Comment on the statement: "Nursing is an art, not a science." Does this mean that there is no such thing as nursing research? Can research be helpful to art as well as to science?

6. In what ways can a theoretical framework or model assist in the conduct of a research study? Does every study need to be based on theories or models?

7. How does research assist in the advancement of theory? Cite some examples from the history of science in which research findings helped to advance the formulation of a theory, principle, or law.

8. In E. Bright Wilson's *An Introduction to Scientific Research* (McGraw-Hill Book Co., Inc., New York, 1962, pp. 30–31), an excellent definition is given of the concept "mathematical model." How can mathematical models be useful in nursing research?

2

THE RESEARCH PROCESS

The conduct of research should be a planned, systematic and logical process. It is this emphasis on a carefully designed and systematic approach that differentiates research from other, less rigorous information-gathering or problem-solving activities such as trial and error. The essence of the research process is closely related to the notion of scientific discipline and its criteria of accuracy, objectivity, thoroughness, and order.

The term "research design" is applied to the plan of research that is developed prior to the actual launching of the study. The research design refers to the methodology for conducting the study. It is an important part of the total research process, which includes a number of steps beginning with the initial formulation of the problem and ending with a report of the findings of the study.

The following six chapters will examine these various steps. Chapter 5 contains an overview of all the steps. Chapter 6 will discuss the principles of research design and will describe the major types of designs that can be applied to research in nursing and patient care. In Chapter 7 the problem of measurement in research will be examined, and in Chapter 8 the major ways in which research data are collected and processed will be discussed. Chapter 9 will discuss analysis and interpretation of research findings, including the reporting of these findings. Finally, Chapter 10 will be concerned with certain practical problems that are encountered in pursuing the research process, such as securing the cooperation of the research subjects, obtaining financial support for the research, and motivating the research team.

The material presented in this part of the book is not by any means the last word on the subject of the research process. The field of research methodology is constantly changing as each new research project adds its experience to existing knowledge. There is no one right answer to many questions of research methodology or one right way of conducting a study in the area of patient care research. However, there are guidelines for the conduct of such research that have proved to be useful in other studies. Without reliance on such guidelines, the pursuit of a research project can degenerate into little more than an exercise in trial and error, often yielding invalid and misleading results.

For the researcher, application of the accepted principles of conducting research, even though these principles may be provisional and subject to change, can enhance the accuracy of research findings. Moreover, these principles can increase the efficiency of the research effort by providing the most valid findings for the least expenditure of manpower, money, and materials. For the consumer of research, knowledge of the key principles of the process of research can aid in interpreting, evaluating, and applying research findings.

The following chapters are organized in the following way. Chapter 5 will provide a brief discussion of the major steps in the research process. Succeeding chapters of this section will contain extended discussions of some of the important principles of research methodology. In the next part of this book, discussions of a variety of actual research projects will portray some applications of these principles and methods to research in nursing and patient care.

Chapter Five

STEPS IN THE RESEARCH PROCESS

CHAPTER 3 of this book indicated that there are a variety of types of research purposes, aims, settings, and subjects. Similarly, there are a variety of ways of conducting a research study. Although there is no one right way to pursue a study, there is a definite sequence of recognizable steps that most researchers take in conducting their projects. Since research is a planned and systematic activity, these steps have to be thought out before launching the actual study. The actual steps to be taken should be described in writing in a document that can serve as the plan for guiding the total research activity. A written research plan, called a research proposal, is mandatory when one is applying for a financial grant to undertake the research or in fulfilling the requirements for a doctoral degree, but it is an extremely valuable document to have in all instances where research is undertaken. By spelling out the research plan in advance, it can be evaluated and possibly improved before the project is actually launched.

This chapter will not be concerned with the actual methods for the preparation of a written research proposal, per se, but rather with the various elements in the research process that have to be considered in developing a research plan. Once determined, these elements then become the specifications by which the study is actually carried out.

Not every research project requires consideration of all the steps in the research process. In methodological and descriptive studies, certain steps do not need to be taken, as will be made clear later.

The twelve major steps in the research process are listed in chronological order:

1. Formulate the problem
2. Review the literature
3. Formulate the framework of theory
4. Formulate hypotheses
5. Define the variables
6. Determine how variables will be quantified

   7. Determine the research design
   8. Delineate the target population
   9. Select and develop method for collecting data
  10. Formulate method of analyzing the data
  11. Determine how results will be interpreted (generalized)
  12. Determine method of communicating results

In the development of the research plan there may be some skipping around among these steps as they are being formulated. As has already been mentioned, all steps are not applicable to certain types of research, but such processes as formulating the problem, reviewing the literature, and defining the variables should occur in all studies. In experimental explanatory research all of the steps will apply.

There is great variation in the amount of time and effort devoted to each step in the actual execution of research studies. In some studies the major part of the research effort may be devoted to the early stages of the research process—the intellectual processes of formulating and defining the problem, the framework of theory, the hypotheses, and the variables. In other studies, little effort may be required for the more reflective stages of research and most of the time is spent on the more active processes of collecting and analyzing the data. Explanatory studies often fall into the first category, whereas descriptive studies are more likely to be of the second kind. In some descriptive studies, particularly nonexperimental field surveys, as much as 90 per cent of the total research effort may be devoted to the collection and analysis of the data.

In developing the research plan all steps in the research process need to be carefully thought out, since the success of the research project heavily depends on the quality of the research plan. The development of the plan is a process of continuous refinement of the various elements of the study. In the first draft of the plan, the researcher outlines the specifications of the various steps in the research process. Then, these are thoroughly analyzed, expanded, and redrafted. When the plan is developed as far as the researcher can take it without actually trying out all or parts of the plan, the *pretest* stage is reached. In the pretest, the methodology for collecting the data is given an actual trial using the same types of research subjects and creating a similar kind of research environment as in the actual study itself. On the basis of the pretest, the various elements in the research plan are again critically examined, revised if necessary, and final polishing is done to the entire plan itself. When the researcher is satisfied that he has gone about as far as he can in perfecting the plan the study is ready to be launched.

Thus, the development of a research plan is essentially a process of moving back and forth through the different steps in research and continuously expanding and polishing these steps until a limit of no further improvement is reached. Needless to say, this limit may not be ideal, since in research—particularly in such areas of study as nursing and patient care—compromises often have to be made in order to attain administrative workability of the research project. For example, if the ideal research plan requires 1,000 patients with a certain disease as study subjects, and if it would take ten years to accumulate data on that sizable a study population, it may be more practical to reduce the number of subjects, even if this meant sacrificing some accuracy in the study results.

It is understandable that in conducting research there is often an urge to complete the passive, often less exciting phase of developing the research plan as quickly as possible. However, it cannot be stressed too strongly that time spent on constructing an efficient and workable research plan can contribute significantly to the success of the research project. A project that is hastily conceived and consequently poorly designed can defeat the entire research effort.

The remainder of this chapter will contain a discussion of the twelve steps in the research process. Later chapters will contain fuller explorations of some of these steps—namely, those concerned with research design and methodology.

1. FORMULATE THE PROBLEM

The very first step in the research process is to select a topic to be studied. It is obvious that the development of the research plan cannot proceed until the topic is selected. Topics for research arise in various ways. One of these is external to the researcher. For the student in school a topic is sometimes suggested by his instructor. Professional researchers who conduct research on request, either as paid employees of the agency initiating the research or as members of a research institute, also perform studies on topics selected by others.

Usually, research is conducted on topics specifically selected by the researchers themselves, although the general area of the research may be suggested and influenced by outside sources. These influences include what the leaders in the field believe to be the most pressing problems for research, or the existence of an authoritative document in the field that expounds research needs, or the availability of financial support for undertaking research.

Some believe that dictated research—the kind where the research topic is selected by others—weakens an important characteristic of a researcher considered to be essential to good research: intellectual curiosity. Only if a researcher possesses this quality, it is argued, can research be pursued in the most creative and productive way. If the content of the research is dictated by others, usually on a contract basis, curiosity and interest are diminished and replaced by a more mercenary, cut-and-dried approach in which the objective is simply to get the job done.

However, many research topics are so complex and present so many difficulties in their design and execution as studies that they cannot be successfully carried out as a singular activity or in a piecemeal fashion. It becomes necessary for a research team to be constituted to pursue the topic. As a member of a research team, the individual researcher may have little influence on the selection of the research topic or on some other important decisions that are made in the course of formulating the research plan. This is a far cry from the very appealing picture that is often evoked of the lone, independent research worker who not only selects his own topic, formulates the problem, establishes the theoretical framework, and so on, but also collects, tabulates, analyzes his own data, and, of course, writes his own final report.

In small, well-circumscribed studies, it is still possible to pursue research as a solo effort. Doctoral dissertations represent one example of this genre, but even here some studies are being conceived as a group activity. A team approach to conducting research is often a necessary and, from the standpoint of efficiency, a desirable form of research organization, particularly where the research deals with complex phenomena, cuts across several intellectual disciplines, requires large amounts of data, and has potential application in a variety of fields. The curiosity and interest of members of the research team have to be generated and sustained by means that may be different from the satisfactions accruing to the lone research worker. How to motivate the efforts of a research team will be discussed in Chapter 10.

Source of Research Topics

Research topics can be suggested by a variety of sources. Some of these, such as authorities in the field or the existence of financial support, have already been mentioned. Another source is review of the literature, particularly literature dealing with the findings of other research. The stimulus for pursuing a research study can be provided by learning what other researchers have found as well as their appraisal of what further research needs to be done. So-called landmark studies often trigger a large number of further studies. Some of these further studies may be repetitions of the earlier study, called replications, having identical research designs for the purpose of confirming or, perhaps, denying the earlier findings. In nursing, in the early 1950's, stimulated by the financial support of the American Nurses' Association and the findings of surveys related to shortages of nursing personnel, a number of studies on a similar topical area (but often different in purpose and methodology) were undertaken. These were concerned with the job activities of nursing personnel and became known as "function" studies, many of which are summarized in *Twenty Thousand Nurses Tell Their Story*.[1]

Another important source of research topics is the researcher's own background and experiences. For example, Hasselmeyer's previous experience included work in the area of the care of premature infants before she undertook her study of the effects on such infants of diaper roll support;[2] Fitzwater was a supervisor in an operating room when she conducted her investigation of the use of surgical instruments;[3] and Belcher was a faculty member of a school of nursing when she became a member of the study team concerned with curriculum research.[4]

Still another source of research topics is that provided by theory and models. In the social sciences, theories pertaining to learning, personality, behavior of small groups, social and occupational roles, perception, and so on, have formed the basis for many different studies. The purpose of these studies has been either to test the theory to see if it really works or to apply it to some new situation among different study populations or settings. In nursing, there are several notable examples of research whose topics were related to some previously developed theory. Role theory played an important part in the research developed by Berkowitz and Bennis in the outpatient department.[5] And some of the studies directed by Flagle at Johns Hopkins have employed linear programming and other statistical and mathematical models that are popular in the field of operations research.[6]

Subject matter areas for research topics in nursing and patient care are vast. Moreover, there are a great number of ways of classifying these areas. These classification schemes could be useful in suggesting topics for research. One type of classification scheme can categorize research in nursing and patient care according to the professional and technical discipline that is primarily concerned with the problem to be studied: sociological, psychological, anthropological, biological, and so on. Another classification might be by the facility in which nursing care is provided: hospital or other type of inpatient facility, outpatient department, physician's office, home. Still another categorization of research topics could place major emphasis on the characteristics of the patients: pediatric, obstetrical, surgical, psychiatric, etc. Another could be procedure-oriented: teaching, observing, physical care, emotional support, and so on. In Chapter 11 of this book a simple classification of research topics is described consisting of only three categories: nursing practice, nursing administration, and nursing education. The first area includes all activities related to the provision of direct and indirect care to the patient—the physical work of the organization. Nursing administration is concerned with all that is done to maintain the organization in operation: staffing, directing, budgeting, coordinating, and so on. Nursing education includes all activities related to the undergraduate and graduate training of students as well as the continuing education of practitioners.

Formulating the Problem

Once a research topic is selected it is necessary to formulate the research problem as specifically as possible. Mere selection of a topic does not provide a sufficient basis for developing a research plan. Just to state that a study is to be done on nursing practice or, even more specifically, on the provision of emotional support to patients with myocardial infarction is not an adequate statement of the research problem, since it cannot provide any specific direction to the research effort. The statement of the problem should serve as the cornerstone upon which the total research plan is based. A problem should represent some situation in need of solution, improvement, modification, or change. A problem may be geared to a practical, real-life situation and as a result precipitate what in Chapter 3 we have described as applied research. Or, it may represent a theoretical situation whose solution may not have any practical consequences, and this would precipitate what has been termed basic research.

In nursing there are a host of problems that could serve as the basis for research. Perhaps the most fundamental of all at the present time is the shortage of nursing personnel. In its broadest sense, this problem can be stated, "Why is there a shortage of nursing personnel?" Stated this way it is questionable whether a research project could be developed to shed light on the problem. First of all, the question is much too broad. It implies that a shortage exists in all fields of nursing, in all areas of the country, in all levels of nursing. Review of the literature will quickly reveal that a shortage is not universal. If study of the nursing shortage is to be successful, it must narrow its scope of inquiry.

Second, what is meant by shortage? If defined as the number of vacant positions in institutions employing nurses, this could lead to a very different type of study than if the concept of "shortage" is defined in a qualitative sense. Third, the problem as stated assumes that a shortage exists—i.e., that the existence of a shortage has been proven in previous research and can be accepted as true in the present research. But this may not necessarily be the case. Perhaps the problem should be restated as, "Is there a shortage of nurses?"

It can be seen that the process of formulating a problem for research is essentially a process of definition of concepts and terms, of narrowing down a broadly stated problem area into one more restricted in scope, and of relating the problem to research findings that have been obtained by others.

A broad topical area when narrowed into a manageable problem can give rise to a large variety of research studies. Some studies might be geared primarily to adding to knowledge (basic research) whereas others might have practical aims, such as the improvement of practice, administration, or education (applied research). Moreover, some of the studies stemming from the same problem area might be experimental in methodology while others might be designed as field surveys or employ some other type of nonexperimental approach.

One of the ways by which a broadly stated problem area can be narrowed down to a more specifically stated one is through the formulation of significant questions about the problem area. Taking the problem, "Why is there a shortage of nurses?" a series of relevant questions can be posed to mold it into a meaningful basis for research:

What is the extent of the shortage?

Is the shortage spread uniformly through all fields and levels of nursing?

Is the shortage related to insufficient numbers of new entrants into the field?

Is the shortage related to the inefficient use of nursing time?

Can the shortage be alleviated by improving working conditions for nurses?

Is the shortage related to lack of adequate numbers of personnel or a deficiency in the quality of services provided, or both?

Does the use of practical nurses and aides contribute to the relief of the nursing shortage?

From further questions like these it is possible to eventually delimit the research problem into something as specific as, "Does the quantity of nursing care available influence the condition of the patient?" Such a question, with additional refinement, definition of terms, and restatement as a hypothesis, has actually formed the basis for numerous studies in the nursing field. Some of these, described in Chapter 14, exemplify explanatory studies whose purpose is to determine optimum staffing patterns for providing patient care. Other studies that have been developed from such questions are more descriptive in nature. The previously mentioned function studies, supported by the American Nurses' Association, are examples of these.

The selection of a research problem or research question is a very important step in the total process of research:

It is the difficulty or problem which guides our search for some order among the facts, in terms of which the difficulty is to be removed. We could not possibly discover the reasons for the inundation of the Nile unless we first recognize in the inundation a problem demanding solution.[7]

And as Merton said, ". . . the experience of scientists is summed up in the adage that it is often more difficult to find and formulate a problem than to solve it."[8] This saying has relevance to the fact that although much highly sophisticated methodology is available for conducting research there is no readily available method for choosing and developing the problem to be studied:

> For no rule can be given by means of which men can learn to ask significant questions. It is a mark of scientific genius to be sensitive to difficulties where less gifted people pass by untroubled with doubt.[9]

Certain guidelines do exist to help decide whether it would be worthwhile to develop a problem into a formal research project. These guidelines can be applied to situations where some difficulty is felt and the question arises as to how best can the difficulty be solved—i.e., through research or some other means? In Chapter 3 it was pointed out that there are several widely used substitutes for research. These include problem solving by logical reasoning, the use of judgment, experience, expert advice, and trial and error. But there are many instances where these substitutes will not be satisfactory. Conversely, there are situations where formal research might not be the most appropriate approach to the solution of the problem. By asking the following questions about the problem it is possible to arrive at a decision as to whether it should be pursued through formal research or some other means:

Guidelines for Assessing Researchability of a Problem

Is it Feasible to Conduct Research on the Problem?   Although many problems offer promising possibilities for development into a research project, it may not be practical to do so. For one thing, appropriate methodology may not be available. Many problem areas cannot be adequately studied at the present time because appropriate tools do not exist. But lack of methodology may present only a temporary obstacle to research. This is made abundantly clear in the developments that are occurring in our efforts to travel to outer space.

A second obstacle to research results from the fact that the study may demand so large a number of study subjects and require so much time for completion as to render the findings out of date and useless. Thus, if we were concerned with the effect of certain nursing procedures on patients with rare conditions, it might take years to accumulate a sufficient number of cases to yield valid findings. During this time the procedures being studied might well become obsolete, and all interest in the findings would be dissipated. Obsoleteness is a distinct possibility in these times when so many changes are occurring in the care of patients.

Another obstacle to the pursuit of a research problem is the possibility of harming the health of the subjects involved in the study. Many drugs, for example, are not tested because they might endanger the life of study subjects. Certain kinds of psychological or sociological research are inhibited by their possible detrimental effects on the emotions and attitudes of the study populations.

Still another obstacle to the pursuit of a research problem is the cost to conduct the project. Some problems would require so much money for their solution through research that their findings would not be worth the effort of a formal study.

In brief, then, feasibility of pursuing a research problem can be evaluated by the following criteria:

Availability of methodology
Length of time needed to complete the study
Possible danger to life, or physical and mental well-being of study
   subjects
Cost of undertaking the research

Is the Problem of Sufficient Importance? As has been indicated, the conduct of research may involve large expenditures of time, effort, and money. The decision to launch a study must balance the expected value of the research findings against these expenditures. If the project can be inexpensively pursued, we can be satisfied with modest results. If the study will require large amounts of time and money, we should expect the importance of the results to be commensurate with the resources expended. If what the study produces will be of little importance yet require a strenuous research effort, other less costly means of achieving the same results should be explored.

The importance of a research problem can be evaluated in terms of various criteria. One of these is the economic effect of the research findings. If a problem is closely related to the expenditure of large sums of money, there is often good justification for undertaking research to solve it. The field of market research is an illustration of this point. Before manufacturers spend large sums of money in developing a new product, they often test its acceptability on a sample of its potential users. In hospitals, research on the application of automatic data processing to the reporting of data on patients is motivated by the amount of time and money that are presently expended on such reporting systems. Justification for studies of the turnover of nursing personnel is based on the large economic cost of the high job turnover of these personnel.

Another criterion of the importance of a research problem is the possible effect of the research findings on the health and welfare of people. Much of the justification for employing research to solve problems in the nursing field can be related to the intimate connection between nursing care and patient welfare. In the field of medicine, the impetus for subjecting new drugs to carefully controlled clinical trials is their vital effect on the health of individuals. The impact of research on peoples' health probably overrides any other criterion in determining whether a problem should be pursued as a formal research study.

A third measure of the importance of a research problem is the frequency of its occurrence. For example, if a public health agency is constantly being faced with a problem of broken appointments in its various clinics, it might decide to investigate formally the problem rather than rely on assessments of the situation based on the judgments of the clinic supervisors, particularly if these judgments were in conflict with each other. Another example: interest in the problem of the relationship between smoking and lung cancer did not precipitate an actual research study until there were dramatic increases in the number of deaths from lung cancer and in the consumption of cigarettes. Of course, wide occurrence of a problem is not a necessary condition for undertaking research. A unique problem may often possess adequate justification for pursuit as a research project if other criteria of importance are present.

To What Extent Can the Findings of the Study of the Problem Be Generalized? Sometimes research is evaluated according to the extent to which its findings can be applied to situations other than the research setting in which it was conducted. This criterion has greatest relevancy to explanatory research where the purpose is to confirm or reject some hypothesis. As will be discussed shortly, hypotheses are statements of relationships among variables that refer to a broader population than just the subjects who participated in the study. There usually would be more justification supporting a research project if its findings would have broad implications than there would be if it produces narrowly restricted generalizations. For many investigators an ideal research problem is one that would lead to "earth-shaking" findings. The danger here, though, is that the desire to make an impact with one's research findings can lead to the neglect of many important research problems that do not have such wide applicability. Also in the attempt to make a "big splash" with one's research findings the scientific integrity of the research itself can be depreciated. Some studies reported in the literature are to some extent motivated by the desire of the researcher to advance his own standing in his professional community rather than to advance knowledge. In the interest of achieving high-quality research, this should be scrupulously avoided.

What Need Will Solution of the Research Problem Meet? To fully evaluate whether a problem merits the effort of a formal research study, the need the solution of the problem will meet should be clearly described. This is sometimes called defining the purpose of a study. If the purpose cannot be defined, the problem is clearly not researchable. By definition, research is a purposeful activity. This purpose may be to add to the fund of knowledge in the field in which the problem lies, or to attain some more immediately practical objective, such as developing a new procedure, method, or product. Sometimes the same problem can lead to different research purposes. Thus, the problem of how best to train professional nurses could be developed into a descriptive study to provide data on the characteristics of graduates of various kinds of educational programs. Or it could lead to an experimental study that would compare the effectiveness of different kinds of educational programs. But whatever purpose is formulated it should meet a real, existing need. Unless it did, research would be a rather sterile activity.

Often, research serves a long-range as well as a short-range need. To the extent that a problem is carefully and completely formulated, both long- and short-range objectives will become clear. To illustrate, assume that the research problem was concerned with the reasons why recent graduates from schools of professional nursing withdrew at such a high rate. The short-range need to be served by the research might be to point out immediate ways of reducing this attrition, such as offering economic or other types of incentives for the young graduate to remain at work. The long-range need to be met by the research might be the shedding of light on the possibility of changing the emphasis on the type of individual recruited to a nursing school or revising the curriculum. These research objectives are long-range because they may take years to achieve. Once achieved, however, the effect on solving the problem of attrition would undoubtedly be more substantial than in meeting the short-range need.

Another illustration of the ways in which research can meet both long- and short-range needs is the fact that while research findings can serve an immediate specific need in solving a practical problem, they can also contribute, although perhaps in a modest way, to the development of a theory, principle, or other generalized knowledge. For example, studies concerned with the determination of optimum staffing patterns for providing patient care may provide concrete information that is immediately useful to administrators of patient care. At the same time, they can contribute to the development of a generalized theory of the relationship between nursing care and patient welfare.

In developing a research problem, therefore, the following question should be continuously raised: What are the long- and short-range needs that will be met by this study? The answers to this question should influence the study during the whole course of its development and execution.

Is the Problem of Interest to the Researcher?   An important criterion in selecting problems for research is that they be of interest to the researcher who will develop and execute the study. This criterion may appear to be so self-evident as not to warrant any discussion at all. However, it can be demonstrated that many studies are conducted by people who do not have sufficient interest in the research problem. It is often these studies that become bogged down and terminate without attaining the research purposes, or produce findings that may be trivial, irrelevant, or invalid. Lack of interest on the part of the researcher may stem from the fact that he chose his research problem not because of intellectual curiosity, but because it was appealing to a grant-giving agency or to the organization that employs him or to the faculty committee for which he is doing his graduate work.

Interest in the problem can serve as a strong motivation for the researcher to pursue his research project to its valid conclusion, energetically, creatively, and with intellectual honesty. Interest can sustain the researcher through the arid stretches of the research when nothing much seems to be happening or through those difficult, arduous, or boring phases that sometimes occur during the repetitive operations involved in collecting data. The idealized picture that is often drawn of the dedicated researcher is one in which he has such a burning interest in his study that he forsakes everything else to spend all of his time on his research.

Does the Researcher Have Competence to Pursue the Research Problem?   Just as interest in the problem is an important and rather obvious characteristic of the researcher, so is his level of competence in the area of the research. This does not mean that the researcher needs to possess all the skills demanded by the research, particularly in research projects that are so large and complex that a team approach is required. For example, a researcher concerned with a problem related to the emotional needs of patients does not need to be an accomplished psychometrician, psychoanalyst, or statistician, if such skills are required in the development and execution of the study. But he should be sufficiently knowledgeable in these areas to make appropriate decisions as to when such expertise shall be called upon either as consultants to the project or as full- or part-time members of the research team.

The qualities that make up a competent researcher are difficult to define. Research as a distinct professional work activity does not exist. It must be related to some subject matter discipline—medicine, psychology, nursing, and so on. One can specialize in certain aspects of research methodology, such as psychometrics, sociometrics, or statistics, but being expert in one of these areas does not automatically qualify one as a competent all-around researcher. The qualities of a competent researcher, although difficult to define, are quite real. They sometimes exhibit themselves in rather subtle ways. One characteristic of the accomplished researcher is the sophistication with which he formulates the research problem. Although research courses as well as the literature on research can enhance the competencies of a researcher, perhaps the most important way in which research competencies are developed is through experience. It is almost ironic that research, which has been described as a very rational and systematic approach to the solution of problems, can probably best be learned by a firsthand experience similar to the process of trial and error. This is so because there is not one and only one way of pursuing a research problem. Instead there are many alternative ways. Moreover, in the course of a research project there are numerous places where decisions have to be made that can significantly affect the total research effort. In making many of these decisions there are no firm rules that will automatically tell the researcher which alternative to select, but rather there are only guidelines based on experience acquired in the execution of previous research. These guidelines allow appreciable room for the exercise of the researcher's own judgment.

It would appear, then, that a competent researcher should possess some technical skill in research methodology, some knowledge of the subject matter field of the research, ability in knowing how to make use of technical experts, some judgment in coping with the many decisions that have to be made in the course of the research process, and last, but indeed not least, sufficient imagination to take advantage of the many opportunities that often present themselves during the research to "try something a little different," which could lead to an unexpected rich payoff, called serendipity.

To recapitulate, in formulating a research problem the researcher should raise the following six questions:

1. Is it feasible to conduct research on the problem?
2. Is the problem important?
3. To what extent might the findings of the research be generalized?
4. What need will be met by solution of the problem?
5. Is the researcher really interested in the problem?
6. Does the researcher have adequate competence to pursue the problem through research?

A final word about formulating research problems concerns a topic that could well have been discussed first: How do research problems arise? In addition, there is the interrelated topic: Where are research problems found? Problems that may eventually form the basis of a research study arise from a large variety of sources. They are found in all areas of human activity. In nursing, research problems can arise from activities involving giving care to patients, administering this care, or teaching people to give the care—the three content areas, already mentioned, of nursing practice, nursing administration, and nursing education. These problems can arise in a multiplicity of ways. They can arise from an actual work situation, as for example, the shortage of nurses that confronts administrators of nursing service when they try to adequately staff their units. Or they can arise from hypothetical situations, such as the problem of what would happen if acutely ill patients were continuously monitored by closed-circuit television. Research problems may also be suggested by experiences encountered in one's personal life. For example, some psychological studies dealing with the problems of children were suggested to the researcher by observation of the behavior of his own children or those of his neighbors. And, of course, there is the famous but somewhat dubious anecdote of how the falling apple started Newton on the road toward the establishment of the laws of gravity.

Arising from real or hypothetical considerations, research problems in nursing can also crop up in any setting in which nursing takes place. Problems related to the provision of nursing care can arise in a hospital, a public health agency, a physician's office, or the home. Problems concerned with the education of nurses can arise not only in schools, but also in work situations as well as in the off-duty, leisure-time segment of life. "Does the after-hours reading of nursing journals really serve the educational purpose of keeping nurses informed about the latest developments in the field?" is an example of the latter type of research question. Finally, researchable administrative problems are especially plentiful, since they can be found in any situation where two or more persons are working together toward achievement of the same goal.

Indeed, the range of problems that can serve as the basis for research in nursing and patient care is potentially limitless. As has been said, there is a great need for the ability to perceive these problems, to evaluate them in the light of the six criteria that have been previously discussed, and to develop them into a research project that would make a significant contribution toward the advancement of knowledge of the field.

In brief, the research process begins with a selection of a topic for study. This signifies the content area and suggests in a general way the nature of the problem. The next step is to formulate the problem. This expresses in rather concrete terms a situation in need of solution. To determine whether the problem should be approached through formal research, such criteria as feasibility, importance, extensiveness of the problem, as well as interest and competence of the researcher can be applied to it. At this stage the purpose of the research that will be developed from the problem should also be crystallized.

Once the problem is more or less formulated, the next step is review of the literature. However, the process of formulating the problem is not really completed until the total research design is developed, since it is subject to continuous definition, revision, restatement, and reformulation.

2. REVIEW THE LITERATURE

In the chronological development of a research project, review of the literature often precedes the formulation of a research problem. Sometimes the researcher may select a topic and then study the related literature to generate ideas relevant to the formulation of the problem. Sometimes the literature review may even precede selection of the topic. This review can often provide useful suggestions for the development of a research topic.

Review of the literature is an essential step in the development of a research project. It can serve several important purposes. First, it can reveal what has been done previously in the problem area, thus relieving the researcher of the necessity of repeating those aspects of the research where sufficient knowledge already exists. Of course, if the knowledge gained in prior research is tentative, equivocal, or incomplete, there is justification in repeating the study in its entirety, called *replication,* so as to confirm or deny the earlier findings. Second, review of the literature can indicate whether it is feasible to do the planned research by revealing difficulties encountered by previous researchers. Third, review of the research design can uncover promising methodological tools, shed light on ways to improve the efficiency of data collection, and obtain useful advice on how to increase the effectiveness of data analysis. Fourth, but certainly not of least importance, literature review can serve as the connecting link between the findings of previous research that has been done in the problem area and the results of the proposed study. Only by relating the findings from one study to the next can we hope to establish a comprehensive body of scientific knowledge in a professional discipline from which valid and pertinent theories might be established.

In recent years nursing has built up a storehouse of information that could be of considerable value to researchers in the nursing field. The journal *Nursing Research* undoubtedly publishes the greatest volume of reports of completed research in nursing. Also, the abstracts of research contained in each issue of this journal provide a useful guide to reports of research published elsewhere. Other journals that from time to time publish reports of nursing and related research include the following.

Administrative Science Quarterly
American Health Care Association Journal
American Journal of Nursing
American Nurse

American Journal of Public Health
American Sociological Review
Cardiovascular Nursing
Health Services Research
Heart and Lung
Hospital Management
Hospital Progress
Hospitals, Journal of the American Hospital Association
Human Relations
International Nursing Review
JAMA—Journal of the American Medical Association
Journal of Advanced Nursing
Journal of Continuing Education in Nursing
Journal of Gerontological Nursing
Journal of Health and Human Behavior
Journal of Neurosurgical Nursing
Journal of Nurse-Midwifery
Journal of Nursing Administration
Journal of Nursing Education
Journal of Psychiatric Nursing and Mental Health Services
Journal of Rehabilitation
Journal of the American Association of Nephrology Nurses and Technicians
Lancet
Medical Care
Modern Hospital
New England Journal of Medicine
Nurse Practitioner
Nursing Forum
Nursing Outlook
Nursing Research
Nursing Research Report
Nursing '79
Pediatric Nursing
Pediatrics
Perspectives in Psychiatric Care
Primary Care
Public Health Reports
The Nursing Clinics of North America

Bibliographic Developments Affecting Nursing

The greater involvement of nurses in research and increased investigations of nursing problems have influenced the bibliographic developments affecting nursing.[10] The U.S. Public Health Service's Division of Nursing regarded the need for access to the literature important and supported two bibliographic projects—a survey and assessment of nursing research by investigators at Yale University and the abstracting of reports and studies in nursing by the Institute of Research and Service in Nursing Education, Teachers College, Columbia University. The Yale survey led to the development of two annotated bibliographies: *Nursing Studies Index*[11] (1900–1959) in four volumes and *Nursing Research, A Survey and Assessment*.[12]

The project on abstracting resulted in two special issues of *Nursing Research*. The abstracting service is now a permanent program of the American Nurses' Foundation and is a regular feature of *Nursing Research*.

The Interagency Council on Library Tools was established in 1960 to exchange information on problems and needs of the nursing literature.[13] Membership includes the American Hospital Association, American Nurses' Association, American Nurses' Foundation, Catholic Library Association, Medical Library Association, National League for Nursing, Yale Nursing Survey Project, and the U.S. Public Health Service.

The Interagency Council on Library Tools, a brain child of Miss Virginia Henderson, came into being because of her farsighted vision. Miss Henderson, a nursing scholar and teacher, has devoted her life to achieving quality nursing practice through her teaching, writings, and pioneering efforts in developing the first comprehensive *Nursing Studies Index*.

As far as orignal research reports are concerned, rich sources are the technical reports of government-sponsored research. It is possible to obtain reports on many of these projects by writing to the investigator that conducted the research. Many of these reports are published and can be identified by title, author, and its research grant number, as for example:

Gerald J. Griffin and Robert E. Kinsinger, *Teaching Clinical Nursing by Closed Circuit TV*—A Demonstration Project of the Department of Nursing, Bronx Community College at Montefiore Hospital in New York City, supported by Research Grant Number NU 00116 from the Division of Nursing, Public Health Service.

It is sometimes difficult to locate reports of government-sponsored research, particularly in fields where the research deals with classified information. An important source of information about reports on government-sponsored research is the National Technical Information Service of the U.S. Department of Commerce. Announcements of new reports are made biweekly in the publication, *Government Reports*. Since 1964 over one-half million reports of research have been compiled by N.T.I.S., copies of which can be purchased from the Service.

In the health field, the Division of Research Grants, of the National

Institutes of Health, publishes a *Research Grants Index*[14] which describes the current research projects being conducted under Public Health Service support. These are listed three ways: by subject matter, by name and address of principal investigator (including publications produced on the research project), and by institute or division through which the grant was awarded. The Bureau of Health Manpower, of which the Division of Nursing is a part, annually publishes a *Directory of Grants, Awards and Loans*. Projects are listed by state and city of location of grantee, institution name, area of support and amount awarded. There is a lag of several years between the issuance of the directory and the time period of the data it contains. For example the 1975 Directory was issued in September 1977 (Publication Number HRA 77–82).

The Division of Nursing has issued abstracts of the research grants it has supported. Two such publications have been prepared. Entitled *Research in Nursing,* one covered the years 1955–1968 and the other 1969–1972. A compilation for the years after 1972 is scheduled to appear in 1979.

In 1962, the American Nurses' Association published a series of monographs containing clinical papers presented during the 1962 convention of the Association. Similar monographs have been published following presentations at subsequent conventions. These are entitled *ANA Clinical Sessions* and contain about fifty papers in each volume.

In 1965 the American Nurses' Association began a series of research conferences funded by the U.S. Public Health Services' Division of Nursing. These were held in different cities and included presentations on a variety of research topics. Papers presented at the conference were put together by the Association in a single volume presented to the Division of Nursing and some papers were later published in various journals. The last conference, held in 1973 in San Antonio, Texas, contained over twenty research papers and reports.

Beginning in 1968, in Salt Lake City, Utah, the Western Interstate Commission on Higher Education in Nursing has sponsored a series of annual research conferences. Initially funded by the Division of Nursing, the conferences are now self-supporting. These conferences have always had a theme. At the 1978 conference in Portland, Oregon, for example the theme was "New Approaches to Communicating Nursing Research." Reports on all the conferences have been published by WICHEN.

Another compilation of papers, some of which deal with research topics, is *The Nursing Clinics of North America* published quarterly by W. B. Saunders. Although not exclusively oriented to reports of research, the material can be of value to those interested in clinical research in nursing.

A recently established information system under the Health Planning and Resources Development Act of 1974 (P.L. 93–641) is known as the National Health Planning Information Center (NHPIC). The Center's primary objective is to provide access to current information on health planning methodology as well as information to be used in the analysis of issues and problems in health planning.[15] The U.S. Public Health Service's Division of Nursing has provided support to the center in order to establish a central source of information on nurse manpower planning. Services available from the center include announcements of relevant documents, which are published by the National Technical Information Service, reference and referral services, and issuance of monographs and bibliographies on subjects relevant to nursing planning. Although established as a tool for planners, the National Health Planning Information Center has considerable value to nurse researchers.

In the education field the U.S. Education Resources Information Center (ERIC) disseminates educational research results, research-related material, and other resource information. Since 1966 the Center has been publishing *Research in Education* on a monthly basis, with annual accumulations. Available from the U.S. Government Printing Office, this is a rich source of education research information.

Other important abstracting services, indexes, bibliographies, and information services relevant to the literature on research in nursing follow.

Abstract Journals. Many journals publish abstracts of the literature in the fields of medicine and the related sciences. These include *Biological Abstracts, Chemical Abtracts, Psychological Abstracts, Human Resources Abstracts, and Hospital Abstracts* to name but a few.

Abstracts of Congressional Publications and Legislative Histories. Congressional Information Service, Washington, D.C., Congressional Information Service, Monthly and Annual Cumulation beginning in 1969.

Abstracts of Hospital Management Studies. Quarterly Index: published by the Cooperative Information Center for Hospital Management Studies, The University of Michigan, beginning with Vol. I, No. 1, Sept. 1, 1964.

Abstracts of Reports of Studies in Nursing. In *Nursing Research,* beginning Vol. 9, no. 2, 1960, and continuing. Abstracts in Vol. 9, no. 2, through Vol. 11, no. 2, prepared under direction of the Institute of Research and Service in Nursing Education, Teachers College, Columbia University; beginning Vol. 11, no. 3, 1962, and continuing through March–April 1974 under direction of the American Nurses' Foundation. Indexed by author and subject and continued by *Nursing Research* through 1978.

American Journal of Nursing indexes:
Annual Index: published separately, available to subscribers on request; sent routinely to schools of nursing.

Cumulative Indexes (five year):
Latest cumulation 1971–75. Earlier cumulative indexes, now out of print but available in many libraries: 1900–1910; 1910–20; 1920–30; 1931–40; 1941–45; 1946–50; 1951–55; 1956–60; 1966–70.

Annual Register of Grant Support. Marquis, Academic Media. Chicago, Marquis Whos' Who, Inc. (Tenth edition 1976–77, published 1976).

Bibliographies on Nursing. New York, National League for Nursing, 1957, 14 vols. Out of print but available in some libraries; still valuable for their wide coverage of book, periodical, and pamphlet materials; film and audiovisual aid lists.

Bibliography of Nursing Literature, 1961–1970. Alice M. C. Thompson, London; The Royal College of Nursing, 1974.

Bibliography of the Socioeconomic Aspects of Medicine. Theodora Andrews. Littleton, Colorado, Libraries Unlimited, Inc., 1975.

Cumulative Index to Nursing Literature. Glendale, Calif., Seventh Day Adventist Hospital Association, Glendale Sanitarium and Hospital, Box 871, beginning in 1956. 1956–1960 plus 1961 supplements in two parts, $30.00; 1961 supplement in two parts, $12.00; continuation supplements annually. An index to periodical literature in nursing and related fields, by subject and author; over 30 periodicals indexed in 1962.

Current Index to Journals in Education. New York, Macmillan Publishing Co., Inc. Index to periodical literature in education from ERIC. Monthly and semiannual cumulations beginning in 1969.

Current Listing and Topical Index to the *Vital and Health Statistics* series 1962–1976. DHEW, National Center for Health Statistics, May 1977. Includes reports from the Hospital Discharge Survey, the National Ambulatory Medical Care Survey, and the National Reporting System for Family Planning Services.

Directory of Health Sciences Libraries in the United States. F. L. Schick and S. Crawford, Chicago, Ill., Medical Library Association, 1969.

Directory of Information Resources in the United States. Library of Congress Washington, D.C., U.S. Government Printing Office, 8th Edition, 1973.

Directory of Special Libraries and Information Centers. Anthony T. Kruzas, Detroit, Michigan, Gale Research Co., 4th edition, 1977.

Encyclopedia of Information Systems and Services. Anthony T. Kruzas Associates. Ann Arbor, Mich., Edward's Brothers, 1974. Describes and analyzes 1750 organizations concerned with information systems.

Facts About Nursing. Kansas City, Mo., American Nurses Association. Sourcebook of nursing statistics, Approximately biannual beginning in 1938.

Federal Library Resources: A User's Guide to Research Collections. Mildred Benton. New York, Science Associates/International, Inc., 1973.

Foundation Directory. Foundation Center New York, Columbia University Press, Edition 5, 1975.

Guide to National and International Associations. Detroit, Michigan. Gale Research Co. Quarterly and Cumulative beginning in 1964.

Guide to the Health Care Field. American Hospital Association, Chicago. Detailed information on all hospitals registered by the American Hospital Association and osteopathic hospitals listed by the American Osteopathic Hospital Associations. Annual beginning in 1964.

Health United States. National Center for Health Statistics. Washington, D.C., U.S. Government Printing Office. Sourcebook of data on health care and health status. Annual beginning in 1975.

Hospital Literature Index. Chicago, Ill., American Hospital Association. Published quarterly with annual and five-year cumulations. Covers literature on administration, planning and financing of hospitals and related health care institutions beginning in 1945.

Index Medicus. National Library of Medicine, Washington, D.C., U.S. Government Printing Office. Bibliography of the Literature of Biomedicine. 2250 of the world's medical journals included, monthly and annual cumulation beginning in 1960.

Indexes to Survey Methodology. U.S. Bureau of the Census, Washington, D.C., U.S. Government Printing Office, 1974. 2,500 entries. Covers nonsampling aspects of survey design and operation, including measurement and control of the nonsampling errors that occur in data collection.

Information Storage and Retrieval Systems for Individual Researchers. Gerald Jahoda. New York, Wiley-Interscience, 1970.

International Classification of Diseases. U.S. Public Health Service. Adapted for indexing hospital records by diseases and operations. Washington, D.C., U.S. Government Printing Office, 8th Revision, Vol. 1 (tabular list), 1969; Vol. 2 (alphabetical index), Dec. 1968, (PHS Pub. No. 1693), DHEW, National Center for Health Statistics.

International Nursing Index:
Indexes approximately 240 nursing periodicals and nursing articles in over 2,000 nonnursing journals published throughout the world. 1966–70; 1971–73; 1974–76.

Introduction to Reference Work. William A. Katz. Vol. I. *Basic Information Sources.* Vol. II. Reference Services and Reference Processes. New York, McGraw-Hill Book Co., 1974.

Medical Socioeconomic Research Sources. Gaithersburg, Md. Aspen Systems Corp. Quarterly and cumulated annually. 1970–

MEDLARS.[16] Medical Literature Analysis and Retrieval System began operation in 1964 and provides a new bibliographic system for the medical literature. MEDLARS is a computer-based bibliographic system making possible "the publication of an index to the medical and related literature and the retrieval of specialized bibliographic information on both recurring and demand bases." The system is based on the *available* published literature.

Access to MEDLARS based at the National Library of Medicine in Bethesda, Md., is available through a nationwide network of MEDLARS Centers at universities, medical schools, hospitals, government agencies, and commercial organizations. There are a number of online data bases available through the MEDLARS network. MEDLINE (MEDLARS on-line) contains references to biomedical journal articles and selected monographs in the United States and foreign countries. TOXLINE (Toxicology Information on-line) includes published references on human and toxicity studies, effects of environmental chemicals and pollutants, and adverse drug reactions. CHEMLINE (chemical dictionary on-line). CATLINE (catalog on-line) contains references to books and serials cataloged at the National Library of Medicine since 1965. SERLINE (Serials on-line). AVLINE (audiovisuals on-line). CANCERLIT contains references to various aspects of cancer. CANCERPROJ contains ongoing cancer research projects. EPILEPSY-LINE contains references to epilepsy. Two subsidiary on-line files are the Name Authority File and the MeSH vocabulary file (information on Medical subject headings).

The Merck Index: An Encyclopedia of Chemicals and Drugs, 9th ed. Rahway, N.J., Merck & Co., 1976.

Modern Drug Encyclopedia and Therapeutic Index, 13th ed., New York, Dun-Donnelley Publishing Company, Sept. 1975.

Multi-Media Materials:
DHEW, National Medical Audiovisual Center Catalog, 1977, *Audiovisuals for the Health Scientist.* Washington, D.C., U.S. Government Printing Office, DHEW Publication No. (NIH) 75–506. *American Journal of Nursing Co.,* Multi-Media Materials 1977–78, Educational Services Division.

Nursing Outlook indexes:
Annual Index: published in December issue each year.
Cumulative Indexes: five-year cumulative indexes, 1953–1957, 1958–1962. Reference Card Service: a current index; annotated reference cards on each article in each issue of the magazine; cards published

monthly. Suggested subject heads and cross references provided with each set of cards. Complete reference card service (*Nursing Outlook, American Journal of Nursing,* and *Nursing Research* cards).

Nursing Research indexes.

Annual index: in final issue, each volume.

Cumulative Indexes: Twelve-year cumulative index 1952–63.

Indexes to Abstracts: In *Nursing Res.,* **8:**129–144A, spring 1959; **9:**107–117, spring 1960; **10:**235–250, fall 1961; **11:**251–264, fall 1962.

Reference Card Service: a current index; annotated reference cards on each article in each issue; published at the time the issue appears. Suggested subject headings and cross references accompany each set of cards. Complete reference card service (*Nursing Research, Nursing Outlook,* and *American Journal of Nursing* cards).

Nursing Studies Index. Virginia Henderson. Vol. I, 1900–1929 (published 1972); Vol. II, 1930–1949 (published 1970); Vol. III, 1950–1956 (published 1966), Vol. IV, 1957–1959. Lippincott, Philadelphia. An annotated guide to reported studies, research in progress, research methods, and historical materials, Prepared by the Yale University School of Nursing index staff under direction of Miss Henderson.

PSRO Information Clearinghouse. Rockville, Maryland, Capital System Group, Inc. Abstracts of materials of interest to groups and individuals concerned with organization and implementation of professional standards review organizations. Materials include evaluation of quality of health care, delivery concepts of peer review, and education and accreditation of health manpower beginning in 1973.

Research Centers Directory. Archie M. Palmer. Detroit, Gale Research Co. 1975. A guide to university-related and other nonprofit research organizations.

Scientific and Technical Libraries. Lucille J. Strauss and others. New York, Becher and Hayes, Inc., 1972.

Smithsonian Institution

Science Information Exchange (S.I.E.), 1730 M St., N.W., Rm. 300, Washington, D.C., is a clearinghouse for information on *current* scientific research actually in progress. The exchange is supported by government agencies having major research and development programs.

The exchange provides broad coverage of basic and applied research in biology, medicine, sociology, psychology, agriculture, and the physical sciences with attention to interdisciplinary reference. For example, all research projects in nursing and health-related fields supported by the federal government are reported by the investigators in the form of a 200-word abstract.

Research investigators associated with recognized research institutions may request information on who is currently working on a specific problem. These questions are answered by a staff of professional scientists who select and forward copies of pertinent notices of research projects.

Research directors and administrators of cooperating agencies may request combinations of data and subject matter information compiled to meet their specific need. This kind of information, furnished only on demand, is developed in each case to meet problems in program management.

To use the exchange write or telephone the exchange, defining the specific research or problem on which information is desired. The exchange will promptly forward pertinent notices of research projects. A concise definition of the problem will insure the best selection of information.

Social Sciences and Humanities Index: formerly *International Index.* Quarterly guide to periodical literature in the social sciences and humanities. 1907/15–74. New York, Wilson, 1916–74. Vol. 1–61.

A cumulative index made up of three parts: (1) permanent cumulated volumes covering four, three, or two years; (2) annual volumes; and (3) current numbers issued quarterly, June, Sept., Dec., and March (frequency varies).

Humanities Index. Vol. 1, no. 1–, June 1974–. New York, Wilson, 1974–. Vol. 1–. Quarterly with annual cumulations. Supersedes in part the *Social Sciences and Humanities Index.*

Subject fields indexed include archaeology and classical studies, area studies, folklore, history, language and literature, literary and political criticism, performing arts, philosophy, religion and theology, and related subjects.

Social Sciences Index. Vol. 1, no. 1–, June 1974–. New York, Wilson, 1974–. Quarterly, with annual cumulations. Continues in part the *Social Sciences and Humanities Index.*

Comprises an author and subject index to periodicals in the fields of anthropology, area studies, economics, environmental science, geography, law and criminology, medical sciences, political science, psychology, public administration, sociology and related subjects.

Social Sciences Citation Index. Philadelphia, Institute for Scientific Information. A citation index of 2,000 selectively covered journals. Triannual cumulated annually beginning in 1973.

Source Book: Nursing Personnel. Division of Nursing. Washington, D.C., U.S. Government Printing Office. Sourcebook of nursing statistics, with emphasis on historical trends. Published irregularly, latest edition 1979, beginning in 1951.

Sources of Information in the Social Sciences: A Guide to the Literature. Carl M. White and Associates. Chicago, American Library Association, 1973.

Standard Nomenclature of Disease and Operations. Edited by E. Thompson and A. C. Hayden. Chicago, American Medical Association (5th edition), 1961.

Statistical Abstract of the United States. U.S. Bureau of the Census, Washington, D.C., U.S. Government Printing Office, Annually. 1879–

Statistics Sources. Gale Research Co. Detroit, Michigan, Gale Research. Guide to sources of numerical data about the United States and foreign countries, 1974.

Studies in Nursing (Clearing House List). New York, American Nurses' Association published only four times between 1955 and 1961. All currently out of print but available in some libraries.

1955   Clearing House for Studies in Nursing, 1950–1953 and Supplement 1954–1955, Vol. 1, Number 1.

1956   Clearing House for Studies in Nursing: Supplement 1955–1956, Vol. 1, Number 2.

1959   Studies in Nursing: Supplement 1957–1958, Vol. 1, Number 3.

1961   Studies in Nursing: Supplement 1959–1961; Vol. 1, Number 4.

Reference Card Service: a current index; annotated reference cards on each article in each issue; cards published monthly; suggested subject headings and cross references with each set of cards. Complete reference card service (*American Journal of Nursing, Nursing Outlook, Nursing Research* cards)

The material gathered in the literature review should be treated as an integral part of the research data, since what is found in the literature not only can have an important influence on the formulation of the problem and the design of the research but also can provide useful comparative material when the data collected in the research are analyzed. In many research reports the literature review occupies an important place, usually in the section of the report where the background of the problem is discussed.

It is sometimes easy for a researcher to become bogged down in the literature review, especially if the area is one where much previous research work has been done. In fact some research never gets beyond this stage, and the reviewing itself becomes the end product. A hard-and-fast rule as to the proportion of time that should be spent on literature review is difficult to state. In a project budgeted for a period of, say, two years, certainly two months should be more than adequate for the review —in many cases a lesser time should be sufficient. With the use of indexes, abstracts, and computerized information retrieval systems the process can be considerably hastened. Also, personnel might be especially assigned to the research project to assist in the search of the literature and the preparation of abstracts.

The objectives of the literature review in the total process of research should always be kept in mind so as not to allow this step to get out of hand. Essentially, the objectives are to see what previous researchers in the same area of study have discovered and to find out which kinds of methodology have proved useful and which have not. Consideration of extraneous material, as interesting as it may be, can be wasteful and can retard the development and execution of the project.

3. FORMULATE THE FRAMEWORK OF THEORY

The formulation of a theoretical basis or framework for a research study is frequently not given adequate consideration in the development of the project. In many studies reported in the literature only passing reference is made to the existence of theory, if at all, and usually little connection is drawn between this theory and the research that has been done. One of the reasons for this lack, particularly in the area of nursing, is the newness of the research effort as well as the recency of attempts to place the discipline of nursing on a scientific, intellectual footing. Much of what composes the body of knowledge known as nursing is a collection of unrelated empirical facts, practical advice, and material borrowed from other fields such as medicine, physiology, and psychology. As nursing matures intellectually, so, hopefully, will theories of nursing evolve.

What are theories and how can they assist the research project? A theory is essentially an abstraction or generalization from concrete phenomena that serves as a summarization and explanation of the phenomena. A theory, contrary to some popular usage, is not a hypothesis, a speculation, or a guess. A theory has been proved to be true either by formal research or some other form of systematic observation.

Years ago a theory was considered to be final and immutable. However, only truly scientific theories, as for example the *theory of relativity,* are stable and widely accepted. By contrast, many theories in the social sciences are tentative, controversial, and subject to revision. This does not mean that theories used in the physical sciences are never modified or even abandoned. One of the functions of research is to revise or reformulate existing theory by providing new knowledge concerning the theory.

To be truly useful theories must correspond meaningfully to that aspect of the real world to which they relate. An important test of the adequacy of a theory is its relevant application to the real world. Many theories in the natural sciences can be tested in terms of how well they work when practically applied. In the social sciences such empirical validation is sometimes not possible. Without validation, theory construction can degenerate into an intellectual exercise that is little more than playing with words.

Role of Theory in Research

The role of theory has been described as:

. . . to summarize existing knowledge, to provide an explanation for observed events and relationships and to predict the occurrence of as yet unobserved events and relationships on the basis of the explanatory principles embodied in the theory.[17]

Theory assists the research process in several ways. First, it can highlight the most promising research avenues to pursue, thereby performing a valuable function in the process of problem formulation. Thus, if the problem selected for research is concerned with the best way of training students for nursing, reference to existing learning theories might suggest the most fruitful approach to developing the problem into a research study.

Second, theories can enrich research by pointing to the way in which the specific findings of isolated research studies relate to some broader and more abstract body of knowledge. For example, individual studies might show that patients in hospitals request relatively fewer sleeping pills or other depressants on weekends than on weekdays. Although interesting and perhaps attributable to the greater number of visitors on those days who perhaps exert a calming (or exhausting) effect on the patient, such findings do not necessarily offer greater insight into how nursing might be improved unless they are cast against pertinent theories of interpersonal relationships.

And just as theories can enrich research, research can contribute to theory:

Any research project, considered in its entirety, may clarify theory, reformulate theory, initiate new theory, or deflect theory entirely, as well as verify theory.[18]

To the degree that a research study can be formulated within a framework of theory, the more valuable function will it serve in promoting the advancement of knowledge.

How a Theory Is Developed

Earlier in this discussion a theory was said to involve abstraction or generalization of concrete subject matter or events. To illustrate what is meant by a theory, suppose it was found in a study of the financial status of a group of otherwise similar hospitals that some hospitals showed deficits while others managed to balance their budgets. This finding is a description of concrete events which by themselves may not be especially instructive. However, further investigation might reveal that hospitals that are better off financially are those characterized by a higher degree of community involvement in their operations, such as maintaining a volunteer program and encouraging broad representation of community members on the governing board. Still further studies might confirm this relationship by indicating that community involvement in the affairs of the hospital encourages more enthusiastic participation in fund-raising activities, greater acceptance of higher charges by patients, etc.

The final step then might well be the pronouncement of a theory of the economic success of a hospital that could be worded as follows: The financial health of a hospital is dependent on the intensity of community participation in its internal affairs. This, then, is an example of a theory. It is phrased in the form of a generalization, not in terms of specific events. Its value lies in the ability it affords to control a specific situation by predicting the outcome of certain changes we might make in the situation. Given this theory it is possible to alter the economic well-being of a hospital by influencing the degree of community participation. We can improve its financial health by providing greater community involvement, or we can weaken it by reducing the level of community involvement.

In formulating research problems it is highly desirable to conceptualize the problem at a level sufficiently abstract as well as sufficiently well-defined so that findings of the study can be related to those from other studies concerned with the same concepts. Studies in nursing that deal essentially with the same problem area and produce findings that reinforce each other could provide a step in the direction of theory development. Failure to take this step is due to the level of abstraction in which these studies are formulated. To illustrate: although a number of studies have dealt with what nurses do in the care of patients, there has been little attempt to integrate their data into a coherent and cohesive body of knowledge. One of the reasons this has not been done is that many of these studies are based upon elementary concepts. No effort has been made to move beyond the specific subject matter into the realm of abstraction and theorizing.

Another limitation to the development of theory from studies in nursing—however tentative these theories might be—is dividing the research effort among a large number of different problems. Few studies have dealt with precisely the same topic. The motivation appears to be to do something new and different each time a piece of research is proposed. Agencies granting research funds as well as educationl institutions offering doctoral programs encourage fragmentation of the research effort by judging the need for the research by its newness. A single study has severe limitations in the development of theory, since it is conducted in a specific setting, it uses selected subjects, it occurs at a specific time period, and it is concerned with a particular, concrete problem. What is urgently needed is the development of a systematic body of knowledge based on a number of replicated studies.

Where Are Existing Theories Found?

This question is much simpler to answer for the natural sciences than for the social sciences. In the natural sciences many generally acceptable theories can be found. In the social sciences most theories are tentative and often quite controversial.

Any reliable textbook in the natural sciences, for example in the field of physics, contains many well-tested theories, laws, and principles. These are usually identifiable by their titles: Boyle's law of gases, Ohm's law of electricity, quantum theory, the laws of mechanics, the special theory of relativity, the law of gravitation, and so on. Likewise, textbooks in the social sciences often catalogue the state of the art in theory development, although many of these are continuously being revised. Social science theory includes learning theories, the theory of small groups, psycho-analytic theory, the theory of the business cycles, and so on. Note that the term "law" is rarely applied in the social sciences. The term "theory" is used in a more speculative, transitory sense than is "law," which is considered to be well established. Moreover, a theory is generally broader than a law, the latter being usually confined to a single relationship.

In addition to textbooks, professional journals are a good source of current material relating to revisions, modifications, and refutations of existing theory. Also, whole books are sometimes devoted to a develop-ment of a single theory. In the social sciences, for example, we have Veblen's economic theory as contained in his *Theory of the Leisure Class,* Toynbee's theory of history contained in his *Study of History,* and Par-sons' all-embracing theory of sociology contained in his *Essays in Socio-logical Theory.*

As has been indicated, few distinctive theories have been developed in the field of nursing. Those that have are largely tentative and embry-onic. Some examples of theories in the areas of nursing and patient care were discussed in Chapter 4. We hope, in the not too distant future, literature in the field of nursing will also contain entire books devoted to the exposition of valid theories.

Models

Related to the role of theories in research is the use of models. The term "models" has a rather recent history. It has appeared in the literature only in the past thirty years, stimulated by developments in the fields of operations research, cybernetics, computer logic, and statistical decision theory. In research, models are symbolic or physical visualizations of a theory, law, or other abstract construct. A model, thus, is an analogy of the actual phenomenon expressed in a format that is more readily grasped and understood than the abstract conceptual scheme it sometimes is used to describe.

A model is an attempt to free oneself from the restrictions, vagueness, and ambiguities that may arise from the use of language when attempting to verbalize a theory, thereby achieving a clarity and succinctness of expression. Freeing the statement of a theory or some other conceptual scheme from the difficulties inherent in the use of imprecise language not only can achieve greater lucidity and precision of thought, but sometimes can make it possible to see additional implications of the theory through its visualization in either a symbolic or physical model. Models based on theories that express relationships among phenomena have a value in making clear the predictive possibilities of a theory. Thus, a schematic model of a patient's needs for nursing care shows that if changes occur in either the patient's self-help ability or in his personal needs, his need for sustenal care will also be affected in a predictable way.[19]

$$N\ Ca\ Sus = f\left[(SHA-) \times (NP)\right]$$

Where: $N\ Ca\ Sus$ = need for sustenal care
           $(SHA-)$ = reduced state of self-help ability
           NP = unsatisfied personal needs
           f = indication that the factors are
                      functionally related to each other

As has been indicated in the discussion of the role of theory in research, only through a process of abstraction and generalization can the findings of different studies be successfully integrated to form a cohesive body of scientific knowledge. The use of models can help the researcher to apply more of the process of abstraction to the development of his research project as well as to the interpretation of its findings. The process of abstraction focuses the attention of the researcher on the need for precise definition of terms included in the study, on the careful selection of those aspects of the real world that he will incorporate into his study, and on clarifying those important phases of the research process concerned with measurement of the phenomenon under study and analysis of the data that have been collected. In relation to the latter point, the following is particularly relevant:

Models are an abstraction of the properties of the data, and the "fit" of models to the data is dependent upon the quality of the process of abstraction.[20]

Naturally, the use of models in research has certain limitations. First of all, although a model can simplify the presentation of a complex idea, it can also oversimplify it. In the natural sciences a brief symbolic formula can sometimes completely and accurately describe complex phenomena, as Einstein's $E = mc^2$. In the social sciences not only are the phenomena very difficult to define in a way that would be universally true, but they are usually the product of a multiplicity of causes. One of the constant problems faced by researchers studying human beings is the necessity of translating complex relationships, concepts, and ideas into simpler representations and, in the process, losing some of the richness and subtlety of the original material. This problem will receive further attention in Chapter 7, in the discussion of measurement of variables.

Bross, in his stimulating book *Design for Decision*,[21] points out another danger in the use of models—the attachment of a researcher to a model to the point where he appears to be "riding a hobbyhorse," so to speak. Some research is indeed characterized by the repetitious "brute-force" approach in the application of the same model or theory to a variety of problems. In some of these applications the model may be completely irrelevant. It is used anyway because the researcher is enamored of it. Thus, in study after study in nursing dealing with disparate problems and subject matter, "role" theory, Maslow's need theory, or some other model or method keeps being used. The application of models should be custom-made to the individual research project. A model should make a truly creative contribution to the conduct of a study and not merely be a crutch or window dressing:

A child may become so devoted to the doll that she insists that her doll is a real baby, and some scientists become so devoted to their model (especially if it is a brain child) that they will insist that the model *is* the real world.[22]

Types of Models

There are a number of different kinds of models that can be of value to researchers in nursing. These fall under the two main headings of *physical* and *symbolic* and include the following major types of models:

Physical models
Lifelike physical representations
Abstract physical representations
Schematic and other diagrams

Symbolic models
Mathematical models
Statistical models

A brief description of each of these models follows:

Lifelike Physical Representations   Before any new product is actually fabricated, an exact physical model is usually prepared. Such models are often scaled to miniature size. We are familiar with the various models that have been made of the spaceships and rockets to be used in the exploration of outer space. Similarly, in hospital construction, a mock-up in miniature of a hospital is usually made of the finished building as well as its equipment and layout. The value of such models is to provide a means for predicting how the finished product will actually work out. In the area of patient care, the kinds of questions that can be answered by such physical models are: Can six beds be placed in an intensive care unit in such a way as to provide maximum visibility from all directions? How much walking will a staff nurse have to do in providing care to her patients? How can a system of record-keeping be best maintained in the completed hospital?

In addition to answering questions concerning physical layout, facilities, equipment, and supplies, concrete physical models can serve other purposes in clarifying problems of nursing and patient care. For example, in research on problems of communications within the hospital, actual models of the work situation might serve to point up likely places where obstacles to the flow of communications can occur. However, as a tool for facilitating the process of conceptualization and abstraction, a lifelike physical model has certain limitations. It is in fact an exact reproduction, usually on a miniature scale, of the actual object of which it is a model. To achieve a higher level of abstraction, abstract physical representations can be employed.

Abstract Physical Representations   Like concrete physical models these are also three-dimensional representations of the object. However, they are not lifelike reproductions, but rather abstractions of the objects they portray. Since models such as these are often used to describe phenomena that are not directly observable, their abstract character is well justified. Thus, the complicated physical model that has been constructed to describe the DNA molecule, consisting of numerous colored balls arranged in an intricate pattern representing the configuration of the atoms, is an abstraction because the actual physical appearance of the molecule may be totally unlike that of the model. No one has actually seen the structure of the molecule. The model is purely a figment of the designer's imagination.

However, abstract physical models can be used to designate concrete subject matter. Thus, three-dimensional abstract models have been used to portray such tangible phenomena as the components of a patient care system in which various three-dimensional symbols rather than exact physical representations were used to designate the various components of the system. The inpatient area was represented by one type of symbol, the outpatient area by another symbol, the patient's home by still another abstract symbol, and so forth.

The value of using abstract rather than concrete models is that the former can be employed as a shorthand method of conveying the essential properties of the object it represents. Thus, in the model of the patient care system, in which the focus might be on the availability of highly specialized technical care, the inpatient component can be designated in terms of a complicated-appearing symbol in contrast to a less complicated-appearing symbol for the home component. By comparison, in an exact physical replica of a patient care system, the different elements, such as a hospital facility, would require great skill to construct properly, but would not readily highlight the greater complexity of services rendered by a hospital in contrast to other facilities as would an abstract model. In research this ability of the abstract physical model can underscore certain characteristics of the phenomena under study as well as reduce a mass of detail into simple, uncluttered symbols. It can also serve the important purpose of clearly bringing to light the essential elements of the problem under study as well as the interrelationships among these elements.

Schematic and Other Diagrams   These are perhaps the most commonly used devices to assist in visualizing the essential elements in a research study. They are also widely used in work situations. In this category of models are found such devices as organization charts, flow charts, process charts, blueprints, and schematic diagrams.

Like the previously discussed three-dimensional models, two-dimensional diagrams may be either concrete or abstract. Thus, a blueprint containing the layout of a new health center is essentially a two-dimensional representation of the exact physical structure of the facility. On the other hand, a flow chart showing how a surgical patient moves through a hospital, organized according to the principles of Progressive Patient Care, can be made abstract by using symbols to represent each area of the hospital.

In research studies schematic diagrams are very popular and can be used in various ways. An organization-type chart can be used to show the total research plan. Flow charts can show how the data will be collected and processed. Schematic diagrams can serve as models to portray the theoretical background for the study. Examples of diagrams used as models for research are numerous. Chapter 4 contains several of these: Figure 4-1, page 76, containing a verbal schematic of the mission, task, and resources of the hospital system, Figure 4-2, page 77 showing the nurse-patient-physician triad, and Figure 4-3 on page 81, the scale of self-help ability and nursing care requirements.

Schematic diagrams are widely used in research because they have numerous virtues. Unlike exact physical models, they can be prepared quickly and are relatively inexpensive. They are also very versatile and can take a great variety of forms, as either verbal, symbolic, pictorial, or some combination of these approaches. Their value to a research study can be to clarify concepts and relationships, suggesting fruitful areas for further investigation, and to reveal the links with previous research.

Mathematical Models   A popular model for research and, indeed, the type that appears to add most to the prestige of a study is the mathematical model. This is considered the purest type of an abstract model. The symbols used in the formulation of a mathematical model do not resemble in the least the actual phenomena they represent. Most mathematical models employ letters of the alphabet, Greek, Roman, or other, to represent the various elements included in the model, while specially devised symbols are used to indicate the mathematical operations (addition, subtraction, multiplication, division, and so on) that are incorporated by the model.

Mathematical models can be used only where the phenomena represented by the model can be quantified. In the model for optimizing the level of patient care in the hospital system developed by Howland:[23]

$$\text{Patient care} = A_1X_1 + A_2X_2 + A_3X_3 + A_4X_4$$

Where: X_1 = sociological factors

$\quad\quad X_2$ = psychological factors

$\quad\quad X_3$ = physiological factors

$\quad\quad X_4$ = physical factors

$\quad\quad A_1, A_2, A_3, A_4$ = respective factor weight determined by expert opinion

This model assumes that each of the factors in the equation, X_1, X_2, X_3, X_4, can be quantified and in its exactness and austerity resembles the equations in which scientific laws are formulated.

Mathematical models express a precise formulation of the quantitative relationships among the factors they include. It is obvious, therefore, that few phenomena in the social sciences can be formulated in such precise, quantitative terms. However, a mathematical model does not have to be a real representation of the phenomena under study. It can be a theoretical, idealized conception of the phenomena. In the real world most phenomena, particularly those concerned with human beings, behave in a probablistic rather than a deterministic way. We, therefore, have to use such terms as "approximately," "on the average," "in the majority of cases," "it is likely that," "the probability of occurrence is," in interpreting the results of the application of mathematical formulations.

The role of mathematical models in most conceivable research topics in nursing is limited. The use of such models must necessarily be very selective, since the phenomena they deal with must be subject to quantification as well as to manipulation by mathematical processes. Also, these phenomena have to be limited in number because the more phenomena that are encompassed by the mathematical formulation, the greater are the amount and complexity of mathematical manipulation required to solve the equation. However, with electronic computers this has become a less important consideration.

The value of mathematical models lies in the ability they afford to predict behavior with a high degree of precision. Thus, if our mathematical model would state that Y (the quality of patient care) is functionally related to X (the quantity of patient care), then by manipulating the quantity of care we can predict the resulting quality of care.

Of course, not all mathematical models are in the form of simple linear, algebraic equations. Other branches of mathematics—such as geometry, set and group theory, and the theory of probability—can also contribute models for research.

Statistical Models   One of the most useful types of models for research in nursing is a statistical model. This is a type of mathematical model that essentially states the relative frequency with which certain events will occur. Statistical models are, therefore, probabilistic. They take into account the actual behavior of phenomena in the real world, particularly those involving human beings. This behavior is characterized by a considerable amount of variability, thus militating against the establishment of exact, invariant relationships. Exact relationships can only be approximated by probabilistic equations in which a measure of variability becomes a part of the equation. Thus, our previous example of the relationship between Y and X, where Y is quality of care and X is quantity of care, becomes more complicated when considered as a statistical model.

In most research concerned with human beings we do not find the simple equation where one factor is totally and invariably related to another factor, but rather a more complex equation expressing the relationship among the factors we have singled out for study plus a residual term representing other influences we have not studied, which can be called "chance" influences. Thus we have as a statistical model: $Y = b_1X_1 + b_2X_2 + b_3X_3 \ldots b_mX_m + C$ in which $X_1X_2X_3 \ldots X_m$ represents each of the factors we have isolated for study, $b_1b_2b_3 \ldots b_m$ the weights of the factors—i.e., a measure of the extent to which each factor influences Y, the quantity being predicted—and C is measure of the residual influences.

This statistical model is known as the general linear hypothesis. It is one of the most important statistical models in explanatory research, particularly where experimental design is employed. It will be more fully discussed in the following chapter, which will present the principles of experimental design.

To recapitulate, whether models are physical or symbolic, mathematical or statistical, they can serve a useful purpose in developing a research project. A model can be used to portray a theory or a part of a theory, to clarify concepts, constructs, or definitions, or to develop typologies, classifications, or methods of measurement. Models can reveal relationships among the phenomena being studied and link phenomena to other studies in which the same phenomena have been included. In essence, then, a model, like a theory, can provide a framework for a study. Moreover, models are related to hypotheses, the next topic to be discussed, for as has been said:

In any research project a model is the set of assumptions, or postulates, not being directly tested. Some efforts may be made to test the model during the research project, but the main objective of the research is to test hypotheses that have been developed from the model. For example, the assumption of the normal curve is frequently part of a statistical model, and this assumption is frequently tested in a preliminary phase of a statistical investigation. The model of one research project may become hypotheses in another project.[24]

4. FORMULATE HYPOTHESES

The actual design of a study begins with the formulation of hypotheses, for they can provide specific guidance for the investigator as to the kinds of data that need to be collected in the study as well as the method for analyzing the data. The previous stages of the research process—that is, selecting the topic, formulating the problem, reviewing the literature, and establishing the framework of theory—can be considered as providing the background for the study. These are, of course, very essential steps in the research process, but they have a less direct impact on the data to be gathered in the study than do the hypotheses that are formulated.

Hypotheses can be defined as *statements of the expected relationship(s) among the phenomena being studied.* In the language of research these phenomena are called variables. A variable can be defined as a *quality, property or characteristic of the persons or things being studied that can be quantitatively measured or enumerated.* Hypotheses then are speculations of how the variables in the study behave. The object of the study is to find out whether this speculation is true or not. Essentially the purpose of the study is to test the hypotheses. Once tested and proven true, a hypothesis may begin to qualify as a law or to be incorporated into a theory. It should be noted that a hypothesis tested and found to be true in a single study does not automatically acquire the status of a law or theory. In most scientific fields of knowledge the corroboration of numerous studies is needed to verify the lawful status of a hypothesis. Each study is in essence a single sample of results. Considerably larger-sized samples than that of a single study are needed to elevate a hypothesis to the level of a scientific law. Moreover, many hypotheses that are tested in research represent only a piece of a whole theory. What is required is the testing of all parts of the theory in a series of studies to provide a composite meaningful whole.

It should be noted that not all research studies are based on hypotheses. As has been indicated in Chapter 3, some research has as its purpose the obtaining of new facts concerning certain phenomena (variables). These studies do not intend to relate the phenomena to each other according to a connecting hypothesis. Such studies are called descriptive studies, in contrast to explanatory studies where the purpose is essentially to find out why something happens, to search out causes, to discover relationships among variables. For example, the problem to which we might direct a study is: What is the extent of usage of home nursing services provided by public health agencies in this country? The variable to be studied is "usage of home nursing services." Since we are not interested in studying it in relationship to any other variable nor in explaining the extent of usage, this is an example of a descriptive study. It is difficult to conceive what the hypotheses might be for a study like this. The research problem is formulated in terms of a straightforward question requiring a factual answer.

After this study was done, suppose we were to find that a much higher proportion of older persons are served in their homes by public health agencies than the proportion of older persons among the total population. This finding might well lead to the development of another study that is explanatory in purpose, concerned with determining why older persons compose such a large share of the home-visiting case load. For this explanatory study, it would be possible to state hypotheses. These would be concerned with the relationship between the variables—age of patients and usage of home nursing services. Whereas the previous study was concerned solely with one variable—usage of home nursing services—we have now inserted into the study the variable "age of patients." Based on these two variables, it would be possible to develop the following hypotheses:

Older patients need more home nursing services than do younger patients.

Older patients require more nursing time than younger patients.

The types of nursing services provided in the home are geared to meet the needs of older patients.

Home nursing care programs are less well publicized to younger persons than to older people.

Chronically ill patients can be cared for more efficiently in their homes than in the hospital.

These do not, of course, exhaust all the possible hypotheses that could be developed concerning the variables "usage of home nursing services" and "age of patients." The hypothesis selected for actual study would be the one most closely related to the problem of greatest concern to the researcher. Also, the hypothesis selected for study should meet the same criteria that were applied in selecting the research problem—namely, those of feasibility, importance, need, interest, and competence of the researcher.

The example of the study of home nursing services illustrates several points concerning hypotheses. First, it shows that a purely descriptive study does not need to be based on a hypothesis. The absence of hypotheses is one of the most common features that distinguishes a descriptive study from explanatory research. However, all other steps in the research process are equally applicable to both types of research. These include the formulation of the problem, its framework of theory, and all of the steps concerned with the collection and analysis of the research data.

Second, the example reveals how a descriptive study can lead to the development of hypotheses that can be tested later in explanatory studies. Indeed, many descriptive studies are essentially explanatory studies having as their central purpose the generation of hypotheses for further study. The U.S. Bureau of the Census' *Decennial Census of the Population of the United States* is essentially a descriptive study. It provides a wealth of data for the formulation of problem areas. On the basis of these problems, specific hypotheses can be developed to guide the undertaking of explanatory studies.

Third, the example illustrates the fact that the same problem can lead to the development of many different hypotheses. One of the attributes of a sophisticated researcher is his ability to select the most productive and worthwhile hypotheses to pursue in an explanatory study.

In addition to descriptive studies, research that is primarily concerned with development of methodology does not usually include hypotheses. However, some researchers believe that all studies possess hypotheses. In descriptive and methodological research, although rarely explicitly stated in the research plan, the hypothesis is that the new facts or methodology that such studies are intended to produce can actually be produced. Since by undertaking the study the researcher is signifying that he believes he will be successful in achieving the goals of his research, it does not appear that such hypotheses serve a very useful purpose.

In explanatory research, hypotheses can serve several useful purposes. As mentioned previously, a hypothesis is a tentative explanation of the relationship among the variables studied and is directed toward the solution of the research problem that has been formulated. Hypotheses serve as guides to the kinds of data that must be obtained to shed light on the research problem. Hypotheses represent a statement of the variables to be studied and indicate what is being measured or enumerated. When defined as explicitly as possible, hypotheses can suggest how the data concerning the variables will be collected as well as the way in which they will most effectively be analyzed.

Examples of Hypotheses

The following is a set of twenty-five examples of hypotheses:

1. A basic degree program produces a more proficient bedside nurse for general hospitals than a basic diploma program.
2. The hours of nursing care available in general hospitals are related to patient satisfaction with nursing care.
3. Democratic administration of nursing services produces lower turnover among nursing personnel in hospitals.
4. Smoking causes lung cancer among adult males.
5. Professional nurses are more heterosexual than female elementary school teachers.
6. Patients in open wards in general hospitals receive more nursing than do patients in private rooms.
7. Academic performance in high schools is a good predictor of success in a school of professional nursing.
8. Premature infants supported by a diaper roll will gain weight faster than unsupported infants.
9. Disposable surgeons' gloves are better than reusable gloves.
10. Nursing aides can be more effectively trained through teaching machines than with conventional methods.
11. People who watch television extensively read fewer books.
12. The length of hospitalization of patients with heart disease can be shortened through good nursing care.
13. Better patient care in hospitals can be provided through the use of intensive care units.
14. It is better not to tell a patient that he has a fatal illness.
15. Mental illness is associated with the growth of civilization.
16. The use of tranquilizers is more effective than shock therapy in treating disturbed mental patients.
17. Professional nurses are poorly paid.
18. Obesity causes heart disease.
19. There is a difference between the personality of surgical nurses and that of medical nurses.
20. It is not necessary to take routine T.P.R.'s.

21. Patients' length of stay in hospitals is related to the intensity of their illness.
22. A public health nurse's case load is increasing.
23. Broken appointments in the outpatient department can be reduced by a good patient education program.
24. Marriage is the main cause of attrition among professional nurses.
25. The school nurse program should be administered by the health department rather than the education department.

Some of the examples were actually tested out in studies. Others are purely illustrative and, as far as is known, have not been studied. Some are fairly well-stated hypotheses, while others are quite poorly stated and would need considerable refinement and definition before serving as a basis for an actual study. All are characterized by a high order of concreteness. Some are oversimplified. In actual studies, hypotheses are often considerably more subtle than these and may be pitched to a rather high level of abstraction. The purpose for presenting these examples at this time is to show the extent to which hypotheses have a common structure. This structure is: *hypotheses contain a statement of the relationship between the independent and dependent variables and, also, the applicable population to which the relationship applies.*

The variables that are spelled out in the hypotheses are called explanatory variables. The distinction between independent and dependent variables is as follows. The independent variable, also known as the *stimulus, treatment,* or *causal variable,* is the one that is manipulated (varied) by the researcher. The effects of the manipulation of the independent variable are studied in terms of the dependent variable, also known as the *response* or the *effect variable,* or the *criterion measure.*

Diagrammatically, the relationship between the independent and dependent variables is similar to the stimulus-response model developed in the field of psychology: A stimulus (S) is applied to an organism (O) and the response (R) in the organism is measured:

$$S \longrightarrow O \longrightarrow R$$

In this model the application of the stimulus is under the control of the investigator. All other stimuli are eliminated. Since the stimulus precedes the response, and since all other stimuli are withheld (controlled), the stimulus can be said to cause the response. This model describes the classical experimental design. It is the fundamental model for those studies whose purpose it is to test a hypothesis. Essentially the purpose of such studies is to understand the relationship between cause and effect, and these terms can be substituted for stimulus and response. In agricultural studies as well as those in the medical field the terms "treatment" and "effect" are usually applied to the stimulus and response variables.

In the social sciences, few studies can authoritatively demonstrate that one variable is totally responsible for the effects observed in the other variable, because of the complexity of the variables studied, the multiplicity of factors impinging on these variables, and the difficulties in maintaining strict control over the total research process. Often the best that can be achieved is to show an association among the variables studied: the variables are related to each other in some predictable way, but not necessarily in terms of cause and effect. For this reason, instead of labeling the variables as cause and effect, it is more appropriate to use the terminology independent and dependent variables.

To assist in the identification of independent and dependent variables in hypotheses, the following designates these variables as well as the applicable population to which they refer, for the odd-numbered hypotheses contained in the previous examples:

Independent Variable	Applicable Target Population	Dependent Variable
1. Type of educational program	Bedside nurses in general hospitals	Proficiency of nurse
3. Type of administration	Nursing personnel in hospitals	Turnover of nursing personnel
5. Type of profession	Professional nurses and elementary school teachers	Degree of heterosexuality
7. Academic performance in high school	Students in schools of nursing	Success in school of nursing
9. Type of glove	Reusable and disposable surgeons' gloves	Quality of glove
11. Extent of television viewing	People	Extent of readership of books
13. Type of nursing units	Hospitalized patients	Quality of patient care
15. Growth of civilization	People	Prevalence of mental illness
17. Type of profession	Nurses and other professional workers	Level of salary
19. Clinical specialty of nurse	Surgical and medical nurses	Type of personality
21. Intensity of illness	Hospitalized patients	Length of stay in hospital
23. Type of patient education program	Patients in outpatient departments	Frequency of broken appointments
25. Type of organizational control	School health programs	Effectiveness of program

It should be noted that many studies are concerned with more than one hypothesis. Some may test as many as a dozen or more. In the case of multiple hypotheses, the research problem is usually so broad that it has to be approached through a set of hypotheses. Sometimes multiple hypotheses contain identical variables, but are directed toward different population groups. For example, hypotheses concerning the relationship between the variables "nursing care" and "patient welfare" could be applied to different types of patients: cardiac patients, maternity patients, acutely ill patients, chronically ill patients, and so on. In multiple hypotheses each should make a distinct contribution to the solution of the overall research problem and not merely be a restatement of the same hypothesis.

In addition, hypotheses often include more than one independent or dependent variable. Such hypotheses may be concerned with the simultaneous effects of multiple independent variables on a single dependent variable. To illustrate, hypotheses about the relationship between nursing care and patient welfare can include as independent variables the "proportion of care" provided by professional nurses and the "method of organization" of the nursing staff (team versus primary). An advantage to studies like these that test hypotheses with multiple independent variables is that not only can the effects of each of the different independent variables be tested separately, known as the main effects, but the effects of combinations of variables, called interaction effects, can also be evaluated.

Similarly, studies may contain hypotheses with a single independent variable and several dependent variables (criterion measures). Thus we may be interested in varying the amount of nursing care provided to patients and measuring the effects on a number of psychological and physiological responses of patients to the differing amounts of care. This type of design was actually employed in studies conducted at the University of Iowa in which the criterion measures of the patient included skin conditions, mobility, mental attitude, physical independence, length of hospitalization, absence or presence of fever, and usage of sedatives, analgesics, and narcotics.[25]

It is also possible to conceive of hypotheses that would contain multiple independent as well as several dependent variables. The problem here is that it would be more difficult to relate the appropriate responses to the appropriate independent variables than it would be in a simpler research design. But, as will be discussed in the following chapter, techniques are available for coping with hypotheses that contain a multiplicity of variables. The problem is that the variables in such hypotheses need to be even more sharply defined and objectively measured than do those in simpler hypotheses.

Explanatory and Extraneous Variables

In discussing the types of variables included in hypotheses, the distinction has been drawn between independent and dependent variables. These have been called explanatory variables and are of primary interest to the researcher. They are often stated in the hypotheses. The explanatory variables are the ones that will be investigated in the study. The independent variable will be varied and the effects measured in terms of the dependent variable. The latter is known as the criterion measure and reflects the change in the independent variable. However, these are not the only variables that will be present in the research. Particularly where human beings are the study subjects, there are literally millions of variables that can enter into the research and affect the findings. The variables that are not of interest to the researcher are extraneous and need to be controlled so that the hypothesis can be validly tested. Ways of controlling these extraneous variables will be described in the following chapter.

Since human beings can generate a multiplicity of variables the researcher must be aware of the possible impact of extraneous variables in formulating his hypotheses. These variables can be classified into two broad categories: organismic and environmental. Organismic variables deal with all the many personal characteristics of human beings as individuals—physiological, psychological, demographic, and so on. Environmental variables relate to the many factors in the setting in which the individual is studied that can impinge on the individual. These include economic, anthropological, sociological, and physical factors. The following is a very brief listing of examples of organismic and environmental variables.

Organismic—age, sex, marital status, education, type of work, personality, height, weight, blood pressure, racial group, nationality, religion, job skill, intelligence, hair color, eye color, political belief, income, level of wellness

Environmental—climate, family composition governmental organization, work organization, physical setting (layout, etc.), ideological climate, community setting

Diagrammatically the relationship between independent and dependent variables can be shown as follows:

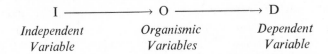

I —————→	O —————→	D
Independent	*Organismic*	*Dependent*
Variable	*Variables*	*Variable*

Thus, in hypotheses concerned with the relationship between nursing care and patient welfare a great variety of organismic as well as environmental variables can influence the relationship. The organismic variable, age of the patient, can have an important effect on the relationship, since older patients may respond differently to nursing care than do younger patients. Similarly, other extraneous variables like sex, type of illness, educational level, and so on, can also affect the relationship as can such environmental variables as the physical layout of the nursing unit and its organization.

As has been said, a major purpose of research design is to control the effects of all possible extraneous variables so that a valid test can be made of the hypothesis under study. Ways of controlling these effects are discussed in the following chapter. One way is to restrict the study population to a certain group, such as patients 65 years of age and over, or patients with hypertension, or patients in intensive care units. Or, instead of eliminating the extraneous organismic or environmental variables they may be brought into the study as additional variables. Thus, the hypothesis could be extended to include the effects of the *type* of nursing care on patient welfare as well as effects of the *amounts* of care provided.

Types of Hypotheses

Hypotheses that are developed from research problems can be concerned with various kinds of relationships. First of all, they can be concerned with causal relationships: the independent variable is the causal factor, and the dependent variable is the measure of the effect of the causal factor. Cause and effect have been defined as follows:

By the cause of some effect we shall understand, therefore, some appropriate factor invariably related to the effect. If A has diphtheria at time t is an effect, we shall understand by its cause a certain change C, such that the following holds. If C takes place, then A will have diphtheria at time t, and if C does not take place, A will not have diphtheria at time t; and this is true for all values of A, C, and t, where A is an individual of a certain type, C an event of a certain type, and t the time.[26]

The testing and establishment of causal relationships represent a most desirable goal of scientific research. If we know with certainty the cause, we can predict the effect and thereby have a means of exerting control over events. Few studies, particularly in a field of research such as nursing, can establish unequivocal causal relationships. The explanatory variables with which such research is concerned are too complex, and the extraneous variables are too numerous.

In the natural sciences, where strict experimental controls can often be exerted over the total research setting, it may be possible to establish causal relationships. In the social sciences the best we can achieve is to establish a second type of relationship, which can be called an "associative relationship." Here we know that a change in the dependent variable *is* related to a change in the independent variable, but we cannot with certainty say that the effect on the dependent variable was directly caused by the independent variable. Many hypotheses tested in nonexperimental studies express associative rather than causal relationships. Thus, we know that smoking is associated with lung cancer, but we have no absolute proof that smoking causes lung cancer. Such a causal relationship has not been established experimentally, at least not among human study populations. It may be that another, more fundamental variable, not tested in the study—e.g., the genetic make-up of a person that affects both the amount of smoking and the development of lung cancer, is the underlying causal agent. If this were true, smoking would not be an independent variable but another dependent variable.

Associative relationships can be most useful for making predictions. To take a rather extreme example, let us assume a study finds that success in nursing school is closely associated with the height of the applicant to the school: all applicants 5 feet 6 inches and under do well, all over 5 feet 6 inches do poorly. It would be useless to say that level of performance in a school of nursing is caused by the height of the student since we intuitively know that performance is a function of such variables as aptitude, personality, interest, motivation. However, with such an association we would have a useful predictive tool in selecting applicants, even though we may have no valid explanation of why students differ in their performance or why shorter students do better than taller ones.

Thus, associative relationships, while potentially useful as predictive devices, may be weak as diagnostic tools. The limitations of associative relationships must be recognized to avoid the fallacy of assigning the role of a causal agent to a variable that may itself also be affected by the true underlying cause. Moreover, in many associative relationships it is not possible to specify with assurance which is the dependent and which the independent variable. Sometimes variables are specified as one or the other as a matter of convenience, not that one is really dependent on the other or that one is the cause of the other. In fact in associative relationships the designations of variables can often be interchanged:

> If we wish to compare the frequency of symptom X in patients with diseases A, B and C, the independent variable is disease, the dependent variable is the symptom (present or absent). If, however, we wish to find the frequency of diseases A, B and C in patients who come to us with symptom X, the independent variable is the symptom, the dependent variable is disease.[27]

Associative relationships are characterized by the fact that the variables being considered are related to the *same* individuals composing the study population. Smoking and lung cancer are variables that are measured in relation to the same individuals. So are heights of individuals and their performance in schools of nursing.

In a third type of predictive relationship, which can be called an "artificial relationship," the variables may not characterize the same individuals but rather represent discrete study populations. Thus, it has been possible to establish a quantitative relationship between the number of freight cars loaded in New York City and the number of deaths from famine in China. When more freight cars were loaded, the number of deaths increased; when freight car loadings dropped, so did the deaths. Superficially there is little logical connection between these two variables. They arise from entirely different study populations. The only factor both have in common is the variable, time. In relationships like these it is often not possible to say which is the dependent and which the independent variable. However, we know that the variables do behave in a related fashion. For predictive purposes, if we know the value of one variable we can estimate the value of the other. In economics, many relationships like these are used in making forecasts. The behavior of certain economic variables, such as prices of securities, is sometimes linked to certain noneconomic variables, such as birth rates, which, although only remotely connected in a logical sense, may be closely related in terms of their performance and thus serve as good predictors of each other.

In associative or artificial relationships the incorrect assignment of a cause and effect relationship to variables is termed a "spurious relationship." A well-known example of a spurious relationship is the study that found a relationship between the number of stork nests contained in the chimneys of different cities and the number of births occurring to residents in the city—the larger the number of stork nests, the greater the number of births. Thus, it can be humorously maintained that births are *caused* by storks. However, it is obvious that the number of stork nests is a function of size of population of a city, and so is the number of births. The larger the population the greater is the likelihood that more stork nests will be found, since there would be more houses in the city. And with increase in population, the greater is the likelihood that there will be more births. Both variables, then, number of stork nests and number of births, are dependent variables, with population the independent variable.

The conditions for establishing true cause and effect relationships are several. First of all, there must be a consistency, directness, and persistency of the relationship between the dependent and independent variables: ". . . if C takes place, then A will have diphtheria at time t, and if C does not take place, A will not have diphtheria at time t. . . ." Second, the time interval between the application of the independent variable and the appearance of an effect in the dependent variable should not be too long. If a disease occurs many years after exposure to its supposed cause, it is difficult to establish a causal relationship because of the possible intervention of other independent variables during the passage of time. Thus, smoking as the direct cause of lung cancer is obscured by the fact that most smokers who have developed lung cancer have been smoking for many years prior to the onset of the disease. During this time many other independent factors, such as exposure to air pollution or to radiation, could have also exerted their influence on the dependent variable.

Finally, in order to establish a valid causal relationship there must be a logical and plausible connection between the dependent and independent variables:

> . . . if we stuck postage stamps to the beds of some patients (without knowledge of patients or staff) and found that all those patients recovered, whereas all those without stamps died, we could nevertheless not attribute the recovery to the postage stamps, because the relationship would not be credible, or conceivable, or rationally acceptable.[28]

Stating Hypotheses

Hypotheses can be stated in a variety of ways. In studies where the hypotheses are to be tested by statistical tests of significance, to be discussed in Chapter 9, the practice is to employ the concept of the "null hypothesis." The null hypothesis states that there is no relationship between the variables studied. For example, in studies of the effect of drugs on patients a null hypothesis would state that there is no difference in the recovery rate of patients who receive the drug and those who do not receive it. Our belief may well be that the drug will have a positive effect on patients. However the null hypothesis is used because our statistical test is geared to either rejecting or accepting the hypothesis by comparing the observed difference in recovery rates among the treated and untreated patients with the difference that should occur if the drug had no effect, which should be no difference beyond that attributable to chance. If the data lead us to an acceptance of a null hypothesis, we have not established a significant relationship between the dependent and independent variables.

In many studies involving statistical tests of the significance of relationships, alternative as well as null hypotheses are formulated. By rejecting a null hypothesis we are accepting one or the other of two main alternative hypotheses that can be formulated. One alternative is that the drug is related to recovery rate in a *positive* way—patients will have a higher recovery rate with the drug. The other alternative is that patients will have a higher recovery rate without the drug. Thus, for each null hypothesis, two main alternative hypotheses can be stated. Actually, many alternative hypotheses are possible since the difference in recovery rates between the treated and untreated patients can be formulated in terms of the actual magnitude of difference expected, not just that one group's rate will be higher than the other's.

A psychological advantage of stating a hypothesis in the null or no-relationship format is the sense of scientific objectivity that pervades such a statement. If the hypothesis is stated as, "It is expected that patients who receive the drug will have a more favorable recovery than untreated patients," the impartiality of the researcher in conducting the study can be questioned, since he appears to have a preconceived opinion of the value of the drug. However, merely stating the hypothesis in the null form is not going to ensure objectivity of the study and lack of bias in the findings. The various techniques collectively known as research design, to be discussed in the following chapter, have been developed to reduce bias in research. In fact, it can be argued that a researcher should state the hypothesis in the form of the relationship among the variables that he expects the data to support. Such affirmative statements might instill more reality into the total study design as well as into the interpretation of the findings.

Sometimes what may appear to be a hypothesis for a study may not be a hypothesis at all. Instead it may be a proven fact, at least to the researcher, and the purpose is not really to test it in an objective study, but rather to demonstrate it—to advertise it so that it could gain wider acceptance and use. Thus, if the real purpose of the study is to promote a certain pattern of nurse staffing, say, the team method of assignment, by demonstrating the benefits it can provide, the project should not be labeled as research. The purpose of such a project is not to test the value of the team method of patient assignment but rather to *demonstrate* the already "proven" merits of the method. A demonstration project is a meritorious activity, but it should be clearly distinguished from research.

One of the qualities of a researcher is the need to have an open mind in relation to what the study findings will show. This is particularly true in studies in which a product, method, or procedure is tested. If the researcher were certain that what he was testing would have no effect on the study population—that is, if he really thought that the null hypothesis were true—it is quite unlikely that he would conduct formal research on the subject.

As we move away from explanatory research, which has as its purpose the testing of a new product, procedure, or method, toward the more basic type of study concerned with explaining why something happened, the need for expressing hypotheses in the null form becomes less critical. Studies of the basic phenomena in the social sciences sometimes contain hypotheses stated in the form of the expected outcome of the data: "Prejudice is more widespread where educational level is low." "High morale is a symptom of good interpersonal relationships." "The degree of social integration in a community is affected by the extensiveness of shared purposes and interests among community members."

Assumptions

In addition to the hypotheses that are actually tested in a study, most studies include assumptions that are not tested in the study. Assumptions can be defined as *statements whose correctness or validity is taken for granted*. Assumptions can be based on several sources. First, they may be so-called universally accepted truths or be so self-evident that they require no additional testing. Thus, in evaluating the effect of nursing care on patient welfare, we can assume that patients require *some* nursing care without which their lives might be endangered. Therefore, we can design our experimental staffing patterns to be above a certain minimum level of staffing. Second, assumptions can be based on theories that are accepted as being applicable in the field in which the research is done. A study of patients' physical reactions to nursing care might well contain assumptions based on theories or laws that are prevalent in the fields of nursing, physiology, medicine, or other related disciplines. Third, assumptions may be based on the findings of previous research, even though such findings may not possess the finality of a theory or a law and be subject to revision. A study of methods of achieving continuity of patient care may use as assumptions findings related to existing practices of coordinating patient care that have been obtained in previous studies.

In formulating research problems and hypotheses based on these problems, assumptions may be stated explicitly in the research plan or, as is true in most research studies, may be implied by the researcher. Only if an assumption has a significant bearing on the rationale for the study does the researcher need to bother to spell it out concretely. As has already been stated, theories, models, and other conceptualizations that provide a meaningful intellectual framework for the research design can enhance the potential usefulness of a study. Similarly, the careful spelling out of all other important assumptions that can significantly affect the course of the study can also be beneficial.

Limitations of the Research

At the time the researcher is considering the assumptions upon which his study is based, it would be well to begin assessing the limitations of the study. Just as few researchers make the effort to state their assumptions explicitly, few concern themselves with evaluating the extent to which their studies may possess certain important limitations. Knowledge of the limitations of a study is essential to an appropriate interpretation of the findings. The limitations of a study are primarily conditioned by the study design. They include restrictions on interpretation of findings due to the nature of the hypotheses—particularly the characteristics of the study population, the variables being measured, the extraneous variables that are not completely controlled, and all other influences that can affect the collection and analysis of the data.

If the investigator is aware of all possible limitations and restrictions on his research, he can perhaps take appropriate precautions to soften their effects. Thus, if the hypothesis is concerned with an area of study in which many extraneous variables are prevalent he can design the study in such a way as to keep them under control. One such control is to enhance the size of his study population to permit statistical analysis of the more important extraneous variables. Moreover, conveying this limitation in the report of the research would put the reader in a more appropriate frame of mind to make a valid interpretation of the data.

From Problem to Hypothesis

Progressing from the formulation of the problem to the establishment of appropriate hypotheses is essentially a process of definition, delineation, refinement, and consolidation. This process continues throughout the total planning stage and is terminated at the point at which the actual data collection phase of the study begins. It cannot be emphasized too strongly that the formulation of hypotheses must be completed before the data are collected. Too often studies are conducted in which hypotheses are formulated after the data are collected, sometimes being suggested by the findings themselves. Such "ex post facto" hypotheses are legitimate if they are to serve as the basis for additional research in which new data are to be collected. They cannot be legitimately tested by the data from the study from which they arose, because the study design, particularly the definition of the variables and the selection and development of the measuring instruments, was not expressly tailored to the "ex post facto" hypotheses. As a result, certain hidden biases may serve to distort interpretations of data concerning the new hypotheses. Furthermore, in statistical tests of hypotheses it is mandatory that these hypotheses be formulated in advance of the data collection to avoid the likelihood of inferring spurious relationships among the variables studied. These errors will be discussed in a later chapter.

To show how a hypothesis may evolve from a broad problem area the following example is presented. As has already been indicated a perpetual problem in nursing and patient care is the shortage of nurses. Early research in this area was descriptive, dealing with attempts to measure the magnitude of the shortage through such criteria as vacant positions in institutions employing nursing personnel or by the probing of attitudes of personnel and patients concerning the existence of such shortages. From attempts to measure the extent of the shortage, studies progressed toward analysis of possible reasons for the existence of shortages. Early explanatory studies attempted to describe the things professional nurses do and to evaluate how much of their work load could be assumed by other personnel—practical nurses, aides, ward clerks, floor managers. Later studies were concerned with determining optimum staffing patterns that would maximize the use of scarce nursing time by integrating other types of personnel into the nursing team.

Today, studies of the problem of a shortage of nurses have progressed beyond a direct concern with such variables as quantity of nursing care provided and the appropriate distribution of duties among different types of personnel to an examination of more complex variables. These variables are becoming more focused on the patients themselves rather than on personnel providing the services. Thus, essentially prompted by the question of how to alleviate the nursing shortage, a number of studies have evolved to test hypotheses of the relationship between alternative kinds of nursing practices and the welfare of patients. These hypotheses have become more patient-oriented in the same way that efforts are being directed to make the provision of nursing care more patient-centered. We hope the results of these patient-centered studies will promote a widespread and lasting improvement in the quality of patient care.

The remaining sections of this chapter deal largely with that phase of the research process known as research design. These topics will be explained in detail in the following five chapters. Only a brief discussion will be presented here. As has already been stated, although the order of presentation of these topics is similar to the order in which they are considered in formulating a research proposal, there is a constant movement back and forth through the various steps as the proposal is being refined and formalized. However, as was indicated in relation to hypotheses, once the actual data collection begins, all the major elements of the research design should remain unchanged for the entire study. Altering any part of the design after the study has been set in motion could radically change the whole course of the study and invalidate the results.

The different elements of research design apply to all types of studies, explanatory as well as descriptive, experimental as well as nonexperimental. The primary purpose of these elements is to ensure the validity of the study and to enhance the efficiency and economy of the research enterprise itself.

It should be noted that the steps in the research process that occur after the problem and hypotheses are formulated, which we have termed research design, are in some studies the responsibility of a specialist. Specialists in research methodology are concerned with such problems as measurement of variables, collection and processing of data, and the statistical analysis of findings. The use of specialists for these tasks depends upon the extensiveness of the study. Large studies are often administered by a research team consisting of full-time specialists from a variety of fields of subject matter and research technology. Small studies are often the responsibility of a single investigator, with possible consultation from technical experts when required. Whether a member of a large research team or an individual worker on a small study, familiarity with all aspects of the research design is necessary for a proper appreciation of the most effective way of pursuing a research study.

5. DEFINE THE VARIABLES

In explanatory studies, the hypotheses contain statements of the dependent and independent variables, known as the explanatory variables. In descriptive studies, in the absence of explicit hypotheses, the research plan should clearly state the variables that will be investigated. In many studies, descriptive as well as explanatory, data are often collected for variables that are not really explanatory variables, but nevertheless are of interest to the researcher. There are usually organismic variables—age, sex, marital status, education, occupation, and so on. In reporting the findings of a study, data on these organismic variables, sometimes called "face-sheet" data by social scientists, provide background information on the composition of the study group. These data can be helpful in interpreting the findings on the main explanatory variables.

It is a good idea to prepare as part of the research plan skeleton outlines of statistical tables for the data that will be collected. Such table outlines, also called dummy tables, will reveal the different variables for which data will be collected. Variables appearing in these tables are those that need to be carefully defined in the research plan.

The definition of variables, of course, should be completed before any data are collected. Defining variables is essentially a process of making them meaningful, concrete, and operational. The goal is to achieve an operational definition of the variables. An operational definition is "the use of a series of words which clearly designate performable and observable acts or operations that can be verified by others."[29]

Thus, the term "patient welfare" by itself is not an operational definition of a variable. It does not designate an observable act that can be verified by independent observers. One operational definition of patient welfare might be the number of times a day the patient rings his call-bell for a nurse. It is possible to make reliable observations of the performance of this behavior. However, the question may be raised as to whether this is a *meaningful* definition of patient welfare. A low frequency of ringing the call-bell might not necessarily be indicative of good patient welfare, nor would a high frequency of ringing always mean that the level of patient welfare was low. Other definitions of patient welfare are, of course, possible—many of them. Some are physiological other psychological, and still others sociological. Ways of determining the most valid, reliable and meaningful definitions of variables will be discussed in Chapter 7. The importance of this step in the research process cannot be stressed too much, since the way the variables in a study are defined determines how they will be measured and how the data concerning these variables will be collected.

6. DETERMINE HOW VARIABLES WILL BE QUANTIFIED

Much research in nursing, as well as in many other fields, deals with quantitative observations of variables. Therefore, it is necessary to define variables in a way that they can be quantified according to a scale of value. By definition, every variable has some theoretical underlying scale of value, varying from one extreme to another. The example of an operational definition of patient welfare described earlier—the number of times a day the call-bell is rung—is in quantitative form. The scale could vary from zero times a day to an upper limit of, say, 100 times a day.

The value of quantifying data in research is almost self-evident. One is the ability to apply meaningful tools of statistical analysis when the data are in numerical form. However, not all research deals with quantified data. Anthropological research as well as some types of sociological studies are often completely devoid of numerical data. Instead they depend heavily upon verbal descriptions and other types of narrative data. Case studies, whether of people, institutions, communities, or whole societies, are largely composed of anectdotal data.

In developing the research plan, quantification of the variables to be included in the study can vary from a very simple procedure, demanding little or no technical skill, to a highly involved process of measurement requiring the help of specialized technicians. At its simplest, quantification of variables is merely a matter of recording the number of times something occurs according to some straightforward classification scale. Thus, in our example of the use of the call-bell as an indication of patient welfare, the classification scale can be conceived as consisting of just two classes: rings bell, does not ring bell. Eact time the bell is rung a recording of this fact can be made. At the end of the day the frequency of occurrences of all bell ringing can be determined for each patient.

At the other extreme, patient welfare can be operationally defined as a complex psychological phenomenon requiring measurement through an involved battery of tests. Such measurement might require the skills of specialized psychometricians, particularly if the tests did not already exist.

For many variables the scale of measurement already exists and, if found to be applicable to his own study, can be used by the researcher even though not developed especially for it. Where the scale of measurement is simply a classification of the variables into discrete categories in which the frequency of occurrence of each class is measured through a process of counting, the scale classes are often established through traditional use and are similar in study after study. Thus, the variable *sex* has two classes: male, female; the variable *marital status,* four classes: single, married, widowed, divorced or separated; the variable hair color, four classes: black, brown, blond, red; and so on. But even if prior studies have not established the classification scale, some variables are so obviously defined for quantification purposes that little difficulty is presented. Thus, if patient welfare is defined in terms of frequency of patient usage of tranquilizing or pain-killing drugs, one does not have to be an expert in measurement to determine how the variable will be quantified.

7. DETERMINE THE RESEARCH DESIGN

The process of defining variables and determining how they will be quantified is essentially another stage in the process of refinement of the research problem. When the variables have been defined as operationally as possible, and the means by which they will be quantified is determined, the researcher can consider the type of research design he will use for his study. This does not mean that definition of variables is completed by the time this stage is reached. As has been mentioned, the goal of the development of a research plan is the achievement of a final, valid and workable plan which can be attained only by carefully polishing the various steps a number of times until no further improvement is apparent. Thus, the definition of variables and the determination of how to quantify them will be influenced by all later stages of the research process and will be modified by decisions that are made concerning these stages.

Determination of the research design is a most important decision in the research process because the type of design employed vitally affects each step of the total research process. Determination of the research design involves the choice of the overall method by which the study subjects shall be selected, controlled, and, in experimental studies, assigned to the various experimental groups. Two main types of research design are available: the experimental and nonexperimental. In the experimental method all the conditions of the study are under the control of the researcher. In nonexperimental research, called "surveys" by some, there is considerably less control over the study subjects and the setting in which it is conducted. Experimental research in its most controlled form is conducted in a specialized research setting—a laboratory, an experimental unit, or a research center. Nonexperimental research is frequently conducted in a natural setting—a school, a public health agency, a hospital, or a patient's home. The major benefit to be gained by the use of a tightly controlled experimental design is the possibility of establishing causal relationships.

There are many variations of nonexperimental research. In one type of design the main elements of experimental and nonexperimental research are combined. These can be called partial experiments or partially controlled nonexperimental designs. Partial experiments may be of the kind where a natural setting is used, say, a nursing unit in a hospital, but the researcher exercises some control in the assignment of the study subjects to the various study groups. Completely nonexperimental designs can be of several types—cross-sectional, retrospective, or prospective. In the cross-sectional design, the researcher dips into the study setting at a given point in time, after the study design is completed, and obtains data on events occurring at that time. A cross-sectional study can be made of the amounts of nursing care that patients receive on a certain day according to a classification of their needs for nursing care. In a retrospective study, data are collected on events occurring in the past—before the study design is completed. A retrospective study could be made of what happened to patients who were discharged from the hospital during the past year. In a prospective study, the events upon which data are collected also occur after the study design is completed, but the study continues over a relatively long period of time into the future and not just for a brief period as in the cross-sectional type of study.

A prospective nonexperimental study could be made of what happens to patients who are discharged from the hospital during the next year. Studies like these are sometimes called follow-up or cohort studies and are most useful in studying the relationship among independent and dependent variables where the effects of the independent variable may be of a long-term nature.

Prospective and retrospective studies are sometimes called longitudinal studies because they extend over a long period of time in contrast to a cross-sectional study, where the time period is of short duration. However, since in retrospective studies the events have occurred prior to the initiation of the study and in some types of retrospective studies the data concerning the events have also already been collected, such studies are often simply a matter of bringing together the data either by means of questionnaires or through existing records. Thus, it is possible to collect longitudinal data reflecting a patient's medical history spanning many years of his life in the one or two hours that it takes for him to fill out the questionnaire. Likewise the personnel office of a health agency contains data in personnel records that might be useful in research covering a number of years of an employee's work experiences.

By definition, all experimental studies are prospective. Among the advantages of prospective studies is the possibility of manipulating the research variables and observing the effects. In the retrospective study of what happened to patients after they were discharged from the hospital, there was no control by the researcher over the course of action pursued by the patient. In the prospective study, the patient's action can be influenced by establishing as part of the research a referral system, which may be the independent variable being tested.

Another limitation of retrospective studies is that the researcher has less control over the definition and measurement of the variables being studied. In a retrospective study of patients' needs for nursing services using data contained in existing records and based on the hospital's own classification of needs, the investigator has to accept the definition of needs established by the hospital, which could present certain serious limitations to the research. Moreover, retrospective studies are limited by the availability of the data. We could not conduct a retrospective study of patients' needs if the hospital had not recorded data on this variable in the first place. Similarly, we are limited in questioning the job or health history of a person by the recall ability of the respondent.

Research design is basically concerned with controlling and even eliminating the many biases that can produce fallacious data. Among these biases are those attributable to extraneous variables. In studies on human beings such variables are especially abundant. One of the ways to control the influences of these variables is through the process of randomization. This process is a key element in experimental design, and much of the technical writing on this subject is devoted to methods of achieving it. These methods will be discussed in the subsequent chapter, as well as ways of controlling other sources of possible bias in the design of research.

The decision to employ one type of research design or another is often not a matter of free choice for the researcher. Certain kinds of research problems cannot easily be approached through the experimental process, if at all. Also the time and effort required to conduct a true experiment are often considerably greater than for a nonexperimental approach to the same problem. The advantage of the experimental approach is, of course, the possibility of its being able to establish causal relationships that are more valid than those obtained through the nonexperimental approach.

8. DELINEATE THE TARGET POPULATION

A research study must establish a population, or a "universe," to which its findings are applicable. This target population may consist of human beings; parts of human beings, such as limbs, teeth, hair; or human characteristics, such as personality, job activities, education. The population can also be inanimate objects like refrigerators, schools, or hospitals; abstract concepts like community attitudes, professional ethics, forms of government; and so on. Moreover, a study population can consist of animals, plants, or other living matter. The individual members of this total population are called "sampling units." Each unit must be a discrete entity and independent of all other units. A study usually is done on a fraction of all the sampling units in the total population, and this fraction is known as a sample. The process of selecting the sample is known as sampling.

Delineating the target population is still another step in narrowing down and tightening up the research problem. By focusing on the composition of the target population the researcher is forced to analyze the extent to which the findings of his study can be extrapolated beyond the actual sampling units included in the study. Does the study refer to all patients in the United States? To all patients in one state? To all patients in one hospital? To only male patients in one hospital? To only male patients aged 65 years and over in one hospital? To only male patients aged 65 years and over with coronary artery disease in one hospital?

The notion of a target population is an elusive concept. Even if we were to study all patients in the United States, or in the whole world, we could do this only during a specific time period, and so our target population would be limited in terms of the scope of the time period to which it refers. Although the findings of a study today may hold true tomorrow, next year, and perhaps even for the next ten years, we must be aware of the limitations imposed by the current relevance of a research study in interpreting the results of the study. We must recognize that the findings of a single study are restricted by the fact that we have included a limited study population, that we have conducted the study in a particular geographic location and at a particular time in history.

9. SELECT AND DEVELOP METHOD FOR COLLECTING DATA

The next step after delineating the target population is to determine how the data will actually be collected. Two important decisions have to be made during this step in the research process. The first is concerned with how the study population (sampling units) will be selected from the target population. The second decision is concerned with how the data will be collected from the study population.

Selection of the study population is done by a procedure known as sampling. This is a technical procedure and one that is the subject of numerous books and articles in the field of statistical methodology. In many studies no distinction is drawn between the target and the study population, so that the process of sampling is not considered in the development of the research plan. What actually occurs in studies like these is that the target population is not clearly defined, and the study population represents a "chunk" of an ill-defined larger population.

In selecting a sample, the aim is to obtain a study population that is as representative of the total population as possible. The more representative the study population is of the target population, the greater is the accuracy with which generalizations can be made from the sample to the total population.

A large number of techniques are available to the researcher for the collection of data. Choice of the technique to employ in a particular study depends on the nature of the problem, the kinds of variables included in the study, the type of research design, and the type and number of sampling units. Since, in the actual conduct of a study, collection of the data is often the most expensive and time-consuming of all the various research steps, it is essential that decisions concerning this step be carefully made well in advance. Even if all other steps in the research process were carried out as perfectly as possible, imperfections in the data-collecting instruments could invalidate the findings of the study.

10. FORMULATE THE METHOD OF ANALYZING THE DATA

After the data are collected they need to be processed in a way that would permit a valid analysis of their meaning. In small studies processing of the data can be a simple task consisting of combining by hand the data collected on each sampling unit with the data obtained from all other sampling units. In larger studies, where the number of sampling units is very large, or where the number of variables upon which data have been collected are many, it may not be possible to process the data by hand. Various kinds of equipment are available to speed up the data processing. The most sophisticated of these are the electronic computers, which can also perform complex mathematical computations, if required, for the analysis of the data.

It is essential that the method by which the data are to be processed is decided on in advance of the actual collection of data, since it can influence the way in which the data are to be collected. For example, if the data are to be processed through punched cards, the data-collecting form could be set up to facilitate the transference of data from the form to the punched card.

Analysis of data collected in a research study consists of converting the raw data into an orderly and "digestible" body of knowledge that can be interpreted meaningfully. Analysis of data includes a wide variety of techniques—from the simplest to the most complex. Among the simple techniques are the summarization of data in tables and charts and the computation of summary measures of central tendency and variation of the data. The more complicated techniques include the computation of statistical tests of significance and errors of estimation.

Sometimes researchers may become overly preoccupied with the statistical analysis of their data and consequently actually overanalyze their data. The importance of the statistical arithmetic that is performed in the analysis of the data may have been exaggerated out of proportion to its real importance. In some studies, it may be more fruitful to treat the data with the simpler technique of summarization in appropriate statistical tables, rather than to apply complicated statistical methods that are not appropriate to the data. A logical approach to understanding what the data mean can then be used.

11. DETERMINE HOW RESULTS WILL BE INTERPRETED

Interpretation of the data consists of relating the findings of the study to the research problem, the hypotheses, if appropriate, and the theoretical framework for the study. If the study is a descriptive one, concerned with the problem of describing the characteristics of patients in nursing homes, interpretation may proceed from a series of questions. What can we conclude from the data we have collected about the age of the patients, their economic status, the reasons they are in nursing homes, and other pertinent facts that will contribute to our understanding of the problem?

If the study is a test of the hypothesis that seriously ill cardiac patients who are placed in intensive care units have a lower mortality rate than do patients in conventional units, what is the statistical significance of the difference in the rates we have found? What is the practical significance of the difference? To what extent can we generalize the findings to the target population? To other target populations? To what extent can we generalize our findings into the future? What is the need for additional tests of the same hypothesis to support our own findings or, perhaps, to disprove them?

Interpretation of the data, then, consists of drawing meaning out of the data. In interpreting his data the researcher takes a stand on what he feels the data say, their significance and their importance. In interpreting his data the investigator can refer to data from other research, and he can relate his findings to existing theories, laws, and hypotheses. In fact, an important function of the process of interpretation is to link the findings of the study to the mainstream of scientific knowledge in the field. During the process of interpretation, the researcher should be most sensitive to the needs for additional research in his area of study. Assessment of the significance and limitations of his own findings will suggest gaps in knowledge that should be met by additional research. This step in the research process may require the greatest amount of intellectual activity on the part of the researcher to assure that the value and meaning of his findings are maximized. If this is not done, it is possible that important findings might be lost forever.

12. DETERMINE METHOD OF COMMUNICATING RESULTS

The end product of a research study is a report of the findings. This can take many forms. It may be a brief, typewritten paper that simply contains the main findings of the study, or it may consist of a lengthy published book that reports in great detail on all stages of the study.

Unfortunately, a considerable amount of completed research is never written up or published. One reason for this is the fact that many otherwise highly competent researchers seem to freeze up when they approach the task of writing a report and having other researchers challenge their findings. It is obvious that a research study can make no impact if its results are not communicated to members of the professional field, particularly in periodicals. This communication should take the form of at least one published article in a professional or scientific journal reporting on the highlights of the study as well as a complete report, published and available for all interested persons to read, which covers all phases of the design and execution of the study.

One of the reasons that some researchers seem to find preparation of the final report such a burdensome chore is that the entire writing task is left to the very end, a time when a great deal of energy has already been expended and interest in the project might have waned. One way of avoiding the difficulty of writing the entire report at the end is to prepare intermediate reports—working papers—at the conclusion of each of the major stages of the project. For example, a working paper could be prepared on the research problem, another on the review of the literature, another on the research design. Such working papers can serve a dual purpose. Some of the material can become a part of the final report, thus making its preparation less burdensome. Also, the working papers can serve as a vehicle for critically reviewing the various stages of the development of the research project, thereby improving the total research project. Sometimes, individual working papers like those concerned with reviewing the literature or developing a conceptual framework for the study are of such value that they may find their way into the published literature prior to the completion of the total study.

Another reason why there may be a lack of enthusiasm for reporting on a research project is that the study may not have produced conclusive findings or may even have yielded negative findings—i.e., contrary to the researcher's expectations. It should be stressed that any findings from a study should be communicated to the members of the professional field. Perhaps it was the peculiarity of the study population, or some deeply hidden bias in the design, that produced the inconclusive or contrary findings. By permitting the study to be scrutinized by others, we are more likely to obtain constructive explanations of the perplexing findings than if they were hidden from view.

Indeed, a researcher has a fundamental obligation to communicate to the members of his professional field on the methodology and findings of his study. Only through such communication and the resultant accumulation of facts, ideas, interpretations, and analyses can a body of scientific knowledge and theories in nursing be developed.

Summary

The twelve major steps in the research process have been discussed. Although the development of a research project usually proceeds in chronological order from the first step—selection of a topic and formulation of the problem—to the last step—writing the final report—there is a great deal of going back and forth through the various steps as the total research plan is tightened, polished, and formalized. As has been pointed out, not all types of studies include the twelve stages of the research process. For example, descriptive studies may not include hypotheses. Methodological studies may omit certain phases of data collection.

The next several chapters of this book will contain more detailed discussions of those stages of the research process devoted to the design of the research, measurement of variables, collection, tabulation, analysis, and interpretation of data. As a review of the topics discussed in this chapter and as a guide to reviewing a completed research plan, the following questions can be used to focus on the main components of the research process. The answers to these questions, when applied to an actual research proposal, can point up possible shortcomings in the plan and suggest areas where the research may be strengthened, clarified, or simplified. These questions can also be used to assess the weaknesses and strengths of a completed research project.

GUIDE QUESTIONS FOR EVALUATING A RESEARCH PLAN OR A COMPLETED RESEARCH PROJECT

1. The Problem

Is it feasible to conduct research on the problem? Is the problem important? To what extent can the findings of the research be generalized? What will the solution of the problem achieve?

Is the researcher really interested in the problem? Is the researcher adequately competent to pursue the problem through research? Can the research best be labeled as basic or applied? If applied, what are the possible practical outcomes of the research?

2. Review of the Literature

Have all possible sources of related literature been investigated? Are the findings of previous studies that are relevant to the research being considered? What practical problems have previous researchers encountered?

Does the review of the literature provide supporting evidence to show the need for carrying out the research? In what ways does the research being considered go beyond what already has been found in previous studies? Does the research make provision for consultation with experts in the field when they are needed?

3. The Framework of Theory

Does any applicable theory exist in the field of knowledge in which the research is being done? Can the problem area in which the research is being done be conceptualized in the form of a model of some kind? Is the model useful in clarifying concepts and relationships contained in the research?

If the research deals with statistical data, what is the statistical model for the analysis of the data? Are the theories or models used in the study meaningful and helpful to the study, and not just used as window-dressing?

4. Formulation of Hypotheses

Are the hypotheses stated clearly and unambiguously? Do they contain a statement of the dependent and independent variables and the target population to whom the findings will be generalized?

Do the hypotheses deal with causal or associative relationships? Is the study concerned with artificial relationships, and if so, are there dangers of inferring spurious relationships from the data?

Are the independent and dependent variables operationally defined?

Are these variables meaningful and realistic in terms of their possible application outside of the experimental situation?

Does the design recognize the extraneous variables that may affect the results of the study? How will these extraneous variables be controlled or eliminated? What are the major organismic and environmental variables that are involved in the study?

If the hypothesis is stated as a null hypothesis, what are the alternative hypotheses?

Are the major assumptions underlying the study stated explicitly or implicitly? Are the bases for these assumptions, theories, laws, common sense, generally accepted facts, or findings from previous research? Have they been documented by references in the literature?

5. Definition of the Variables

What is the scale of classification for the explanatory variables? Do valid scales or instruments already exist for measuring the variables? Are the variables defined clearly and concretely enough so that they are readily understood?

6. Quantification of the Variables

Are the variables to be studied capable of being quantified? Is the quantification meaningful, valid, reliable? Has the quantification of variables been established in previous studies, or does the research establish original quantifications of the variables? Does the research deal with any variables that can not be quantified, and if so, how are these handled in the analysis? Are expert consultants needed to develop variables that can be quantified?

Do the measures of the variables have a practical application in the real world?

7. The Research Design

Is the choice of the design—experimental or nonexperimental—appropriate for the research problem? Is the setting for the study natural or artificial?

What controls over possible hidden biases have been set up for the study? If appropriate, will random assignment procedures be used to allocate the sampling units to the different groups under study?

If an experiment is conducted, is the length of the experiment adequate for drawing valid conclusions?

Can the data from the experimental setting be generalized to other settings?

8. The Target Population

Has the target population been clearly designated by the research? Is the target population reasonable, or is it too ambitious?

What type of sampling units does the target population consist of—people, things, ideas, etc?

Can an appropriate sample be drawn of the target population? Will it be possible to draw a valid sample of the target population that is representative of the population?

9. Collecting and Analyzing Data

Is the target population to be sampled randomly? Will the size of the study population be adequate for drawing valid generalizations?

Are the methods that will be used to collect the data and the measures that will be derived from them valid and reliable? Do these measures have any practical application in the real world?

Have the data-collecting instruments been carefully pretested? Have they been used in previous research, or have they been developed purposely for the research?

Does the study clearly indicate the ways in which the data will be tabulated? Will the tabulations permit a meaningful and comprehensive interpretation to be made of the data?

Has sufficient time been allowed for the period of data collection? Have provisions been made to ensure completeness of data?

If needed, have provisions been made to hire sufficient personnel (field interviewers, observers) to assist in the collection of data? Is specialized equipment needed to tabulate the data, and are provisions made to obtain it?

Is the budget allowed for the study adequate for the amounts and kinds of data to be collected, for the method of collecting the data, and for the time allowed to do the research?

Are the statistical methods that will be used to analyze the data clearly indicated? Are these methods appropriate to the kinds of variables that will be studied, the kinds of data that will be collected concerning these variables, the methods of collecting these data, and the nature of the study population? Does the analysis of the data relate in a relevant way to the research problem and to the hypotheses under study?

Are the data analyzed in such a way as to yield maximum information from the findings?

10. Interpretation of the Data

If tests of statistical significance are included in the design, what levels of significance are being used? Are these appropriate to the kinds of data with which the study is concerned?

Apart from a statistical significance that might be obtained from the study data, what might be the practical significance of the findings?

What is the scope of the generalizations that can be made from the data—as to length of time for which this generalization might apply, the nature of the applicable population, geographic coverage?

Does interpretation of the data lead back to the hypotheses, theoretical framework, research problem? Does the interpretation relate the findings to the general body of knowledge in the field? Does it show what the study has contributed to the advancement of knowledge in the field?

11. Communicating the Research

Have adequate provisions been made to communicate the method and findings of the research to the audience most likely to be interested in and concerned with the research? Is the format for reporting the research appropriate to the content of the study? Does the researcher convey any sense of interest and enthusiasm in pursuing his research study?

Does the report contain a clear statement of the problem and purpose of the research and the framework of theory? Is the methodology adequately described?

Have the limitations of the study been carefully spelled out in the report? Does the report contain appropriate cautions in interpreting the data?

In the presentation of the statistical data, are detailed source tables placed in the appendix or some other part of the report where they will not interfere with the flow of the reading? Are the findings clearly presented and in an interesting style? Does the text point up in an interpretative way the important facts contained in the statistical tables and not just merely restate the data from the table?

Is the report related to previous research in the field? Is appropriate credit given to findings, theories, concepts, and methods used from other studies? Does it contain suggestions for further research that should be undertaken? Does it suggest how the findings of the study might be applied?

Does the report clearly indicate what the researcher has accomplished?

12. The Research Plan as a Whole

Looking at the research design as a whole, what are the limitations of the study? In view of these limitations, was it (or will it be) worthwhile to go forward with the study? What modifications, if any, could be made in the research design to improve it without significantly increasing the time and money required to carry out the study? Would a nonexperimental research design be more appropriate to achieve the aims of the study than an experimental approach, or vice versa? Will it be possible for other researchers to replicate the research design of the study?

References

1. Everett C. Hughes, Helen MacGill Hughes, and Irwin Deutscher, *Twenty Thousand Nurses Tell Their Story*. Philadelphia, J. B. Lippincott Co., 1958.
2. Eileen G. Hasselmeyer, *Behavior Patterns of Premature Infants*. U.S. Public Health Service Publication No. 840, Washington, D.C., Government Printing Office, 1961.
3. Janet Fitzwater, "The Selection of Instruments for Major Operations." *Nursing Res.,* **9:**129–136, summer 1960.
4. Mary S. Tschudin, Helen C. Belcher, and Leo Nedelsky, *Evaluation in Basic Nursing Education*. New York, G. P. Putnam's Sons, 1958.
5. Norman H. Berkowitz and Warren G. Bennis, "Interaction Patterns in Formal Service-Oriented Organizations." *Admin. Sc. Quart.,* **6:**25–50, June 1961.
6. Charles D. Flagle, *The Problem of Organization for Hospital Inpatient Care*. Preprint No. 55 of a paper presented at the 6th Annual International Meeting of the Institute of Management Sciences, September 1959.
7. Morris R. Cohen and Ernest Nagel, *An Introduction to Logic and Scientific Method*. New York, Harcourt, Brace and Co., 1934, p. 199.
8. Robert K. Merton, "Notes on Problem Finding in Sociology," in Robert K. Merton *et al.* (eds.), *Sociology Today*. New York, Basic Books, 1959, p. ix.
9. Cohen and Nagel, *op. cit.,* p. 200.
10. Lois B. Miller and Edith N. Rathbun, "Growth and Development of Nursing Literature." *Bull. Med. Library Assoc.,* **52:**420–426, April 1964.

11. Virginia Henderson, *Nursing Studies Index,* Vol. IV. Philadelphia, J. B. Lippincott Co., 1963, subsequent volumes are Vol. III (1950–1956) published 1966; Vol. II (1930–1949), published 1970; Vol. I (1900–1929), published 1972.

12. Leo Simmons and Virginia Henderson, *Nursing Research—A Survey and Assessment.* New York, Appleton-Century-Crofts, 1964.

13. Miller and Rathbun, *op. cit.,* p. 425.

14. National Institutes of Health, Division of Research Grants, *Research Grants Index.* U.S. Public Health Service Publication No. 925, 1963 edition. Washington, D.C., Government Printing Office, Vols. I and II, 1963.

15. Division of Nursing. *The National Health Planning Information Center.* DHEW Publication No. (HRA) 76–33. Washington, D.C., Health Resources Administration, 1976.

16. Edith N. Rathbun, "MEDLARS," Research Reporter. *Nursing Res.,* **12:** 251–252, fall 1963.

17. Claire Selltiz *et al., Research Methods in Social Relations.* New York, Holt, Rinehart, and Winston, 1962, p. 481.

18. James M. Beshers, "Models and Theory Construction." *Am. Sociol. Rev.,* **22:**32, February 1957.

19. Faye G. Abdellah, *et al., Patient-Centered Approaches to Nursing.* New York, Macmillan Publishing Co., Inc., 1960, p. 58.

20. Beshers, *op. cit.,* p. 35.

21. Irwin D. J. Bross, *Design for Decision.* New York, Macmillan Publishing Co., Inc., 1953.

22. *Ibid.,* pp. 171–172.

23. Daniel Howland, "A Hospital System Model." *Nursing Res.,* **12:**232, fall 1963. For a discussion of cybernetic models in health care see Alan Sheldon, "Adaptive Cybernetic Approaches to Health Care," in Larry I. Shuman, R. Dixon Speas, and John P. Young, *Operations Research in Health Care.* Baltimore, Johns Hopkins Press, 1975.

24. Beshers, *op. cit.,* p. 34.

25. Myrtle K. Aydelotte and Marie E. Tener, "An Investigation of the Relation Between Nursing Activity and Patient Welfare." Iowa City, State University of Iowa, Utilization Project, 1960 (U.S.P.H.S. Grant GN 4786).

26. Cohen and Nagel, *op. cit.,* p. 248.

27. Donald Mainland, *Elementary Medical Statistics.* Philadelphia, W. B. Saunders Co., 1963, p. 17.

28. *Ibid.,* p. 95.

29. Pauline V. Young, *Scientific Social Surveys and Research,* 2nd ed. Englewood Cliffs, N.J., Prentice-Hall, 1949, pp. 133–134.

Problems and Suggestions for Further Study

1. Make a list of ten topics that might be fruitful to develop into research problems. Apply the guidelines for assessing the researchability of a prob-

lem to the topics and determining the degree to which they meet the criteria of the guidelines.

2. Review some reports of research in nursing that have appeared in such journals as *Nursing Research* to see if it is possible to distinguish those conducted by a research team from those conducted by an individual investigator. Can any conclusions be drawn concerning the nature of the research (e.g., the kind of problem studied, the methodology used, the scope of the study) when it was the product of a team approach as compared to the efforts of an individual researcher?

3. What is the difference between the research problem and the research purpose? Why is it important to state the purpose of a study?

4. Carefully distinguish the following six terms: problem, theory, postulate, law, model, hypothesis. Show how a problem can be evolved into a hypothesis. How can a hypothesis become a law? Are you familiar with any scientific laws applicable to your field?

5. Read the article by Peter Blau, "Operationalizing a Conceptual Scheme: The Universalism-Particularism Pattern Variable" (*Am. Sociol. Rev.* **27:** 159–169, April 1962). How does the author define an operational definition? Does the variable "universalism-particularism," as defined by the author, have any relevance to research in nursing? What is meant by the term "framework" as used in this article?

6. Discuss the assertion, "Not all research has to be based on hypotheses." What role do hypotheses serve in research? Can an explanatory study be undertaken without a hypothesis?

7. Examine the list of hypotheses on page 135–36. Assess these hypotheses in terms of the criteria of feasibility, importance, and need. Select a few of these hypotheses and explain how you would go about testing them in a research study. How would the hypotheses have to be restated, if at all, to make them researchable?

8. Operationally define the following variables in quantifiable terms:
   Patient's needs for nursing services
   Patient's mobility
   Quality of patient care
   Intensity of illness
   Nursing procedure
   Patient satisfaction with care received
   Nurse-patient relationship

9. Is it possible to define adequately "cause and effect"? Are the terms "stimulus and response" simpler to define? What characteristic about an independent variable makes it independent?

10. Can you distinguish between a mathematical and a statistical model? Why is it necessary to have quantified data before these models can be applied in a research study? Does all research have to be based on quantified data? If not, cite examples where this would not be true.

11. Define what is meant by a spurious relationship among variables. Can you give some examples of spurious relationships other than those described in this chapter? Why might any of the following be an artificial or even a spurious relationship?
   a. High cholesterol intake produces heart disease.
   b. Female patients are more demanding than male patients.

    c. The rate of personnel turnover is higher in larger hospitals than smaller ones, therefore morale may be lower in larger hospitals.

    d. The death rate from tuberculosis is higher in Arizona than in any other state.

    e. The need for public health nurses in relation to population has not increased appreciably for at least 20 years because the ratio of public health nurses to population has remained stable.

    f. A nursing student with a superior I.Q. will not do as well in school as a student with an average I.Q.

12. Why is it important to explicitly state the major assumptions and limitations of a study? Can you conceive of any studies that would have no assumptions or limitations? If a study has many assumptions and limitations, is it worthwhile doing?

13. What is the value of being able to predict the behavior of one variable through knowledge of the other variable even though the variables are not causally related? Can you think of any predictive relationship that you could make use of in your work, studies, or home life?

14. For the even-numbered hypotheses on page 135, state the independent and dependent variables and the applicable target population. Which of these hypotheses do you think would lend themselves best to the establishment of causal relationships?

15. In testing a hypothesis, why is it desirable for the researcher to be impartial about whether the data he collects will prove or disprove the hypothesis? Is it possible for a researcher to be completely neutral in his belief concerning the existence or lack of existence of the relationship expressed by the hypothesis?

16. Read the article, "Problems of Ambulation and Traveling Among Elderly Chronically Ill Clinic Patients," by Schwartz, *et al.* (*Nursing Res.,* **12**:165–171, summer 1963). Describe the target population for this study. To what extent do you feel that the findings of this study can be applied generally to the care of elderly, chronically ill clinic patients?

17. Select a completed research study in your area of interest. Evaluate it by applying the guide questions beginning on page 157. What is your overall evaluation of the study on the basis of your answers to the specific questions?

18. What is meant by interpreting the results of a study? Is this process different from analyzing the data from the study?

19. Read Chapter 8, "How to Think," in Hans Selye, *From Dream to Discovery: On Being a Scientist* (New York, Arno, 1975). Discuss the following statement by the author:

> There is a great difference between a sterile theory and a wrong one. A sterile theory does not lend itself to experimental verification. Any number of them can be easily formulated, but they are perfectly useless: They could not possibly aid understanding; they lead only to futile verbiage. On the other hand, a wrong theory can still be highly useful, for, if it is well conceived, it may help to formulate experiments which will fill important gaps in our knowledge. Facts must be correct; theories must be fruitful. A "fact," if incorrect, is useless—it is not a fact—but an incorrect theory

may be even more useful than a correct one if it is more fruitful in leading the way to new facts. (p. 280.)

20. Read Chapter 4 (pp. 63–98) "Finding the Facts" in Jacques Barzun and Henry F. Graff, *The Modern Researcher*. New York, Harcourt, Brace and Jovanovich, Inc., 1977. Develop a study idea in which the data would come from existing sources. What are the advantages to conducting a study from already collected data? What are the disadvantages?

21. Chapter 6 (pp. 73–97) in *Scientific and Technological Communication* by Sidney Paasman, Oxford, Pergamon Press, 1969, discusses "The Secondary Literature." Survey the secondary literature in nursing and name the various kinds of literature that exist (i.e., indexes, abstracts, state-of-the arts review, etc.).

Chapter Six

RESEARCH DESIGN

RESEARCH DESIGN is concerned with the overall framework for conducting the study. Although the design of a study actually begins when a topic for research is first selected, the detailed work of determining the study format usually takes place after the problem has been concretely formulated and the hypotheses, if any, have been stated.

The essential question that research design is concerned with is how the data are to be collected. This does not mean the specified method for collecting the data—e.g., questionnaire, interview, or direct observation—but rather the more fundamental question of how the study subjects will be brought into the scope of the research and how they will be employed within the research setting to yield the required data.

Basically, there are two types of research design, the experimental and the nonexperimental. The main difference between the two types is that in experimental research all major elements of the design are largely under the control of the researcher. These include the research setting, the explanatory variables, the study subjects—particularly the assignment of these subjects to the different study groups—and the method for collecting the data from the study subjects. In nonexperimental research, sometimes called surveys, the researcher does not have as strict control over the various elements of the design.

EXPERIMENTAL RESEARCH

Experimental research is particularly well suited to the purposes of diagnosis and explanation. Although numerous examples of experimental research can be cited from the field of the physical sciences where the purpose of the experiment is purely descriptive—as, for example, a microscopic analysis of the characteristics of the chromosomes in the egg of a frog—the most powerful application of the experimental technique is undoubtedly for the purpose of explanation: what happens to A when B occurs. Experimental research probably finds its greatest application today

166

in evaluating products, programs, techniques, tools, or methods of procedure. These evaluations can be called comparative experiments, in which the effects produced by the independent variable are compared in terms of some criterion measure to find out which produces the most desirable effect.

The comparative experiment is basically a more sophisticated as well as a more efficient form of the method of trial and error. In the trial and error approach to problem solving a change is introduced and the effects produced by the change are observed. If the introduction of the change has not solved the problem, another change is introduced and the effects observed. The process is continued until the problem is finally solved. Thus, if arthritic patients complain of severe pain, we may first try physical means to relieve the pain. If that does not work, we may try a pain-relieving drug. If that still does not work, the surgeon might recommend surgery. When relief is finally obtained we would ascribe the cure to the last method employed.

Instead of applying different methods of treatment, we might have begun by giving the patient a certain dosage level of a drug, and if that did not work, the dosage could be increased until a level was reached where pain was relieved. The worst approach of all (from a research point of view): all methods of treatment would be varied simultaneously for the same patients, thus completely clouding the issue of which factor was responsible for improvement, if any.

There are several obvious drawbacks to the trial and error method. First is the fact that when we have produced the desired effect we cannot be certain that it is totally or even partially attributed to the last treatment, since the effect may be *cumulative,* one treatment reinforcing the other. Or the effect may even be a delayed action, due to an earlier treatment whose impact would be completely masked by later treatments.

In addition to the crudities of the trial and error approach as an evaluative device, it is obvious that it is inefficient. Many unnecessary trials may have to be carried out by such a testing method. This can be financially wasteful. Of even more concern, it can be harmful to the well-being of the study subjects.

The experimental approach to testing is ideally one in which all factors except the one being tested are held under strict control, so that only the tested factor will be able to exert an effect on the study subjects. Experimental research, thus, should be able to accurately relate the effect to its appropriate cause with an economy of research effort.

The field of comparative experiments—where the purpose is to test out some procedure, or program—is a young one. Early comparative experiments were conducted in the agricultural field, where the effects on crop yield of different levels of such variables as chemical fertilization, depth of plowing, and moisture were experimentally studied. The study of experimental design as a systematic statistical method for carrying out comparative experiments dates back to the 1930's with the publication of Sir Ronald A. Fisher's famous treatise, *The Design of Experiments*.[1] Most of the major books on the subject have been published since the 1950's: Cochran and Cox, Kempthorne, and Federer—writing about the design of agricultural experiments; Edwards—psychology; Chapin—sociology; Chew—industry; and Finney—biology and medicine.[2-8]

Not only is the experimental approach a powerful tool for testing alternative ways of doing things, but it is also a valid approach to the understanding of causal connections between phenomena. Thus the experimental method when applied to problems of a more fundamental nature than the evaluation of products or methods has made important contributions to the advancement of basic scientific knowledge.

Cause and Effect

The previous chapter presented a definition of cause and effect, which stated that the *cause* of a certain *effect* was some appropriate factor that was invariably related to the effect. The experimental method that has been developed in the attempt to discover causal connections between phenomena stems from John Stuart Mill's five rules or canons of experimental research contained in Book III of his *System of Logic*.[9] Two of the fundamental rules of Mill's method of experimental inquiry are his *method of agreement* and *method of difference*. Mill describes these rules as follows:

> The simplest and most obvious modes of singling out from among the circumstances which precede or follow a phenomenon, those with which it is really connected by an invariable law are two in number. One is, by comparing together different instances in which the phenomenon occurs. The other is by comparing instances in which the phenomenon does occur, with instances in other respects similar in which it does not. These two methods may be respectively denominated, the Method of Agreement, and the Method of Difference.[10]

Method of Agreement   The method of agreement states that if the circumstances that lead up to the occurrence of a given event, *B,* have during every occurrence of the event only one factor in common, *A,* then *A* is probably the cause of *B*. This is a useful principle, particularly in the development of hypotheses. However, it has certain limitations. First, we must be sure that the event, *B,* is defined in such a way as to have a constant meaning during each occurrence. This problem is a major difficulty encountered in research on the cause of cancer. It is now recognized that cancer may not be a single, circumscribed entity with one well-defined cause, but rather a variety of entities each with its own causal agent.

Second, in applying the method of agreement we must be sure that we can confine the circumstances leading up to the occurrence of *B* to a single, isolated factor, *A*. Thus, if everyone who develops lung cancer also smokes, we cannot say smoking caused lung cancer unless we can be sure that there were no other factors common to all those who developed lung cancer—such as genetic makeup or a personality characteristic.

Method of Difference   The method of difference states that if two or more sets of circumstances are different in respect to only one factor, *A,* and if a given event, *B,* occurs only when *A* is present, then *A* is likely to be the cause of *B*. Thus, if two groups of patients are provided with identical kinds of nursing care in identical settings, except that in one group the team method of assignment is used and in the other group the functional method is employed (one nurse is responsible for all the medications, another for all patient teaching, and so on), and if patients in the team assignment group appear to get well faster than those in the other group, we might say that we have demonstrated the truth of the hypothesis that the higher recovery rate is caused by the team method of assignment.

However, there is a serious shortcoming to this approach. We cannot be sure that the two sets of circumstances—the nursing care, the environment, and, most important of all, the patients—are different in respect to only one variable, the type of organization for providing care. Perhaps in terms of some subtle, difficult to perceive characteristic the patients in the two groups are really different, and this characteristic is actually the cause of the difference in recovery rates. Or, maybe it is not the method of patient care organization per se that influences recovery rates but some deeper sociopsychological factor that is intrinsic to the form of organization employed.

Such pitfalls as these in the application of the method of difference have given rise to the principles of statistical design of experiments. An essential aspect of these principles is the technique of randomization, to be discussed later in this chapter. Through randomization the groups under study can, theoretically at least, be equated on all factors. Except for chance differences that are attributable to randomization itself and measurable by statistical methods, the only difference between the groups should be the independent variable manipulated by the researcher.

Joint Method of Agreement and Difference   A third canon of experimental research, called the joint method of agreement and difference, combines the two methods in an attempt to make a more valid assessment of cause and effect. In the joint approach, the method of agreement is applied first to discover the one characteristic, *A,* that is common to all occurrences of the phenomenon, *B*. Then the method of difference is applied to determine that *B* does not occur when *A* is absent. Thus, if we first show that the team method of assignment is the one characteristic common to all instances where high recovery rates among patients are found, and that the team plan is never employed where low recovery rates among patients occur, we would say that the team plan was the cause of higher patient recovery rates. However, we are again faced with the problem of the equalization of the groups on all factors except that of the independent variable—type of nursing care organization. Again the method of randomization is the most reliable way of achieving this.

Concomitant Variation   A fourth rule of experimental research is that of concomitant variation. As formulated by Mill the canon states that whenever two phenomena vary together in a consistent and persistent manner, either the variations represent a direct causal connection between the two phenomena, or else both are being affected by some other common causal factor.

In essence this rule is merely a broadening of the notions contained in the previous canons. However, here the phenomena (the independent and dependent variables) are variables that differ in degree and can assume a wide range of values, whereas the previous canons were concerned with independent variables that differed in kind—team plan versus functional assignment—or were of the all or nothing variety—smoke, do not smoke.

Of course, as has been pointed out in the previous chapter, three main types of relationships can be found among dependent and independent variables—causal relationships, where the dependent variable is causally related to the independent variable; associative relationships, where both variables stated in the hypotheses are causally related to some third independent variable; and artificial relationships, where the variables included in the hypotheses are statistically related to each other, but they may not even be causally connected to the same independent variable. Thus, the rule of concomitant variation, while a useful model for explanatory research, has its limitations as a method for causal discovery.

As Cohen and Nagel[11] have stated:

Even very high correlations, especially in the social sciences, do not necessarily signify an invariable connection. For the phenomena between which such correlations can be established may be in fact unrelated in any way which would warrant our believing them to be invariably connected. A little statistical skill and patience make it possible to find any number of high correlations between otherwise unrelated factors. We do not discover causal connections by first surveying all possible correlations between different variables. On the contrary, we suspect an invariable connection, and then use correlations as corroborative evidence.

Method of Residues   Mill's fifth canon of experimental research is called the method of residues. This method requires that use be made of previously established causal relationships. It thus seeks to discover causes by a process of elimination. The method of residues states that when the factors that are known to cause a part of some phenomenon are isolated, the remaining part of the phenomenon is the effect of the residual factors. The eliminative approach in seeking the causes of certain phenomena is especially applicable in research on human beings where the effects that are observed are frequently due to a multiplicity of causes and not a single factor. Thus, lung cancer may be related to other factors as well as inhalation of cigarette smoke because some persons who die of lung cancer do not smoke cigarettes. Conversely, many cigarette smokers do not die of lung cancer. Similarly it is not possible to demonstrate that there is a complete and invariant relationship between nursing care and patient welfare, since many factors in the patient care situation in addition to nursing care impinge on patient welfare, not the least of which are the staggering number of organismic variables found in the patients themselves.

Mill's five canons have been most useful in providing a logical basis for pursuing explanatory research—that type of research which has as its ultimate purpose the discovery of causal connections among the variables studied. Research design is essentially the means by which such research can be pursued most efficiently and validly. And as has been said, the most valid way of pursuing causal connections among variables is by the kind of research design known as an experiment.

Experimental Design

In the classic design of an explanatory experiment the researcher establishes two groups from his study population. The groups are equalized in terms of all possible extraneous variables. This can be done by some deliberate matching procedure or by random assignment to one of the two groups or by a combination method. Then, one of the groups, called the experimental group, is exposed to the independent variable, which may be a treatment, method, procedure, or some other factor that is being tested. The other group, called the control, contrast, or comparative group, does not receive the independent variable. Or the experiment may consist of applying different levels of the independent variable to the groups (e.g., different dosages of a drug). After an appropriate period of time has elapsed the effects of the independent variable on the two groups are compared in terms of some criterion measure (dependent variable). Differences in the values of the criterion measure for the two groups are compared with an estimate of the differences attributable to the randomized extraneous variables to assess the significance of the effects produced by the independent (causal) variable. To the degree that these effects are significantly greater than would be expected by chance alone, as well as to the degree that we are sure that all relevant extraneous variables have been accounted for, the greater is the confidence that a causal connection has been established between the independent and dependent variables.

Thus, modern experimental design, building on the foundation of Mill's canons, has added the features of randomization to equalize the groups studied and statistical assessment of differences produced among the groups through application of probability theory. Modern experimental design incorporates the following canons of Mill:

1. The method of difference is applied in setting up the two study groups, the experimental and the comparison group, so that they are identical in all important respects, except in regard to the independent variable manipulated by the researcher. Thus, according to this canon, any response in the dependent variable must be attributable to the independent variable. Moreover, by equalizing the characteristics of the experimental and the comparison group, thus starting with a clean slate, so to speak, it can be clearly demonstrated that the application of the independent variable preceded the response measured by the criterion variable.

2. The rule of concomitant variation is the basic underlying statistical model for experimental research. In its fundamental form this model is the general linear hypothesis, which states that $Y = f(X)$, where Y is the dependent variable and X is the independent variable. The model states that any change in Y is associated with a change in X.

3. By different experiments concerned with the same explanatory variables the method of agreement can be shown to apply in the drawing of causal inferences from the data. Thus, if it is found in repeated trials that similar effects are produced by a common factor, this common factor may be designated as the causal agent.

4. Repeated verifications of the same hypothesis in identically performed experiments (replications) will serve to uphold the relationship among the variables as an invariant relationship.

5. By a series of experiments, each testing different independent variables as possible causes of the phenomenon, we apply the method of residues. Each experiment can eliminate independent variables that have no relationship to the dependent variable. In cases of multiple causality— an effect being the result of a number of factors—we can see the extent to which each partially causative variable contributes to the explanation of the dependent variable.

Essentially then, experimental research is a highly controlled, forward-looking study often conducted in a specially created setting in which the researcher has himself consciously manipulated the independent variable and has applied it in such a way to his study subjects that he can be confident that he has controlled any possible extraneous variables that could affect the dependent variable. By contrast, in an nonexperimental explanatory study the independent variable is not manipulated by the researcher. He must accept it as it naturally occurs in the study population in its normal environment. Often, a nonexperimental explanatory study looks back to the past in that the researcher first observes the effects in the dependent variable and then traces back to the possible independent variables that could have caused the effects he has observed. Thus, in a nonexperimental study the independent variable has often been applied before the actual study was begun, whereas in an experimental study application of the independent variable always precedes measurement of the dependent variable:

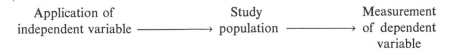

Application of   Study   Measurement
independent variable ——————→ population ——————→ of dependent
                                                     variable

In nonexperimental explanatory research, measurement of the dependent variable may precede the time at which application of the independent variable is observed:

Measurement of   Study   Observation of
dependent variable ——————→ population ——————→ independent variable

The antecedent nature of the application of the independent variable and the resultant control over extraneous variables are essential characteristics of the experimental method's ability to establish causal relationships, since cause and effect implies a temporal relationship in which cause always precedes effect. In the nonexperimental method it is not possible to exert as high a degree of control over the extraneous variables, nor is it always possible to demonstrate that the application of the independent variable preceded the response measured in the dependent variable. Thus, the best that we can often hope to achieve in such research is to establish an associative relationship which may be very useful for predictive purposes, although weak for purposes of explanation, diagnosis, and fundamental understanding of the nature of the phenomena we are studying. What has to be guarded against in nonexperimental research is that the relationship we establish among variables is not an artificial or a spurious one.

Advantages and Disadvantages of the Experimental Design

The advantages of the experimental design over the nonexperimental approach for conducting research can be summarized as follows:

1. Where the purpose of research is explanation it may be possible to establish causal relationships among the explanatory variables in an experiment, particularly when inanimate objects compose the study population, and the variables are narrow, well-defined and easy to control.

2. In descriptive studies, the experimental approach can yield a higher degree of purity in observations by providing a controlled environment in which to conduct the research.

3. It is possible to create conditions in an experimental setting that would be impossible to find in a natural setting. Thus, if we want to test a new procedure, technique, or product, we must of necessity deliberately manipulate the independent variable that we are testing.

4. Through the experimental approach we can often create conditions in a short period of time that might take many years to occur naturally. For example, in genetic studies we can experimentally breed certain strains of animals in a fraction of the time that it would take if left completely to the forces of nature.

5. The experimental approach to research, particularly when conducted in a laboratory, experimental unit, or other specialized research setting, is removed from the pressures and problems of the actual real-life situation. Thus removed from possibly contaminating and disturbing influences the researcher can pursue his study in a more leisurely, careful, and concentrated way.

However, the experimental design is not free of certain disadvantages. Some of these are so severe that the selection of this design may be automatically ruled out in certain types of studies. In brief, the main disadvantages are:

1. Although theoretically the experimental approach can yield insight into the causes of certain kinds of phenomena, in research involving human beings the phenomena being studied are usually so complex and often derive from such a plurality of causes that the simple experimental model, $Y = f(X)$, does not apply at all. Instead what may be required is a much more complicated multivariate nonlinear model, which might only with great difficulty be amenable to the experimental approach.

2. For many important human variables—as, for example, patient welfare or level of wellness—there are no valid criterion measures available at the present time. Therefore, the use of the refined, experimental approach in studies involving such variables represents in essence a mismatch of study design and measuring instrument. Likewise in many studies the independent variables may be so crude or gross—as, for example, the variable "nursing care"—that a mismatch between degree of refinement of design and of the measurement of the explanatory variables would create a situation reminiscent of the old saying of "shooting flies with an

elephant gun." Where variables are crude and not well-defined it may be better to use the more flexible nonexperimental approach.

3. For certain research problems, because of the possible danger to the health and well-being of the members of the study population, it is not feasible to conduct experiments on humans. Certain drugs or treatments are so dangerous that we dare not try them on human beings. Instead we would use animals for our study population, realizing that it might not be possible to make valid generalizations from the animal to the human population. Or even if our independent variable is not dangerous to physical health, it may be psychologically harmful to the study subjects and would create difficulties in securing and maintaining the cooperation of these subjects. Examples of such variables are those included in studies of sensory deprivation.

4. In some research it might not be possible to create experimentally the conditions to be studied. This is particularly obvious in a field like astronomy where the uniqueness of the subject being studied—say, the effect of solar radiation on the development of life on Mars—makes it impossible to create the study conditions in a laboratory setting. In patient care research we might be interested in studying the effects on patient well-being of a global independent variable like the organizational and physical structure of a hospital, which would be totally impractical to attempt experimentally.

5. Experiments are often impractical where the effect of the independent variable being studied may require a lengthy period of time before it makes itself evident in terms of the criterion measure being studied. For example, in studies of the possible causal relationship between smoking and lung cancer, there is a long time lag that occurs between exposure to smoking and the development of lung cancer making it difficult to keep the study population intact and under control for the length of time required for the experiment. This situation is very pertinent for many of the variables that could be studied in the patient care and nursing areas. One of the main drawbacks to conducting experiments on the effects of nursing care on acutely ill hospitalized patients is the fact that the patients are discharged from the hospital in such a short period of time that there is little opportunity for the effects we are studying to occur. Only by a difficult and costly procedure of following up discharged patients in their homes is it possible to observe experimental results.

6. Another limitation of the experimental design is the difficulty frequently encountered in enlisting the cooperation of study subjects. Participation in an experiment usually imposes much more of a burden on subjects than other types of studies. Therefore, in experiments with human subjects it is desirable to keep the study population as small as possible and consistent with the requirements for obtaining sufficient and mean-

ingful data. With small-sized study populations assigned to the different study groups it becomes especially important that the members of the groups be kept intact. Drop-outs from a group, as well as the possible contamination of one group by members of the other group, can destroy the validity of an experiment. The administrative problems in securing and maintaining the cooperation of study subjects are indeed formidable. They can sometimes discourage the selection of this type of design as the method for a study.

7. Because the study population for experiments involving human beings is often kept very small, there is a question as to how representative the finding of such studies can be. If the target population is very diverse, if the explanatory variables are complex, if the extraneous variables are numerous, and if these extraneous variables can exert spurious influences on our dependent variable when uncontrolled, there is some question as to whether a small number of study subjects can provide findings that are meaningful for a larger population even if they have been carefully selected and kept intact during the course of the study.

The use of experimental design is ruled out in many research problems because the number of study subjects required to provide meaningful data would be impractically large. Consequently, in order to be approached experimentally, many research problems have to be delimited to permit the use of small-sized study groups. Such narrowing down, of course, restricts the importance of the study findings in relation to their application to the real world. In basic research, they may make only minute contributions to the advancement of scientific knowledge. Experiments can be so restrictive in scope that they could become nothing more than a sterile exercise.

8. The entire matter of artificiality can be raised concerning the application of the experimental method to many problems in the area of patient care research. To what extent can findings be generalized from an essentially unnatural setting in which the variables being tested are artifacts, created by the researcher and manipulated by him among study subjects who may not represent the population at large? These limitations are especially restrictive where the aim of the research is a practical application of the findings. Many experiments conducted in the social sciences suffer from artificiality because, first of all, they often use a specially selected study population, such as students or patients in hospitals. Such subjects are not broadly representative of any larger target population. It is difficult to say to what extent data collected in experiments like these can be generalized at all. Second, the setting in which such experiments are sometimes conducted—a classroom, a laboratory, or some specially devised experimental unit—may not have any resemblance to reality, thus making it difficult to justify an application of the findings to a real-life

setting. Third, the independent variable being manipulated experimentally, say the size and composition of the nursing team, may be so artificial as to make application to an actual nursing situation impossible.

The limitations inherent in the experimental approach are greatest where the experimental subjects are human beings. Since most conceivable patient care studies will involve humans, the use of the experimental method in such research will not be widespread. However, this method serves as the ideal model for all types of studies where the aim is to discover causal relationships among variables. Indeed, some aspects of the experimental method can be incorporated into the nonexperimental design to improve the quality of data collected.

Advantages and Disadvantages of Nonexperimental Design

Perhaps the greatest distinguishing feature between experimental and nonexperimental explanatory research is the fact that in the latter the investigator does not actually manipulate the independent variable. That is to say, its application to the study subjects is not under his direct control. In fact, in many retrospective studies the application of the independent variable has occurred prior to the time when the study is initiated. Regardless of this limitation the nonexperimental approach to research does have certain advantages:

1. Generally, the nonexperimental design, particularly the retrospective survey, is less expensive to conduct than is the experimental method. In the survey types of research the subjects are not brought together in a specially designed study unit, but remain in their natural settings. Often, mailed questionnaires are used to gather the data, or the data may be obtained from already existing sources. The per unit cost of collecting data is much lower than in an experiment.

2. A survey can usually be completed in a much shorter period of time than can an experiment. A retrospective study of the variables associated with deaths from certain diseases can be done in a relatively short period of time, usually less than a year. A prospective study may extend over many years, and may not be completed until all study subjects have died.

3. The problem of obtaining the cooperation of study subjects is generally less formidable in nonexperimental research than it is in an experimental study. Frequently, all that is required from a study subject in a survey is for him to supply some information, which may take a short period of time. On the other hand, an experimental subject not only may have to devote a considerable amount of time to participation in the research but may also have to expose himself to unusual, unpleasant, or even burdensome conditions during the course of the study.

4. The nonexperimental approach is the method of choice where there is a large time lag between the application of the independent variable and the appearance of a response in the dependent variable. It is easier to keep track of study subjects when they are able to function in their normal setting rather than in the highly controlled environment demanded by the experimental approach.

5. Nonexperimental studies involving human beings can often attain a greater reality in relation to the total content of the research—particularly the variables studied and the setting for the research—than can an experiment. Thus, the translation of nonexperimental research findings beyond the boundaries of the research setting can be more readily apparent as well as more acceptable to the consumers of the research.

6. In general, the findings of nonexperimental studies are more broadly representative of a larger target population than are findings from experimental studies. In some experiments the subjects are brought into the study as a matter of convenience and are not representative of any larger target population. Because it usually is less expensive and less burdensome to collect data in a nonexperimental study, the number of study subjects can be much larger than in an experimental study, thereby increasing the representative character of the research. Moreover, it is usually possible to obtain much wider geographic representation of study subjects through the nonexperimental approach by the use of mailed questionnaires and other means of data collection that cannot be employed in a highly controlled experiment. Greater representation of study subjects means that the findings of nonexperimental research often have greater applicability than do the findings of experiments.

But there are certain drawbacks to the use of the nonexperimental approach in research. The most serious of these are:

1. The nonexperimental method cannot establish causal relationships with the same degree of confidence as can the experimental method. As has been pointed out, the main attribute of the experimental method is the higher degree of control that can be obtained over the extraneous variables that could confound the relationship among the explanatory variables being studied. Often the best that can be achieved in a nonexperimental study is the establishment of associative relationships. These, of course, are useful for predictive purposes but may be weak for diagnosis and explanation. This is not to say that with the experimental approach it is always possible to establish cause and effect relationships. In many studies the extraneous variables are so large in number and so potent in their effects on the explanatory variables that they cannot be entirely eliminated, even by such experimental procedures, to be discussed

shortly, as randomization. However, the danger that exists in nonexperimental research to a much greater extent than in experimental studies is the erroneous ascribing of a causal relationship among variables that may only be artificially or spuriously related.

2. It is obvious that the nonexperimental approach, particularly the retrospective or cross-sectional, cannot be easily applied to test out a newly developed product, program, or procedure. A nonexperimental study has its greatest usefulness where the variable being studied is already established. By contrast, the essence of the experimental approach to evaluative research is innovation—the trial of something new.

3. The nonexperimental approach is usually not as useful in the development of new theories, ideas, principles, as is the experimental method. Experimentally we can create the appropriate conditions necessary for an investigation of some theoretical construct. Nonexperimentally, we do not create the conditions but must take them as they exist naturally. These natural conditions may not serve as very efficient raw materials for a theoretically oriented investigation.

4. Among some people, only a study based on the experimental method is considered true research. Nonexperimental studies are often given the title "surveys" to distinguish them from so-called real research. Thus, acceptance of the findings of surveys may be less enthusiastic, more qualified, than the findings of experimental studies. In other words, a stigma is sometimes attached to nonexperimental research which may make it difficult to gain financial support to undertake the study. Moreover, there may be hostility toward acceptance of the findings of such studies as making a valid scientific contribution to the advancement of knowledge.

Comparison of Experimental and Nonexperimental Design

The advantages and disadvantages of both methods of research design have been discussed. As a summary of the main features of the two methods the following illustration is provided to show how the same problem can be approached by the different types of research design.

Suppose someone were interested in making a study to find out whether a graduate of a basic degree program in nursing is more proficient as a bedside nurse in a general hospital than a graduate of a basic diploma program. Whether this study were to be conducted experimentally or nonexperimentally, certain common elements in the design of both types of studies would have to be considered. First, the total population to which the study findings will apply would have to be specified. Second, the method for selecting the subjects who will be included in the research would have to be determined. Third, the alternative versions of the independent variable that will be tested—the basic degree curriculum and the basic diploma curriculum—would have to be defined. Fourth, the criterion measure that will be used to evaluate the effects of the two types of nursing programs—proficiency as a bedside nurse—would have to be developed. Finally, the methodology for the statistical analysis of the results of the study would have to be determined.

If the study were conducted experimentally, a group of high school graduates would be selected, randomly assigned to an experimentally developed and administered diploma or degree program. They would be followed up after they had graduated from their program and been employed as graduate nurses in hospitals. Then, their proficiency as nurses would be measured to see whether there was a difference in proficiency between the graduates of the two types of programs.

If the study were conducted nonexperimentally, a random sample of graduate nurses in hospitals would be selected, their proficiency as bedside nurses would be measured, a determination made of whether they had attended a degree program or a diploma program, and a statistical analysis performed to test the difference in proficiency scores between graduates of the two types of programs. The study, if carried out experimentally, might take a minimum of five years and require much money and effort. If carried out nonexperimentally, it could possibly be done in about a year and with considerably less expense. However, the experimental approach would provide data that would permit the drawing of inferences about the effect of type of curriculum on proficiency that would more likely be free from the impact of such uncontrolled variables as the innate ability of the study subjects, their values, goals, and ideals, the quality of teaching in the two types of programs, and other extraneous organismic and environmental variables.[12]

The main differences between the two types of design as illustrated by this example is, first, the greater degree of control over the character of the independent variable in the experimental approach—the type of educational program. In the experimental design such relevant variables as content of curriculum, physical facilities, quality of instruction, could conceivably be standardized and controlled. In the nonexperimental approach, these environmental factors are not manipulated by the researcher but must be accepted by him as they naturally exist in the real world. The only type of control the researcher can exert over these environmental variables is through an "ex post facto" approach by sorting out his data according to these variables after they are collected, assuming such "cross-tabulation" would be possible to do retrospectively.

For example, if quality of instruction were considered to be a potentially significant extraneous variable that could affect the proficiency scores, perhaps even overriding the effect of type of program, data could be collected so as to control it. Thus, each study subject, in addition to supplying data on the type of program in which she took her training, would also be asked to rate the quality of the instruction she received.

Or, if the subject's rating were not considered to be a valid and reliable measure of instructional quality, it might be possible to make an independent evaluation of faculty quality by going back to the school attended by the subject to obtain a rating of the faculty either by the head of the school or by a panel of outside experts. This latter procedure would, of course, substantially increase the expense and difficulty of the conduct of the study, perhaps to the point where an experiment would be the better approach.

The value of the use of "ex post facto" data on important extraneous variables can be demonstrated by the following data which, of course, are fictitious. Suppose in the nonexperimental study of the comparison of nursing proficiency of graduates of diploma and degree programs the following average proficiency scores were obtained for samples of 1,000 graduates from each program (assume a range of scores of 0 to 100 per cent, where 100 per cent represents excellent proficiency and 0 poor proficiency):

Type of Program from Which Graduated	*Proficiency Scores*
Average, both types of programs	75%
Degree	90
Diploma	60

These data would make it appear that the degree graduate was considerably more proficient than a graduate of a diploma program. Therefore, we may be secure in inferring that a degree program prepares a better nurse than does a diploma program. But the difference in scores may not be causally related to type of program at all but to some other variable, such as the quality of instruction received. This variable could be the major influence on proficiency regardless of the type of program pursued by the graduate. Thus, if we were able to obtain ratings of the quality of faculty and introduce this variable into the tabulation we might find the following relationship:

	Proficiency Scores by Quality of Instruction		
Type of Program from Which Graduated	*Average, Both Types of Instruction*	*High-Quality Instruction*	*Poor-Quality Instruction*
Average, both types of programs	75%	95%	57%
Degree	90	95	55
Diploma	60	97	58

We see that when quality of instruction is accounted for, diploma graduates surprisingly score at least as well as degree graduates in both categories of instruction—high and poor quality. Thus, a very different interpretation can be drawn from these data than when only the variable "type of program" is considered. This interpretation is: the graduate of a diploma program is at least as proficient as a degree graduate when their schools are standardized for quality of instruction.

The following question may well be raised concerning the data just presented: How can the average proficiency scores for the two types of instruction *combined* indicate a greater proficiency for the degree program graduate, whereas the diploma graduate scores higher in proficiency than does the degree graduate in *each* category of quality of instruction? The solution to the problem becomes evident when the number of study subjects in each category is tabulated:

Type of Program from Which Graduated	Number of Nurses by Quality of Instruction		
	Total, Both Types of Instruction	High-Quality Instruction	Poor-Quality Instruction
Total, both types of programs	2,000	950	1,050
Degree	1,000	850	150
Diploma	1,000	100	900

We see from the number of nurses in each of the categories that there are as many nurses who graduate from degree programs with high-quality instruction as there are graduates from diploma programs with poor-quality instruction. Thus the average proficiency scores, when quality of instruction is not considered, is weighted by these highly skewed distributions.

In brief, from these data we see that the quality of instruction is related to the type of nursing program. Degree programs are characterized by high-quality instruction, diploma programs by lesser quality. It may well be that the "cause" of high or low proficiency scores is not type of program, per se, but the more specific and operationally definable variable, quality of instruction. If we want to raise the level of proficiency of graduates, we do not necessarily have to eliminate the diploma program, but rather raise the level of the quality of instruction in these programs. This would indicate that the independent variable, "type of nursing program" is much too broad. It must be redefined to take account of the significant elements that really distinguish a diploma and a degree program.

A second difference between the experimental and nonexperimental research design is the greater control over organismic variables that is obtained by the experimental approach through random assignment of the study subjects to the different groups included in the sudy. The purpose of random assignment is essentially to equalize the composition of the different study groups in terms of all relevant organismic variables. If the groups are not equalized it may well be an uncontrolled organismic variable that could influence the dependent variable rather than the independent one, as in the case of the environmental variable, quality of instruction, illustrated previously.

In nonexperimental research there is no equalization of the groups under study by the process of random assignment of subjects. Actually, the groups have been formed through a process of self-selection.

Thus, in the nonexperimental approach to evaluate the proficiency of diploma and degree graduates, the study commences at the point at which the subjects are already graduated from nursing school and are practicing as graduate nurses. They themselves had selected the type of educational program they pursued.

Although a random process can be said to be operating in the selection by random sampling of the study subjects for inclusion in the study, an organismic variable may be present, highly correlated with the type of nursing program selected, that actually influences the difference in proficiency scores. One such variable could be the intelligence level of the student. This could be correlated with the student's selection of an educational program: high I.Q. students choose a degree program, lower I.Q. students select a diploma program. Moreover, high I.Q. nurses may score better on the proficiency scale than do low I.Q. nurses, irrespective of the type of educational program they attend. Consequently, it is intelligence that determines proficiency, not the type of program attended.

There are several methods by which the various comparison groups being studied can be equated in a nonexperimental design according to the relevant organismic and environmental variables to avoid inferring spurious relationships. One of these ways is to elaborate the analysis of the data by treating all important extraneous variables as additional independent variables. This would mean that data would be gathered on all these additional variables and they would be cross-tabulated with the criterion measure. Analysis by this method of all significant organismic and environmental variables could lead to a standardization of the various groups under study similar to what is hopefully achieved through the process of random assignment.

A third difference between experimental and nonexperimental research designs is the fact that an experiment is generally easier to reproduce than a nonexperimental study. Reproducibility is a valuable characteristic of an experiment. It permits other researchers to conduct a repetition of the identical study which can serve to confirm the findings of the original study. Such confirmation is important in the establishment of a scientific body of knowledge, since the results of a single experiment cannot be considered as conclusive evidence.

An experiment is easier to reproduce—or, in statistical terminology, to replicate—because the elements of the study are so well controlled and standardized. The protocols for the experiment—the document containing the detailed design for the study—could serve as the plan for repeated studies. In nonexperimental studies, where there is less control over the research elements, exact replication of the total design by other investigators is more difficult to attain. For example, since the independent variable is not manipulated by the researcher, it is difficult to achieve a uniformity of definition of the alternative study groups from one study to the next. Referring again to the study of the relationship between type of educational program and proficiency of the graduate nurse, it is impossible to assure that the alternative groupings for the "type of program" variable—degree and diploma—would be the same from study to study even if the replicated study were conducted in the same schools. Because of this lack of control over the independent variable, certain significant changes could be made in the programs offered by these schools from one study to the next that could make them noncomparable.

Basically, then, the main virtue of the experimental approach to research lies in the degree of control over the various elements in the study— the setting, the subjects, and the variables being studied. The particular advantage of this method lies in the researcher's ability to control the extraneous variables—the variables that are not of interest to him, but which if uncontrolled could exert a significant and perhaps misleading influence on the dependent variable under study.

Variables in Explanatory Studies

To recapitulate the nature of the variables that are present in every explanatory study, we can say that these variables fall into two major categories: (1) the explanatory variables, those among which the researcher is seeking to find a relationship, and (2) the extraneous vari-

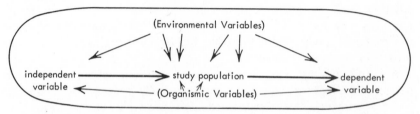

Fig. 6–1. Schematic representation of variables in explanatory studies.

ables, those that the researcher is not interested in and he attempts to keep under control through the application of an appropriate research design:

A. Controlled Extraneous Variable(s)

1. By random assignment of study subjects to the different comparison groups representing alternative versions, levels, gradations, or types of the independent variable.
2. By random assignment of study subjects to the comparison groups with matching of the subjects on relevant organismic variables.
3. By random assignment of study subjects with the application of the covariance technique to the analysis of the data.
4. By limiting the target population to subjects with certain specific characteristics, thus reducing the number of different organismic variables present among the study subjects and providing for greater homogeneity among them.
5. By limiting the study settings to a small number of homogeneous units.
6. By ex post facto standardization of the study groups through elaboration of the data by cross-tabulation with additional variables—essentially a process of introducing additional independent variables and relating them to the criterion variable.

B. Uncontrolled Extraneous Variable(s)—the variables that are confounded with the explanatory variables and can result in spurious relationships among these variables.

TYPES OF EXPERIMENTAL DESIGN

In its simplest form the essential objective of an experiment is to vary the independent variable among the study subjects while holding all other relevant organismic and environmental variables constant, and to measure the effect of this variation in terms of a measure of the dependent variable. The major design problem lies in the phrase, "holding all other relevant organismic and environmental variables constant." Numerous experimental designs have been developed to accomplish this as well as provide efficient ways of analyzing the data after they are collected. These designs are summarized in Table 6–1. A brief explanation of each of them follows.

One-Group Design

The weakest of all types of experimental designs is the one in which a stimulus is applied to a study population and the response then measured in the dependent variable. To illustrate, we may decide to institute a program of self-medications for hospitalized patients to be included in the study. Patients are given a supply of the medications that have been prescribed, excluding those where an error would have serious consequences,

TABLE 6-1

Types of Experimental Design

I = Application of independent variable to the group of study
subjects
D = Measurement of the dependent variable before application of
the independent variable
D = Measurement of the dependent variable after application of
the independent variable

Type of Design	Structure of Design	Form of Data Analysis
1. One-group	I D	Evaluate magnitude of D
2. One-group, before-after	D I D	Compare change from D to D
3. Two-group	Study group: I D_1 Comparison group. D_2	Compare difference between D_1 and D_2
4. Two-group, before-after	Study group: D_1 I D_1 Comparison group: D_2 D_2	Compare difference between change D_1 to D_1 and change D_2 to D_2

Designs with Random Assignment to Alternative Groups

5. Two-group with control group	Experimental group: I D_1 Control group: D_2	Compare difference between D_1 and D_2
6. Multiple comparison groups, single independent variable	Experimental group 1: I_1 D_1 Experimental group 2: I_2 D_2 Experimental group 3: I_3 D_3 etc.	Compare difference between D_1, D_2, D_3, etc.
7. Multiple comparison groups, multiple independent variables	Exp. group 1: I_1 I_1' I_1'' D_1 Exp. group 2: I_2 I_2' I_2'' D_2 Exp. group 3: I_3 I_3' I_3'' D_3 etc.	Compare difference between D_1, D_2, D_3, etc., in terms of main effects of each of the independent variables as well as the interaction among the variables

Note: Subscripts (e.g., D_1, D_2) signify the different study groups.

and allowed to take them according to the required dosage and time
schedule. The criterion measure to evaluate this procedure might be the
frequency with which patients correctly follow their medication regimen. If
we found a very high level of cooperation among the patients as well as a
very low rate of medication errors, we would probably regard the new
system as a success. If medication errors were high, we would evaluate the
system as a failure.

In this example the one-group type of design might be workable because we have an implicit standard of comparison in which to evaluate the effect of the change in the medication procedure. This standard is one which says that the system is workable if it operates with perfect or nearly perfect accuracy. However, consider a different type of study. Suppose we desired to measure the effect of a new drug on the rate of a patient's recovery. If we gave a group of patients the new drug and then observed the percentage of patients who recovered from the illness, we would not be able to attribute this effect to the administration of the drug because we have no knowledge of what would have happened to the patients if they had not been given the drug at all. Assuming that the illness was not one that was invariably fatal, we can expect that some patients would recover even in the absence of the drug. In order to validate the impact of the drug we would need to have some standard of comparison that would tell us what the patients' recovery rate would be without the drug. Another example of the one-group design is an attempt to influence people to obtain polio immunization by distributing a pamphlet aimed at achieving this purpose and aftreward measuring the level of immunization in the community. The problem in evaluation here is that if the level is low we would probably be correct in saying that the educational campaign was a failure. But if we find that the level is high we cannot validly attribute this to our independent variable because we do not have any assessment of the change in the immunization level that resulted as a direct consequence of the health education program. The level may have been high initially.

A final example concerns the reorganization of the nursing unit to include ward secretaries and then measuring the "effect" of this reorganization in terms of the proportion of time the professional staff spends in providing direct nursing care to patients as opposed to indirect activities like charting. If we found that the staff was spending a fairly high proportion of time on direct care to patients after the introduction of the ward secretary we would not then be able to attribute this effect to this independent variable because: (a) we do not have a basis for comparison to tell us what proportion of time would be spent on direct care in the absence of ward secretaries (it might be higher because with more pressure on her time the nurse might make better use of it), and (b) even if a standard of comparison did exist to indicate an improvement in the expenditure of time on direct care, it would be difficult to attribute this to the independent variable—the use of ward secretaries—because we have not controlled any of the possible extraneous variables that could also influence our dependent variable—time spent on direct nursing care. These extraneous variables might be any of a whole host of uncontrolled organismic variables, such as the educational level of the staff, their personality, their perceptions of their jobs.

Thus, because the study subjects we selected have insight into how to schedule their time, they devote to patient care most of the time that has been freed from clerical work by the provision of ward secretaries. However, such insight may not be typical of nurses in general, in which case we might well be incorrect if we inferred that the use of ward secretaries would typically permit nurses to spend more time on patient care.

Another type of extraneous variable that can confound the findings of studies like this one can be labeled the sociopsychological reaction that human beings often exhibit to the process of change itself, which may be stronger than the reaction to the independent variable we are testing. Doing something for a patient that seems to indicate that you are interested in him and want to be helpful to him can produce a positive reaction independently of the substantive nature of what it is you are doing. Giving a patient a back-rub may well have a more important psychological impact on him than a physical one. Therefore, in bringing together a group of persons in a specialized research setting, we may create a group feeling among the subjects and generate interactions among them that can cause them to respond in unexpected ways to the independent variable we are testing.

Reaction to a novelty introduced by a study was first observed in the classic experiments at the Hawthorne plant of the Western Electric Company in Chicago, during the late 1920's and early 1930's, and has become known as the "Hawthorne effect."[13] In this study the experimenters were interested in measuring the effect on the quantitative production of telephone relays of experimentally varying among a group of specially selected subjects certain independent variables such as the physical environment in which they worked. Contrary to the expectations of the researchers, no direct relationship was found between productivity and physical working conditions. However, the experiment pointed out a most important methodological principle that has been of great value to the development of research design. As described by French[14] the principle is as follows:

From a methodological point of view, the most interesting finding was what we might call the "Hawthorne effect." In order to manipulate more precisely the physical factors affecting production, the experimenters had set up a special experimental room for a small group of girls who were wiring relays. This wiring room was separated from the rest of the factory, and the girls working in it received special attention from both outside experimenters and the management of the plant. Careful studies of this wiring group showed marked increases in production which were related only to the special social position and social treatment they received. Thus, it was the "artificial" social aspects of the experimental conditions set up for measurement which produced the increases in group productivity.

In the one-group type of design the "Hawthorne effect" is especially troublesome, because there is no way of either controlling this effect or measuring its impact on the study subjects. For this reason alone, it should be ruled out as a design for most studies. Moreover, except where standards are already established from other studies or similar authoritative sources, it does not provide its own basis of comparison for assessing the changes that may be produced by the independent variable. Finally, we cannot be sure that the changes produced in the study would hold true beyond our study population, because we have no control over or even any assessment of the effect of certain important organismic variables related to the specific characteristics of the particular subjects included in our study.

In brief, the one-group design is essentially not a research design at all. It is nothing more than the trial and error approach. Like trial and error, it is inefficient and subject to spuriousness.

One-Group, Before-After Design

This type of design makes a modest improvement over the simple one-group design. Here a measurement is made of the dependent variable before the independent variable is applied. The independent variable is then applied. After an appropriate period of time has elapsed the dependent variable is measured again. The main distinction between this type and the previous design is that an initial measurement is made which can serve as a basis for comparing the terminal measurement after the independent variable has been applied. In the analysis of the data the difference between the initial and terminal measurement represents the effect of the independent variable.

To illustrate this design, suppose we were interested in the same research problem mentioned previously, that of measuring the effect on the population of a community of an educational campaign to convince people to obtain immunization against polio. Our criterion measure is the percentage of the total population that is immunized against polio. Our independent variable is the distribution by mail to every home in the community of an attractive pamphlet describing the value of polio immunization and urging everyone to obtain it. We measure the rate of immunization prior to the distribution of the pamphlet by sending a mailed questionnaire to all residents of the community asking if they have been immunized against polio. We repeat this questionnaire six months after the pamphlet has been distributed. If we find that the rate of immunization has increased significantly, can we attribute this to the educational campaign?

Actually this design is not much superior to the previous one where only an "after" measure is taken. Although in this design we do have some standard of comparison—the "before" measure—we do have certain real biases. Because of the weaknesses in this design, we cannot draw causal inferences with assurance. There are at least four important kinds of extraneous variables that could have influenced the change in the rate of immunization in the positive way that it occurred in this study.

First is the fact that the residents of the community might have been exposed to some other stimulus during the period of study that we have not controlled; it may be the real basis for the increase in the immunization level. Such an event could be the presentation on one of the popular fictionalized television programs dealing with medical or nursing themes of a moving account of the suffering that a family undergoes when one of its members contracts polio. Of the many people viewing this program some may be stimulated by its content to obtain immunization against this disease for themselves and their families. Therefore, it could well be that the increase in the immunization rate that was observed was largely attributable to this TV program and not to the pamphlet that was distributed. Without the influence of this program, the immunization rate might not have shown any significant change.

A second type of extraneous variable that could be operating in this situation can be labeled the effect of the passage of time. With passage of time certain uncontrollable forces related to aging and maturation of the study subjects can exert significant influences on the dependent variable being studied. These can override or mask the effect of the independent variable. Thus with the passage of time a predisposition to obtain immunization that had its origin well before the study began may reach its peak during the study period. It would therefore contribute to an increase in the rate of immunization, although it was totally unrelated to the independent variable being tested. For example, the birth of a baby to one of the families in the study population during the study period may reinforce a long-standing intention to obtain immunization for all members of the family. This event may influence immunization behavior independently of the educational material. In before and after research on patients this extraneous variable is especially important to control. In studying the effect of nursing care on patients in which we observe the patients over a long period of time, changes in the patient that are purely a function of the passage of time must be sorted out and controlled so that they are not confounded with the effects of the nursing care that we expect to measure. Thus, we know that over time patients with various types of illnesses undergo many changes in their physiological as well as psychological states that are associated with the maturation of their illness process and not necessarily with the care they receive.

A third type of extraneous variable that can confound the findings of before and after studies is exposure to the measuring process itself. In the study described, the subjects are asked in a questionnaire about their immunization status prior to being exposed to the educational campaign. The act of asking people whether they are immunized or not can serve as a stimulus for those who would otherwise not seek immunization. Thus, the success of the distribution of the educational pamphlet can be exaggerated, since part of increase in the immunization level may be attributable to the questionnaire. Another aspect of this type of spuriousness is the use of the same psychological test to obtain before and after measurements in a study. Initial exposure to the test can make the subject "test-wise." As a result the terminal responses may be more closely related to this factor than to the application of the independent variable being evaluated. Even physiological measurement can affect behavior. As described by Campbell:[15]

In general, any measurement procedure which makes the subject self-conscious or aware of the fact of the experiment can be suspected of being a reactive measurement. Whenever the measurement process is not a part of the normal environment it is probably reactive. Whenever measurement exercises the process under study, it is almost certainly reactive. Measurement of a person's height is relatively nonreactive. However, measurement of weight, introduced into an experimental design involving adult American women, would turn out to be reactive in that the process of measuring would stimulate weight reduction.

A fourth source of bias in this type of design can result from the previously discussed Hawthorne effect. The design makes no attempt to either control or measure its effect. Thus, the comparison of the values of the before and after measurements might well be merely measuring the socio-psychological reaction of the process of change introduced by the application of the independent variable and not to the variable itself. If we give patients a drug to relieve pain and assess the level of pain before and after taking the drug, we cannot be sure that any reduction in pain that may be observed is attributable to the attention the patient received from the nurse rather than to a true physiological reaction to the medication.

Two-Group Design

This design is a decided improvement over the two previous ones. Unlike design one there is a comparison group against which any change in the study group can be evaluated, and unlike design two this comparison group is an external one and not the study subjects themselves. Thus, we can select two communities for our study of the effect of an educational pamphlet on the level of polio immunization and distribute the pamphlet to the residents of one community and withhold it from the other community. Then, after an appropriate lapse of time we can measure the rate of immunization in both communities. If, however, in comparing these rates we find a difference, can we attribute it to the effect of the educational program?

There are a number of reasons why we cannot. First, we do not know what the initial levels of immunization were in the two communities. The level may well have been much higher in the community in which the pamphlet was not distributed. Therefore, the effect of our educational campaign might be masked unless we can, on an ex post facto basis, standardize our two communities in terms of initial level of immunization. But even if we can retrospectively standardize the two groups this way, we are still faced with the problem of the differential effect of our independent variable among groups that have different immunization patterns to begin with. Assume that before we distribute the pamphlet, the community receiving it has a much higher rate of immunization than the community where we withhold it. It would undoubtedly be more difficult to raise the immunization level by the distribution of the pamphlet, because the few who are not immunized might well include those individuals who would resist any appeal. Conversely, with a low immunization level in the community receiving the educational material, an extravagant improvement might occur because there is potentially greater room for improvement.

Furthermore, in this design there are a number of other important extraneous variables that could well affect the dependent variable in addition to the independent variable that we controlled. Thus, if the city in which we distributed the pamphlet contained a more highly educated population than the other city, we might find that we achieved greater success with our program than we would have with a less educated population. It has long been demonstrated that the appeal of a health education program is greatest among those whose educational level is, in general, high.

Moreover, this type of design is also afflicted by the biases of the Hawthorne effect. We cannot be sure that any effects produced in the study group—even having available to us the criterion measurement for the comparison group—were related to certain extraneous sociopsychological variables rather than to the educational program. Finally, there is the bias that could arise from the uncontrolled occurrence of an event (the television drama that is shown in only one of the cities) that could influence the dependent variable in ways unknown to the researchers.

The one advantage this design has over the previous one—the one-group, before-after—is that it eliminates the possible bias attributable to exposure to the measuring process itself. Considering the many limitations of this design, this is a small virtue, indeed. As an experimental design it is very weak and, consequently, is rarely used in prospective studies.

Actually, this particular design is a widely used model for retrospective nonexperimental studies. Thus, two groups may be found to differ in terms of a particular variable. Through the application of Mill's method of difference, the groups may also be observed to differ in terms of another variable. If there appears to be a logical connection between these two variables, one may be designated as the independent and the other as the dependent variable. Thus, if we observe a high rate of attrition in one school of nursing and a low rate in another, and upon further investigation we find that the school with the high drop-out rate has poor physical facilities while the other school does not, we may then infer that quality of physical facilities is related to drop-out rates in schools of nursing. The shortcoming of the approach is that for the "method of difference" to apply we have to be sure that the schools are more or less identical in terms of all relevant variables except that of physical facilities. In short, we have to be sure that we have controlled for all the biases that could occur in the presence of uncontrolled extraneous variables.

Two-Group, Before-After Design

This type of design attempts to correct the grave weakness of the previous one—that of making comparisons among study groups that are not equalized according to important extraneous variables. In this design lack of initial equalization of the groups is compensated somewhat by the fact that in the data analysis we can compare the change that has taken place in both from the time preceding the application of the independent variable to the time following its application. In the analysis the differences in the before and after measures for each group are calculated. Then, the changes in each of the groups are compared to see if the change in the study group is larger than that in the comparison group. If it is, it might be attributed to the independent variable. Thus, if the difference in the before and after rate of immunization is larger for the group that received the educational material than it is for the comparison group, we would be in a better position to attribute this effect to the educational program than in the case of the previous designs.

This design corrects many of the faults of the three previous designs by controlling most of the extraneous variables that could influence our dependent variable. In the immunization study the immunization levels of both groups would be tested initially so that effects of extraneous variables —such as the measuring process, the passage of time, etc.—would appear equally in both groups. If these extraneous variables were to exert an influence on the level of immunization, this influence could be estimated by the difference in the before and after immunization rates for the comparison group. To illustrate, assume we had collected the following data:

	Total Population	Number Found to Be Immunized Initially	Number Found to Be Immunized after Educational Campaign
Study group	1,000	400	700
Comparison group	1,000	600	700

If we had used design one (one group only), all we would have known is that after the educational campaign 70 per cent of our study group was immunized. In the absence of any comparative measure there would be no meaningful way to evaluate this statistic. If we had used design two (one-group before-after), we would have been able to compare the 70 per cent terminal rate with the 40 per cent initial rate and would perhaps have attributed this significant rise in the immunization level solely to the program of health education, which, of course, may not be a valid inference. In design three (two-group), we would compare only the terminal measures, 70 per cent for both groups, and undoubtedly conclude that the educational campaign had no effect.

But if we had used design four (two-group, before-after), we may be able to come closer to the truth. In this design we can estimate the increase in immunization level attributable to extraneous factors as: the increase in the immunization rate in the comparison group. We can then estimate the increase attributable to the explanatory variable as: the increase in the immunization level of the study group *after* subtracting the increase attributable to extraneous factors. Thus, in the comparison group there were 400 persons who were *not* immunized at the time of the initial measurement. At the terminal measurement, 100 of these had become immunized. Therefore, the percentage of the 400 who had become immunized during the course of the study was 25 per cent: $(100 \div 400) \times 100$. This percentage can be considered as an estimate of the effect of the extraneous variables. Applying it to the number in the study group who were initially not immunized—600—we can say that 25 per cent of these, or 150, were influenced to seek immunization during the study period as a result of the uncontrolled factors, and the remaining 150 of the 300 who were immunized during the study period were influenced by the educational campaign. Our conclusion from a study using this design would be that the campaign was *more* effective than was found in the two-group after-only design where all we knew was that both groups had the same level of immunization at the terminal measurement, but that it was *less* effective than was found in the one-group before and after design where the 300 immunizations that occurred during the study period were all attributed to the educational campaign.

The two-group, before-after design is perhaps the most widely used design in partially controlled experiments in the social sciences, particularly in those conducted in natural settings. It is unquestionably superior to the three designs previously discussed, but it does have a serious shortcoming. It assumes that both groups have been equalized for all important extraneous variables. For this design to yield valid data it is important that if an extraneous factor significantly affects one group it should also affect the other group. Even with the before and after measurements for both groups, if the study group had been exposed to that television program previously mentioned between the taking of the initial and the terminal measurements and the comparison group had not (and this could happen if the two groups were located in different cities and the program were shown only in the city where, say, the study group were located), then the 150 people immunized during this period whom we have attributed to our controlled independent variable—the educational campaign—might well have been influenced by this uncontrolled environmental variable.

Second, the composition of the two groups may differ so widely in terms of relevant organismic variables as to override any effects of our explanatory variable. Thus, if the study group consisted of more highly educated people than did the comparison group, we might attribute a larger number of immunizations to the educational campaign than if the two groups were more alike educationally.

Finally, the Hawthorne effect is not eliminated by this type of design and, as has been said, could be particularly troublesome in patient care studies. For example, if instead of an educational campaign our independent variable were some nursing procedure, we would have no way of measuring how much of a change in our dependent variable is related to the procedure itself and how much to the Hawthorne effect, even if we used this design. If the Hawthorne effect cannot be kept from influencing the study group, we need a way of also exposing the comparison group to it so that its influence would be measured along with the other extraneous variables in the before-after evaluation.

In partially controlled experiments and in nonexperimental studies there is great difficulty in equalizing the groups being compared in terms of all the relevant organismic and environmental variables that can influence the study results and lead to spurious inferences. These difficulties have given rise to the development of what are considered to be "true" or fully controlled experimental designs, in which maximum control over all extraneous variables is achieved. The key element in these designs is *random assignment* of the study subjects to the alternative groups. Through such assignment, equalization is achieved for extraneous organismic variables, although it is not always perfect. A measure of the effects of the randomized extraneous variables, known as the experimental error, can be computed. To control the influences of environmental variables, the study setting is kept as identical as possible for the different groups, and external events are prevented from affecting the groups differentially. Certain techniques are employed to keep the Hawthorne effect from biasing the study.

Ideally, then, the true experimental design creates conditions for both the study and comparison groups, called the experimental and the control groups, in which the two groups are identical in every respect, except in terms of the independent variable. Thus, any difference that occurs in the values of the dependent variable for the two groups can be attributed to the independent variable. The fully controlled experimental designs will now be discussed.

EXPERIMENTAL DESIGNS WITH RANDOM ASSIGNMENT

Two-Group with Control Group

This is the classical experimental design and the basic model for more complex types of highly controlled experimental designs. In this design the target population is first delineated. A random sample of study subjects is selected from the target population, and these are further subdivided into the experimental and control groups by a process of random assignment. (Methods for selecting a random sample from the target population will be described in Chapter 8, and methods of random assignment of the sample will be discussed later in this chapter.) Random assignment essentially means that neither the investigator nor the study subjects shall deliberately determine whether a particular subject is assigned to the experimental or the control group. This randomization procedure equalizes the composition of the two groups in the same way that tossing a coin yields, over the long run, the same number of heads and tails.

The independent variable in the fully controlled experiment may be of the all-or-nothing variety in which the "all" alternative (an educational campaign, a nursing procedure, a drug) is applied to the experimental group while the control group receives nothing. In other fully controlled experiments the independent variable may be graded so that, for example, the experimental group may get one dosage level of a drug whereas the control group would receive a different dosage level. In still other studies the independent variable may involve different versions of some phenomenon such as different types of teaching methods: the experimental group might be exposed to a teaching machine whereas the control group would be taught by conventional methods. More complex designs consist of more than two groups, as in experimenting with a variety of nursing staffing patterns (the team, functional assignment, case method, primary nursing). Still further complicated designs involve the simultaneous testing of a number of different independent variables. Thus instead of the terms "experimental and control groups," it may be desirable to use a more general terminology such as "contrast groups" or "comparison groups," since in many experiments each group receives some positive value of the independent variable.

Randomization   As has been indicated, the purpose of randomization is to attempt to equalize the composition of the various groups under study so that they would be identical in respect to all pertinent organismic variables. The groups, then, would differ only in terms of the explanatory independent variable. Any differences found among the groups in the values of the criterion measure could then be ascribed to the influence of the independent variable, since in all other respects the groups were identical. Randomization requires the allocation of the subjects to the different study groups according to the laws of chance—as, for example, placing the names of all our sample subjects on slips of paper, putting the slips in a hat, mixing them up, then picking the first slip, which is placed in the experimental group, picking the second, which is placed in the control group, assigning the third to the experimental group, and so on. Thus, in our immunization study if we had a total sample of 2,000 subjects, half to be placed in the experimental group to receive the educational campaign and the other half in the control group from whom the educational campaign would be withheld, by random assignment to the two groups we should allocate about the same number who have already been immunized to each group, as many highly educated people to each group, the same number of older people, and so on.

Randomization therefore attempts to control the bias from extraneous organismic variables that could influence our comparisons among the groups by making these groups similar in composition. We know, however, that randomization will not completely eliminate these influences, particularly if the size of our groups is small.

Random assignment has another important value. Through the use of randomization we compute the value of the "experimental error" by using appropriate statistical techniques. This in essence is a measure of the effect of the extraneous variables that we have attempted to randomize among the groups being studied. This measure is analogous to the illustration in design four, where the effect of the extraneous variables was estimated by the change in the before and after measure for the group in which the educational campaign was withheld.

The extent to which the differences we find among our experimental and control groups are actually attributable to the independent variable we have controlled can be evaluated by comparing the observed differences in the values of the dependent variable for the experimental and control groups with the value of the experimental error in a statistical test known as the "t-test." In this comparison we actually divide the value of the observed difference by the experimental error, and the magnitude of the resulting quotient is essentially an index of the extent to which the observed difference can be attributed to the independent variable we have controlled.

The model for analysis of data from experiments, known as tests of significance, to be discussed in Chapter 9, has the following format:

Level of significance
of difference ob-
served (probability
that observed differ-
ence could have
arisen by chance)

$$\text{Level of significance} = \frac{\left(\begin{array}{l}\text{Value of measure of} \\ \text{dependent variable for} \\ \text{experimental group}\end{array}\right) \text{ minus } \left(\begin{array}{l}\text{Value of measure} \\ \text{of dependent variable} \\ \text{for control group}\end{array}\right)}{\text{Value of measure of experimental error}}$$

A third benefit to be derived from the use of random assignment is the fact that it can be used in more complex, highly sophisticated types of designs in which very efficient and sensitive tests of significance can be applied to the data. In the following designs that will be discussed briefly, a test known as the "analysis of variance," where more than two alternatives of the independent variable are tested simultaneously or where the experiment involves more than one independent variable, can be used to provide valuable information concerning not only the effects on the dependent variable of each independent variable (main effects), but also the effects of combinations of these variables (interactions). For our immunization study we could simultaneously test numerous independent variables—the pamphlet, the educational level of the study subjects, age of subjects, and so on. Through the analysis of variance we would be able to test the effects of each of these variables separately as well as the combined effects of several variables (e.g., does exposure to the pamphlet among poorly educated subjects have less an effect on immunization level than exposure among highly educated subjects?).

As would be expected, the practical application of randomization is not without its limitations. Foremost among these is the already mentioned drawback common to all highly controlled studies—the difficulty of actually putting and keeping people in one or another of the alternative groups.

In drug studies it may be very difficult to withhold the drug being tested from a patient in a control group who might benefit from it. In the study of the impact of health education on the level of polio immunization, how practical would it be to assign our study subjects to one group or another and still keep them uncontaminated by outside influences, such as one group interacting with the other? Randomization works best with inanimate objects or with animals in the laboratory setting. In partially controlled settings, where a classroom, a patient's unit, or a physician's office is used as the site for the experiment, it may be possible to randomly assign the subjects to the alternative groups of the independent variable, but it may be very difficult to control the environmental variables. Thus, if two patients are side by side and one is in the control group and the other in the experimental, they will interact with each other, and this interaction may significantly influence the values of the criterion measure.

A second limitation of random assignment is the fact that while it can promote equalization of the characteristics of the members of the various groups, it cannot *guarantee* it. In fact it is possible, but not too likely, that random assignment will do a bad job in equalizing the composition of the groups on relevant organismic variables. After all, the probability of shuffling a deck of 52 playing cards (randomizing them) and dealing a perfect bridge hand to each player (13 cards of the same suit to each player) is highly remote, but it is as equally likely as dealing out any other specific distribution of cards that may be stipulated in advance by the dealer. In other words, sometimes by randomization we might not achieve the effect we desire—that of shuffling our study subjects so that all of one kind do not end up in one group.

Several techniques have been developed to provide added assurance that alternative groups will be equalized in terms of all relevant characteristics beyond that provided by randomization. These three techniques are *pairing, balancing,* and *covariance.* Sometimes these techniques are embraced under the general heading of "matching."

Pairing Perhaps the most commonly used method of equalizing the experimental and control groups is to determine the important extraneous variables for which the study subjects in the two groups are to be matched and, then, to assure that these variables are equally represented among the study subjects in the two groups by a method that combines purposive assignment with randomization. Pairing is described by Cochran[16] as follows:

Matching of the experimental and control samples with respect to the covariables can be accomplished in a number of ways. Conceptually, the simplest is the method of pairing. Each member of the experimental samples is taken in turn, and a partner is sought from the control population which has the same values as the experimental member (within defined limits) for each of the covariables. One way of doing this is to perform a multiple classification of the control population by the variables. We then examine the first member of the experimental sample, pick the cell which contains all control members having the desired set of covariables, and choose as the partner one control member at random for this cell. This procedure is repeated for each member of the experimental sample.

If an occasional cell is found to be empty, it is usually preferable to choose the control partner from a neighboring cell, rather than to omit the experimental member. If numerous cells are found to be empty, this is a danger signal. Either the limits of variation allowed in the covariables are too narrow or the control population is not satisfactory.

The analysis of the results is very simple. The difference (experimental-control) is computed for each pair, and any t-tests are applied directly to this series of differences.

An ideal type of pairing that has been used in a few studies in the psychological area is the so-called co-twin control, in which one twin is assigned to the experimental group and the other to the control group.

The method of pairing subjects in establishing experimental and control groups was employed by Hasselmeyer[17] in her experimental study of the effect of the diaper roll on the behavior (crying, sleeping, eating, etc.) of premature infants. In this study the variables selected for matching the infants were birth weight (4 groups), sex (2 groups), and race (2 groups). A total of 16 cells were established ($4 \times 2 \times 2$). For each of the cells there was an even distribution of experimental and control subjects. The placement of a specific infant into either the experimental or control group was determined by chance, thus providing the randomization necessary to justify the computation of experimental error and the application of statistical tests of significance of differences between the experimental and control groups.

There are several drawbacks to the use of the matched pair design. One of these is the subjectivity introduced in the selection by the researcher of the variables upon which the pairing will be based. The variables selected should be those organismic variables most likely to affect the dependent variable and confound the results of the study if proper equalization of the experimental and control groups is not achieved by randomization. Use of unimportant variables in pairing will not contribute in the least to the control of extraneous influences on the data and will only add an unnecessary burden to the research design. In patient care studies typical matching variables for patients might be diagnosis, age, sex, educational level, and severity of illness.

Another disadvantage to the use of pairing is that it complicates the design of the study and can slow down its progress, particularly where the size of the study groups is large and where there are a number of matching variables, each having numerous subdivisions. The process of pairing can then become tedious and difficult. Also, where the experiment extends over a long period of time there is danger of loss of some of the study subjects, which can spoil the balanced pattern of the pairs—an experimental member of a cell might lose its mate. A missing member of a pair means that the data collected for the unmatched member must be discarded.

With all of its drawbacks, pairing is a helpful device in matching the composition of the experimental and control groups on important organismic variables. It can be particularly helpful and usually easy to administer in patient care studies where, if uncontrolled, some of the organismic variables can have a significant impact on the behavior of the dependent variable.

Balancing   The purpose of balancing is similar to that of pairing. The difference between the two methods is that matching by balancing is accomplished in terms of the groups as a whole rather than in terms of the individuals composing the groups, as in matching by pairing. Thus if age is one of the balancing variables, the assignment of members to the two groups is arranged so that the average age of the group is identical. If sex is another matching variable, the percentage of males (or females) assigned to the alternative groups is the same. The assignment of a specific study subject to either of the groups, of course, is still accomplished through a random process. However, unlike unrestricted random assignment there is a deliberate attempt to match the groups as a whole in terms of those extraneous organismic variables deemed to be of sufficient importance to be specially controlled.

Balancing is generally easier to accomplish than is pairing and provides about the same amount of precision in equalizing the two groups. However, in testing the statistical significance of the differences in the values of criterion measures for the experimental and control groups a more complicated type of analysis has to be used than pairing.[18]

Covariance The analysis of covariance is another procedure that is applied to the data to take account of important extraneous variables (called in statistical terminology, covariables). Unlike the two previous methods, where matching of the groups is obtained by actually assigning individuals to the study groups on the basis of certain covariable characteristics *before* the independent variable has been applied, covariance analysis is a procedure for adjusting the data to equalize the groups *after* the independent variable has been applied to the subjects and measurements have been made of the dependent variable.

Actually the analysis of covariance combines the two statistical techniques of regression analysis and the analysis of variance. The computations involved in the analysis of covariance are rather complicated, especially if the number of covariables is large. However, as a device for ex post facto matching of groups it can be extremely useful, particularly when it is not feasible to match the groups during the assignment process by either pairing or balancing. Sometimes the covariable used in the analysis is an initial measure that is made of the dependent variable. In essence then, covariance analysis becomes a type of "before and after" design with the "before" measures used to adjust the "after" data. Thus, if we were studying the effects of a drug on weight reduction, and our experimental group consisted of subjects who were given the drug and the control group of subjects from whom the drug was withheld, we would make weight measurements of the study subjects before application of the independent variable. These measurements would be used in the covariance analysis to adjust the data obtained on the "after" measurement of the subjects.

Other Matching Methods Another method of equalizing the study groups is really not a formal method at all but a restriction of the study population to subjects with homogeneous characteristics. Thus, if we wished to evaluate the effects of a referral system on reducing the rate of patients' readmissions to the hospital, we might restrict the study population to patients in a particular age group, with a particular diagnosis, and in a certain income group, so as to eliminate the effects of these variables and insure that our experimental and control groups would be closely matched. Naturally, restriction of the study population means that the target population has also been narrowed in scope, thereby limiting any generalizations that can be made from the data that are collected.

Still another method of matching the groups under study, widely used in nonexperimental research although applicable to experimental studies as well, is the already mentioned cross-tabulation of the data in terms of relevant organismic and environmental variables. Like the covariance technique this too is an ex post facto approach, although these variables should be determined in advance of actual data collection. Stipulation in advance is, of course, a necessary procedure in order to insure that data pertaining to these variables will be collected from the study subjects and available for analysis when that stage of the research process is reached. In the previously discussed study of the effect of an educational campaign on immunization levels, not only can the data be tabulated to show the immunization levels *after* exposure to the educational campaign according to whether the individual was or was not exposed to the campaign, but they can also be analyzed in terms of the age of the subjects, their educational level, income, sex, and other organismic variables deemed to be important in influencing immunization behavior.

It is through randomization that the "two-group with control group" design equalizes the groups under study according to the extraneous organismic variables and prevents them from exerting a spurious influence on the relationship between the independent and dependent variables studied. In fully controlled experimental research, extraneous environmental influences are controlled by standardizing the study setting for both experimental and control groups. All external disturbances are fully eliminated or at least equalized for both groups.

But there still remains the one problem of the Hawthorne effect—the sociopsychological reaction of the subjects to the study situation itself. Coupled with this is the need to control the biases originating in the collection of the data, known as observer bias. In experimental studies of the effects of drugs on patients, called clinical trials, these problems have been resolved by the development of two techniques for controlling psychological biases. These are known as the "placebo" and the "double-blind technique."

Placebo   The term placebo, which in Latin means "I will please," is used in clinical trials of drugs to describe an inert capsule, tablet, or injection that is disguised to serve as an imitation of the drug actually being tested. While the subjects in the experimental group receive the true drug, the placebo is given to the subjects in the control group to induce a psychological reaction that parallels the psychological reaction of the experimental subjects who actually receive the drug. Any difference in the values obtained on the criterion measure for the experimental and control groups should be above and beyond the psychological reaction to the study situation itself. The difference should provide a real measure of the true physiological effect, if any, of the drug itself.

In studies not concerned with testing drugs, it is possible to conceive of a "dummy" treatment that could be applied to the control group to induce among members of this group a psychological reaction to the study conditions. In essence this reaction would provide a measure of the Hawthorne effect. For example, in a study testing out a new nursing procedure on a group of patients, the amount of professional nursing time that would normally be spent with patients would be increased for patients in the experimental group because of the new procedure. Therefore, instead of only withholding the procedure from the control group, added nursing time should also be provided to the subjects in the group to equalize the attention both groups receive from nursing personnel. In other words, for every exposure to the independent variable given experimental subjects, an equivalent "dummy" exposure should be provided to the control group. In this way we can be surer that the difference we measure between the two groups is more purely related to the independent variable we are testing and is unconfounded by extraneous social or psychological factors.

Double-Blind   The placebo is employed to provide a further control that the experimental and control groups are identical in every way except in terms of the independent variable that is being tested. Whereas randomization attempts to equalize the groups at the start of the study by controlling biases that could arise from organismic variables, the placebo equalizes them by controlling any psychological biases arising from the subjects' reaction to the process of receiving the medication, apart from any therapeutic benefits it might have. A further control on the psychological biases that could arise during the course of an experiment is the double-blind technique. Through the use of this technique, neither the research workers who are in actual contact with the study subjects nor the subjects themselves are aware of which subject is in the experimental group and which is assigned to the control group.

In the double-blind approach the randomization of subjects to the alternative groups is done by someone who will not have any contact with the study subjects. In drug trials using placebos, neither the subject nor the investigator should know whether the subject is receiving the actual drug or the placebo. Concealing the fact of whether the patient is in the experimental or the control group in studies like these can eliminate the bias that could occur where, for example, an otherwise well-meaning nurse might interfere with the course of the study by giving a patient in the control group the drug being tested rather than the placebo because she felt that to deprive him of the drug would cause undue suffering. Similarly, if a patient knows which group he was assigned to he might react psychologically in a way that might bias the measurements of the dependent variable. He might be fearful or upset if he knew he was in the control group and thought he was being deprived of a potentially beneficial drug. Or, conversely, aware of being in the experimental group he might be concerned as to whether he was being exposed to a potentially harmful drug.

In studies other than tests of drugs or of similar types of independent variables where a placebo can be developed that disguises the fact that the subject is receiving a "dummy" treatment rather than the real thing, it is not possible to use the double-blind approach. For example, in measuring patient responses to a nursing procedure it is not possible to conceive of a "dummy" alternative that could be applied to the control group. Also, in studies testing out alternative versions of some variable—say, different methods of obtaining information from patients (structured interviewing compared with nondirective interviewing)—the double-blind approach is totally inapplicable and in fact may be unnecessary, because each of the alternative groups receives a "treatment" of some kind.

The use of placebos and the double-blind technique have their greatest applicability in experiments in which an experimental group receives a treatment, drug, or stimulus of some kind, while the control group receives nothing. However, in all types of studies the researcher must be on guard against possible sources of psychological biases that could arise during the course of the study, from either the subjects themselves or the investigators that could distort the relationship among the explanatory variables being studied. It should be constantly borne in mind that the paramount objective is the attainment of ideal experimental conditions in which the comparison groups are identical in every respect except in terms of the independent variable being studied. Practically, this ideal is rarely achieved outside of strictly controlled laboratory studies where the subjects are inanimate or are animals, or in agricultural field experiments where the subjects are plots of land.

In studies of human beings, because of the vast number of extraneous variables present in a study, we can only hope to approximate this ideal. We should be continually alert during the entire course of human experiments to the possible sources of such biases so as to keep them under control. If we cannot eliminate these biases, at least we should be aware of the limitations they impose on the quality of our data. With such awareness we can then make a more valid and meaningful interpretation of the data we collect.

Multiple Comparison Groups, Single Independent Variable

In many studies, the independent variable can be grouped into more than just two categories as previously discussed. Some variables can be scaled according to a quantified continuum in which many relevant gradations are possible. One example that might serve as the independent variable for a patient care study is hours of nursing care available to patients. Another is the dosage level of a drug. Still another might be size of nursing unit (number of patients) or size of hospital, school, or community.

Other types of independent variables with multiple categories are those that are scaled according to some qualitative distinction. Thus the variable "patient observation method" might consist of such categories as direct observation by the professional nurse, indirect observation by the professional nurse through the use of television, or monitoring by electronic devices attached to the patient. The variable "educational program for training in nursing" might consist of four groupings: practical nurse training, associate degree preparation, diploma education, and college education.

Problems of scaling both the independent and dependent variables in a research study will be discussed in the following chapter. From the standpoint of research design the main advantage of the multiple comparison group design is that it provides more information than does the two-group design. The two-group design, particularly the experimental-control group, all-or-nothing variety, is relevant only where there are no meaningful alternatives to the one tested in the experimental group, or as in the case of drug studies, where it is not certain that the drug being tested will have any beneficial effect at all, regardless of the dosage level used. The latter, the two-group, all-or-nothing design, can serve as a prescreening trial study. If in such a trial, the drug or other dichotomized variable being tested appears to have promising therapeutic benefits, further research can test out finer gradations of the variable to determine the optimum therapeutic level.

When the independent variable can be scaled according to quantitative gradations, the analysis of the relationship among the independent and dependent variables can be expressed in the form of a mathematical equation that can be refined to reveal that value of the independent variable that produces the maximum or optimum value of the dependent variable. In nonexperimental research concerned with the relationship among independent and dependent variables that can be scaled quantitatively, such studies are sometimes called correlational studies, and in many fields of knowledge are very popular. In experimental research, since the elaboration of the study to include additional groupings of the independent variable increases the number of subjects required for the study, and since the cost of increasing the number of subjects to be studied is considerably higher than in nonexperimental studies, such correlational studies are less frequently undertaken.

However, the one-group before-after design is frequently elaborated to vary the independent variable according to certain graded levels to determine which level produces the best effect. Thus, the dosage level of a drug may be gradually increased until optimum patient response is noted. The danger in the use of this design, in addition to all the limitations of the before-after design discussed previously, is the cumulative confounded effect on the patient of repeated applications of the independent variable. Since each treatment is not really independent of previous treatments, it may not be possible to ascribe any specific effect observed to a particular level of treatment.

A drawback, then, to the use of multiple comparison groups is the need to expand the study to include additional study subjects. This, of course, adds to the expense of the study. Moreover, with additional comparison groups the problem of equalizing the composition of the various groups so that everything is at least theoretically held constant, except the independent variable being tested, is compounded. However, through the use of such a technique of statistical analysis of experimental data known as the analysis of variance, the multiple comparison groups design can yield more information per unit cost of conducting the experiment than can the simpler, two-group design. As such it is a more efficient design.

Latin-Square Design   A type of experimental design involving multiple comparisons that has been developed to make efficient use of the study subjects in an experiment is the so-called latin-square design. In this design the number of times each alternative of the independent variable is replicated is equal to the number of comparison groups. Thus, if we were studying the effect of four different patterns of nursing care (team plan, functional assignment, etc.) on patient satisfaction, each pattern would be replicated four times among different study groups to provide 16 measures of our dependent variable. The assignment of study groups to each of the replications would, of course, be by a random process.

The latin-square design originated in the agricultural field, where it offered a means not only of efficiently analyzing the results of the study, but also of randomly assigning the plots of land to be studied to the alternative versions of the independent variable. Suppose, for example, four kinds of fertilizer were to be tested, each containing different proportions of nitrogen, phosphorus, and potash (5–10–5, 10–6–4, 10–10–10, 20–10–5). The experimental field would be divided equally into four equal parts north to south (rows), and four equal parts east to west (columns), making a total of 16 equal-sized plots. Each of the four types of fertilizer would be randomly assigned to four plots, a crop planted on all plots, and the yields of the plots measured and compared to see which produced the greatest output. The latin-square method of assignment of the four kinds of fertilizer to each plot would be such that each kind would appear only once in each of the four rows and once in each of the four columns, thus fertility variations in both directions are randomized. If each type of fertilizer were labeled A, B, C, D, the method of assignment to the plots might be as follows:

A	C	B	D
D	B	C	A
C	A	D	B
B	D	A	C

Fig. 6-2. A randomized latin-square.

Now instead of this randomized latin-square pattern of assignment, suppose it were decided to systematically assign the different types of fertilizers to the plots. R. A. Fisher told the anecdote, which will be somewhat altered for simplicity, of the experimenter who thought the systematic type of allocation of treatment to the experimental subjects would be better than the random method, so instead of using a randomized latin-square he deliberately assigned the different fertilizers along the diagonal of the field. He felt he would thereby achieve better representation of the fertilizers among the different parts of the field:

A	B	C	D
D	A	B	C
C	D	A	B
B	C	D	A

Fig. 6-3. A systematic latin-square.

He went ahead and conducted the experiment in this fashion. He observed the yields, compared the results, and discovered that the plots treated with type A fertilizer had a very much greater crop yield per plot than the ones fertilized with any other type. Fertilizer A was then marketed and extravagant claims were made for its effectiveness in producing rich yields of wheat.

Some time later, complaints were received by the fertilizer company concerning the fact that fertilizer A was not living up to the claims made for it. The experimenter went back to his experimental plots to recheck the design. To his dismay he made the following discovery. On a closer examination of the geography and soil conditions of the 16 plots, he discovered that an underground stream ran in a perfect diagonal straight through the four plots he selected for fertilization with Type A. Thus, his dependent variable—crop yield—was at least as much affected by this uncontrolled independent variable, moisture content of the soil, as by the independent variable he actually controlled—chemical fertilization. If he had used a truly randomized latin-square design, which would have randomly allocated the plots to the alternative groups, he most likely would have eliminated the effect of this extraneous, confounding factor.

Multiple Comparison Groups, Multiple Independent Variables

Perhaps the most efficient of all is this design, which tests the simultaneous effects of several independent variables. Such a design may also involve multiple alternatives for each of the independent variables. These designs are known as *factorial designs* and were originally used in research on nonhuman subjects, such as studies in the fields of agriculture, botany, and genetics. Although potentially useful in studies of human beings, factorial designs still have their widest use in the physical and biological sciences rather than in the social sciences.

In an agricultural experiment using the factorial design, our dependent variable might be the yield of a crop; our subjects, plots of land; our independent variables (factors), depth of plowing, amount of fertilizer used, and amount of irrigation of the plots. Assignment of the plots to each of the numerous combinations of these variables would be strictly on a random basis. Each of the many possible combinations of factors would be represented by at least one of the plots.

The number of possible combinations in a factorial experiment is equal to the product of the number of alternative groupings of each of the independent variables tested. If the depth of plowing factor had two alternative groupings, the amount of fertilizer three groupings, and the amount of irrigation four groupings, the number of different comparisons (combinations of factors) would be $2 \times 3 \times 4 = 24$.

Applied to research in nursing, a possible factorial design might be a study of the effects on quality of care (assume a valid quantitative measure of this dependent variable existed) of such factors as size of hospital (small, medium, large), layout of the unit (large open ward, a ward consisting of all semiprivate units, a private ward), and amount of nursing care (high, medium, low). In this experiment, known as a 3^3 factorial, the number of combinations that can be formed from the different factors is $3 \times 3 \times 3 = 27$. To conduct this experiment as a fully controlled one, patients would be randomly assigned to one of the 27 groups upon admission to the hospital. Each group would represent a different combination of factors. Assuming that we would want 20 patients in each of the 27 comparison groups, the allocation of the patients would be as in Table 6-2. As can be seen, the number of patients exposed to each of the three variables as a whole, as well as to the alternative versions of each variable, is the same, or, in experimental design terminology, perfectly balanced. In fact this type of design is part of a family of experimental designs, like the latin-square, called a balanced design. Essentially it is a design in which the study subjects are matched according to exposure to the different combinations of the various independent variables. One of its major virtues can be seen from Table 6-2. Whereas each of the basic 27 comparison groups consists of 20 patients, which would be a sizable sample to make a meaningful statistical analysis, for each of the three main variables as a whole, there are 180 subjects: there are 180 patients in each of the three different amounts of nursing care groups, 180 patients in each type of nursing unit, and 180 in each size hospital. Similarly, for each combination of two of the variables, there are 60 patients in each of the comparison

TABLE 6-2

**Number of Patients Assigned to Each Combination
of the Independent Variables**

Hospital Size and Type of Nursing Unit	Amount of Nursing Care			
	Low	Medium	High	Total
Small hospital				
Private unit	20	20	20	60
Semiprivate	20	20	20	60
Ward	20	20	20	60
Medium hospital				
Private unit	20	20	20	60
Semiprivate	20	20	20	60
Ward	20	20	20	60
Large hospital				
Private unit	20	20	20	60
Semiprivate	20	20	20	60
Ward	20	20	20	60
Total	180	180	180	540

groups: 60 patients in private units of small hospitals, 60 in private units of medium-sized hospitals, 60 in private units of large hospitals, and so on for a total of 9 groups. Finally, for each combination of three variables there would be 20 patients in each of the 27 groups.

If, instead of a factorial design we had designed the study to test the effect of only one independent variable, say, amount of nursing care, on our dependent variable, quality of care, we might well have needed 60 subjects in each of the three comparison groups to produce valid findings. With this design, we would have only been able to make three comparisons —among the three levels of amounts of nursing. Through the factorial design with just *three* times the number of study subjects, we can make *nine* times the number of comparisons. Moreover with the factorial design, not only can we compare the effects of each of the three main variables themselves, known as the main effects, to see which, if any, exerts the greatest influence on our dependent variable, but we also have important information on the interactions between these variables. As Edwards[19] says:

> This in turn means that the outcomes of the experiment provide a sounder basis for generalizing about the effectiveness of the experimental variables, since they are tested not only in isolation, but in conjunction with the effects of other variables.

The factorial design is a very efficient form of experimental design, perhaps the most efficient that has been developed to date. With the use of the analysis of variance to analyze the data, the amount of information yielded by the study as well as the precision of the data analysis is maximized. In the sample cited we would learn not only whether providing higher hours of nursing care produces higher quality of patient care, but also whether hours of care in conjunction with (interaction with) size of nursing unit and size of hospital affect quality.

Consideration of the effects of several variables simultaneously is a more sophisticated approach to explaining why something happens than is the approach to understanding causation by examining only one variable at a time. This is particularly true in research concerned with human beings, where, as has been discussed, there usually is not a single explanation for the occurrence of an event but rather a multiplicity of causes.

However, one drawback exists in the application of factorial designs to human subjects. A balanced design, like the factorial design, is a symmetrical design and requires the assignment of the same number of study subjects to the alternative groups. If, as so often can happen in research on humans, a subject drops out of the study, the quality of the data is threatened. Even with techniques available to estimate missing values for lost cases, attrition of subjects remains a serious problem not only in factorial designs, but in all types of experimental designs. And, as Mainland[20] points out, statistical analysis of data obtained by experimental designs in which multiple comparisons are made—the analysis of variance methodology—is most efficient and (some say) only applicable where the dependent variable is a quantitative variable having a finely graded numerical scale and not a qualitative variable with broad, crudely defined classes.

HOW TO CONDUCT AN EXPERIMENT

The previous discussion has provided a rather rapid overview of the various types of experimental designs, beginning with the weak type of only partially controlled designs without random assignment of study subjects to the alternative groups, moving through the fully controlled designs with random assignment, and ending with the highly sophisticated factorial design, in which the effects of several independent variables are studied simultaneously. Understanding of the experimental approach can be acquired only through further study of the subject by reading some of the specialized literature in the field, as well as obtaining personal experience in conducting experiments. The material presented here can be considered only as an introduction to the subject. While these designs provide the structure of an experiment, determination of the design to use in an actual study is only one of the 12 important steps in the experimental process. The major steps in conducting an experiment are chronologically and substantively nearly identical with the 12 steps in the research process outlined in the previous chapter. The following is a very brief review of these steps with special emphasis on the experimental approach to research.

1. Formulate the experimental problem. A clear, precise statement of the problem is especially urgent in experimental research where large expenditures of time, effort, and money are often required in collecting data. Determine the purpose of the experiment—is it to advance knowledge or to test a product, program, or procedure? Raise questions as to the *need* for the experiment, its *feasibility,* the *importance* of the problem as to requiring an experimental approach, the degree to which findings of the experiment can be *generalized,* the *interest* of the experimenter in the subject matter of the experiment, and his *competence* to pursue the experiment.

2. Review the literature. In some areas of study little experimental work has been done previously. In other areas, the literature in the field is vast. Much is to be gained from learning about another experimenter's firsthand experiences in attempting to approach a research problem experimentally. Such experiences are sometimes communicated in the literature.

3. Formulate the framework of theory. An experiment will have greater meaning as well as importance if it can be placed within a theoretical framework. Even very practical studies on a specific subject such as evaluating alternative procedures or methods can usually be placed within a broader conceptual base. Linking a study to theory can contribute to the accumulation of a comprehensive body of scientific knowledge instead of just providing some isolated facts.

4. Formulate hypotheses. Most experiments are explanatory in nature, seeking insight into the causation of observed phenomena. For such experiments the formulation of clearly stated hypotheses is essential. The hypothesis should contain a statement of the expected relationship among the variables studied as well as the population for whom such relationship maintains.

5. Define variables. In experiments comparing the effects of an independent variable or variables on a dependent variable, the alternative groups of the independent variable being tested must be clearly differentiated. The criterion measure by which these alternative groups will be evaluated must be meaningful and consistent. All variables need to be defined operationally in terms of performable acts and in such an objective way that they can be consistently and accurately observed by independent observers.

6. Determine how variables will be quantified. The analysis of the results of experiments employ highly sophisticated statistical techniques that require the data to be in a quantitative form. Moreover, the use of perhaps the most refined statistical tool for analyzing experimental data—the analysis of variance—requires that the dependent variable have a numerical scale of measurement, most desirably with a finely graded continuous scale—as for example, temperature, weight, blood pressure, time, and other scientific scales.

7. Select the research design. A fully controlled, explanatory experiment requires the establishment of comparison groups representing the alternatives of the independent variable being tested, the assignment of the experimental subjects to the alternative groups on a strictly random basis, and the keeping of the conditions constant during the entire course of the experiment for the various alternative groups so that the only differences are in the independent variable. Greater efficiency in experimental design can be achieved by testing the effects of several independent variables simultaneously and by employing more than just an all-or-nothing version of the independent variables. Among the more complex designs are the latin-square and the factorial. The main objective in an experiment is to control the effects of any possible extraneous variables, organismic or environmental, that could bias the relationship among the explanatory variables being studied. In partially controlled experiments, randomization of study subjects to alternative groups might be omitted. Also, in such studies after the application of the independent variable to the subjects and before measurement of the dependent variables, there might not be complete control over the experimental conditions. Lack of randomization can lead to a mismatching of the characteristics of the alternative groups with possible biasing of results by extraneous organismic variables. Lack of complete control over the uniformity of study conditions can invite the spurious influence of extraneous environmental variables.

8. *Delineate the target population.* For an experiment to have value beyond its actual subjects and setting, the subjects must be drawn from some larger population, called a "target population." This selection should be made in such a way as to insure that the experimental subjects are validly representative of the members of the target population. The greater the extent to which the findings of an experiment can be generalized, the greater is the contribution of the findings to the body of scientific knowledge existing in the field.

9. *Select and develop the method for collecting the data.* Numerous methods are available for collecting data from experimental subjects. In many experiments the data are obtained directly from the subjects through the use of human observers. In data collection, as well as in the entire process of exposing the study subjects to the experimental conditions, the sociopsychological biases—called the Hawthorne effect—that can result when human beings are placed in novel situations or are treated in a special way must be controlled. The use of such techniques as the *control group* from which the experimental treatment is withheld and the *placebo* or *dummy treatment* given to the subjects of this group are examples of these controls. The *double-blind* technique, to completely disguise which subject receives the real treatment and which the dummy treatment, can also help control psychological bias in many types of experiments such as drug trials, or those in which the independent variable consists of the all-or-nothing variety.

10. *Formulate the method of analyzing the data.* In comparative experiments, using random assignment of subjects to the alternative groups studied, the statistical analysis of the data is well-defined and fully described in numerous textbooks on statistical methodology. In comparing the values of criterion measures for two groups, a test known as the "*t*-test" evaluates the actual difference found in the measures in relation to an estimate of the effect of the randomized extraneous variables, called experimental error. In making multiple comparisons a technique known as the analysis of variance is used in which the evaluation of the effects of the various experimental alternatives is accomplished by means of an "F-test."

11. *Interpret the results of the experiment.* The statistical tests of the results of an experiment—such as the *t*-test and F-test—give a measure of the statistical significance of the findings—i.e., the extent to which the differences found among the alternative groups exceed that which can be

attributed to chance (randomized) factors. The practical or substantive meaning of the data can be extracted only through the interpretative skills, sophistication, and the subject matter expertise the experimenter brings to bear on the data. Interpretation of results must be tempered by due recognition of the limitations of the experiment.

12. Communicate the results of the experiment. A single experiment cannot provide the final word on any conceivable research problem. The findings of one experiment are limited by the fact that it is generally based on a small group of subjects and is conducted in a specific place at a specific period of time. Publication of the method and findings of an experiment can serve to stimulate replication of the experiment by others as well as providing a link with the total body of scientific knowledge existing in the field.

Some Practical Problems in Conducting an Experiment

Not all of the decisions that need to be made in conducting an experiment are technical, theoretical, or statistical in nature. An experimenter is continually faced with a large variety of very practical problems. The solutions to these problems often depend on the experimenter's accumulated practical experience and wisdom as well as his intuitive grasp of the implications of the decisions made concerning these problem areas. Some of the more important of these problems will now be discussed.

1. Choice of experimental setting. Ideally, the most desirable setting for an experiment is one especially developed for that purpose, such as a laboratory or some other type of experimental unit. It is generally easier to exert control over extraneous influences in such settings. In animal studies or experiments concerned with inanimate objects, such specialized facilities are highly desirable, but for use in experiments with humans they may be limited. One drawback is the difficulty in obtaining the cooperation of people in being placed in an unnatural environment. A related, and perhaps more important, limitation is the difficulty of controlling the psychological biases that can result when human beings are placed in a strange and novel setting. The Hawthorne effect actually was first identified in the atmosphere of an artificial experimental situation. Finally, the artificiality of a specially constructed experimental setting puts restraints on the extent to which findings can be generalized to real-life situations. Nursing care provided to a patient in a "far-out" setting may have little relevance to the care actually provided in a real hospital.

Of course, the content of many experiments requires specially devised settings. The independent variable might be such as to necessitate radical alterations of the normal setting. A study of the use of television in monitoring patients would require significant changes in the usual facilities of the hospital. Likewise the extensive use in a study of a complicated mechanical instrument to measure the dependent variable—as, for example, a cardiotachometer—would represent an "unnatural" environmental factor.

The main concern in the choice of an experimental setting has been described as the degree to which the possible disturbing influences of extraneous variables can be kept under control. Fortunately, a high degree of control can be exerted in many types of settings that could be used for research in nursing and patient care. In hospitals, such facilities as operating rooms, intensive care units, recovery units, and nurseries can serve as highly controlled settings for studies involving patients as experimental subjects. Other types of highly controlled natural settings of possible use in experimental research in nursing include classrooms, outpatient clinics, and employee health units.

The problem in controlling the influences of extraneous variables introduced by the study setting varies directly in magnitude with the time lag between the application of the independent variable and the observation of the effect in the dependent variable. If the time lag is very short, as in an experiment concerning alternative ways of assisting a patient with his feeding as evaluated in terms of both nurse and patient acceptance of the method, extraneous environmental influences have little opportunity to bias the experiment. In such studies natural settings can be used without fear of loss of control over the experiment. If the time lag is very long, however, extraneous influences have more opportunity to affect the experiment. Thus, if we attempted to experimentally test in the natural setting of the patient's home the effect of teaching family members how to provide certain elementary nursing services to the patient, there might be a lag of several weeks or even months before the effect (skill at providing such services) can be expected to be observed. During this time many outside variables could influence this dependent variable and might well confound the effect of the independent variable. Of course, the longer the time lag between stimulus and response, the more difficult and impractical it is to conduct a fully controlled experiment. There are definite limits as to how long a "captive audience" can be expected to remain cooperative.

2. How many subjects shall an explanatory experiment include? The number of subjects (replications) to be included in an experiment is not a simple, cut-and-dried determination. Other things being equal, the larger the size of the study population (the sample of the target population), the more precise will be the findings of the experiment. But, of course, size of sample must be balanced against the practical problems involved in obtaining cooperation of subjects to enter the experiment and in keeping them intact after the experiment has begun. As has been indicated, attrition from an experiment can seriously damage the data. This would suggest the desirability of keeping the size of the sample sufficiently small to be practically manageable yet large enough to provide definitive findings.

Discussion of methods for determining the appropriate number of experimental subjects is contained in Chapter 8. Briefly, the size of the sample depends upon six factors:

a. A primary consideration in determining size of sample required in an experiment is the amount of precision desired in the results. This precision, which in testing hypotheses is called the level of statistical significance, is essentially a measure of the confidence that can be placed in the fact that any difference in the values of the criterion measure found among the comparison groups is truly related to the independent variable tested and not to extraneous factors. Generally, greater precision in study results requires that a larger number of experimental subjects be studied.

b. The uniformity of the members of the target population in relation to significant organismic variables influences the number of subjects needed for an experiment. If there are large differences among the members of the population in important extraneous variables such as age, health status, education, and so on, a larger sample would generally be required to assure representation of the target population than if there were greater uniformity among members. It is obvious that if all members of the population were exactly alike—a highly unlikely situation—one subject in each of the comparison groups would suffice to be representative of the target population.

c. With a greater degree of control over all possible confounding environmental variables, a smaller sample of experimental subjects can be used to achieve the same level of accuracy than when more environmental variables are uncontrolled. Thus, a perfectly controlled experiment would be more efficient than one that is less perfectly controlled, since it could yield just as precise findings with fewer subjects studied.

d. Size of sample is usually influenced by the size of the difference among the comparison groups that we would accept as being of practical, substantive significance. If we established a large difference as being practically significant, we would generally need a larger sample to support the fact that it is also statistically significant than if we accept a small difference as being practically significant. A larger sample is more likely to demonstrate the statistical significance of experimental findings, but the practical meaning of these differences also needs to be considered.

e. The sensitivity of the measuring instrument used to evaluate the effects of the independent variable can also influence the size of sample required. With a crude instrument having only a few gross gradations it might be necessary to use a larger sample to detect both statistically as well as practically significant differences among the comparison groups than if a more finely calibrated, sensitive instrument were employed. Of course, whether sensitive or gross, the measuring instrument must yield valid and reliable data to assure the veracity of the experiment.

f. With greater numbers of independent variables and more alternative groups for each variable, the number of experimental subjects required will be larger than in simpler experiments. But, as has been mentioned, factorial experiments involving the simultaneous testing of several independent variables are much more efficient than designs with single independent variables, since the amount of information to be gained substantially exceeds the increase in sample size required.

3. How are the experimental subjects randomly assigned to each of the comparison groups? Through randomization, neither the experimenter nor the experimental subject deliberately determines to which of the groups the subject shall be assigned. Many procedures are available for achieving a truly random allocation of experimental subjects. These include tossing a coin, drawing names as in a lottery, and shuffling cards. Perhaps the best method of randomization is the use of a table of random numbers. Such a table can be found in the inexpensive publication by Arkin and Colton, *Tables for Statisticians* (New York, Barnes and Noble, Inc., 1959). The use of this table is very simple. Suppose in a study of different methods of infant feeding we wanted to divide 40 infants who were in the nursery into two groups, A and B, each receiving a different method of feeding. We would write the names of each infant (or its number) on a separate index card. We would then shuffle all the cards. Next, we would open the book containing the random numbers to any particular page (at random), select a two-place digit from anywhere in the table (at random), and write the digit down on the first card. We would proceed to copy down consecutive two-place digits on succeeding index cards by moving in any particular order in the table of random numbers—up or down, to the right or left. After we had assigned a random number to each of the cards, we would arrange them in order of magnitude of the random numbers (from 00 to 99). The first 20 lowest numbers would then be assigned to group A, and the 20 highest numbers to group B. Thus by what may appear as a rather involved but actually very simple procedure we have accomplished the assignment of our infants to each of the groups in a completely random fashion. Such random allocation would increase the likelihood that the two groups of infants were equalized in terms of extraneous variables as well as enabling the computation of a measure of the influences of such randomized variables.

4. How long shall the experimental subjects be exposed to the independent variable? The answer to this question, of course, depends upon the nature of the independent variable being studied. For some variables that elicit a quick response from the subjects, short exposure may be sufficient. For others, where reactions are slower to develop, a longer period of exposure might be required. Suppose we were experimenting with the most desirable way (i.e., the cheapest, the most efficient, providing the highest quality of care) to organize a hospital. Our independent variable might consist of the two alternatives: the Progressive Patient Care type of organization and the conventional hospital organization. In such an experiment, it might require a period of study extending over a number of years for the two alternative systems to be in effect before any differences could be detected in the criterion measures. Such a lengthy period is required because the influences exerted by such complicated independent variables as these are subtle and indirect. Also, it will often take long periods of time for the experimental subjects to settle down within the experimental situation and begin to respond normally to the independent variable itself rather than to the novelty of the experimental situation.

5. *How long a time lag shall there be between exposure to the independent variable and measurement of its effect on the dependent variable?* Like the previous question, the answer to this one depends on the nature of the explanatory variables studied. Generally, a strong independent variable will produce a quicker effect than a weaker one. Similarly, a very sensitive dependent variable should be able to detect the effects of the independent variable in a shorter period of time than a less sensitive one. As has been indicated, there is danger in too great a lag between exposure of the experimental subjects to the independent variable and measurement of response in the dependent variable. Problems of attrition of subjects are magnified, as well as the greater likelihood that intervening extraneous variables will enter the study.

6. *Can an experiment include several dependent variables as criterion measures?* Many experiments include numerous dependent variables to measure the effect of the independent variable. For example, a study of methods of organizing a hospital (Progressive Patient Care versus conventional organization) can have as criterion measures: an evaluation of the hospital's financial status, a measure of personnel satisfaction, an audit of the quality of patient care, and a comparison of patient mortality. Hasselmeyer[21] in her study of the effect of the use of a diaper roll on the behavior of premature infants used six criterion measures: time required to regain initial birth weight, sleep behavior, crying behavior, bodily movements, and eating ability. Where multiple criterion measures are employed each should make distinctive and substantial contributions to the understanding of the independent variable. They should not merely be duplications of the other dependent variables. When studies contain multiple dependent variables they are usually analyzed separately in terms of their relationship to the independent variable. However, techniques are available in an area of statistical methodology known as *multivariate analysis,* in which these criterion measures are analyzed as simultaneous responses and each can be weighed against the other.

7. *How can the experimental groups be kept intact during the whole course of the experiment?* There are no hard and fast rules for maintaining the cooperation of the study subjects throughout the course of the experiment. Some subjects might have to drop out because of circumstances beyond anyone's control. In patient care studies we are continually alert to the fact that some of our subjects may have to leave the study because of their illness or even death. In out-of-hospital studies, people move, change jobs, or otherwise alter their status, which removes them from the scope of the study. One approach to the drop-out problem is to motivate the subjects toward the study and to see that they fully understand its aims, methods, and importance.

THE USE OF THE EXPERIMENTAL APPROACH IN STUDIES OF PATIENT CARE

With increasing frequency the experimental method is being applied to problems in nursing and patient care. Chapter 14 contains several illustrations of such studies. In general it can be said that research employing the experimental approach has been limited to narrowly defined problems conducted in settings where experimental controls could be feasibly applied: the team method of assignment on a hospital ward, the use of a diaper roll as a support for premature infants, closed-circuit television as a method of teaching nursing students, and so on. Such narrowing of the research problem is required by the nature of the experimental method.

Close analysis of the studies that have employed the experimental method will frequently reveal lack of full control over the experimental situation. At best, most experiments in nursing and patient care can be classified as partially controlled experiments. In few studies has the random assignment of the subjects to the alternative groups been attempted. Also, most experimental studies in nursing have been conducted in natural settings where control over extraneous environmental variables has been difficult to achieve. Moreover, for most of the independent variables included in nursing studies it is difficult to control sociopsychological biases. The double-blind method of assignment and the placebo treatment are difficult to apply in such studies.

The problem of applying rigorous controls in experiments involving human beings can be illustrated by examining a rather well-publicized study to test the comparative pain-relieving effects of five popular aspirin-containing analgesic preparations.[22] The five drugs included two containing aspirin alone, one with aspirin and additional ingredients to avoid a gastrointestinal upset, and two containing aspirin and other pain-relieving ingredients. As a control on psychological biases, a sixth comparative group was established in which a placebo was given. In the administration of the drugs the double-blind method was used.

The study contained three phases. In phase 1, the analgesic potency and rapidity of onset of relief from pain was studied among a group of postpartum patients. In phase 2, the gastrointestinal side effects were tested among a group of elderly patients. In phase 3, a group of nine arthritic patients were studied in relation to the effects of the drug on pain relief and gastrointestinal disturbance.

In none of the phases of the study were the subjects selected at random from some larger target population. Consequently, it is not possible to make *statistical* generalizations of the results of the study beyond the study population. However, in all phases of the study the drugs were randomly assigned to the patients. In phase 1, medications were randomly and "blindly" administered to the patients upon their request. Patients were interviewed prior to administration and seven times after the drug was administered, beginning 15 minutes after the drug was first given and ending four hours afterward. When interviewed the patients were asked to rate their pain as absent, slight, moderate, severe, or very severe. A quantitative score was applied to these ratings indicating a change from one level of severity to the next. One of the criterion measures used was the percentage of patients reporting complete pain relief at selected intervals. The data for the one- and three-hour intervals are as follows:

	Per cent of Patients Reporting Complete Pain Relief after:	
	1 hour	*3 hours*
Buffered aspirin	71	67
Combination of ingredients I	67	73
Plain aspirin I	59	60
Plain aspirin II	52	59
Combination of ingredients II	49	67
Placebo	24	40

Statistical analysis of these data (the well-known "chi-square test" discussed in Chapter 9) revealed that for both one- and three-hour intervals there was no significant difference among the five drugs in the percentage of patients reporting complete relief. However, the percentage was significantly greater for all drugs than for the placebo.

In phase 2, a 6 by 6 latin-square design was employed in which 60 patients were randomly divided into 6 groups of 10 patients each. Concurrently each group was given a different drug for a period of five days until all groups had received all five drugs and the placebo. One hour after a drug was given to a patient he was interviewed to find out whether he had experienced a gastrointestinal disturbance. The following occurrences were reported:

Drug	Number of Doses Given	Percentage of All Doses Given in Which GI Upset Reported
Buffered aspirin	812	0.6
Placebo	833	0.8
Plain aspirin I	818	1.1
Plain aspirin II	829	1.1
Combination of ingredients I	799	2.9
Combination of ingredients II	760	4.5

According to the researchers the incidence of upset stomach was significantly higher for the combination of ingredients than for the three other drugs and the placebo. No statistical significance was found among the rates of upset stomach for these three drugs and the placebo.

In phase 3, a group of nine arthritic patients who had been receiving regular doses of aspirin three times a day over a long period were given the five drugs in random order and interviewed afterward in relation to pain relief and gastrointestinal upset. No differences were found in the patients' reactions to the drugs.

Here, then, is a clear example of the use of the experimental method in pursuing a research problem among human beings directly concerned with patient care. That the problem is of sufficient importance to warrant an elaborate experiment is easy to demonstrate. The use of aspirin is more widespread than the use of any other drug. As the authors remark, "Analgesic compounds have assumed a leading position among the proprietary drugs that are most widely and most stridently advertised."

In the conduct of the experiment, every possible control was employed, including random assignment to the alternative groups, the placebo, and the double-blind. Control over extraneous environmental factors was attained by the very short lag between administration of the independent variable (the different pain-relieving drugs) and measurement of the dependent variable (pain and gastrointestinal upset).

We have in this research the elements of an experiment involving human beings where a very high degree of control can be achieved, perhaps, higher than can be attained in most conceivable patient care studies. Yet with all its controls it still possesses certain weaknesses in design which would make it not completely free of the influences of extraneous variables. The lesson to be learned from this study is that it is extremely difficult, if not impossible, to conduct a fully controlled experiment among human beings.

Among some of the weaknesses of this experiment are:

1. There is no target population to which the findings can be statistically generalized. The study subjects—hospitalized patients—are unquestionably very different from the typical aspirin user: an out-of-hospital,

ambulatory, otherwise healthy individual. However, this does not preclude the experimenters from generalizing the data beyond the experimental setting if they are convinced by their knowledge and experience that their findings would apply to other people, in other places, and at other times.

2. In phase 1, randomization was used without any further attempt at matching the groups. We have no assurance, then, that the influences of extraneous organismic variables were equalized among the groups. However, in phases 2 and 3, the use of balanced designs essentially matches the groups, since each subject in each group receives each of the alternative drugs being compared.

3. The criterion measures used, the patients' own evaluations of the occurrence of pain and gastrointestinal upset, are highly subjective measures. Because of their subjectivity, their validity and reliability can be questioned. However, it can be argued that these variables represent highly subjective phenomena and that self-reporting is the only realistic and meaningful type of measurement.

4. Although the double-blind approach was employed in the experiment, there is some question as to whether the identity of the drugs could really be completely disguised. Physically, the drugs tested do differ in appearance, and although this difference may be slight, it could introduce psychological bias into a study of this kind.

5. Some question can be raised as to the cumulative effect on the experimental subjects of the application of the independent variable. In phase 2, for example, the drugs were given three times a day for a period of five days. Repetitive dosage may build up in the recipient of the drugs an effect differing from that of a one-time or at least short-term use, the most common type of use. Therefore, the findings of the experiment might not be directly relevant to the research problem that precipitated it—that of the widespread use and advertisement of analgesic compounds.

6. In all phases of the study, repetitive measurements were made of the dependent variable. In repetitive measurements there always exists the danger that the measuring process itself will introduce psychological bias. Although, of course, the use of the placebo serves as a control and a measure of the influence of such bias, the unnaturalness of the experimental situation is thereby increased.

NONEXPERIMENTAL DESIGNS

Nonexperimental designs, sometimes called *surveys,* are probably the most widely used type of designs in research involving human beings. Descriptive studies, where the aim of the research is to generate new facts, are largely nonexperimental. Nonexperimental design is especially suited to such studies, since description implies natural observation of the characteristics of the research subjects without deliberate manipulation of the variables or control over the research setting. If we are interested in determining descriptive facts about the nursing needs of home care patients, we will attempt to observe and record these needs in their actual setting under real-life, not artificial, conditions.

Nonexperimental explanatory research, also called analytical surveys, have the same objectives as explanatory experiments: to discover causal patterns or relationships. As has been said earlier, nonexperimental research can rarely establish causal relationships. Because of the lack of control over all possible extraneous variables that can confound the relationship between the explanatory variables, the best that can generally be achieved is the establishment of associative relationships in nonexperimental studies. Such studies can be very useful in making predictions as well as in suggesting controlled experiments which may ultimately lead to causal explanations.

The model for nonexperimental explanatory research is, of course, the controlled experiment. The essential difference between the two types of designs is the absence of deliberate randomization of the study subjects to the alternative groups being compared. Thus, while in the experimental design the experimenter manipulates the independent variable through actual assignment of subjects to the various alternative groups, the manipulation of the independent variable in the nonexperimental design is done by bringing subjects into the study who already possess that quality of the independent variable. In other words, in the nonexperimental approach to explanatory research the subjects have been exposed to the independent variable by forces other than deliberate assignment to the alternative groups through a random process.

In nonexperimental explanatory research there are several methods available for achieving the equalization of groups that in experimental research is accomplished by random assignment and the matching techniques of pairing, balancing, and covariance. One of these has features of some of the matching methods in that the comparison groups are selected so as to be alike in as many important extraneous variables as possible. To illustrate, assume we wanted to nonexperimentally study differences in the rate of readmission to a hospital between patients discharged from a hospital with a home care program and those discharged from a hospital without such a program. We would attempt to select the alternative hospitals so that except for the home care program they would be similar in respect to all important extraneous variables, such as amount and type of nursing care available, the educational level, economic status, and diagnoses of the patients, and the characteristics of the patients' home environment.

Another way of enhancing the comparability of the groups is to restrict the target population to homogeneous subjects. A nonexperimental study of the effect of different patterns of outpatient department care on the general health status of patients could limit the patients to those in certain age, economic, education, and diagnostic groups. Such restrictions of the target population, of course, limit the scope of generalization of the findings of the study.

Basically there are two kinds of nonexperimental designs: cross-sectional and longitudinal. In addition, a longitudinal design may be either retrospective or prospective. These designs will be briefly discussed.

Cross-sectional Design

A cross-sectional survey can be thought of as analogous to the taking of a snapshot of some situation and analyzing it. We "stop" the action as of a specific point in time and examine it. Most descriptive surveys are of this type. Thus, when a nurse renews her license to practice she supplies certain data concerning her age, employment status, and field of practice. These data are then compiled to provide a composite picture of the characteristics of the registered nurse as of a given point in time. Similarly, the American Hospital Association routinely collects data from a panel of short-term general hospitals concerning the utilization of the hospitals as of a certain time period. Every two years the United States Public Health Service surveys the number and educational preparation of public health nurses employed in the United States as of January 1 of that year.

The cross-sectional design can also be applied to explanatory surveys. In a study of the relationship of the amount and type of nursing care available in hospitals, a sample of hospitals was selected that included hospitals with different staffing patterns (the independent variable).[23] Evaluation of the adequacy of nursing services provided at that time was obtained from patients and personnel in each of the hospitals (the dependent variable). The two variables were analyzed to see if there was a relationship between them.

It can be clearly seen that in the cross-sectional design the researcher has not randomly assigned the subjects to the various alternatives. In the study just cited, the patients and personnel were not allocated at random to the different staffing patterns. Although theoretically a sort of random process is in operation in that the distribution of the patients to the different hospitals can be considered to be a function of chance factors, we cannot be sure that all conditions are more or less equivalent for the different groups being compared.

Retrospective Design

One of the most popular types of nonexperimental designs, particularly in explanatory studies, is retrospective. The dependent variable is observed first and then traced back and related to relevant independent variables that are hypothesized as being associated with the dependent variable. For example, in a study of birth injuries reported on the birth certificate, it was noted that the incidence of injuries appeared to be higher in some hospitals than others. In following back to the hospitals it was found that those hospitals with a higher rate of birth injuries had more poorly designed and equipped delivery rooms than did hospitals with lower rates of birth injuries. Also, the early studies of the relationship between smoking and lung cancer originated from observation of an increasing incidence in the number of deaths from lung cancer among men. A sample of these cases were followed back to determine their smoking habits. As a "control group" the smoking habits of a group of men who died from causes other than lung cancer were also traced back. Comparison of the two groups indicated a much higher percentage of cigarette smokers among the men who died of lung cancer than among those who died of other causes.

Retrospective studies are popular because they are relatively inexpensive and are easier to administer than other types. Basically, a retrospective explanatory study is the reverse of the experimental design. In experimental explanatory studies, exposure to the independent variable precedes observation of the dependent variable. In the retrospective method the dependent variable is observed first, and then the independent variable that may have caused the behavior of the dependent variable is sought.

Retrospective explanatory studies are essentially longitudinal in that the relationship between the dependent and independent variables extends over a period of time. For such variables as smoking and lung cancer, a lengthy period of time has elapsed. A limitation of this approach is the great lack of control over the research setting, subjects, and variables being studied. Consequently there are difficulties in establishing relationships among the variables studied that are free of spuriousness. Moreover, retrospective studies often make extensive use of data originally collected for a purpose other than that of the researcher's, such as data contained in birth and health records, health histories, patient records, and personnel records. Or, they may use data that are heavily dependent upon the respondent's ability to accurately recall some past event. Such data are not as valid and reliable as that collected in prospective studies. The advantage of retrospective designs is, of course, the relative ease and inexpensiveness of collecting the data. As hypotheses-generating, exploratory-type studies, retrospective studies can be most valuable.

Prospective Design

Prospective explanatory surveys are similar to experiments in that the study begins with alternative groups of study subjects who are followed up over a period of time and compared in terms of some criterion measure.

We may, for example, follow up two groups of premature infants after discharge from the hospital, one group from a formally organized premature nursery, and the other from an ordinary nursery, to see if any differences occur over a period of time in their physical development. Or we may follow two groups of high school students, one in which future nurse clubs are organized in the school they attend and the other where no such schools exist, to determine whether there are any differences in the proportion of subjects in each group choosing nursing as a career.

The major difference between the prospective nonexperimental and experimental designs is the absence in the former of random assignment to the comparison groups. Also there is looser control in the survey—in fact, no control at all—over the many variables to which the subjects are exposed during the study period.

Prospective nonexperimental studies are very popular in following up a group of subjects over a long period of time to observe what happens to them. Studies that focus on the same group of subjects over time are also known as *cohort* studies. The term "cohort" refers to a set of study subjects who are grouped together according to certain characteristics and observed longitudinally. In explanatory studies these characteristics would be the independent variables. Thus, we can select a group of graduates from a degree program in nursing and another from a diploma program and observe them at regular intervals over a long period of time to see how many remain in nursing and how many leave the field. Of those remaining in nursing we can find out how many become supervisors and administrators and how many remain as staff nurses and, of those leaving, how many are housewives and how many take jobs in other fields. The experience of the subjects over time can be related to their cohort characteristic, which in this example is the type of nursing program pursued.

Cohort studies are very widely used in the field of demography where, for example, the mortality or morbidity experience of a group of individuals may be observed over a long period of time. In one type of cohort study "life tables" are produced which statistically quantify the experience of the cohort groups. Thus, we can take a group of individuals who have some disease like cancer, follow them up over a period of time, and record the number of deaths that occur at different time intervals: one year after onset, two years, three years, etc.

Cohort studies like the ones described are essentially a series of cross-sectional studies involving the same subjects that are repeated over a period of time. Subjects from a given group are tested at regular intervals and measurements of the same phenomena made. The cohort-type study, particularly where there is only one group involved, is similar to the "before-after" type of experimental design in which control over possible confounding organismic variables is achieved by restricting the study to the same study subjects.

Mixed Designs

In actual research practice, mixed types of design are sometimes employed. Thus, we may begin our study as an experiment and then employ a prospective, cohort-type nonexperimental study. For example, the experimental phase of the study might consist of randomly assigning one group of hospitalized cardiac patients to a very comprehensive program of patient teaching while another group would receive no formal teaching at all. After discharge from the hospital, the patients in both groups (the cohorts) would be followed up to determine whether there is any difference in their mortality experience. Due to the many intervening variables that could exert an influence on the mortality rates, however, it would be difficult to demonstrate a causal relationship among the variables studied.

Another common type of mixed design is one that incorporates a cross-sectional approach and an experiment. Through this approach certain relevant clues may be obtained in a cross-sectional survey concerning the variables of interest to the researcher, and these may be incorporated into an experimental study. Likewise, a retrospective study often precedes a prospective one, the former serving as an exploratory phase to generate hypotheses and to suggest fruitful avenues of approach in the forward-looking study.

Historical Research in Nursing

Historical research in nursing is a neglected area and yet it should be one of highest priority for the researcher.

Research into present day problems without adequate search into the past to examine the course of events which produced the present problems, or to bring to light past investigations of the same or similar problems by nurses or others, results in research which only scratches the present surface and may even duplicate previous work.[24]

Historical research is sometimes referred to as documentary research and is recognized as an appropriate method of inquiry. Such research goes beyond the collection of facts and dates and considers the relationship of facts and incidents to current and past issues and events. "A major contribution of historical inquiry is in the development of a broader, more complete perspective to enhance our understanding of the present and our approach to the future."[25] It is different from the scientific method only in that historiographers are concerned with "the conscious or thought-side of human existence."

The historical method has similarities to the methodology of the natural sciences in that both must deal with the discovery, verification, and categorization of facts.

Criteria of Historical Research

Historical research must pass the same rigorous tests of validity and reliability as other forms of research. The historiographer seeks to establish truth, ascertain facts and form the basis of all conclusions and generalizations. Christy[26] points out that historiographers have evolved two separate processes for the critical examination of data. The first is external criticism which establishes the validity of documents such as manuscripts, letters, and books, and internal criticism which determines the reliability of the information contained within the document.

All important is that the historiographer compare documents with the originals and whenever possible use primary sources. This is the best way to establish fact. If available, two independent primary sources that corroborate should be used. If only one primary source can be found and there is no contrary evidence, the evidence can be considered probable.

Fitzpatrick[27] identifies the following key criteria used in evaluating historical research:

1. Nature, adequacy, and completeness of sources. The historiographer uses a systematic approach in collecting and verifying data. Primary sources are used and are not limited to one. Further, varied sources are used—documentary materials (letters, minutes, proceedings) as well as published materials.
2. Completeness with which the identified subject is treated. Are the important components addressed? Are varied and key questions asked? Are limitations stated? Are explanations of why different approaches were or were not used provided?
3. Recognition of bias in selection of hypotheses. Is the researcher directed to certain data and issues without consideration of alternatives? Is information provided that leads to preconceived judgments? Does the researcher recognize the complex nature of the area being researched?
4. Contextualism. Historiographers must have concern for context and time that make events unique.
5. Interconnectedness. The historiographer is concerned with the relationship of parts to the whole; the weaving together of disparate parts to form a coherent explanation that communicates meaning.
6. Organization.
7. Clarity.
8. Logical sequence.
9. Originality of interpretation.

SELECTED EXAMPLES OF HISTORICAL RESEARCH IN NURSING

The National Organization for Public Health Nursing, 1912–1952: Development of a Practice Field by M. Louise Fitzpatrick.[28]

This superb example of historical research makes a significant contribution to the all too few efforts of historians in the field of nursing. The author provides a fully documented and scholarly report of the origin, development, and activities of the National Organization for Public Health Nursing from 1912 to 1952. Particularly important is the author's unique approach to describing public health nursing as it was reflected in the interests and activities of the National Organization for Public Health Nursing. A span of 40 years is covered in which the work of NOPHN contributed to the advancement of public health nursing and the educational preparation of public health nurses.

A Cornerstone for Nursing Education by Teresa E. Christy.[29]

Historical research contributes a valuable perspective to the analysis of current activities by providing a sense of continuity over time through the analysis of persons, movements, events, and concepts. Through the process of reconstructing events of the past and the analysis of why events occurred as they did, the historian has the capacity to assist professional groups in measuring, evaluating, and predicting social change.[30]

This was the sentiment expressed by Eleanor Lambertsen in describing the Christy historical research:

"The author provides a history of the Division of Nursing Education of Teachers College, Columbia University, and places the main events in juxtaposition with parallel events at the beginning of the twentieth century. The historical presentation is not limited to the history of one institution but particularly important is the thorough documentation. . . of the broad movement toward better, more uniform education for nurses. The international influence of M. Adelaide Nutting and Isabel M. Stewart is clearly portrayed."

Mary Adelaide Nutting: Pioneer of Modern Nursing by Helen E. Marshall.[31]

This is a biographical study in which the author attempted to trace the development of nursing as a profession by reporting the achievements of one of its great leaders, Mary Adelaide Nutting. The author had access to Miss Nutting's papers preserved by Isabel Stewart and Mary Roberts. Miss Virginia Dunbar collated the correspondence between Miss Stewart and Miss Nutting and indexed the Nutting family papers. What resulted in Dr. Marshall's biography of Miss Nutting is a very personable account of a leader in the nursing profession.

Watch-Fires on the Mountains: The Life and Writings of Ethel Johns by Margaret M. Street.[32]

The biography of a pioneer nurse of the Canadian west whose leadership helped to shape American nursing. Of particular importance is the historiographer's approach to relating events of the first half of the twentieth century to nursing affairs at the local, national, and international levels.

From Nightingale to Eagle: An Army Nurse's History by Edith A. Aynes.[33]

An example of the experience of an army nurse before, during, and after World War II. She portrays her personal experiences and documents these with significant events of the times, thus producing a historical document with a personal assessment and point of view.

The Lamp and the Caduceus. The Story of the Army School of Nursing by Marlette Conde.[34]

A well-documented account of the history of the Army School of Nursing. Several notable leaders who were graduates of this program have had great influence on American nursing. The author had access to a number of primary documents such as army and alumnae records.

A School of Nursing Comes of Age. A History of the Frances Payne Bolton School of Nursing, Case Western Reserve University, By Margene O. Faddis.[35]

An excellent example of how the history of a professional school can become an important part of the history of a profession. The development of the Frances Payne Bolton School of Nursing clearly reflects the evolution of nursing toward a true profession. Primary sources were used from the university archives, the archives of university hospitals and alumnae records.

HISTORICAL RESEARCH TOOLS AND RESOURCES

Manuscripts and Oral Histories

The historiographer has available both the tape-recorded interview and the historical record but these research tools are not without their problems.

Manuscripts continue to be the main resources for the historiographer. These may include letters, drafts, a variety of historical records exclusive of archives and other documents.[36] Oral tape-recorded interviews have come to be an accepted historical record and research tool and now fall within the range of primary research materials. Oral histories may serve as single historical documents or one aspect of the total research effort.

The historiographer using the oral history "attempts to capture the recollections and interpretations of those participants in the development of contemporary medicine who are judged to be knowledgeable about the subject under study."[37] Thus the oral history can provide information related to a specific subject or an autobiographical memoir. The oral history has one major limitation in that it lacks the footnote or citation considered basic to scholarship. Interpretations by other historians are limited, and additional verification of the facts and opinions on tape may be needed.

Thus, related historical documents to verify the facts in the oral history become extremely important. Historiographers using the oral history as a research tool should preserve primary records for possible future research. Such histories can also extend the usefulness of manuscripts.

Oral history materials to be used by researchers must be cataloged and administered by qualified personnel in historical libraries. The historian will find *The American Archivists, The Journal of the Society of American Archivists,* helpful in that it publishes an annual bibliography covering subjects related to archives and manuscripts. Also helpful is *Library Trends.*[38]

A unified manuscript-oral history approach has merit for the historiographer in that a single and combined catalog of related subjects would be available.

Significant progress has been made at the National Library of Medicine (medicine is used here in the generic sense as it refers to all health literature) in developing and handling archival material. Sizable manuscript collections housed at the National Library of Medicine have cataloged together manuscripts and oral histories.

THE NURSING ARCHIVES AT THE NATIONAL LIBRARY OF MEDICINE

At a historical meeting on April 6, 1973, the Executive Director and the president of the National League for Nursing (NLN), Deputy Chief of the History of Medicine Division, Dr. Peter D. Olch, and Chief Nurse Officer of the USPHS met to discuss the establishment of a nursing archives at the National Library of Medicine. At this meeting it was agreed that the NLN would transfer the material in their archives to the National Library of Medicine. This material, which included early records of the NLN, the American Society of Superintendents of Training Schools, and the National Organization of Public Health Nurses, was received on December 12, 1973. At the meeting, participants also agreed that the NLN should make an effort to identify the location, content, and accessibility of manuscript items important to the history of nursing in the United States. In those instances where materials could not be adequately processed and preserved at the parent institution, the representative of the National Library of Medicine would discuss with a designated NLN committee the advisability of transferring the material to the National Library of Medicine.

Recognizing the importance of the preservation of manuscript materials documenting the history of the American nursing profession, the repository at the National Library of Medicine has welcomed the receipt of the NLN collection and hopes their action will stimulate other individuals and nursing organizations to seriously consider the preservation of their personal papers and records in this or other repositories where they can be organized and made available for scholarly research.

A catalog entry of the NLN collection appears in the 1976 volume of the *National Union Catalogue of Manuscript Collections* which originates in the Descriptive Cataloging Division of the Library of Congress.

Reference inquiries pertaining to NLN material in the library will be answered, but it is important to realize that MEDLINE has no information about any manuscript collections within the library.

Steps are being taken by the Public Health Service to encourage faculties at Teachers College, Columbia University, Wayne State University, Boston University, and other universities to have a historian or archivist develop registers for special collections. These registers could then be made available at the National Library of Medicine for cross-reference. Thus, historians would have a total picture of what is available at the National Library of Medicine as well as at the on-site location of private collections.

At the present time historical documents of the Federal Nursing Services cannot be accepted at the National Library of Medicine due to a regulation published in the *Code of Federal Regulations,* Title 41, Public Contracts and Property Management, Chapter 101 (Revised July 1, 1974), which requires records of the Federal Nursing Services to be filed with the federal archives. After full exploration, it was found that 85 to 90 per cent of records submitted to the National Archives are destroyed and a separate nursing collection is not maintained. For this reason, other avenues are being explored that will permit the Federal Nursing Services to submit their historical documents so that they can be added to the nursing collection at the National Library of Medicine. At present the National Library of Medicine can only accept private collections such as the National League for Nursing (NLN) historical documents. The preservation of important historical nursing documents is critical and every use should be made of the superb resources at the National Library of Medicine located in Bethesda, Maryland.

BIBLIOGRAPHIC INFORMATION NETWORK FOR SCIENCE AND TECHNOLOGY

The National Library of Medicine developed a program for gaining access to the biomedical literature nearly 100 years ago. *Index Medicus* was first published in 1879. Starting in 1962 the library initiated a number of computerized systems both nationally and internationally to gain access to the biomedical literature.[39] These will be described briefly to encourage the researcher to use these valuable tools.

MEDLARS is a computer system which has been operational since 1964 and is a medical literature analysis and retrieval system. It is a computerized system for the production of *Index Medicus*. To use the system a qualified health professional submits a written request describing the details of the information needed. The request is then translated by a trained analyst and coded into the vocabulary of MEDLARS for input into one of the computers. A request takes approximately three to four weeks to process.

MEDLINE (Medical Literature Analysis and Retrieval System On-Line) is a data base maintained by the National Library of Medicine containing references to approximately half a million citations from 3,000 biomedical journals. MEDLINE contains the current year's citations and the prior two previous years. Ancillary files date back to 1969. Citations on a given subject from MEDLINE can be retrieved by entering terms from article titles and/or abstracts or by entering any of 12,000 medical subject headings listed in the MEDLINE-controlled vocabulary, MESH.

CHEMLINE (Chemical Dictionary On-Line) is the National Library of Medicine's on-line, interactive chemical dictionary built by the toxicology information program in collaboration with the chemical abstracts service. It provides a mechanism whereby 270,000 chemical substance names representing 76,355 unique substances can be searched and retrieved on-line.

CATLINE (Catalog On-Line) is a data base maintained by the National Library of Medicine containing nearly 140,000 references to monographs and serials cataloged since 1965.

AVLINE (Audio Visuals On-Line) is a test data base maintained by the National Library of Medicine containing references to audiovisual instructional materials in the health sciences. The materials are professionally reviewed for technical quality, currency, accuracy of subject content and educational design. AVLINE became operational September 1975 and will allow teachers, students, librarians, researchers, practitioners, and other health science professionals to retrieve citations that will aid in evaluating audiovisual materials.

CANCERLINE (Cancer On-Line) is the National Cancer Institute's on-line base of approximately 37,000 citations dealing with cancer therapy and chemical, physical, and viral carcinogenesis from 1963 to current year. Also included are *Carcinogenesis Abstracts* and *Cancer Therapy Abstracts*. The data base will be expanded to include all other aspects of cancer research as well as abstracts and protocols of on-going cancer research projects.

HOW TO CONDUCT NONEXPERIMENTAL RESEARCH

The 12 steps in the research process discussed in the previous chapter provide the sequence of activity involved in developing a nonexperimental as well as an experimental study. We begin with formulation of the problem and end with reporting the findings. While the steps involved in developing all types of research studies are identical, the emphasis on certain of the steps differs somewhat for the various designs. The main differences are as follows:

1. In nonexperimental research more effort is usually devoted to the statement of the problem than in an experiment. Many nonexperimental studies come to grips with thornier, more broadly conceived problems than do experiments. Hypotheses in such studies are often less specific and may not lend themselves to simple statistical tests.

2. In nonexperimental studies the variables are usually less clear-cut, the relationships among them more complex, and the need to consider the impact of extraneous variables more pressing than in experimental studies.

3. In an experiment much more concern is usually expended on the specific design of the study, particularly the randomization procedure, the form of statistical analysis of the data, in fact, the total mechanics of administering the study, than is devoted to similar matters in the nonexperimental approach.

4. More time is spent in nonexperimental studies analyzing data through statistical tables and in interpreting them above and beyond their statistical significance.

5. In a nonexperimental study more concern is usually devoted to the method of random selection of study subjects from the target population. An experiment is more concerned with the random assignment of the subjects to the alternative groups being compared.

6. Collection of data is often different for the two approaches—the experimental approach usually involves direct collection of data through observation, interview, or use of mechanical instruments. The nonexperimental approach is more likely to employ indirect methods like the mailed questionnaire.

7. The types of criterion variables are frequently different in the two approaches. The experimental method often employs more refined tools of measurement, often using scientific instrumentation. The nonexperimental is more apt to employ more crudely measured variables.

HOW TO DECIDE WHETHER TO USE AN EXPERIMENTAL OR NONEXPERIMENTAL DESIGN FOR THE RESEARCH

One type of research design can often serve as a substitute for another type. The actual choice of design for a study depends on the evaluation of numerous factors. Many of these have been discussed in an earlier section dealing with pros and cons of the two types of design. To recapitulate, briefly these factors are:

1. *Nature of the research problem.* Some research problems do not lend themselves to the experimental approach because they cannot be set up outside of an uncontrolled natural setting. Similarly, other problems may not be capable of study nonexperimentally because the ingredients of the research may not exist in nature and may have to be experimentally constructed.

2. *Amount of resources available to do the research.* Generally speaking, it is more expensive in money, manpower, and materials to conduct an experiment than a nonexperimental study on the same subject.

3. *Amount of time available to do the research.* An experiment will generally require a longer period of time for completion than will a nonexperimental study concerned with the same problem. Many retrospective or cross-sectional studies can be completed in a matter of several months. In an experiment this length of time may be needed just to plan the study.

4. *Possible danger to health or safety of people.* Some research cannot be pursued experimentally because of potentially harmful effects on the subjects. These harmful effects may not always be physical in nature; they can also be emotional. Nonexperimental studies are far less likely to have such negative consequences on the study population.

5. *The exploratory nature of the study.* In a field where little research has been done previously and where it may be presumptuous to launch a full-blown, highly structured experiment, a nonexperimental study can be very useful in exploring the field, clarifying concepts, developing hunches, and formulating the problem and the hypotheses.

6. *The degree of refinement of the measurement of the variables.* The success of an experiment is heavily dependent upon the ability to clearly and operationally define the various alternatives of the independent variable that will be tested as well as upon the availability of valid, reliable, and sensitive criterion measures.

7. *The extent to which we can enlist the cooperation of our study subjects.* Generally, it is easier to obtain cooperation from study subjects in a nonexperimental study than in an experimental one. This is so because fewer demands are likelier to be made of the subjects in a nonexperimental study. This factor must be given serious attention in the choice of a design, since the validity of an experimental study can be severely damaged by high attrition of study subjects.

8. *The degree to which we hope to explain causality.* The major attribute of the experimental method is the greater likelihood that we will be able to discover causal relationships. If the explanation of the cause

of some effect is the aim of our research, the closer we can model our design after the experimental method, the greater is the assurance we will have of achieving it.

Summary

The aim of the experimental method is to control the influences of all extraneous variables that could bias the data we are gathering in the study. In experiments involving human beings, total control of all extraneous variables is seldom achieved. Nevertheless, it is the goal to which the task of designing a valid experiment is dedicated. The means for controlling the major sources of bias in explanatory experiments are shown in Figure 6-4. In this diagram of an "ideal" experimental design involving two comparison groups, one of which receives the actual treatment and the other a placebo or dummy treatment, the four major ways in which the design controls the influences of extraneous variables are as follows:

1. The experimental subjects are drawn at random from the target population in order to insure representativeness of subjects as well as

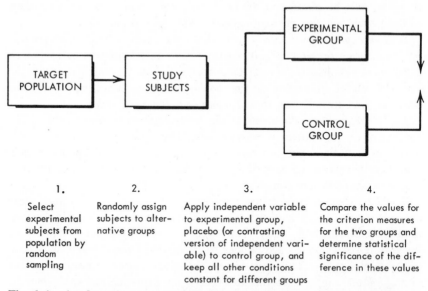

1.	2.	3.	4.
Select experimental subjects from population by random sampling	Randomly assign subjects to alternative groups	Apply independent variable to experimental group, placebo (or contrasting version of independent variable) to control group, and keep all other conditions constant for different groups	Compare the values for the criterion measures for the two groups and determine statistical significance of the difference in these values

Fig. 6–4. A schematic representation of the experimental method for explanatory research (showing four stages of experimental control). (*Courtesy* Greenberg, B. G. "The Philosophy and Methods of Research." In Harriet H. Werley (ed.): *Report on Nursing Research Conference.* Walter Reed Army Institute of Research, Washington, D.C., 1961.)

to be able to quantitatively estimate the extent to which the subjects are an adequate sample of the total population.

2. The subjects are randomly assigned to the alternative groups to insure equalization of the characteristics of the subjects composing the groups. By the techniques of pairing, balancing, and covariance analysis, additional control over the matching of the composition of the groups can be achieved.

3. After the administration of the treatment, all environmental variables are also controlled, so that the only difference between the alternative groups is in terms of the independent variable. By the use of a dummy treatment (placebo) and the double-blind technique, sociopsychological biases (Hawthorne effect) can be controlled.

4. The differences found in the criterion measures for the alternative groups are compared to the differences attributable to extraneous (chance) factors computed by taking into account the number of subjects in the study group (size of sample) and their variability in relation to the criterion measure. The resulting index is a measure of the degree to which the actual differences exceed that which can occur due to chance alone. This procedure assesses the statistical significance of the differences we have found in the study.

Even with all these safeguards against bias, there is always the possibility that our experiment may produce results that can be erroneously interpreted, a problem to be discussed in Chapter 9. Moreover, a critical area of control not included in the four controls mentioned is that concerning the definition and measurement of the explanatory variables. No matter how well the experiment is otherwise controlled, weaknesses in measurement can seriously damage the validity of an experiment. Therefore, all conclusions based on a single experiment, particularly among such variable subjects as human beings, should be considered as tentative until confirmed by replicated experiments.

Nonexperimental research generally lacks some of the important controls found in an experiment. It is, therefore, weaker in control of extraneous variables. Although nonexperimental explanatory studies may employ random sampling of study subjects from the target population, the researcher does not randomly assign the subjects to the alternative groups being studied. In other words, he does not deliberately manipulate the independent variable except through his bringing into the study subjects already assigned to the alternative groups or by an ex post facto sorting of the subjects into the alternative groups through statistical manipulation of the data (cross-tabulation). An important value of nonexperimental research is the broader scope that such studies can have, since it is less costly to use large samples of study subjects than in experiments. Therefore, more independent variables can be studied, with perhaps a greater depth of analysis possible than in an experimental approach to the same problem. Moreover, the artificiality of the experimental situation is eliminated, thereby providing findings that can have more relevant application to the real world. Nevertheless, the experimental approach to research remains as the ideal model for establishing a body of trustworthy scientific knowledge.

References

1. R. A. Fisher, and G. T. Prance, *The Design of Experiments.* Darien, Conn., Hafner, 1973.

2. W. G. Cochran, and Gertrude M. Cox, *Experimental Designs,* 2nd ed. New York, John Wiley and Sons, 1957.

3. Oscar Kempthorne, *The Design and Analysis of Experiments.* New York, Robert E. Krieger Publishing Co., Inc., 1973.

4. W. T. Federer, *Experimental Design: Theory and Application.* New York, Macmillan Publishing Co., Inc., 1955.

5. A. L. Edwards, *Experimental Design in Psychological Research.* 4th ed. New York, Holt, Rinehart and Co., 1973.

6. F. S. Chapin, *Experimental Design in Sociological Research.* Westport, Conn., Greenwood Press, 1974.

7. Victor Chew, *Experimental Designs in Industry.* New York, John Wiley and Sons, 1958.

8. D. J. Finney, *Experimental Design and Its Statistical Basis.* Chicago. University of Chicago Press, 1955.

9. John Stuart Mill, *A System of Logic.* New York, Harper and Brothers, 1873.

10. *Ibid.,* p. 222.

11. Morris R. Cohen and Ernest Nagel, *An Introduction to Logic and Scientific Method.* New York, Harcourt, Brace and Co., 1934, p. 263.

12. Adapted from Eugene Levine, "Experimental Design in Nursing Research." *Nursing Res.,* **9:**203–212, fall 1960.

13. Elton Mayo, *The Human Problems of an Industrial Civilization.* New York, Macmillan Publishing Co., Inc., 1933.

14. John R. P. French, Jr., "Experiments in Field Settings," in *Research Methods in the Behavioral Sciences,* Leon Festinger and David Katz (eds.). New York, The Dryden Press, 1953, Chapter III, p. 101.

15. Donald T. Campbell, "Factors Relevant to the Validity of Experiments in Social Settings." *Psychol. Bull.,* **54:**297–312, 1957.

16. William G. Cochran, "Matching in Analytical Studies." *Am. J. Pub. Health,* **43:**684–691, June 1953.

17. Eileen G. Hasselmeyer, *Behavior Patterns of Premature Infants.* U.S. Public Health Service Publication No. 840. Washington, Government Printing Office, 1961.

18. Bernard G. Greenberg, "The Use of Analysis of Covariance and Balancing in Analytical Surveys." *Am. J. Pub. Health,* **43:**692–699, June 1953.

19. A. L. Edwards, *op. cit.,* p. 233.

20. Donald Mainland, *Elementary Medical Statistics.* Philadelphia, W. B. Saunders Co., 1963, p. 17.

21. Eileen G. Hasselmeyer, *op. cit.*

22. Thomas J. DeKornfeld, Louis Lasagna, and Todd M. Frazier, "A Comparative Study of Five Proprietory Analgesic Compounds." *J.A.M.A.,* **182:**1315–1318, December 29, 1962.

23. Faye G. Abdellah and Eugene Levine, *Effect of Nurse Staffing on Satisfactions with Nursing Care.* Hospital Monograph Series No. 4. Chicago, American Hospital Association, 1958.

24. Mildred E. Newton, "The Case for Historical Research." *Nursing Res.,* **14:**1:20, winter 1965.

25. Lucille E. Notter (editorial), "The Case for Historical Research in Nursing." *Nursing Res.,* **21:**6:483, November–December 1972.

26. Teresa E. Christy, "The Methodology of Historical Research: A Brief Introduction." *Nursing Res.,* **24:**3:189–192, May–June 1975.

27. M. Louise Fitzpatrick, Critique of Philip and Beatrice Kalisch's paper: "Congress Copes with the Nurse Shortage, 1941–1971: Dynamics of Congressional Education Policy Formulation." Ninth Nursing Research Conference, Kansas City, Missouri, American Nurses' Association, 1973.

28. M. Louise Fitzpatrick, *The National Organization for Public Health Nursing, 1912–1952: Development of a Practice Field.* New York, National League for Nursing, 1975.

29. Teresa E. Christy, *Cornerstone for Nursing Education.* New York, Teachers College Press, Teachers College, Columbia University, 1969.

30. *Ibid.,* p. vii.

31. Helen E. Marshall, *Mary Adelaide Nutting: Pioneer of Modern Nursing.* Baltimore, The Johns Hopkins University Press, 1972.

32. Margaret M. Street, *Watch-Fires on the Mountains: The Life and Writings of Ethel Johns.* Toronto, University of Toronto Press, 1973.

33. Edith A. Aynes, *From Nightingale to Eagle: An Army Nurse's History.* Englewood Cliffs, N.J. Prentice-Hall, Inc., 1973.

34. Marlette Conde, *The Lamp and the Caduceus: The Story of the Army School of Nursing.* Washington, D.C., Army School of Nursing Alumnae Association, 1975.

35. Margene O. Faddis, *A School of Nursing Comes of Age: A History of the Frances Payne Bolton School of Nursing, Case Western Reserve University.* Cleveland, The Alumni Association of the Frances Payne Bolton School of Nursing, 1973.

36. T. R. Schellenberg, *The Management of Modern Archives.* Chicago, The University of Chicago Press, 1965.

37. Peter D. Olch, "Oral History and the Medical Librarian." *Bulletin of Medical Library Association,* **57:**1–4, January 1969.

38. Robert L. Brubaker, "Manuscript Collections." *Library Trends,* **13:**226–256, October 1964.

39. David B. McCarm, and Joseph Leiter, "On-Line Services in Medicine and Beyond." *Science,* **181:**318–324, July 27, 1973.

Problems and Suggestions for Further Study

1. Discuss the following statement by Camilleri ("Theory, Probability and Induction in Social Research," *American Sociological Review*, **27**:173, April 1962): "A fundamental criticism of Mills' methods of experimental inquiry is that to use them to discover the causes of a phenomenon or to prove that a particular factor is the cause of a phenomenon requires the *a priori* assumption that all the possible causes are known and examinable."

2. Select five hypotheses from pages 135–36. Briefly outline how research would be conducted to test these hypotheses experimentally and nonexperimentally. What are some of the practical problems in pursuing this research experimentally? Would it be possible to establish causal relationships for the variables stated in the hypothesis if the research were conducted nonexperimentally?

3. What kinds of studies can be done experimentally that cannot be done nonexperimentally? Conversely, what kinds, if any, can be done nonexperimentally that cannot be done experimentally?

4. Is it ever possible in research on human beings to conduct a completely controlled experiment? How would a researcher know that he had controlled all possible extraneous variables?

5. A dictionary definition of "chance" is "something that befalls as the result of unknown or unconsidered forces." Does the term "forces" in this definition mean the same as "extraneous variables" as used in research design? Look up the definition of the term "random" and discuss its relationship to "chance."

6. Explain the following mathematical terms:

a. Linear equation	g. Exponent
b. Function	h. Stochastic process
c. Nonlinear equation	i. Nonparametric
d. Slope of a line	j. Algorithm
e. Parameter	k. Subjective probability
f. Coefficient	

7. How does random assignment differ from random sampling? How are these procedures alike? Why is the use of a table of random sampling numbers a better way of randomizing than a lottery-type drawing of names?

8. Read the book *Explanation in Social Science* by Robert Brown (Chicago, Aldine Publishing Co., 1963, 198 pp.). How many different methods of explanation about social phenomena does the author present? Comment on the following statement by the author, "Most work in the social sciences, like most work in history and in the natural sciences, is not directly concerned with the furnishing of explanations. It may well be true, as is so often said, that the tasks of any empirical science are to explain, predict, and to apply. But in any such field these tasks are embedded in a workload that may be referred to as identification, classification, description, and measuring and reporting as well." (p. 47.)

9. The following eight references report on studies that have at least some aspects of an experimental design. Read them and determine which of the designs summarized in Table 6-1 were employed in each of the studies:

    a. Peter K. New, Gladys Nite and Josephine Callahan, *Nursing Service and Patient Care: A Staffing Experiment.* Kansas City, Mo., Community Studies, Inc., 1959.

    b. Mildred Struve and Eugene Levine, "Disposable and Reusable Surgeon's Gloves." *Nursing Res.,* **10:**79–86, spring 1961.

    c. Phyllis A. Tryon, "The Effect of Patient Participation in Decision Making on the Outcome of a Nursing Procedure" in Monograph No. 19 of papers presented at the clinical sessions, of the 1962 American Nurses' Association Convention. New York, American Nurses Association, 1962, pp. 14–18.

    d. Therese K. Cheyovich, Charles E. Lewis, and Susan R. Gortner. *The Nurse Practitioner in an Adult Outpatient Clinic.* DHEW Publication No. (HRA) 76–20, Washington, D.C., U.S. Government Printing Office, 1976.

    e. M. R. Kinney, "Effects of Preoperative Teaching Upon Patients with Differing Modes of Response to Threatening Stimuli," *Int. J. Nurs. Stud.,* **14:**49–59, 1977.

    f. Loretta T. Zderad, "A Study of the Effectiveness of a Cooperative Group Method in Teaching Basic Psychiatric Nursing." *Nursing Res.,* **2:**126–137, February 1954.

    g. Mark Mulder and Al Stemerding, "Threat, Attraction to Group, and Need for Strong Leadership." *Human Relations,* **16:**317–334, November 1963.

    h. Sally O'Neil, "The Application and Methodological Implications of Behavior Modification in Nursing Research," in *Communication Nursing Research: The Many Sources of Nursing Knowledge.* Boulder, Col. The Western Interstate Commission for Higher Education, November 1972, pp. 177–191.

10. Why is it important to equalize the composition of the comparison groups in an experiment? Discuss the various methods for achieving such equalization in an experiment. Is it ever possible to obtain perfect equalization of the groups? Discuss methods for equalizing the groups in an explanatory survey and in this connection read Chapter 7 of Hyman's *Survey Design and Analysis* (Glencoe, The Free Press, 1955, pp. 295–329), "The Introduction of Additional Variables and the Elaboration of the Analysis."

11. In experimental studies of patient care, what are some of the sources of sociopsychological biases? What are the methods by which they can be controlled? Is it really possible to eliminate completely the "Hawthorne effect" from the usual kinds of patient care studies that are conceived?

12. Comment on the following statement by R. A. Fisher in his *The Design of Experiments* (London, Oliver and Boyd, 1935 ed., p. 8): "Experimental observations are only experience, carefully planned in advance, and designed to form a secure basis of new knowledge. That is they are systematically related to the body of knowledge already acquired, and the results are deliberately observed and put on record accurately."

13. What are the advantages and disadvantages of introducing more explanatory variables into an experimental study? What are some guidelines that a researcher can use in determining the most pertinent explanatory variables for his study? Why is a "factorial design" considered to be an efficient experimental design?

14. A factorial experiment in which each factor is tested at two levels is called a 2^n factorial experiment. If the number of different factors is 3, there would be 2^3 different combinations possible or 8 ($2^3 = 2 \times 2 \times 2$). If the factors are tested at 3 levels it would be called a 3^n experiment. How many different combinations would be possible in an experiment that consisted of 6 factors: 2 of which have 2 levels, 2 have 3 levels, and 2 consist of 4 levels? Does the term "interaction" mean the same as "combination" as used here? (Note: see a book such as Cochran and Cox, *Experimental Designs*. New York, John Wiley and Sons, 1957, Chapter V, "Factorial Experiments," for a discussion of interaction in factorial designs.)

15. Obtain a copy of a table of random numbers, such as in appendix b of Phillips and Thompson *Statistics for Nurses* (New York, Macmillan Publishing Co., Inc., 1967). Using the table, create a hypothetical experiment in which 100 subjects are randomly allocated into four comparison groups.

16. Discuss the statement that a cohort study is "actually a series of cross-sectional surveys repeated over a period of time for the same study population." Give five examples of well-known cross-sectional surveys that are conducted in the health field. By definition are all experimental studies prospectively longitudinal? Are they also cohort studies?

17. Critique the study conducted by Lenn, Gurel and Lenn, "Patient Outcome as a Measure of Quality of Nursing Home Care" (*Am. J. Public Health,* **67**:337–344, April 1977). What techniques were used to control extraneous variables? What extraneous variables would affect patient outcome?

18. Read Chapter 3 of Philip J. Runkel and Joseph E. McGrath, *Research on Human Behavior: A Systematic Guide to Method.* New York, Holt Rinehart, and Winston, Inc., 1972, pp. 35–80. Discuss some of the practical advice the authors give in relation to planning a study.

19. Read Theodore X Barber's *Pitfalls in Human Research: Ten Pivotal Points.* New York, Pergamon Press, Inc., 1976. Which of the pitfalls are most serious? Which of the pitfalls can be controlled by careful research design?

20. What are some of the difficulties in long-term longitudinal research? What are some of the advantages of this type of research? In this regard read Lucille Knopf's *RN's One and Five Years After Graduation.* New York, National League for Nursing, 1975. What was the attrition rate among study participants? Was this a high rate as compared to other longitudinal studies?

Chapter Seven

MEASUREMENT OF VARIABLES IN RESEARCH

THE SUCCESS of a research study is dependent upon how well the various steps in the research process have been formulated. These steps are like links in a chain. If one is defective the entire chain may fail. Often, the weakest link in the chain of steps composing the research process is the definition and measurement of the variables included in the study. Deficiencies in this area can destroy the validity of the total research effort, particularly in explanatory research. The purpose of this chapter is to discuss ways of defining and measuring the variables being studied, to describe criteria for evaluating this process of definition and measurement, and to give examples of some measures of variables useful in patient care studies.

DEFINITION OF VARIABLES

In descriptive research no distinction is usually made among the variables studied according to which are dependent variables and which are independent. Where quantitative data are to be collected concerning these variables it is important that the plan for the descriptive study contain a skeleton outline of the statistical tabulations, called dummy tables, to be made of these data. These dummy tables serve to indicate the nature of the variables included in the study. Their preparation in advance of the actual study will assist in sharpening up the definition of the variables as well as indicating how they are to be measured.

Explanatory research is usually concerned with testing a hypothesis about a relationship between an independent variable (causal, treatment, stimulus variable) and a dependent variable (effect, response, or criterion variable). In explanatory research the independent variable is manipulated by the researcher. The effects produced by these manipulations among a group of study subjects are evaluated in terms of some measure of the response in the dependent variable, called a criterion measure. In addition to these variables, explanatory research also includes variables that are not of specific interest to the researcher but are present in the research situation and can, if uncontrolled, influence the findings concerning the relationship among the explanatory variables. These are called extraneous variables. They are of two major types: organismic variables related to the characteristics of individual research subjects themselves, and environmental variables that are related to the characteristics of forces external to the study subjects.

While it is generally necessary to identify only the major extraneous variables in a study, it is essential that all explanatory variables be operationally defined. As has been stated previously, an operational definition is the use of a series of words that clearly designate performable and observable acts or operations that can be verified by others. Thus if our hypothesis is that the quality of nursing care (independent variable) is related to patient welfare (dependent variable), we must be able to define each variable operationally. Quality of nursing care must be defined as certain actions on the part of the nursing staff that can be consistently observed and evaluated by independent observers. Patient welfare must be defined in terms of some objective indicator of a patient's response to the care he receives.

Direct and Indirect Definition of Variables

In defining variables in research we need not always use literal constructs. It sometimes may be more advantageous to define variables indirectly. A literal definition of patient welfare might be the degree to which the patient is well—that is, free from illness. However, a valid measure of this variable is not available at the present time, so that we could not use it in a study. Therefore, we might use a more indirect definition as the basis for valid measurement of this variable. Thus, patient welfare might be defined as the extent to which a patient requests a tranquilizing, sleep-inducing, or pain-relieving drug. This may not be a direct measure of patient welfare if defined as the degree of freedom from illness, but it may well be a correlated variable, so that low usage of such drugs is consistently associated with a high degree of freedom from illness, and vice versa.

Indirect measures of variables are widely used in psychological measurement. Thus, the variable "personality" can be assessed in terms of literal evidence as the way in which the subject responds to such questions as, "Do you like to be with other people?" "Do you like members of the other sex?" "Would you rather be a politician or a hermit?" "Do you like to watch fires?" Personality can also be assessed in terms of nondirective measures such as the thematic apperception test, where the respondent describes what he sees in a series of pictures, or in terms of even more nondirective measures, as the Rorschach test in which the subject describes what he sees in inkblots.

The variable "creativity" is currently being given considerable attention because of the search for people with scientific talent. Literal measures of this variable assess a person's capability to produce something original. Originality can be measured, for example, by asking the respondent to provide titles to a synopsis of a movie plot, or to create new things from such disparate items as a nail and a stick, or a piece of string and a stone. Somewhat more nondirective is the type of measure of creativity based on a respondent's reaction to such questions as, "What would happen if there were no longer any nighttime?" "What would happen if people lost their ability to speak?" "What would happen if money became value-less as a medium of exchange?"

Defining the Independent Variable   The independent variable repre-sents the characteristic by which the alternative groups we are studying are distinguished. Usually the independent variable is divided into a few discrete groups distinguished from each other in some meaningful way. Thus, in the hypothesis linking smoking to lung cancer, the independent variable may be divided into two categories, smoker or nonsmoker, with a smoker being defined as someone who smokes at least one cigarette a day. For greater refinement more than two categories can be established—as, for example, nonsmoker, light smoker, moderate smoker, and heavy smoker. Definition of these categories might be nonsmoker: no cigarettes smoked; light smoker: less than 15 cigarettes smoked a day; moderate smoker: 15 to 30 cigarettes a day; heavy smoker: more than 30 cigarettes a day.

In the hypothesis relating type of nursing education program to pro-ficiency as a graduate nurse, the independent variable might consist of the categories: diploma program, associate degree program, and baccalaureate degree program. For the hypothesis testing the relationship between nursing care and patient welfare, the independent variable could be various arrangements of the nursing team: 25 per cent professional nurses, 25 per cent practical nurses, 50 per cent nursing aides, or 50 per cent professionals, 25 per cent practical nurses, and 25 per cent nursing aides.

In some studies the independent variable might be numerous finely graded classes of the variable, such as different dosage levels of a drug, different amounts of caloric intake of food, or varying amounts of ex-posure time to a medical treatment, an education program, or some other stimulus.

There are three important objectives in defining the independent vari-able. First, the various subdivisions or categories of the variable should be sharply distinguished from each other. Moreover, they should be mutually exclusive. This means that a subject could be placed in only one category of the variable with no overlapping possible. Thus, if our independent variable is the amount of cholesterol intake in the subject's diet, and if the variable has three categories—high, medium, and low—it should only be possible to classify a study subject in one of the categories and none of the others.

Second, the distinction between the categories should be meaningfully directed toward the research problem. Thus, if we are interested in measuring the effect on patient recovery of various types of physical facilities in hospitals, such as intensive care units versus conventional units, the alternative versions of the independent variable being tested—types of patient care facilities—should be defined so as to truly and completely represent the different facilities. The definition should not refer to just one aspect of the variable, such as the ready availability of certain supplies and equipment, or to some other variable altogether, such as nurse staffing pattern.

Third, the definition of the independent variable must remain constant throughout the period in which the study subjects are exposed to it, as well as during the analysis of the data. If we were to shift definitions, so that some subjects are exposed to one definition and other subjects to another, we would in effect be introducing a new variable. To illustrate, if experimentally we wanted to test the effect of a certain dosage level of a drug on the responses of patients, and if after a series of trials we were to find no response among the patients, we might be tempted to increase the dosage level if we felt it was not sufficiently potent. By increasing the potency we have in fact established a new alternative of the independent variable. Unless we treat it as such, we might not make the proper interpretation of our data.

More subtly, in a partially controlled experimental study of the effect of a new method of ordering and delivering drugs on the incidence of medication errors, some of the physicians and nurses might not obey the protocols of the study and continue to order and deliver drugs in the same old way. In such a situation another alternative version of the independent variable is actually present in the study and is being tested. If the investigator were unaware of this situation, the relationship he discovers between the independent variable he thinks he is testing and the dependent variable might be a spurious one.

Defining the Dependent Variable   While the independent variable is applied to the study subjects as a group, with all members of a group receiving the same alternative, the response in the dependent variable is measured for each subject separately. While our concern with the independent variable is primarily one of definition, with the dependent variable we have to consider the dual problem of definition and measurement.

To illustrate this point we can begin by stating that the fundamental design for explanatory research is one in which differences in the independent variable—usually just a few fixed groups (values)—are assessed in terms of differences in the dependent variable—often numerous values. Thus, in testing the effect of an appetite-depressing drug on weight reduction, we might give one group of subjects the drug and the other group a placebo. After a period of time we measure the body weight of *each* subject in the alternative groups and compare the amount of weight change occurring in the two groups. The independent variable in this example possesses just two values—administering the weight-reduction drug and withholding the drug. On the other hand, the dependent variable, defined as change in body weight, possesses many values and is measured in terms of a highly refined, multivalued scientific scale such as body weight.

In some studies the dependent variable may have as few groups as the independent variable. Thus, in the study discussed in the last chapter in which the effects of a health education program on the polio immunization rate were evaluated, the independent variable had two categories—exposed to the educational material and not exposed to the material—and so did the dependent variable—vaccinated, not vaccinated. The main difference between the two variables is that while both had to be carefully defined—What is a health education program? What do we mean by vaccinated?—it was the latter variable that was "measured," the measurement consisting of counting the number of people in each of the two categories of the vaccination scale.

The remainder of this chapter will deal with the problem of definition and measurement of the dependent variable. Known in explanatory research as the *criterion measure,* definition and measurement of this variable are the most crucial phases of this important type of research.

QUANTIFICATION IN RESEARCH

The definition of the variables in a study provides a framework for determining how the variables in the study will be measured. Measurement depends on the gradations, levels, or degrees of difference possessed by the variable we are studying. In the process of measurement we are essentially determining into which of these graded categories the phenomenon we are observing belongs. These categories may be of a qualitative nature—as, for example, the statement that the patient feels warm. Here the variable is body temperature, and the gradations of our measuring device, called a scale, may simply be below normal, normal, warm, hot. Or the measuring device may have a quantitative scale and be graded into finely distinguished numerical values, ranging from 94.0° F. to 109.9° F, a total of 160 different scale points, not merely 4, as in the qualitative scale.

Both types of scales provide a means of obtaining numerical values for the observations made of the variable. In a qualitative scale we observe the subject, and on the basis of the definition of the variable we place him into one of its categories. We observe the next subject and place him into the applicable category, and so on. If we applied the qualitative temperature scale to a group of 100 subjects, we could accumulate data like these:

Temperature	Number of Patients
Total	100
Below normal	5
Normal	70
Warm	20
Hot	5

Thus, through a process of counting, we have derived some interesting quantitative data which serve as a measurement of the condition of our subjects. As a summary of the data we can say that 70 per cent of our subjects have normal temperatures.

Qualitative scales of measurement like these are sometimes called *enumeration scales*. The numerical data they yield are called *frequency data*. They show the frequency with which the subjects studied possess each of the discrete categories of the scale.

Variables such as body temperature can be measured by a scientific instrument. The temperature instrument is called a thermometer. Its scale is in quantitative form, ranging perhaps from 94.0° F. to 109.9° F. Such quantitative scales are sometimes called *measurement scales* because of the wide and continuous range of values to which a subject can be assigned and because the properties of the scales are such that we can assess the meaning of the intervals along the scale. That is to say, with the qualitative temperature scale we cannot objectively evaluate differences in temperature. In comparing a subject classified in the "hot" category with one in the "warm" group, we know one is hotter than the other, but the term "hotter" is highly subjective. However, we can say that a subject with a temperature 104° F. is 5° hotter than one with 99° F. This 5° difference has an important significance in evaluating the health status of the two patients.

The quantitative data yielded by the measurement scale for body temperature would be recorded as follows:

Temperature in Fahrenheit	Number of Patients
98.1	1
98.2	3
98.3	0
98.4	4
98.5	5
98.6	12
98.7	9
98.8	8
98.9	4
99.0	6
99.1	4
99.2	3
99.3	5
etc.	

These data, for convenience in analysis, can be grouped as follows:

Temperature Total	Number of Patients 100
Under 98.6	13
98.6–99.6	61
99.7–100.9	19
101 and over	7

Whether the scale is a verbal or a numerical one it can yield numerical data that can be of value in a study. The verbal scale yields a qualitative classification value for each study subject and numerically provides a count of the total number of study subjects possessing each of the qualitative values contained in the scale. The numerical scale provides a quantitative measurement value for each study subject and can also provide a count of the total number of study subjects possessing each quantitative value in the scale.

Use of Nonquantitative Data in Research

Not all research requires data to be in quantitative form. Certain types of descriptive research, such as case studies, contain for the most part verbal descriptions of the subject encompassed by the study. Anthropological research is largely of this type, and so is psychologically oriented research employing the psychoanalytic approach.

Most studies use both quantified and nonquantified data. Narrative descriptive statements are often included in the analysis of the data not only to add more interest to the report of the study, but to provide more meaning and insight into the interpretation of the data.

One of the most frequent uses of narrative data is the quotation of verbatim statements by individual study subjects. An example of such a quotation, from a study of nurses' attitudes toward the people they work with, illustrates the usefulness of quotations in clarifying the meaning of variables and other concepts employed in the study.

Another recurrent theme in these early talks with nurses was deep concern about "the move away from the bedside." But there was by no means complete agreement about what this meant or what should be done about it. Some were worried because nurses did not have, or would not take, enough time for individual and intimate contact with patients. One typical head nurse, assailed with increasing paper work and administrative duties, was waiting for the proverbial day when the utilization of ward clerks or floor managers would free her to devote more time to her patients and her nursing staff. One supervisor, taking another tack, blamed the training of present day graduates for their "carelessness about details" and "their lack of devotion"; she felt that "something fine had gone out of nursing."[1]

Sometimes verbal descriptive data are used as a substitute for quantitative data. This is done to avoid overwhelming the reader with excessive amounts of numerical data or to guide the reader's attention to the main interpretative points the writer wishes to make. A typical statement of this kind is:

In those services for which there are few incidents reported, the medication load is relatively light and most of the medicines are given by graduate nurses and doctors. The close correspondence between the proportion of medicines given by student nurses and the proportion of incidents they reported suggests that the job classification may not be as important a variable as the medication load or other factors associated with a particular service.[2]

Where such verbal presentation is employed, the numerical data are often also included. Thus, the nonquantified data do not replace quantified data but serve as a embellishment of them. It is rare that nonquantified data can provide the total data for a study.

One of the deficiencies of nonquantified data is the lack of objectivity resulting from the use of many evaluative terms in analyzing data of this kind. To illustrate, we can discuss the data on the body temperatures of the 100 research subjects as follows: "A few subjects had below normal temperatures, the majority had normal temperatures, some were warm, and a small group had temperatures that could be described as hot."

A shortcoming of this statement is that terms like "a few," "some," "a small group," and even "the majority" may mean different things to different people. Such terminology lacks the precision that is obtained from the use of numerical data. And in research the aim should be to maximize the precision of the analysis of the findings through the use of as sensitive data as are available. Nonquantitative data should be used very selectively. They can be most useful in enriching the analysis of the research and in providing insights into the meaning of the phenomena being observed:

> The inspection of nonquantified data may be particularly helpful if it is done periodically throughout a study rather than postponed to the end of the statistical analysis. Frequently, a single incident noted by a perceptive observer contains the clue to an understanding of a phenomenon. If the social scientist becomes aware of this implication at a moment when he can still add to his material or exploit further the data he has already collected, he may considerably enrich the quality of his conclusions.[3]

The Importance of Quantification in Research

The use of quantification in research enables us not only to state that a subject's temperature is warmer or colder than normal, but to state how much different from normal it is. Being able to state the extent of difference can provide us with a sensitive and perceptive description of the variables we are studying. As Cohen and Nagel[4] have remarked:

> Both in daily life and in the sciences, however, it is often essential to replace propositions simply affirming or denying qualitative differences by propositions indicating in a more precise way the degree of such differences. It is essential to do so in the interest of discovering comprehensive principles in terms of which the subject matter can be conceived as systematically related. Thus we may believe that there is more unemployment this year than last, or that winters during our childhood were more severe than those during the past few years. But it may be important to know how much more unemployment there is, or how much less severe the winters have become; for if we can state the differences in terms of degrees of differences, we not only guard ourselves against the errors of hasty, untutored impressions, but also lay the foundation for an adequately grounded control of the indicated changes.

Quantification in research provides the following important benefits:

1. It enhances the preciseness and objectivity of the data. Evaluative statements like "after treatment the patient's temperature became warmer" or "most patients were discharged after a short stay in the hospital" can mean different things to different people. But statements like "after treatment the patient's temperature rose from 99° F. to 101° F." and "90 per cent of the patients were discharged from the hospital in 7 days or less" not only are more exact but have a certain universality of meaning. Indeed, numbers are a universal language. It could well be possible to understand the statistical data contained in a research report written in a foreign language even if the text were incomprehensible.

2. Quantification performs the function of a type of shorthand in the collection, tabulation, and analysis of data. How cumbersome it would be, for example, if the observations made in a research study, in which

the criterion measure was body weight, were in a qualitative rather than quantitative form. How would we record such observations, and how would we analyze the data if we did not use numbers? It is unquestionably simpler to record our observations as 156 pounds, 190 pounds, 210 pounds, etc.

3. Highly developed statistical techniques are available for analyzing numerical data. Such techniques permit us to obtain the maximum amount of information from the data. Quantification thus provides for efficiency and economy in the conduct of research.

4. When data are in numerical form a researcher can compare his results with those obtained in other studies. Quantification thus provides a means of linking up the data from different studies to provide the basis for the accumulation of a body of scientific knowledge.

5. When data are in quantitative form the investigator has greater control over the research than if nonquantitative data are used. For example, certain checks can be performed to test the reliability of the data which depend on mathematical models requiring numerical data such as the normal curve of error.

6. When a relationship is found among variables that can be expressed in quantitative form, a high degree of control over the behavior of the dependent variable is available. Through such a relationship we know when we change the independent variable a certain quantitative amount we will also thereby change the value of the dependent variable by a certain predictable amount.

SCALES UNDERLYING VARIABLES

The notion of the scale underlying the variable has been introduced in the example of the qualitative and quantitative evaluation of patients' temperatures. In the qualitative scale a set of verbal categories are established, each distinguished from the other in terms of certain meaningful characteristics. For the variable "temperature" we developed four categories: below normal, normal, warm, and hot. Each class should be described in such a way as to permit the user of this scale, the observer, to unequivocally place a subject being rated into one of the alternative classes on the scale. This could be accomplished by the observer's touching of the subject's brow or by some other means that would provide the observer with sufficient information to make a suitable rating.

The quantitative scale for determining a patient's body temperature consists of an instrument whose scale is calibrated in finely divided numerical gradations. When the instrument is applied to the subject it provides a reading of the quantity of temperature possessed by the subject.

There are several differences between the two types of scales:

1. In the qualitative scale the assignment of the subject to the appropriate category depends on the observer's ability to interpret the characteristics distinguishing one class of the scale from another. For many qualitative scales such characteristics may be subjective in that appropriate distinctions depend on the observer's senses—touch, in the case of temperature—or other judgmental and interpretative factors which may not easily be standardized and may vary from observer to observer in unpredictable ways. In the quantitative scale, a so-called scientific measuring instrument is used. By the use of this impersonal instrument, objectivity of measurement is enhanced through the elimination of the influence of the observer's personal judgment in determining the class to which the subject belongs. But even a quantitative measure is not free of observer bias. The instrument still has to be read by the observer, and in this reading process, as many studies have shown, certain subjective elements associated with the ability, attitudes, and personality of the observer may create bias.

2. A qualitative scale usually has only a few discrete categories, while a quantitative scale has many gradations. Theoretically these gradations are infinite, since numbers can be expressed not only in whole units but in fractions of whole numbers as well. Thus if our thermometer were refined enough we might be able to read a subject's temperature as 98.66754° F. in contrast to another subject's temperature of 98.66755° F. Naturally, for all practical purposes these temperatures are identical. But this illustration indicates the potential power of the quantitative scale in making very refined distinctions.

Many qualitative scales consist of just two categories: male-female, dead-alive, sick-healthy, nurse-nonnurse, inpatient-outpatient, and so on. However, there are qualitative scales that contain as many as hundreds or even a thousand categories. Studies of the functions of professional nurses, for example, have developed a classification of over 400 distinct activities. And the *Standard Nomenclature of Diseases and Operations* lists thousands of distinct diseases known to human beings.

3. A major advantage of a quantitative scale is that it provides a means for determining not only that one subject is different from another in terms of the variable being scaled, but also *how much* different he is. A subject who weighs 180 pounds is 30 pounds heavier than one who weighs 150 pounds. Additionally, we can say that the first subject is 20 per cent heavier than the other. In a qualitative body weight scale consisting simply of the categories underweight, normal, and overweight, we cannot say how much different a subject classified in one category is from one classified in another. A quantitative scale thus provides more discriminating information than does a qualitative one.

4. Perhaps the major advantage of a qualitative scale is its descriptive value. Particularly to the consumer of research findings it is often more meaningful to state that "40 per cent of the patients went from over-weight to normal after being subjected to a weight reduction program" than to report that "the average reduction in body weight for the patients in the program was 22.5 pounds." Sometimes, in reporting the results of research, data originally collected by use of a quantitative scale are transformed into a qualitative scale. Data collected by a thermometer might be reported as "70 per cent of the patients had normal temperatures after treatment, while 30 per cent of the patients had elevated tempera-tures after treatment." Thus two qualitative classes, normal and elevated, have replaced a wide range of numerical values.

TYPES OF SCALES

We have used the terms "qualitative" and "quantitative" to distinguish the two major types of scales that are used to measure the variables in research studies. With a qualitative scale we can "measure" by determining how many subjects possess each discrete scale category. With a quantitative scale we can measure the numerical extent to which each subject possesses the variable studied. As has been hinted, these scales are not worlds apart but actually represent different phases in the development of a measuring instrument. Thus, we may in the early stages of development employ a crude, qualitatively differentiated scale to distinguish between the objects we are classifying. In the early history of nursing care, the fact that a patient had fever or not was determined in the way previously described, by touching the patient and making what essentially is a subjective evaluation of whether the temperature was elevated or not. Over the years, with the perfection of scientific instrumentation a numerical scale became available in the form of a thermometer, which when applied to a body cavity gives a quantitative measurement of body temperature.

For many variables for which today only qualitative scales are available, a numerical scale might be developed at some future time. Thus, the variable sex is usually differentiated in terms of two classes—male and female. However, it may be possible to develop a quantitative measure of the degree of maleness or femaleness based on measurement of some biological or physiological characteristic that when applied to a subject would supply a numerical value similar to that provided by a weight scale or a thermometer. The variable hair color is usually scaled in terms of four qualitative categories: black, brown, blond, red. Since color can be measured quantitatively in terms of the wavelength of the light it emits, it is possible to scale hair color (or eye or skin color) numerically.

Similarly we have shown that quantitative scales are often transformed into qualitative scales. This is done to clarify the meaning of the data as well as to put them into a form that would be operationally more useful. Every numerical scale can thus be recast in the form of a verbal one. But to accomplish the reverse procedure requires the availability of appropriate measuring instruments.

In the present stage of development many of the criterion measures employed in patient care research are qualitative in nature, particularly those related to psychological or sociological phenomena. Only when physiological variables are being measured can a significant number of quantitative criterion measures be found.

Scaling theorists have identified four distinct types of scales. Two of these are qualitative and two are quantitative. Each will be briefly discussed.

QUALITATIVE SCALES

Nominal Scale

This is the most fundamental and, particularly in descriptive research, one of the most widely used scales of all. As its name implies, a nominal scale is essentially a scale in name only. It consists of a number of discrete, mutually exclusive categories of a variable, each possessing a distinctive attribute in terms of the variable, but otherwise there is no necessary relationship between the categories. In applying such a scale, an individual is assigned to the appropriate category according to the definition of the category. Among the many variables found in studies in nursing that possess nominal scales are: occupational field, race, marital status, religion, nationality, type of illness, and cause of death. Nominal scales vary in size from those having just two categories to those with numerous categories. An example of the former is the variable "sex": male-female. An example of the latter is "type of illness."

Quantitative data are generated with the use of nominal scales by counting the number of subjects that are classified in each of the categories contained in the scale. Such data, called frequency or enumeration data, are usually summarized in terms of the percentage of subjects in each of the categories: the number of subjects in each category is divided by the total number of subjects being rated and the resulting number (the quotient) is multiplied by 100.

Sometimes numbers are assigned to represent the different categories. For the variable "marital status," the number 1 might be assigned to married, 2 to single, 3 for widowed, and 4 for divorced or separated. The assignment of these numbers is a labeling procedure known as *coding*. It is essentially a form of shorthand that expedites the tabulation of the data. Such labeling has no other quantitative meaning.

It is possible to relate data on variables possessing nominal scales by a statistical technique known as attribute correlation. For example, suppose we are able to classify a group of patients composing a case load of a visiting nurse association according to their marital status and whether they are receiving service because of cardiovascular illness or some other type of illness. It would be possible to determine if there were a relationship between the two variables (associative, of course, not causal) by a procedure known as cross-tabulating the data:

| | Illness Category | | |
Marital Status	Cardiovascular	Other	Total
Single	5	95	100
Married	50	100	150
Total	55	195	250

Such figures would indicate that for the 250 patients in the study there was indeed a high relationship between the two variables—most patients with cardiovascular illness are married. Of course, such a relationship does not mean that a married person is more likely to acquire a cardiovascular illness than is a single person. The true interpretation might well be that another variable, age, which has not been controlled in the data analysis, is the underlying causal factor, being directly related both to marital status (the older a person is, the more apt he is to be married) and to illness (the older a person is, the more apt he is to have a cardiovascular illness).

As criterion measures, nominal scales leave much to be desired. Many nominal scales often describe invariant properties of people, such as race, sex, nationality. Therefore they cannot be used as criterion measures of whether a change in the dependent variable is indicative of, say, improvement or lack of improvement among the subjects studied. A nominal scale is essentially a sorting device for grouping the subjects into different pigeonholes. Evaluatively, these pigeonholes may have no connection with each other. That is to say, there is no underlying continuum for the scale which links the different categories together in terms of some graded order.

Ordinal Scale

A more highly developed form of qualitative scale is one that actually relates the different categories included in the scale in terms of a graded order. This grading or ranking may be according to some underlying continuum of intensity, as in most intense to least intense; or quantity, as in highest amount to lowest; distance, nearest to furthest; strength, strongest to weakest; emotion, happiest to saddest; preference, love to hate; and so on.

Ordinal scales are utilized in a manner similar to that of nominal scales. Definitions of each scale category are provided, and the observer applying the scale places the subject into that category which the subject most closely fits. Ordinal scales can also be used as self-rating instruments in which the subject places himself in the category he feels is most appropriate. An example of the latter is the typical type of rating scale given to patients to evaluate nursing services: "How did you like the nursing care you received: Excellent, very good, average, poor?"

Most ordinal scales have only a few categories. Very common are scales with three or five categories, a middle, neutral point and one or two classes on the upper and lower ends. Few scales of this type have more than ten groups, since it is difficult to make fine qualitative distinctions beyond that number.

Quantification of data collected with ordinal scales is similar to that employed in the use of nominal scales. Counts are made of the number of subjects in each category. These counts are converted to percentages to show the relative frequency of occurrence of each scale value among the subjects studied. The most typical scale value, an average called the mode, is the one in which more of the subjects are placed than in any other. Also, numbers may be assigned to each scale value to show the rank order of the values (excellent—1, very good—2, average—3, poor—4). Through such ranking procedure it is possible to analyze the relationships between several variables that are ordinally scaled by using a statistical procedure known as correlation of ranked data. To illustrate, suppose we obtained a rating from a group of ten patients, each in different hospitals, of their satisfaction with nursing care and placed these on an ordinal scale having four categories ranked from 1 to 4. At the same time suppose a group of expert judges rated the adequacy of the nursing services provided to the patients, also in terms of a four-point scale. The data we gather might appear as follows (1 = best, 4 = worst):

Patient No.	Rating of Adequacy of Care	Rating of Satisfaction with Care
1	2	3
2	1	1
3	2	2
4	1	2
5	4	3
6	4	4
7	1	1
8	2	3
9	3	3
10	1	2

By inspection it can be seen that there is quite a high relationship (correlation) between the two ratings. For five patients, both ratings are identical. For the others the ratings are never more than one category apart. Statistical techniques are available for actually measuring the magnitude of the correlation between the two variables.

One of the limitations of the ordinal scale is the fact that there is no way of evaluating the interval between one scale category and another. We do not know in the example just given whether the difference between 1 and 2, excellent and very good, is the same as the distance between 2 and 3, very good and average. Nor can we say that the interval between 1 and 3 has twice the value as the interval between 1 and 2, or 2 and 3.

But even with this limitation, ordinal scales can serve useful purposes as criterion measures, since they do provide a means of evaluating the effects of manipulating an independent variable. A scale like the one just mentioned of adequacy of nursing care can be used to evaluate different types of staffing patterns, physical facilities, nursing care provided, or some other kind of independent variable. However, in such uses another shortcoming of an ordinal scale often becomes apparent. This is a lack of sensitivity in a scale that consists of only a limited number of categories. With only four or five, or even seven, scale points it may be difficult to detect fine differences produced by the independent variable. Only by use of more sensitive measuring instruments can such subtle effects be detected.

Ordinal Scales in Social Science Research

Perhaps the most ambitious efforts to develop ordinal scales have been made in the field of social psychology. Primarily concerned with the area of attitude testing, such pioneers as Thurstone, Likert, Guttman, and Stevens have done a great deal of work in developing scales for measuring such variables as morale, prejudice, and political orientation. A brief description of the more widely used of these scaling methods follows.

Graphic Rating Scales In this method the variable is qualitatively scaled along a continuum from one extreme to the other. The rater, who may be the study subject himself, or an expert judge or some other type of observer, places a check mark at that point on the scale which most closely represents his evaluation of the degree to which the object being rated possesses the variable studied. An example of such a scale for evaluating adequacy of nursing care is:

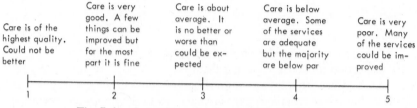

Fig. 7–1. A graphic rating for assessing nursing care.

Although equally spaced, the true intervals between the five scale points have not actually been determined. Therefore, the scale is of the ordinal type. One of the disadvantages of such a scale is the tendency of the rater to avoid the extreme categories. This results in a pile-up in the central classes which reduces the sensitivity of the measuring instrument. One way of avoiding this bias is to omit the central category. This forces the rater to take a position in one direction or the other.

In order to increase the sensitivity of the measurement, some rating scales permit the rater to indicate his evaluation by placing a mark between the categories. The rating might then be scored as a fractional estimate of the distance between the two categories: 2.8, 3.4, 4.1, and so on. The fallacy in such a procedure is that it assumes that the intervals between the scale points are equal, or that they have some quantitative significance. If this assumption were correct, this type of scale would be a quantitative rather than a qualitative scale. However, such scales are indeed qualitative and the only meaning that can be assigned to the numbers on the scale—1, 2, 3, 4, 5—is a positional one. They provide an indication of the rank order of the scale categories. That is to say, they show the ordinal relationship of the categories to each other rather than the quantitative degree to which the object being rated possesses the variable.

Thurstone-Type Scale   In this scale, an attempt is made to establish the quantitative distance between the categories included in the scale. Instead of having a rater make a direct rating on the scale, as in the graphic type of scale, a battery of statements—as many as 20 to 25—is presented to the rater, and he checks those statements which most closely represent his position. Since each statement has a previously established scale value, which of course is not shown on the checklist, it is possible to obtain a numerical rating for the individual rater by computing the average scale value for the statements he checks.

The scale values for the statements included in such a checklist are determined in the following manner, through a method known as "equal-appearing intervals." First, the variable being scaled is clearly defined. Then the scale developer collects as many statements as possible representing different evaluative positions along the continuum underlying the variable. Thus, if the variable were "adequacy of patient care," defined as patient's feelings toward the care he receives, examples of typical statements might be:

1. My nurse is very friendly and pays a lot of attention to me.
2. I feel that I am not told enough about my care.
3. I cannot wait until I am able to go home. This institution is very poorly run.

4. Everybody seems so rushed around here, I often feel that I am imposing on the staff when I request a needed service.
5. The food they serve here is as good as that in some of the best restaurants I have eaten in.
6. I cannot sleep very well; there is too much noise and the light shines in from the hallway.

The procedure for selecting and scaling the items for the final checklist is to have a large number of expert judges sort the items into eleven piles. The piles are considered to be equally spaced in value and represent different scale points along the continuum underlying the variable. Thus for the variable "adequacy of patient care," the first pile would be for the statements representing highest adequacy of care, the second pile for the next highest, and so on down to the eleventh pile, which would contain statements representing the lowest adequacy of care. The sixth, or middle, pile is the center point representing care that is neither adequate or inadequate. For each of the sortings by the judges a statement is assigned a value from, say, 1 to 11, depending upon which pile it is placed into. After all sortings have been completed by the judges, the average value is computed for each of the statements. A final selection of statements is made to compose a checklist consisting of about 15 to 20 items whose average values spread over the scale from one extreme to the other. Statements are selected that have been consistently rated by the individual judges and are clear and unambiguous in meaning. When completed by a respondent the checklist yields a numerical score that is arrived at by summing up the values of the checked items.

Unlike the numbers on a graphic rating scale, which only indicate the rank order position of the categories, a Likert-type scale produces a numerical score that supposedly expresses the degree to which the variable is possessed by the object rated. For this reason it is considered to be superior to an ordinal scale, as it is reputed to be a quantitative scale whose values can be analyzed by refined statistical techniques. However, many authorities in the field of scaling techniques have questioned whether the method of equal-appearing intervals does in fact produce a numerical scale in which the intervals between the scale points have a valid numerical meaning. The main criticism concerns the assumption that the distance between the eleven piles can be quantitatively assessed by the judges:

Even though judges consider the eleven piles as being equal distances apart, this does not mean that the processes inferred from the statements actually change linearly with these perceived equal distances. This places on the unsophisticated judge the responsibility for interpreting not only the relative amount of unfavorableness implied by agreement with certain statements but also the increments of unfavorableness. In other words, he must do, without any knowledge of the problems involved, what the experts have found impossible.[5]

Other limitations of the scale include the extent to which competent and representative judges can be selected to make the sortings of the items, as well as the ability of the scale developer to make an initial selection of items that are meaningful in terms of the variable being scaled. For these reasons, the Thurstone-type scale may be considered as an ordinal scale, although one in which more finely graded categories can be developed than in the graphic rating method.

Likert-Type Scale In this type of scale the variable is also evaluated by a series of statements which when responded to by study subjects can provide a criterion measure of the variable. The Likert scale, unlike the Thurstone, is not based on the notion of equal-appearing intervals but rather is a qualitative, ordinal type scale. The form of the scale is such that the subject is given a battery of statements which can vary in number according to the type of variable being measured. He responds to each statement in terms of a scale expressing favorableness or lack of favorableness toward the statement or agreement or disagreement with it. The scale might consist of three or five or even a larger number of categories. An overall scale value is obtained for the rater by summing the values of the responses to each of the items. An example of a statement from a Likert-type scale for the variable "adequacy of patient care" might be:

The nursing personnel employed by this hospital are trying to do the very best job they can in providing good care to patients:

Strongly Disagree	Disagree	Neither Agree or Disagree	Agree	Strongly Agree
1	2	3	4	5

The method for developing a Likert-type scale is, first, to define carefully the variable to be scaled. Then, many statements are collected concerning the variable. The statements are worded in such a form that a rater can express his evaluation in terms of categories representing agreement—disagreement or favorableness—unfavorableness. The statements are given to a group of study subjects, representative of the target population, who are asked to respond to each statement by rating it according to the applicable scale category. Each statement is scored in terms of a rating that ranges from 1 to 5 (or 1 to 3, depending on the number of scale categories) with the numerical values assigned in a consistent order to represent the degree of favorableness or unfavorableness toward the statement. A total score is computed for each respondent. Responses to each statement are then analyzed to select for the final checklist those items which correlate most highly with the total score, as well as those that consistently discriminate between raters whose total scores are high (very favorable) or low (very unfavorable). Thus, the illustrative item just presented would be considered a good item for inclusion in the final checklist if a rater who marked category 5 for the item—strongly agree—obtained a total score showing a high degree of favorableness toward the adequacy of patient care. Conversely, one who strongly disagreed with the statement should obtain a total score indicating a very unfavorable attitude toward adequacy of care.

The Likert-type scale has several advantages over the Thurstone scale. Among these is the greater simplicity of construction of the scale. A group of expert judges is not required, since the scale is developed among study subjects representative of the target population. Moreover, the content of the statements included in the Likert scale does not have to be as carefully selected as in the Thurstone method, where it is necessary for the validity of the sorting process by the judges to include only statements with comparable subject matter so that they could be evaluatively related.

In the nursing field several Likert-type scales have been developed for research purposes. In an attempt to measure the variable "job satisfaction among nursing personnel," Wright developed a checklist of 215 items concerning job conditions in hospitals.[6] The rating scale for each of the items consisted of four values: agree, disagree, neither agree nor disagree, and don't know. Examples of the items contained on the checklist are:

I like my assignment as well as any other for which I am fitted in the hospital.

There is a lot of confusion around here as to what each kind of personnel is supposed to do.

Our patients get adequate emotional support as well as physical care.

Staff nurses spend too much time doing work that could be handled by clerical personnel.

The teamwork and cooperation among the various departments are good.

Another type of Likert scale was developed in a study of nursing students' perception of patients' needs for nursing care.[7] A four-category scale was used to determine the extent of agreement between patients and students as to the importance of certain aspects of patient care. The scale categories were: very important, important, less important, not important. Among the items were:

To have nurses who are friendly

To have the nurse come promptly when I call

To be able to sleep
To understand why I am getting my medicines
To know that a nurse will come when I need her

In a study of patient and personnel satisfaction with nursing care provided, a variation of the Likert-type scale was used.[8] Instead of having the rater respond to the statements in terms of a scale of favorableness, importance, or agreement, the scale categories represented frequency of occurrence of the items: this happened today; this happened some other day; this did not happen. Among the items included on the patient check-list were:

Nurse did not seem interested in me.
Got waked up too early for temperature taking.
Not propped up, making it hard to enjoy my meal.
My nurse was especially nice to me.
Air in room was poor.
My nurse is always in a hurry.

In an example of the use of an ordinal scale to measure a physiological phenomenon, Hasselmeyer[9] employed the following graded scale to describe different stages of the variable "sleep behavior" as applied to premature infants:

Asleep
Eyelids slit
Undecided
Awake

Guttman-Type Scale   This scale is of the variety known as cumulative scales. It consists of a set of statements to which the rater indicates agreement or disagreement. But unlike the Likert or Thurstone scales, the statements are related to each other in such a graded fashion that a positive response by a rater to item 2 should also be accompanied by a positive response to item 1. Likewise, a positive response to, say, the fifth item in the graded series should also indicate a positive response to the preceding four items. And, a positive response to the tenth item means positive responses to all nine preceding items. A main purpose of Guttman's technique, called scalogram analysis, is to test whether the items form a unidimensional scale. It is actually more useful for this kind of analysis than in constructing a scale for use as a research instrument.

The concept of unidimensionality of a scale refers to the fact that the variable being studied is considered to exist in a single plane if it can be scaled cumulatively. Thus, the scale for assessing adequacy of patient care would be considered to be unidimensional if a series of statements concerning this variable could be graded in such a way that a score of three favorable responses in a series of ten graded statements would invariably —or in most applications of the scale—indicate a favorable response to the first 3 items and negative responses to the succeeding seven items. Similarly, a score of seven would indicate a favorable response to the first seven items in the series. As other investigators have pointed out, however, it is highly unlikely that the variable "patient care" would meet the test of unidimensionality.[10]

However, by selecting one aspect of patient care, say the friendliness of the nursing staff, it may be possible to establish a graded series of statements that would have a cumulative property. An example of a series of four statements pertaining to the friendliness of the nursing staff in which the patient might respond in terms of agreement or disagreement might be:

The staff usually says "Good morning" to me.

I know the names of most of the nurses.

The nurses seem interested in me even though they have a lot of work to do.

My nurses spend a lot of time talking to me and cheering me up.

The cumulative property of these items is such that agreement on any item should also mean agreement with all preceding items. To the degree that this is not so, the items cannot be considered to have formed a scale in the scalogram sense. In other words, they do not describe the variable "friendliness of nurses" in an unidimensional sense. The goal in scalogram analysis is to derive a series of items that will.

Q-Sort   This technique was originally developed, not as a scaling method, but rather as a device to explore the personality of individuals.[11] However, it has become widely used in research as a device to derive an ordinal scale for measuring certain kinds of variables. The procedure for conducting a Q-sort resembles that of the development of a Thurstone scale. The rater is given a set of statements, often numbering 100 or more, related to the variable being scaled. He is instructed to sort the statements into a given number of piles, usually 7, 9, or 11, in terms of some graded scale. Thus, if the statements are concerned with adequacy of patient care, the scale categories might represent degrees of adequacy ranging from very adequate to very inadequate, and each pile would represent a different category.

One difference between the Thurstone method and the Q-sort is the already mentioned fact that the sorting process for the Q-sort is often employed to determine the rater's own attitudes toward the object being rated whereas the Thurstone sort is aimed at obtaining an expert judge's rating of the degree to which the *content* of the statement itself reflects favorableness or unfavorableness toward the object being rated.

A second difference between the two sorting methods is that in the Thurstone approach only the number of piles into which the statements are to be sorted is specified. The number of statements that can be placed in each pile is not specified, so that, theoretically, the sorter could put them all into one pile. In the Q-sort approach the number of statements to be placed in each pile is specified, and the sorter can put no more or less in each pile. The number to be placed in each pile in the Q-sort generally follows "the normal curve" in that few statements can be placed in the extreme piles, with the numbers increasing as the center pile is approached. Thus in a sort of 50 statements into five categories, the number of statements that could be placed into each pile would be:

Pile:	1	2	3	4	5
Number of statements:	4	12	18	12	4

One advantage of stipulating the number to be placed in each pile is that it forces the rater to distribute the items over all scale values. As has been mentioned in the case of the graphic rating scale, there is often a tendency for a rater, when he uses an ordinal scale to choose the center or least controversial or extreme position on the scale. To counteract such a tendency, "forced choice" methods have been developed, like the Q-sort technique.

Another forced choice method is Thurstone's method of *paired comparisons*. In this approach every item is evaluated in terms of every other item according to the scale criterion. The result of these comparisons would form a graded scale. To illustrate, suppose we wanted to determine which components of patient care were the least adequate, and which the most adequate. For simplicity, since each additional item to be compared greatly expands the number of comparisons, assume we select five components for study:

A. Efficiency of admitting procedure
B. Friendliness of the nursing staff
C. Quality of the food
D. Cheerfulness of the room
E. Opportunity to rest

We could pair off each item with every other item and instruct the rater to check the one item of the pair that was the more adequate. The following paired comparisons would be possible: AB, AC, AD, AE, BC, BD, BE,

CD, CE, DE. In mathematical terms the number of different combinations of five items taken two at a time would be:

$$\frac{5 \times 4 \times 3 \times 2 \times 1}{(2 \times 1) \ (3 \times 2 \times 1)} = 10$$

Assume a rater responded as follows by underlining the member of the pair he felt to be more adequate: AB, AC, AD, AE, BC, BD, BE, CD, CE, DE. The items would then fall into the following rank order in terms of adequacy of service.

1. Friendliness of the nursing staff
2. Cheerfulness of the room
3. Opportunity to rest
4. Efficiency of admitting procedure
5. Quality of the food

A widely used example of the technique of paired comparisons is the Edwards Personal Preference Test. This is a measure of the personality of the respondent and consists of items that provide scores for numerous personality variables.

QUANTITATIVE SCALES

Interval and Ratio Scales

True quantitative scales are those that measure the numerical extent to which the object the scale is applied to possesses the variable being measured. Quantitative scales are often called *measurement* scales, since they can provide a numerical value for the variable they are measuring. On the other hand, qualitative scales are called *classification* scales, since they serve as a means for placing the objects to which the scale is applied into discrete classes that are distinguished in terms of some qualitative criterion.

Although, as has been indicated, qualitative scales use numbers to distinguish one class from another, they do not have a real quantitative meaning. In nominal scales the numbers may be a shorthand way of designating the different categories, called the process of *coding*. In ordinal scales, the numbers designating the different classes will show the rank order of the categories included in the scale so that in a scale representing adequacy of nursing care, a value of 1 could indicate more adequacy than a value of 2, a value 2 more adequacy than 3, and so on, but we have no way of assessing how much more.

If we can measure the distance between the scale points—that is, if we can actually say how much more a value of 1 is, say, than a value of 5—then we have a true numerical scale. Thus a thermometer will tell us not only that Mr. Jones' temperature is above normal (an ordinal ranking), but it will also tell us that it is three degrees (or intervals) higher than normal if the thermometer reads 101.6° F. In a five-point ordinal scale of adequacy of nursing care, ranging from 1 as the most adequate rating to 5 as the least adequate, with 3 as the middle, it would not be too meaningful to say that Mr. Jones' evaluation of adequacy of care, which he checked as 1, is two intervals above the middle, since we have no way of interpreting this distance except in terms of the qualitative distinctions we have established for the five categories on the scale.

If the quantitative value of the intervals between the scale points on an ordinal scale can be determined, and that is the aim of the Thurstone "equal-appearing intervals" method, then we have upgraded it to a numerical scale, called an *interval* scale. A major advantage of the interval scale over an ordinal scale is its greater sensitivity. An ordinal scale consists of just a limited number of discrete scale points. These cannot be subdivided any further, since the distance between the points is unknown. On an interval scale the distance between the points is equal, so we can justifiably break the intervals down into finer subdivisions which will provide us with more refined distinctions among the objects we are measuring.

The ability to make more refined distinctions in the measurement process has been particularly helpful in research in the scientific field. To illustrate, we can take the variable "time." This variable is measured in a quantitative scale by the familiar instrument known as a clock. The usual clock ranges over a span of 12 hours, with the smallest subdivision being 15-minute intervals. Large clocks have been developed where the smallest scale intervals are in single minutes. For more refined breakdowns, stop watches have been developed where the total range might be as small as one minute and each subdivision represents a single second. For many measurement needs where time is the variable, instruments such as these are adequate, since refinement beyond, say, one-tenth of a second would be totally unnecessary. However, in the field of atomic physics, where reactions may occur in one-billionth of a second or even quicker, more sensitive "clocks" are needed. Such "clocks" are electronic instruments employing highly responsive circuitry, since the ordinary mechanical clock with its many sources of friction is much too crude an instrument to provide the needed precision.

Quantitative scales possess two properties. One, common to all quantitative scales, is that the intervals between the scale points can be measured. The other, not present in all quantitative scales, is that the scale contains a zero point—a point at which the variable being measured can be said to be totally absent. A quantitative scale without a zero point is called an *interval scale*. One with a zero point is called a *ratio scale*. A ratio scale is so named because having a scale point of absolute zero—the total absence of the variable—it is possible to determine not only *how much* greater one measurement is from another, but also *how many times* greater it is.

The scale for the variable "time" is a ratio scale, since it has a zero point. If we measure how long it takes for nursing aide A to make a patient's empty bed, we might find that it took her three minutes. Nursing aide B took two minutes for the same task. Thus, we can say that it took aide A one minute longer to make the bed than aide B. We can also say that aide A took one and a half times as long to make the bed as did aide B (the ratio 3/2).

The scale for the variable "body temperature" is an interval scale, since it does not have a zero point, but usually begins at about 94° F. If we measure patient A's temperature, we might find it to be 100.5° F. Patient B's temperature might be 99.5° F. We can say that patient A's temperature is one degree higher than patient B's. However, we cannot say that A's temperature is 1.010 warmer than that of B (The ratio 100.5°/99.5°), since in the absence of a true zero point such a ratio is somewhat meaningless in an absolute sense. Moreover, we need to bear in mind that the numbers assigned to the body temperature scale are purely a matter of convention. This is made clear by the fact that there are other types of numerical scales for measuring temperature.

On the centigrade scale, patient A's temperature would be 38.05° C. and B's would be 37.50° C., a difference of 0.55 degrees. Superficially, this would seem that the difference between the two patients' temperatures is less than that found when the Fahrenheit scale was used, where the difference was a whole degree. Yet in terms of a ratio comparison of the temperatures, A's temperature seems to be 1.015° "warmer" than B's (the ratio 38.05°/37.50°) as compared to only 1.010° "warmer" on the Fahrenheit scale.

In ratio scales, even when different types of numerical scales are used for measuring the variable, the ratio of two values on the same scale is identical with the ratio of the corresponding values on the other type of scale. Thus, for the variable "weight," either the avoirdupois or the metric scale can be used, both being a true ratio scale. On the avoirdupois scale two pounds is twice as heavy as one pound. The corresponding values on the metric scale would be 908 grams (2 pounds) and 454 grams (1 pound) also a ratio of 2 to 1.

In interval scales the ratio of two *differences* in scale values (not the values themselves) on one type of scale is identical with the ratio of two *differences* in the corresponding scale values on the other type of scale used to measure the same variable. To illustrate: a rise in temperature on the Fahrenheit scale from 99.5° to 101.5° is numerically twice as much as a rise from 99.5° to 100.5°, the ratio of the *differences* being 2/1. A rise in temperature on the centigrade scale corresponding to a rise from 99.5° to 101.5° is 37.5° to 38.6°, a difference of 1.1°. The rise corresponding to 99.5° to 100.5° on the Fahrenheit scale is 37.50° to 38.05° on the centigrade scale, a difference of 0.55°. Thus on the centigrade scale the ratio of the differences is also 2/1 (1.1/0.55). In interval scales, then, it is possible to speak of ratios of *differences* in scale values even though the ratios of the actual scale values themselves are not meaningful.

Actually, it is possible to construct a temperature scale with a true zero point. *Absolute zero* temperature is at −273.1° C. and −459.6° F. It is possible to transform these scales so that on the centigrade scale, for example, instead of having the zero point at the temperature where water freezes (or ice melts), it could be at absolute zero, defined as the total absence of heat—when all molecular action ceases. Such a scale would be a true ratio scale.

Most quantitative scales are of the ratio type. These scales are often called scientific scales because many of them have been developed in the "hard" scientific fields of physics and chemistry. A distinguishing characteristic of such scales is that they are generally in the form of highly sophisticated, and sometimes highly complicated, mechanical apparatus. Most ordinal and nominal scales, by contrast, are not mechanical instruments but are generally rather simple, "paper and pencil" types of questionnaires, tests, or scales.

In the area of patient care, many scientific scales are available for making quantitative measurements. Table 7-1 lists some of the most common types of instruments and briefly describes their uses. Table 7-2 shows some of the scales developed in the social sciences that have been found useful in nursing research. Many of these scales are essentially qualitative.

A major advantage of quantitative scales, in addition to the already mentioned ones of accuracy, objectivity, sensitivity, is their versatility, since one quantitative scale can serve many different research needs. A weight scale for measuring body weight not only is a clinical diagnostic tool, but can serve as a criterion measure for a wide variety of studies, each directed toward quite dissimilar research problems. For example, it has been used in psychological research to test the effects of psychotherapy on weight reduction and in research on space travel to measure the effects of simulated conditions of weightlessness. A weight scale has also been used as a criterion measure in evaluating the influence of nursing care on premature infants.

Patient outcome indicators (physical, psychological, social) can be most useful in descriptive, experimental, and analytical explanatory studies. Indicators can link appropriate background theory with empirical research

TABLE 7-1

Examples of Some Quantitative Measuring Instruments Used in Patient Care, the Variables They Measure, and Their Uses

Name of Instrument	Variable Measured (Indicators) Physical*	Uses
Arteriography	Identifies site of arterial damage	Useful for patients with transient ischemic attacks to determine surgical accessibility and treatment
Audiometer	Hearing	Tests the power of hearing
Balance	Weight	Increased weight due to edema often associated with congestive heart failure
Biophotometer	Dark adaptation of eye	Indication of vitamin A deficiency
Calorimeter	Metabolism: rate of basal metabolism expressed in calories per hour per square meter of body surface in a subject at absolute rest, 14–18 hours after eating	Diagnosis of diseases of the thyroid gland
Cardiac catheterization	Intracardiac pressure	To secure blood samples
Cardiograph	Heart movements: measures the force and form of the heart's movements	Detection of cardiovascular heart diseases
Cardiotachometer	Heart beats: counts the number of heart beats over long periods of time	Useful in detecting arrhythmias that occur periodically
Clock	Time: beats of pulse per minute	Indicator of state of vital function of the heart
Computed tomographic (CT) scanner	X-ray of head and body using CT scanner	Used in field of diagnostic radiology for early detection of tumors in head and body
Electroencephalography (EEG)	Measures electrical activity of the brain that may be caused by structural or biochemical lesions	Useful in distinguishing between cerebral and brain stem lesions
Electrometrogram	Uterine contractions: records uterine contractions	Measurement of progress of labor
Electromyography	Electric potential of muscle: use of needle electrodes into the muscle to determine if muscle is contracting	Detection and location of motor unit lesions; recording electrical activity evoked in a muscle by stimulation of its nerve, as following a laminectomy or in a paralytic patient
Erythrometer	Color scale for measuring degrees of redness	Useful in diagnosis of erythromelalgia, a disease affecting chiefly extremities of the body marked by bilateral vasodilation
Goniometer	Angles	Measurement of the degree to which a patient can raise or lower a limb, as following a mastectomy or laminectomy

TABLE 7-1 (cont.)

Name of Instrument	Variable Measured Physical Indicators*	Uses
Kinesimeter	Movements: quantitative measurement of movements	Useful in exploring the surface of the body to test cutaneous sensibility
Kinesthesiometer	Muscular sensibility	Study of muscular sensibility as in Hasselmeyer's study of premature infants
Kinomometer	Motion in fingers and wrist	Useful in measuring progress being made by the patient following cerebral vascular accidents
Mecometer	Length of fetus or an infant	Accurate measure of human who cannot stand
Optometer	Measurement of the power and range of vision	Used in diagnosis of eye diseases
Oxyhemoglobinometer	Oxygen content of the blood	Various forms of anemias
Ruler	Distance: holding ruler between the eyes and the printed page	To test binocular and stereoscopic vision
Sphygmomanometer (two types—the mercury and the anaeroid [spring])	Blood pressure: the force of the pressure exerted within the arterial vessels during each of the phases of cardiac action—contraction and relaxation—(Normal—120/80)	A marked increase or decrease in the differential is an indication of disturbed physiological homeostasis as in the hypertensive cardiac patient or shock
Spirometer	Respiratory volumes	Separates total gas content of the lung into tidal volume, inspiratory reserve volume, expiratory reserve volume and residual volume. Used to assess pulmonary function in patients with pulmonary disease.
Telethermometer	Body functions	Records body functions as temperature, pulse, respirations, blood pressure
Thermometer	Temperature (Normal 98.6°F. or 37°C. on a clinical thermometer)	To measure the balance of heat maintained between that which is produced and that which is lost from the body. Disturbance in homeostasis is a measurable deviation in body temperature above or below the established norm
Vital capacity	Air in lungs: the number of cubic inches of air a person can forcibly expire after a full inspiration	Ability of the blood to absorb oxygen from the lungs and carbon dioxide from the tissue

* Physical indicators are measurable signs and symptoms and can be used as nonintrusive evaluative tools.

TABLE 7-2

Examples of Some Measuring Instruments Developed in the Social Sciences Used in Patient Care and Measurement of Human Behavior,* the Variables They Measure, and Their Uses

Name of Instrument	Variable Measured (Psychological Indicators)	Uses
Measurement of Patient Care		
Williams and Leavitt (1947) sociometric index	Leadership performance	Identification of leaders in ward groups
Zeleny scale (1940)	Social status: measurement of satisfaction and moral	Assessment of environmental settings
Patient satisfaction (1953)	Adequacy of nursing care	Assessment of patients' needs
Patient classification (1957)	Degree of illness	Grouping of patients in areas where they can receive nursing care best suited to their needs
Simon (1957) sociometric scale	Mental attitude of patient	Assessment of mental attitude as one criterion of patient welfare
Wooden (1962)	Patient independence	Degree of independence used as a basis for carrying out a program of family-centered care
Dumas (1963) stress scale	Stress prior to and after surgery	Use of nursing care as a way of reducing postoperative vomiting
Meltzer-Pinneo-Ferrigan (1964)	Degree of cardiac damage following coronary: assessment of both physical and psychological factors that might contribute to cardiac damage	Useful in predicting arrhythmias associated with coronary occlusion
Measurement of Human Behavior		
Aptitude tests	Aptitude and ability	To predict success in nursing
Stanford-Binet's test	Mental age of subject; evaluation of overall intellectual level	Mental capacity of children and youth
Wechsler test		
Projective techniques Rorschach test	Human behavior: (a) measurement of personal and spontaneous impulses; (b) signs of insecurity and anxiety; (c) response to promptings from within or without	Provides clues to maladjustment, balance, and control of personality structure
Murray thematic apperception test (T.A.T.)	Deep-lying roots of personality	Gives some understanding of human motivations and inner needs
Self-inventories	Traits, likes and dislikes, attitudes, emotional tendencies	Helps to determine the meaning with which individuals respond to a situation
Self-rating scales	Traits and behavior patterns easily overlooked	Encourages self-analysis and improvement

TABLE 7-2 (cont.)

Name of Instrument	Variable Measured Physical Indicators*	Uses
Standardized tests	Comprehension; facts and skills	Used in nursing curriculums to measure program content
Multiple-choice Completion Alternative-response Simple recall Matching analogies		
Minnesota multiphasic personality inventory (M.M.P.I.)	Personality	Helpful in measuring tendencies toward different kinds of psychiatric difficulty
Stimulation program (Brown and Hepler, 1976)	Provision of sensory and perceptual stimuli experienced by normal full-term newborns	Stimulation used in the care of the critically ill newborn, particularly the premature to provide contact of infant and mother

* For additional examples see: Tyler, Leona A., *Tests and Measurements*. Englewood Cliffs, New Jersey, Prentice-Hall, Inc., 1963.

methods, thus facilitating the development of an appropriate research design within a selected frame of reference.*

Generally, ordinal and nominal scales do not have this versatility. They are frequently developed for a single study and, being tailor-made, are not used again. In using such scales developed in other studies great care must be taken to see if they do have applicability beyond their original purpose. Indiscriminate use of such instruments can weaken the design of a study.

Another important advantage of a quantitative scale is the greater variety of statistical techniques that can be applied to the data. Quantitative measurements permit the use of more high-powered methodology than can be applied to qualitative scales. One such technique, mentioned in the previous chapter on experimental design, is the analysis of variance, a very efficient method for maximizing the amount of information that can be obtained from the data. Another technique applicable to quantitative measurements is regression analysis, which is very useful in analyzing the mathematical relationships among variables.

DEVELOPING A QUANTITATIVE SCALE FROM A NOMINAL SCALE

In the social sciences, most scales that have been developed for measuring psychological or sociological phenomena are of the ordinal or nominal

* University of Alberta School of Nursing, *Development and Use of Indicators in Nursing Research*. Proceedings of the 1975 National Conference on Nursing Research. G. N. Zilm, S. M. Stinson, M. E. Steed, and P. Overton, (eds.). Edmonton, University of Alberta School of Nursing, 1975

type. Such variables as attitudes, personality, perception, aptitudes, and abilities still await the measuring refinement found among variables common to the physical sciences. Considerable effort is being expended to quantify some of these highly complex variables.

As an illustration of the effort to quantitatively scale a variable of interest to nursing research we can examine the development of a scale to measure patients' needs for nursing services, a methodological tool that will be discussed in detail in Chapter 12. The most rudimentary method for classifying such needs is diagnostic categorization according to the patient's illness. Classification by diagnosis can be very detailed. As has been mentioned, the total list of diseases contained in the *Standard Nomenclature of Diseases and Operations* has over a thousand classes. Diagnostic classification can also be in broader classes, as the typical service categories of a public health agency: cardiovascular illness, cancer, communicable diseases, mental illness, etc. Or it can be in still broader classes, as in the typical grouping of patients in a hospital: medical, surgical, obstetrical, pediatric.

These classifications are clearly nominal scales. There is no underlying continuum that connects the different categories. Although they are related in that each represents a distinctive type of illness—a departure from health—the scale provides no quantitative assessment of the extent of this departure nor does it provide any indication of the amount of nursing services required by patients in the different categories.

Taking the variable "nursing needs" it is possible to construct a scale in which the underlying continuum would be a graded scale representing intensity of needs. As discussed in Chapter 12, many such scales have been developed. In one of these, developed at Johns Hopkins Hospital, patients' requirements for nursing service can be assessed according to a scale that possesses three categories: intensive care, intermediate care, self-care. This is an ordinal scale which provides a more analytical evaluation of the needs of patients than does the nominal scale of classification by diagnosis or service category. To illustrate this, suppose we select two hospitals, each with 100 patients. By the conventional classification of patients we might find the following distribution:

Service Category	Number of Patients	
	Hospital A	*Hospital B*
Total	*100*	*100*
Medical	30	40
Surgical	40	30
Obstetric	20	15
Pediatric	10	15

Examination of these data would reveal little understanding of the nursing needs of the patients in the two hospitals. We might conjecture that hospital A's patients have more needs, since it has a larger number of surgical patients. However, this is offset by a smaller number of pediatric patients. Nothing definitive could be said about nursing needs until a scale that measures these needs is applied to the patients. Such a scale might reveal the following data:

Nursing Needs *Category* *Total*	*Number of Patients*	
	Hospital A *100*	*Hospital B* *100*
Intensive care	10	25
Intermediate care	70	50
Self-care	20	25

These data show a picture concerning patients' nursing needs somewhat different from what was conjectured by analysis of the data yielded by the nominal scale. Hospital B has in fact a larger share of patients with more intensive nursing needs than does hospital A. The use of the ordinal scale has thus provided more meaningful data concerning the variable being investigated than did the nominal scale.

The next stage in the development of a scale to assess patients' nursing needs would be to advance from an ordinal to a quantitative type scale. At Johns Hopkins Hospital some progress has been made in this direction. By detailed study of groups of representative patients it was possible to determine the average amounts of nursing care required by patients in each of the three categories. On the basis of these data, a crude quantitative scale was established that provides a value of the interval between the three classes. The following scale shows the quantitative relationship among these classes:

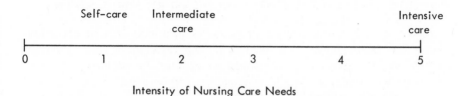

Fig. 7-2. A quantitative scale for assessing intensity of nursing care needs.

This means an intermediate care patient requires twice as much nursing care as does a self-care patient. An intensive care patient has five times the requirements of the self-care patient. These values provide a method for quantitatively assessing the needs of patients which could yield useful data for research as well as for administrative purposes.

The highest stage in the development of a scale to measure the nursing care needs of patients would be to develop a truly comprehensive quantitative measure of a patient's total care needs. Such a measure might well be part of a larger concept of the measurement of a person's level of wellness. Although it is difficult to conceive of such a scale as possessing unidimensionality, since we can speak of wellness in terms of physical, psychological, or sociological factors, it may be possible to develop an abstract measure that would synthesize these various factors.

The importance of a wellness scale to nursing is that it would be concerned with a person's total health status. Present patient classification methods are directed primarily toward his needs as a patient who has some morbid condition in need of correction. A wellness scale would be valuable not only as a criterion measure for many different kinds of studies concerned with assessing the impact on patient welfare of different methods, procedures, or programs, but also as a tool for planning and evaluating patient care.

There is, indeed, a long way to go in applying exact quantitative measurement to the study of human beings. Although some progress has been made, there are still many obstacles to overcome. As Cochran[12] has remarked:

> In the study of human beings many of the problems of measurement are formidable. Not only have we to measure fairly concrete attributes like the state of disease in the individual (which the doctors will assure us is not easy to measure well) but we need to classify and if possible to measure many things that are hard enough to define in the first place, like motives, morale, intentions, feelings of stress. This means a vast undertaking that has had to start from the ground with crude homemade tools. Thus far, for want of anything better in sight, we have obtained our raw data mainly from what the individual tells us. And the recording instrument has usually been another individual.

HOW TO SELECT A CRITERION MEASURE FOR A STUDY

The type of criterion measure or measures used in an explanatory study is, as has been indicated, influenced by the research problem and the hypotheses that have been developed to explore the problem. The hypothesis is a statement of the explanatory variables with which the research will be concerned. After defining these variables as concretely and operationally as is possible, the researcher must decide how the dependent variable will be measured—whether to use a direct or an indirect measure. This decision will be influenced by the ease with which the variable can be directly measured and the extent to which a subtler measure might yield more meaningful data. Also in many instances indirect measurement of a variable may be simpler to accomplish than direct measurement of the phenomenon.

But indirect measurement may be more efficient than direct measurement. For example, it is rather simple to measure the density of liquids on the basis of the law that expresses density as a constant function of the ratio between the weight and the volume of the particular liquid, but it would be tedious and less precise by direct procedures. By a direct procedure we might, for example, use a standard set of solid bodies, which we would place in the various liquids. We would agree to call one liquid more dense than another if we could find a solid body which would float in one but not in the other. Following this procedure systematically for all liquids, we would assign the numbers 1, 2, 3, 4, 5, etc., to designate the position of the liquids in the density scale. Clearly, the direct procedure is more cumbersome and less precise than the indirect procedure.[13]

In some studies the researcher has available to him a variety of criterion measures of his dependent variable. If his variable can be measured in terms of some physiological response there are available many scientific measuring instruments, yielding highly refined numerical measurements, that might serve as criterion measures.

If his variable is some psychological or sociological phenomenon there are also available many satisfactory tests and scales that he can employ. Such variables as personality, motivation, perception, creativity, abilities of all types, intellectual and mechanical aptitudes, as well as a great variety of social attitudes such as prejudice, authoritarianism, and morale, can be measured in terms of ordinal scales by standardized paper and pencil instruments. Furthermore, for many important variables, useful nominal scales exist that can serve the needs of a researcher. A variable like type of illness has been developed into a highly refined nominal scale.

In retrospective studies, of course, the researcher has to accept the measures of the variables as developed by others, since he is using data that were originally designed for another purpose. With data like these care must be taken that they can actually fulfill the needs of the research in which they are used. If our criterion measure in a retrospective study is rate of patients' recovery from their illness, and we obtain our data from hospital charts, we might find large gaps in these records. Moreover, the definitions used might differ from our own. Such deficiencies can seriously weaken the measurement process and can damage the total research effort.

Many studies, of course, have to develop their own measures of the explanatory variables—namely, the dependent variables. In the case of highly complex variables, measurement can be a difficult task, requiring the assistance of experts. There are specialists in the field of measurement, and a researcher should not hesitate to enlist their services when deemed necessary. Most researchers, however, follow a "do-it-yourself" course in developing criterion measures. For many variables this task does not present too much difficulty. For others, it can represent a formidable effort, perhaps the single most time-consuming and difficult step in the entire research process.

Review of the literature in the field can often be very helpful in the development of a criterion measure for a research study. Much of what appears in the research literature is concerned with the measurement of variables. A researcher can sometimes find a measure in the literature that he can use either directly or with some adaptation in his own study. If it is necessary to develop his own measure, useful ideas on how to proceed can sometimes be suggested by the literature.

In the literature of the physical sciences, information on new measurement apparatus is found in the many journals in the different fields. A journal like *Science* sometimes carries such information. Knowledge about existing instrumentation that can be used for research measurement is available from textbooks, manuals, encyclopedias, and similar types of reference works. For example, a good textbook on physiology will contain descriptions of the more common types of measuring apparatus in this field. In the social sciences several specialized journals exist which deal with problems of measurement. These include *Psychometrika, Sociometry, Mathematical Biosciences,* and the *Journal of Mathematical Psychology.* Occasionally, the literature in the statistical field includes material on measurement. Information pertinent to patient care research is most likely to appear in such statistical journals as *Biometrics* and *Biometrika.*

CRITERIA FOR EVALUATING SUFFICIENCY AND EFFICIENCY OF CRITERION MEASURES

Whether the method for measuring the variables in a study has been designed by others or developed fresh by the researcher, the measures that are used in the study must meet certain tests in order to be considered acceptable. Four of the most important criteria for evaluating the adequacy of measures are validity, reliability, sensitivity, and meaningfulness. These criteria will be briefly discussed.

Validity

The criterion of validity is perhaps the most important of the four tests just mentioned. If a measure is not valid, it does not really matter that it meets other tests—it is not a satisfactory measure. The concept of validity, which can also be called relevance, simply means does the measure actually measure what it is supposed to? If a measuring instrument is supposed to measure patient satisfaction with nursing care, does it really measure satisfaction in the way it has been operationally defined, or is it actually measuring some other variable, or nothing at all? As a check on whether a variable like patient satisfaction is operationally defined, the following questions can be raised. What is satisfaction? Is it something vague and unreal, or does it have substance and meaning so that it manifests itself in terms of observable, tangible behavior? Such behavior might be, for dissatisfied patients—vocal complaints including a firm resolve never to return to the hospital; for satisfied patients—unsolicited compliments.

A succinct and humorous illustration of what is meant by validity is given by the following quotation:

We hear of a museum in a certain Eastern city that was proud of its amazing attendance record. Recently a little stone building was erected nearby. Next year attendance at the museum mysteriously fell off by 100,000. What was the little stone building? A comfort station.[14]

In other words the museum was using the number of persons entering the museum as a measure of interest in its exhibits. This measure was invalid because what attracted many people to the museum was actually some other purpose than viewing the exhibits.

The object of measurement is to determine the true value of the variable for the individual being measured. Thus, if we measure satisfaction with patient care and we find differences among the patients whom we include in the study, we would hope that these differences reflect true differences in the level of satisfaction of the patients: that those with higher scores are actually more satisfied than those with lower. However, we must recognize that there are certain sources of variation in measures that do not reflect true differences in the variable we are measuring. In the discussion of research design, we have mentioned two of these—the extraneous organismic and environmental variables. To illustrate, patient care studies have indicated that age is related to how a patient responds to the scale of satisfaction with adequacy of nursing care—older people generally react favorably to their nursing care regardless of its real quality. Thus in an explanatory study of adequacy of patient care in which different groups were compared, it is possible that more older patients would be assigned to one group than to the others. If we were unaware of the relationship between age and satisfaction and we examined only the average satisfaction scores for the groups as a whole, we might conclude that the group with more older patients was receiving more adequate care, when, in fact, by some other criteria it really was not. Errors due to the intrusion of these variables can be largely controlled by such techniques as randomization, balancing, and pairing, which would tend to distribute them so that they would offset each other. However, some effects of extraneous organismic and environmental variables, hopefully slight, are always present in a study no matter how well controlled.

In addition to the variation in measurement attributable to extraneous variables there are the errors that arise from the measuring process itself, which can also affect the validity of the findings. These can arise from defects in the measuring instrument itself—a weight scale with a spring that goes out of order occasionally, an achievement test that contains ambiguous items that are misinterpreted by some respondents—or from errors that are made by the observer who reads the instrument or the rater who scores a test. Such inconsistencies in the measurement process, known as unreliability, can also harm the validity of the measure.

Thus, validity of a measure can be influenced by errors arising from the subjects themselves, from outside influences on the subjects, and from inconsistencies in the measuring process. An otherwise quite valid measure can have its relevance destroyed by these sources of error. However, even if all these sources of error were controlled, we would still have no guarantee that our measure was valid.

Validity of a measure must be assessed independently on its own merits. To illustrate, assume we used a measure like patient's blood pressure as a criterion of the variable "patient well-being" in an experimental study of alternative types of nurse staffing patterns. Further, assume we kept all possible sources of error under control—we randomized our experimental subjects to the alternative groups, the environment in which the patients were kept was identical, and we employed expert observers using the best available apparatus to make consistent measurements of patients' blood pressure. The results of such a study could still be invalid because blood pressure may not be a relevant measure of patient well-being. That is to say, variations in blood pressure measurements might not truly reflect variations in the well-being of the subjects. When an indirect measure is used as a criterion measure of a dependent variable, special care must be taken to see that it is relevant.

For many variables it is possible to make an empirical check of the validity of the measure. This is done by testing the accuracy of predictions based on the measure. In this procedure we correlate the results obtained by the measure with some outside criterion. An example of the empirical validity of a measure is contained in a study of job satisfaction of nursing personnel in which an ordinal scale was developed based on a battery of 215 items representing different aspects of the work situation.[15] A group of representative nursing personnel responded to the items and were ranked according to those with high job satisfaction and those with low satisfaction. Job turnover was selected as the validity criterion, since it was assumed that personnel with low satisfaction would leave the organization at a higher rate than those with high satisfaction. Some correlation was found between turnover behavior and job satisfaction, but it was not high enough to validate satisfactorily the job satisfaction scale in terms of the variable "turnover behavior." Perhaps an outside validation criterion other than turnover would have been better predicted by the satisfaction measure.

Most desirably, validation of a measure should be done empirically by correlating it with some independent behavioral criterion—a criterion that describes some meaningful, objective, observable action. If we are measuring the variable "proficiency as a nurse" by a pencil and paper instrument we should be able to validate it in terms of the behavior of the nurse in actual practice. For many measures, particularly those dealing with somewhat vague sociological or psychological concepts, this type of validation cannot be done too easily, if at all. Let us look at the previously mentioned variable, satisfaction with nursing care. What practical behavioral criterion can we use to make predictions from the measure?

As a substitute for empirical validation of variables like these we can use the technique of validation by a body of independent expert judges. The judges can observe the patients who ranked low on the measure of satisfaction with nursing care and, by using a set of objective criteria, can decide whether they are different in some meaningful way from those who ranked high. This procedure is more subjective than correlating the measure with a behavioral criterion, but if the only other alternative is no formal validation of the measure at all, it should be given consideration.

Reliability

This criterion is also known as the reproducibility or the repeatability of a measure. It refers to the consistency or precision of the measure. A measure is considered to be reliable if it is consistently reproducible.

The concept of reliability can perhaps be best understood when it is considered that variation in measurement can arise from two main sources, assuming control of all extraneous organismic and environmental variables. If we measure a patient's temperature at two different time periods, we might note a rise in the reading. This could be due to two factors: a real rise in his temperature level due to some physiological change in his body, or a false rise due to either a mistake by the observer in reading the thermometer or some failure of the instrument itself. A false reading due to either observer or instrument error would be indicative of lack of reliability of the measuring process. If both errors occur frequently during the course of a study, we say the measure is unreliable. In this example, temperature may well be a valid measure—that is, it relevantly describes the variable under study—but it might not be a reliable one.

Stated the other way, if measurement of an object is made over a period of time, and if the variable being measured has undergone no real change, the measure is considered to be reliable if the observer reports that no change has occurred. Thus, in repeated measurements of a patient's temperature in which no real change has occurred, the measure would be deemed reliable if the measurements likewise indicated no change. Or if in repeated measurements a real change does occur, reliable measurements should also reflect this change.

Perhaps the most likely source of error that would render a measure unreliable is that due to the observer. Mechanical instruments, especially if they are of a high quality, are generally stable. Some can be calibrated and adjusted to account for deterioration over time. Many electronic instruments have controls to adjust for the aging of components, changes in temperature, variations in the electric supply, and so on. Scientific instruments like thermometers, weight scales, and clocks can be checked for accuracy and consistency either by comparing readings obtained with the instrument against another known to be exact or by subjecting the instruments to analysis by test equipment especially made for assessing their reliability.*

Reliability of physiological and sociological instruments can be checked by such techniques as the split-half or odd-even method, in which the score on half of the items included in an instrument is compared with the score on the other half. Since the items are distributed randomly, it can be assumed that the scores on the two halves should be identical. To the degree that they are not is an indication of the unreliability of the measure.

Still another way of checking the reliability of tests and scales is the test-retest method. For variables whose measures for a given individual should remain stable over a period of time, such as intelligence, personality, interest, and certain basic attitudes, repeated measurement should yield approximately the same scores. To the extent that values are different is an indication of the lack of reliability of the measuring instrument.

Observer error in reading scientific instruments can be checked by having independent observers read the same instrument simultaneously and then compare the readings. Reliability is measured by the extent to which the readings of the different observers agree. Unlike the method of repeated measurements over time which tests reliability in terms of the stability of the instrument, comparison of simultaneous measurements eliminates the possibility of differences in the measure related to the passage of time. Thus in a study of the reliability of blood pressure readings by nurses, Wilcox[16] employed a double stethoscope having one head and two different sets of earpieces. Two observers, using a single, accuracy-checked sphygmomanometer, could make simultaneous readings of the same patient's blood pressure. Three pairs of nurses read the blood pressure of the same patient over a brief period of time. The findings revealed

---

* The National Bureau of Standards, Office of Technical Information, Gaithersburg, Md., will test an instrument for its reliability and when possible standardize it (there is a charge for this service).

considerable variation (lack of reliability) in blood pressure readings of the same patients, both systolic and diastolic, among the nurse observers.

Observer error in other methods of data collection, such as an observer making narrative recordings of what she sees, can be similarly checked for reliability through a comparison of recordings made simultaneously of the same events by independent observers. To illustrate, a check of the reliability of a patient classification instrument consisted of having two observers, the head nurse and her assistant, both possessing an equal amount of information about the patient, make simultaneous independent ratings of the same patient's needs for nursing care. The two ratings were compared, and a high level of argeement was found, particularly on those items reflecting physical care needs of patients. A similar reliability check was made of an instrument for gathering data on the activities of nursing personnel. Here, too, independent observers reported on the same events, and the results of their observations compared.

Simultaneous measurement can also be made of the same phenomenon using different instruments. This would tend to check the consistency or equivalence of the different measuring instruments.

Errors in measurement will not disturb the validity of the measurements made of large groups of study subjects, if these errors are randomly distributed, since they would tend to offset each other. Only when they are consistently piled up in one direction can they bias the findings of a study. However, when measurements are needed for individual cases, as in diagnosis of a patient's illness, unreliability cannot be tolerated, since wrong measurements may negatively affect the course of treatment the patient receives.

Reliability of measurements can be controlled if the sources of error are known. The following summarizes the main causes of unreliability in measurements:

1. Defects in the measuring instruments—usually mechanical in the case of physical instruments; wording and other structural defects in the case of pencil and paper instruments.
2. Lack of adequate training and/or experience of the observer in reading the instrument or in scoring or interpreting the results of a pencil and paper test.
3. Psychological biases on the part of the observer which affects her reading of the measure.
4. Errors arising from the person being measured—as, for example, misinterpreting instructions on a test, thereby responding to it in an incorrect way.

It is important to note that if an instrument is highly reliable there is no guarantee that it will also produce a valid measure of the variable. For example, half a dozen experts independently reading the same electrocardiograph measurements could arrive at the same precise interpretation, but their interpretation would be quite irrelevant if the apparatus were defective and produced normal readings for patients who actually had abnormal heart conditions, and vice versa. On the other hand, unreliable measurements can seriously harm the relevance of findings based on a measure that is essentially a valid one.

Sensitivity

This test refers to the ability of the measure to detect fine differences among the subjects being studied. One of the limitations of many types of ordinal and nominal scales is their crudeness. Possessing just a few global categories these scales may not be able to distinguish real, significant differences in the dependent variable, thus masking what may be important effects of the independent variable we are studying. If we use, for example, a scale consisting merely of two categories—improved, not improved—to measure the effects on patients of some nursing procedure we may be lumping together in the improved category patients whose conditions actually vary widely, some showing considerably more improvement than others. However, dividing such a scale into too many categories may not really increase the sensitivity, since some of the categories may represent distinctions that are too fine for the measure to detect properly. Thus, if the improved class were subdivided into "much improvement, moderate improvement, little improvement," we would have to be sure that the specifications for each of these scale values was of sufficient clarity and distinction to permit the use of the scale with a high degree of reliability. Moreover, we would also have to be certain that these more refined categories would have practical significance. That is, they should add substantively to our knowledge of the independent variable being evaluated.

With psychological and sociological phenomena there is often the temptation to expand an ordinal scale by treating it as an interval scale. The intervals between the scale points are subdivided into smaller and smaller segments, and the scale is then treated as a numerical one. To illustrate, assume that a five-category graphic rating scale consisting of the following classes is developed to measure the attitudes of the respondents toward some phenomenon:

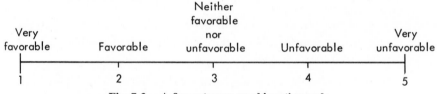

Fig. 7-3. A five-category graphic rating scale.

To introduce greater sensitivity the researcher might subdivide each of the four intervals into five equal parts and instruct the respondent to check the scale at the point that represents his feelings most closely. The researcher might then treat these data as being truly quantitative and expose them to the full battery of statistical methods. With such "refinement" the number of values on the scale has been increased four times:

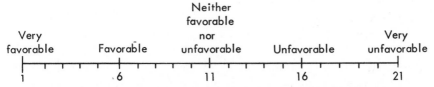

Fig. 7–4. A five-category graphic rating scale with further subdivisions.

That this type of refinement is somewhat unreal becomes obvious when it is considered that the numbers on this scale have no quantitative meaning, per se. They are purely positional, and indicate the rank order of the subject's response. We can say that a respondent with a value of 1 has greater positive feelings toward the phenomenon being rated than one with a value of 4, but we cannot say how much greater his feelings actually are.

The addition of the refined subdivisions has probably not increased the sensitivity of the measurements, since most users of the scale would not be able to make these distinctions validly. In fact, confused by such a large number of choices, they might be inclined to make erroneous ratings. Refinement in a case like this can actually reduce the reliability of an instrument.

With true numerical scales a high degree of sensitivity can be achieved. Theoretically such scales can be infinitely subdivided. A thermometer with gradations for each tenth of a degree can be scaled in terms of one-hundredth of a degree, if such sensitivity were required by the research. However, for readability a much bigger scale would be needed than the one commonly used. The instrument then might become impractical. Also, enlargement of a numerical scale might result in unneeded refinement. In most studies it makes little difference if a patient's temperature is read at 98.60° F. or 98.61° F. Refinement of a scale, even where mathematically justifiable, must be tempered by the practical significance of the very small differences in values obtained by such refinement.

Meaningfulness

The concept of meaningfulness of a measure can also be called the pragmatic test of the measure as a whole. Does the measure have any practical, real-life meaning and application? If an instrument is employed to measure patient satisfaction and it is found that by varying the in-dependent variable—say, hours of nursing care available—the scores on the patient satisfaction instrument are increased, does this mean that the patients are more well off when increased care is provided? What is meant by "well off"? Do they have better recovery rates? Do they live longer? Do they become more productive? Are they able to enjoy life more? In other words, the researcher should be able to translate the criterion of satisfaction, and the scale used to measure this criterion, into something tangible and meaningful.

Meaningfulness of a measure is related to the three previous tests of validity, reliability, and sensitivity. If a measure of a variable is not valid, it certainly cannot be meaningful. If the measure is not reliable, it cannot yield meaningful results, and if it is insensitive, it loses some of its mean-ingfulness.

The quest for a meaningful criterion measure is perhaps the most diffi-cult and the most important aspect of the design of nursing research. Un-less the criterion measure used in a study meets the tests of relevance and practicality, the findings may be ineffective and sterile.

It is difficult to find relevant and practical criterion measures in nursing research. How much simpler a task the medical researchers often have in this regard. Salk demonstrated the effectiveness of his polio vaccine by showing an impressive reduction in the incidence of this disease among children who were vaccinated. His criterion was not only relevant, it was practical and meaningful in a most important way—in a life and death way.

The social sciences have been accused of attempting to measure mean-ingful variables by scales that reduce them to meaningless and artificial constructs. Thus Krutch[17] attacks the attempt to measure a variable like "happiness" as follows:

> Misguided attempts to deal quantitatively with so complex a thing as happi-ness are the enemies of literature and perhaps of happiness itself because they encourage us to assume both that one kind of happiness is the same as another and that they are equally valuable. In fact nothing is more important, pruden-tially or morally, than the realization that whether or not the pursuit of happi-ness is a legitimate chief aim depends upon which of the many happinesses one chooses and upon the means used to pursue it. Taken seriously, statistical studies are all too likely to teach us only how to become dismally "adjusted." Is it safe to take seriously a study in which you put in the same category every-one who says that he frequently feels "on top of the world," even though feel-ing on top of the world may mean anything from the friskiness of a puppy to the joy celebrated in the Ninth Symphony?

Direct meaningful measurement of variables like "happiness" or "pa-tient care" may not be possible because, for one thing, they may not be unidimensional. Instead they might consist of numerous subvariables each having its own distinct underlying continuum. Moreover, like the difficulties encountered in attempting to measure directly the density of water, such complex variables may be measured more meaningfully through indirect methods. Thus, it was found that the variable "job morale" was assessed more adequately, not by constructing the scale from items whose content referred to the specifics of the actual work situation (my pay is not adequate, my supervisor does not treat me fairly, etc.), but rather from items oriented to the total life situation of the worker (my neighborhood is a pleasant one to live in, I enjoy playing with my children, etc.).

SUMMARIZATION OF RESEARCH DATA

In research, measures for individual study subjects obtained through the use of qualitative or quantitative scales are frequently combined and a summary measure computed for the total group. Comparisons are then made of the summary measures for the different groups. Thus, research largely deals with group measures rather than with measures of individuals, although in certain techniques, mentioned previously in the discussion of research design, data for individuals composing the alternative groups are directly compared individual by individual.

It is not the purpose of the following rather brief discussion of some of the more common summary measures to be definitive. Excellent statistical textbooks are available which provide a thorough explanation of these measures. Some of these texts are cited in the bibliography. The purpose of this discussion is to provide some insight into how the individual measures made in a study can be summarized in a meaningful way.

Qualitative Scales

As has been noted, the summarization of data obtained from qualitative scales (nominal or ordinal) is not as mathematically sophisticated as summarizations of measurements obtained from quantitative scales. Qualitative scales produce counts of the number of study subjects in each scale category. One of the most effective ways of summarizing such data is in the form of percentages. For example, for a group of 275 hospitalized patients who were classified into three categories according to their nursing care needs, the following distribution was found: intensive care 31, intermediate care 177, self-care 67. To convert these figures into percentages, each figure can be multiplied by 100 to move the decimal point two places to the right, which puts the data into manageable whole numbers, and each is then divided by the total, 275. The following percentage distribution is obtained:

| | Per Cent |
Total	*100**
Intensive care	11
Intermediate care	64
Self-care	24

* Note: adds to 99 because of the
process of rounding off the figures

Percentages are a type of summary measure known as a rate. A rate
expresses the relative frequency of occurrence of the particular scale value
for which it is computed. For the 275 patients in the example cited, the
relative frequency of occurrence of intensive care needs is 11 per 100
patients.

In a rate the denominator represents the total "group at risk," so to
speak, to exposure to the variable being studied. The notion of "at risk"
comes from the field of vital statistics where such rates as death rates,
case fatality rates, prevalence rates, provide a summary measure of the
number of individuals enumerated in a specific class of the variable out
of the total group "exposed" to the variable.

In a death rate the denominator represents the total group exposed
to the risk of dying. The scale for this variable consists of two alternative
categories: died, did not die. The numerator expresses the number out
of the total who were exposed to death who actually died.

As an illustration, suppose we are interested in computing the death
rate among the patients composing the active case load during the year
of a home nursing care program. We would multiply the number of deaths
occurring among the total case load by 100 (or some multiple of 100)
to have the resulting rate in a whole number, and then we would divide
the figure by the total case load. If the total case load were 26,433 and
the number of deaths 619, the death rate, called a case fatality rate,
would be 2.3 per 100 cases (619 × 100 ÷ 26,433), or in whole numbers,
23 per 1,000 cases. This rate could be refined even further. The total
case load could be divided into specific disease categories—cardiovascular,
cancer, communicable diseases, and so on—and the case fatality rate
computed for each category by dividing the number of deaths occurring
among patients having the specific disease by the total number of cases
in the disease category.

A true rate (relative frequency) has the following basic formula:

$$\frac{a}{a + b}$$

Where:

    a = Number of individuals in a specific category of the variable
    b = Number of individuals in all other categories of the variable

In a true rate the numerator is included in the denominator. If the summary measure does not possess this property, it is not a true rate. The so-called sex ratio shows the number of males in the group for every 100 females. To illustrate, if the number of males in our total home care case load is 10,415, and the number of females is 16,018, the sex ratio is 65 males for every 100 females: $\frac{10,415 \times 100}{16,018}$. It is obvious that this is not a true relative frequency, since the numerator (number of males) is not part of the denominator. If it were we would have a true rate. Such a true rate would show the percentage of the total case load that consists of males: $\frac{10,415 \times 100}{26,433} = 39$ per cent.

Table 7-3 contains some of the most widely used rates in the field of vital statistics. In these rates the total group at risk is usually the entire population of a community, city, state, or nation as a whole. However, the denominator could also consist of a group of study subjects (patients in a hospital, students in a school, residents of a housing development). The rates shown in Table 7-3 have been frequently used as criterion measures in research studies in the health field. Death rates, for example, have played important roles as criterion measures in research like that linking smoking to cancer of the lung. Incidence rates were widely used in research on polio vaccine.

The use of rates as summary measures of qualitatively scaled variables has several important advantages in research:

1. They are true relative frequencies and as such can be subjected to statistical tests of significance (see Chapter 9). In experimental studies of the effects of different methods of treatment on the survival rates of patients (similar to death rates except the numerator consists of the group who lived rather than died), a test of the significance of differences in rates can be applied to evaluate them statistically as in the following data:

Treat-ment Groups	Total in Group	Number Living After 1 year	1-year Survival Rates (in per cent)
Group I	176	114	64.8
Group II	191	119	62.3
Group III	183	101	55.2
Group IV	166	113	68.1

2. Rates reduce large numbers which are difficult to interpret into simpler, more digestible data. In the following data the first column, showing the number of graduates from schools of nursing in the United States

TABLE 7-3

Rates Used in Vital Statistics

Name of Rate	How Computed
1. Prevalence rate	$\dfrac{\text{All cases of specific disease at given time} \times 1{,}000}{\text{Population at given time}}$
2. Case fatality rate	$\dfrac{\text{Deaths from specific disease in given period} \times 100}{\text{Cases of specific disease in given period}}$
3. Annual death rate	$\dfrac{\text{Deaths from all causes in calendar year} \times 1{,}000}{\text{Population of July 1}}$
4. Annual age specific death rate	$\dfrac{\text{Death from all causes for given age group in year} \times 1{,}000}{\text{Population for given age group, July 1}}$
5. Annual death rate from specific cause	$\dfrac{\text{Deaths from specific cause in year} \times 100{,}000}{\text{Population of July 1}}$
6. Annual case incidence rate of a specific disease	$\dfrac{\text{New cases of specific disease in year} \times 1{,}000}{\text{Population of July 1}}$
7. Annual birth rate	$\dfrac{\text{Live births in year} \times 1{,}000}{\text{Population of July 1}}$
8. Stillbirth rate	$\dfrac{\text{Stillbirths in year} \times 100 \ (\text{or } 1{,}000)}{\text{Total births in year}}$
9. Infant mortality rate	$\dfrac{\text{Deaths under one year of age in year} \times 1{,}000}{\text{Live births in year}}$
10. Neonatal mortality rate	$\dfrac{\text{Deaths under one month of age in year} \times 1{,}000 \ (\text{or } 10{,}000)}{\text{Live births in year}}$
11. Maternal mortality rate	$\dfrac{\text{Maternal deaths in year} \times 1{,}000 \ (\text{or } 10{,}000)}{\text{Live births in year}}$

in 1961 according to their performance on state board exams, is much more difficult to interpret than the corresponding percentages:

Total	Number of Graduates (35,328)	Percentages of Graduates (100.0)
Passed	29,647	83.9
Failed	5,681	16.1

3. Rates are especially advantageous as summary measures in comparing data for different-sized groups. The rates, expressed in terms of per 100, per 1,000, or some other base, reduce the data to comparable units. Thus, a comparison of only the number of deaths among the patients in two hospitals that differ greatly in size can give the misleading im-

pression that the occurrence of death was greater in the larger hospital when in fact on a relative frequency basis the reverse was true:

	Total Number of Patients Admitted During the Year	Number of Deaths Among Patients Admitted	Death Rate per 1,000 Patients
Hospital A	21,415	419	19.6
Hospital B	7,631	184	24.1

4. Rates can be viewed as statements of probability of occurrence, and as such can be useful in making predictions.

Quantitative Scales

For many quantitatively scaled variables the values of measurements made for the individual subject would follow what is known as a bell-shaped curve if plotted on a chart. In such a chart the vertical axis, known as the Y-axis, would represent the number of study subjects possessing the values measured, and the horizontal axis, the X-axis, would represent the values of the scale. The bell-shaped curve indicates that the majority of the subjects cluster together and possess about the same scale value, while fewer and fewer subjects possess the more extreme values. The ideal bell-shaped curve is called the normal curve, the normal frequency distribution, or the Gaussian curve, after its discoverer the German mathematician Karl F. Gauss. Such a curve, shown in Figure 7-5, has a single peak where the majority of subjects measured cluster. As the values of the measures fan out symmetrically from the central peak, the curve tapers off to the extremes, where only a few subjects are found.

In actual studies, the distributions of measurements do not precisely follow the shape of the normal curve. Measurements of some variables are better described by other types of curves. In general, though, these curves will also have the property of a single peak, and the values do taper off at each side of the peak, but perhaps not symmetrically. For many quantitatively scaled variables, the normal curve provides a rough approximation of the distribution of the measurements of the variable among the subjects studied. It can be used without greatly violating statistical theory as the model for the analysis of many variables employed in research studies.

Distributions of measurements obtained from variables having quantitative scales can be described by two summary measures. One, known as the measure of central tendency, or the average, is the measure of the value that is most typical of the values of all the individual measurements that have been made. In a normal curve it is the value on the X-axis that

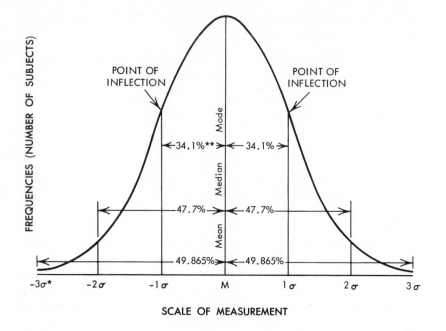

*σ represents standard deviation

** Indicates percentage of total subjects
   possessing the measurement values

Fig. 7–5. The normal, bell-shaped distribution.

lies beneath the peak of the curve (in Figure 7-5, it is the value labeled M). The other summary measure is that of the variation of the values of the individual measurements around the average value. This is known as the measure of the dispersion of the individual values.

Theoretically, measures of central tendency and variation are applicable only to data obtained from quantitatively scaled variables. However, they are also often used for qualitatively scaled variables. For example, achievement and other types of psychological tests, which essentially yield ordinal type data because it cannot be demonstrated that their underlying scales have equal or measurable intervals, are often scored and analyzed, not by rates as for qualitatively scaled data, but by the measures of central tendency and variation specifically developed for quantitatively scaled data. Thus a teacher will often compute the average score for all the students who took an achievement test as well as analyze the variation among the scores.

In addition, rates obtained for qualitatively scaled variables are often averaged. For example, the percentage of the population immunized against polio could be computed for each of the various communities studied. These individual percentages can be combined in terms of a summary measure that expresses the average percentage of the population immunized in all communities studied. In a sense the individual percentages for each community are quantitative measures of the extent to which the members of each community are immunized. Therefore, they can be treated as values arising from a quantitative scale.

Measures of Central Tendency

The three main summary measures that describe the central tendency of a distribution of measures of a quantitative variable for a group of study subjects are the *mode, median,* and *mean.* These summary measures are known as averages. When the individual measures form a normal curve, the values of the three summary measures are equal. In distributions that depart from normality these values are different.

To illustrate the differences in the three measures, assume we are experimentally testing the effects on their blood pressure of giving patients an extra amount of tender loving care. Our experimental group can be labeled A and the control group receiving the usual amount of T.L.C. is labeled B. We randomly allocate 30 patients (and the personnel, too) to the two alternative groups, 15 in each group. We then apply the extra T.L.C. to Group A and after a suitable period of time measure the blood pressures for the 15 patients in each group:

Patient No.	Blood Pressure	
	Group A	*Group B*
1	130	161
2	139	112
3	149	155
4	120	101
5	118	176
6	130	97
7	138	137
8	160	128
9	110	185
10	145	248
11	148	133
12	123	129
13	105	114
14	155	179
15	130	104

Mode   The mode is the most common or typical value in a distribution of measurements. It is found by inspecting the distribution and finding that value which occurs most frequently. In Group A the most common value is 130, since it was recorded for three patients. For Group B no value appears more frequently than another; thus there is no modal value.

As a descriptive as well as an analytic summary measure the mode is less frequently used than the other two averages. One of its shortcomings is the fact that it is sometimes incalculable. Also it may be an arbitrary value. This is particularly true when the individual measurements are grouped into classes, to be discussed shortly, and the value of the mode is influenced by the grouping of values the researcher selects.

Median   When the values of the measurements are arranged in order of magnitude, the median is the value that is larger than half of the values and smaller than the other half. It is thus the middle value of a distribution. To determine the median blood pressure values for our two groups of 15 patients we would first arrange the individual values in order of size:

Group A	Group B
105	97
110	101
118	104
120	112
123	114
130	128
130	129
130	133
138	137
139	155
145	161
148	176
149	179
155	185
160	248

The median blood pressure reading for Group A is 130 and for Group B it is 133. These values are the middle values among the groups of readings: they are the eighth values among the 15 readings when they are arranged in order of magnitude. They exceed seven of the values and are exceeded by seven. Thus in a series of measurements arranged in order of size consisting of an *odd* number of measurements, the median value is actually the middle value. If a series of measurements consists of an even number of items, the median would be found lying between the *two* middle values. For example, if Group B consisted of only 14 values (assume the last reading, 248, is omitted), the median would lie between 129 and 133. In practice these two values are added together and divided by 2 to obtain a single value for the median, which in this example would be 131: $(129 + 133)/2$.

The median is a very useful summary measure of central tendency, particularly where the distribution of measures departs significantly from the model of the normal curve. Such asymetrical distributions are called "skewed" distributions. The median is simple to calculate, although it does require the individual values to be arranged in order of magnitude.

Mean Unlike the two previous summary measures, which depend upon the most frequently occurring value (mode) or the value located in the middle when the values arranged in order of magnitude (median), the mean is calculated by taking account of the actual value of each of the individual measurements. The mean is simply the sum of all the values divided by the number of values. For Group A the mean is $2,000/15 = 133$. For Group B it is $2,159/15 = 144$.

The mean is probably the most widely used measure of central tendency. One of the reasons for this is its mathematical properties, not possessed by the mode or median, which make it very valuable in statistical analysis of the data. These properties are:

1. If the value of each individual measurement is subtracted from the mean and the differences (deviations) are then added, with the plus and minus signs of the deviations considered, the sum of the deviations will always be zero.

2. If these deviations are squared (the value of each deviation multiplied by itself) and then summed up, the value of this sum will be smaller than the value of the sum of the squared deviations of each value from any quantity other than the mean.

Because of these properties, as well as the fact that the actual value of each measurement is considered in its calculation, the mean provides more information about a set of measurement values than do the other averages.

Measures of Variation

The second most important type of summary measure is the measure of variation of the individual values. This tells us the extent to which the values obtained for the study subjects are different from each other. Such a measure complements the measure of central tendency, since it is obvious that two sets of measurements could have identical values for their measures of central tendency, yet be very different in terms of the spread of the individual values. For simplicity, take two groups of five patients in which the following body temperatures are recorded:

Group A	Group B
98.6° F.	96.6° F.
98.6°	97.6°
98.6°	98.6°
98.6°	99.6°
98.6°	100.6°

The mean and median would be identical for both groups—98.6° F.—yet it is obvious that the two distributions of temperatures are very different. In Group A there is no variation among the patients whereas in Group B there is a considerable amount of difference in the temperatures recorded.

There are many summary measures of variation. Three will be briefly described: *range, percentile,* and *standard deviation.*

Range   This is the simplest measure of variation to compute. It consists of the lowest and highest values in the set of measurements. Sometimes the range is considered as the difference between the lowest and highest values. Thus in our blood pressure data the range is 105–160 for Group A. For Group B it is 97–248. This would indicate that Group B's measurements have greater variation than do Group A's. A shortcoming of the range is that it is greatly influenced by extreme values. In Group B, the reading of 248 is considerably out of line with the rest of the measurements. If it were excluded, the range would be 97–185, much closer to Group A's range.

Percentile   The notion of percentiles, which should not be confused with the concept of percentages, is an elaboration of the median. A percentile is a positional value that is found by lining up the values in order of size. The median is the fiftieth percentile. To find any other percentile we would follow the same procedure as in locating the median. To find the tenth percentile we find the value that exceeds 10 per cent of the measurements and is exceeded by 90 per cent of them. Conversely, the ninetieth percentile is the value that exceeds 90 per cent of the values and is exceeded by 10 per cent of them. For the blood pressure data it would be difficult to calculate percentiles, since there are so few values. Percentiles are best calculated when the number of measurements is large, preferably in the hundreds. Roughly, however, the tenth percentile for Group A lies somewhere between 105 and 110 and for Group B is between 97 and 101.

Percentiles have many interesting uses both descriptively and analytically. They have been widely applied in the field of psychological tests and measurements. As a measure of variation the percentile has an advantage over the range in that it tones down the effects of extreme values. One such measure is called the interquartile range. This is the range between the twenty-fifth percentile (the first quartile) and the seventy-fifth percentile (the third quartile—the median is the second quartile). To illustrate how to calculate the first and third quartiles for our two groups of patients we would find those values that exceed 25 per cent of the values and are exceeded by 75 per cent—the first quartile—and those that exceed 75 per cent of the values and are exceeded by 25 per cent—the third quartile. For Group A the interquartile range is 120–148. And for Group B it is 112–176, indicating considerably greater variation of the values of individual measurements for this group of patients. In fact the interquartile range for Group B patients extends over twice the magnitude, 64, of the range for Group A, 28.

Standard Deviation　By far the most widely used measure of variation of a set of measurement values is the standard deviation. This measure is complementary to the arithmetic mean. In statistical analysis these two summary measures often accompany each other. Briefly, the computation of the standard deviation is as follows: The difference between the values of each individual measurement and the mean is determined. Each deviation is then squared. The sum of all the squared deviations is divided by the number of measurements. The square root is then found of the resulting quotient (that number which when multiplied by itself will yield the quotient), which is the value of the standard deviation. For Group A the standard deviation is *16* and for Group B it is *40*.

It is obvious that the value of a standard deviation provides a meaningful indication of the extent of variation among the values of the individual measurements. If there were no differences among a set of measurements, the value of the standard deviation would be zero, as in the example of the five patients in Group A who had identical temperatures of 98.6° F. The greater the value of the standard deviation, the greater the variation among the values of the measurements.

Like the arithmetic mean, the standard deviation has several valuable mathematical properties. Among these is the fact that in measurements that are distributed approximately like the normal curve, deviations of the value of the standard deviation from the arithmetic mean include the following percentage of all the values of the measurements found among the study subjects:

Plus and minus one standard deviation from the mean = 68 per cent of all the values

Plus and minus two standard deviations from the mean = 95 per cent
of all the values

Plus and minus three standard deviations from the mean = 100 per cent
of all the values

These ranges apply best where the number of measurements is large. In
small groups of measures they are only approximate. To illustrate: in
Group A the mean ± 1 standard deviation gives the range 117 to 149
(133 ± 16). This range actually includes 11 of the 15 values, or 73
per cent of them. And ± 3 standard deviations from the mean gives the
range 85 to 181, which includes 100 per cent of the 15 values.

The various summary measures that we have computed for the quantitative measurements of the variable "blood pressure" for our two groups
of 15 patients are recapitulated as follows.

Central Tendency	Group A	Group B
Mode	130	Nonexistent
Median	130	133
Mean	133	144
Variation		
Range	105–160	97–248
Quartile range	120–148	112–176
Standard deviation	16	40

These summary measures provide a succinct and meaningful picture of
the distribution of the individual measurements.

Grouped Data

When the number of individual measurement values is large, it is advantageous to group the measurements into broader scale categories. From
a descriptive standpoint the grouped data are often more meaningful than
ungrouped data. The detail provided by the individual measurements may
be unnecessary, since small differences in values may not indicate substantive differences in the variable measured. From an analytical viewpoint, grouping the data may reveal the shape of the distribution of measurements being analyzed. Thus in grouping the data on the blood pressure
measures we find that A patients appear to follow the pattern of the bell-
shaped curve while the B patients' measurements can best be described by
what is called a U-shaped curve.

Blood Pressure (grouped)	Group A	Group B
Total	15	15
Less than 120	3	5
120–139	7	4
140–159	4	1
160 and over	1	5

It is not difficult to compute the summary measures from measurements that are grouped. When the number of measurements is very large it is often quicker to compute the summary measures from the grouped data than from the individual measurements. Methods for such computations are contained in the statistical texts cited in the bibliography.

THE ROLE OF CRITERION MEASURES IN RESEARCH IN NURSING

Measurement of patient care in terms of valid and reliable criterion measures is a crucial part of research in nursing. Because of the multidimensional nature of patient care, it is difficult but not impossible to measure this variable. Measurement of patient care can be approached by evaluating the adequacy of the facilities in which patient care is provided, the effectiveness of the administrative and organizational structure of the agency providing patient care, the professional qualifications and competency of personnel employed to provide the care, and the evaluation of the effect on the consumers of care—the patients.

Patient care in hospitals is being appraised by four techniques.[18] The first is the examination of the prerequisites for adequate care, such as the minimum and optimum levels of facilities, equipment, professional training and distribution of personnel, and the organizational structure of the institution.

Second is the evaluation of performance, particularly of tasks related to patient care. Here such observable quantitative measures can be used as the time nursing personnel spend on activities with patients, the utilization rates for specific procedures, length of patient stay, use of chest x-rays, laboratory and other diagnostic procedures, autopsy rates, pathological reports on surgical specimens, and correlations between preoperative and postoperative diagnosis.

The development of rating scales to measure levels of adequacy of patient care is the third way of measuring the quality of care. Scales need to be developed which provide appropriate yardsticks to estimate qualitative levels of care. Most desirably such scales should be quantitative.

The fourth way of measuring quality is direct measurement of the patient by clinical evaluation. This can become highly subjective and less relevant than the three previous methods, but in many respects it is the most ideal measure, since it focuses on the product of patient care.

Criterion Measures of Patient Care

Criterion measures of nursing practice must derive from the dependent variables that indicate the effects of practice upon patient care.

The criterion measures of patient care may be categorized into four main groups.

Group I. Criterion measures of patient care related to preventive care needs.[19] These measures are observable in all patients. The patient's ability:
1. To maintain good hygiene and physical comfort
2. To achieve optimal activity, exercise, rest, and sleep
3. To prevent accident, injury, or other trauma and prevent the spread of infection
4. To maintain good body mechanics and prevent and correct deformities

Group II. Criteria of patient care related to sustenal and restorative care needs. This group of criterion measures of patient care relates to normal and disturbed physiological body processes that are vital to sustaining life. The patient's ability:
5. To facilitate the maintenance of a supply of oxygen to all body cells
6. To facilitate the maintenance of nutrition to all body cells
7. To facilitate the maintenance of elimination
8. To facilitate the maintenance of fluid and electrolyte balance
9. To recognize the physiological responses of the body to disease conditions—pathological, physiological, and compensatory
10. To faclitate the maintenance of regulatory mechanisms and functions
11. To facilitate the maintenance of sensory function

Group III. This group of criterion measures of patient care involves those related to rehabilitative needs, particularly those involving emotional and interpersonal difficulties.
12. To identify and accept positive and negative expressions, feelings, and reactions
13. To identify and accept the interrelatedness of emotions and organic illness
14. To facilitate the maintenance of effective verbal and nonverbal communication
15. To promote the development of productive interpersonal relationships
16. To facilitate progress toward achievement of personal spiritual goals
17. To create and/or maintain a therapeutic environment
18. To facilitate awareness of self as an individual with varying physical, emotional, and developmental needs
19. To accept the optimum possible goals in light of limitations, physical and emotional

Group IV. This group covers those criteria of patient care related to sociological and community problems affecting patient care. The patient's ability:

20. To use community resources as an aid in resolving problems arising from illness
21. To understand the role of social problems as influencing factors in the cause of illness

Measurable Components of Patient Care

At present, the components of patient care that are easiest to measure fall into Group II—those observations that report disturbed physiological and body processes. These include vital signs such as T.P.R., blood pressure, EKG, oxygen content in the blood.

Difficulties in Identifying Criterion Measures

Nurses themselves cannot agree upon measurable criteria of effective nursing care. A scientific body of knowledge that is uniquely nursing has yet to be identified to provide a theoretical basis against which nursing practice can be measured. Unlike the use of criterion measures in controlled laboratory research in which the organism being studied is in a controlled environment such as a test tube or a cage, in nursing they must be employed in the framework of the patient's complex environment. Since there are so many extraneous variables in the situation, both organismic and environmental, it is exceedingly difficult to keep them under sufficient control.

The difficulties in identifying criterion measures in nursing have directed much of the research in nursing into areas that are more easily researchable. To illustrate, the study of the nurse—what she does, how much time she spends on patient care—can only provide us with empirical knowledge. This knowledge has value in that it helps to discern problem areas that need to be studied in more depth. Ultimately, how the nurse functions must be measured against the effects (criterion measures) of nursing practice upon the patient.

Likewise, studies of the role of the nurse have value in giving direction to the nursing profession. These studies are indeed important but will have little decisive impact on the improvement of patient care if there are no adequate criterion measures to evaluate effects of changed practice upon patient care. Therefore, we may surmise falsely that we have improved nursing care, but we really may not know what effect this care has upon the patient. We may be meeting the hospital's, the physician's, and the nurse's needs, but not the patient's!

The lack of criterion measures in nursing places a partial blindfold on the nurse as she provides nursing care. Her practice thus becomes one of trial and error instead of one based upon tested practices proven to be scientifically effective.

Donabedian in a paper, "Some Basic Issues in Evaluating the Quality of Health Care," presented at the ANA, National Invitational Conference, "Issues in Evaluative Research," 1975, stated that there is not enough knowledge at present to base any program of quality assessment assurance exclusively on any one structure, process, or outcome. All three have to be used simultaneously. The system also needs to be designed to show the relationships among the three. Desirable outcome criteria related to health care are controversial and some not economically feasible. They are also time-dependent—outcomes taking different times to become apparent. The identification and equalization of risk factors are necessary preconditions to the assessment of outcomes.

Progress Made in the Measurement of the Quality of Nursing

Research in nursing can produce new knowledge, better methods of caring for people, and sounder rationales for tested nursing practices. Nurses may undertake studies that throw light on patient problems or reveal characteristics of the community setting of health problems. Thus, research is an important means of improving quality nursing practice.

The first significant early attempt to measure quality nursing care was made by Reiter and Kakosh in 1950.[20] They identified 12 components of nursing care to define some standards for appraising observed nursing care. These components are:

1. Control of environment
2. Mental adjustment
3. Condition of skin and mucous membranes
4. Elimination
5. Posture, position, and exercise
6. Rest and sleep
7. Nutrition
8. Observation of signs and symptoms
9. Administration of laboratory tests
10. Administration of medicines
11. Administration of treatments
12. Teaching health

Each component was defined in operational terms and an observational guide was developed to record these observations.

Six qualitative categories were next developed and defined to form criterion measures that might be quantitatively scaled. These are:

Dangerous: The patient's health or welfare is endangered by the nursing care he received.

Safe: No harm comes to the patient for having had nursing care; patient's life and values protected.

Adequate: To the extent that it is possible, the patient's standards and customary way of living are kept as normal as possible; that he recovers to the greatest extent his former state of health at his own rate of recovery.

Optimum: The patient's integrity is respected and he is helped to improve his state of health and is better able to care for himself.

Maximum: The design of patient care is based on the best known scientific advances to date.

Ideal: Patient care is examined and evaluated for the purpose of improvement through controlled research in nursing.

Quality nursing practice is based on scientific findings that emerge from a study of nursing practice itself. Quality nursing practice has been defined as follows:

For the patient it means that the best present nursing practice is not good enough and for the nurse it means incorporating research in nursing into the practice of nursing. The components of such care not only include the conscious and continuous search for the reasons underlying the nursing care but also the creation of new ways of care.[21]

Recent Attempts to Measure Quality

Several other direct attempts have been made to measure quality nursing practice. A few significant ones will be mentioned.

A long-range study was initiated in 1955 by Aydelotte and Simon[22] at Iowa in which measures of skin condition, mental attitude, and mobility were developed. Simon[23] continued the work by studying activity patterns of hospitalized medical and urological patients with the aim of deriving patient activity indices that might be used as measures of patient welfare. Sampling was carried out by nurse observers who used a special code to record what each patient was doing at the moment he was observed. Twenty-eight different indices were computed for each patient, each representing the proportion of time the patient spent in a given category of activity. These indices were correlated with other patient welfare measures and were found to be significant.

A four-year study of nursing care of the hospitalized patient with a diagnosis of myocardial infarction was undertaken by Nite and Willis[24] at Community Studies, Inc., Kansas City. A nurse and a social scientist participated in giving direct care to patients and were able to identify some of the "measuring rods" that could be used in evaluating a special type of care given to these patients. The conceptualization underlying this research is that nursing practice can be therapeutic when it is directed toward correctly identified problems of specific patients, and when administered to the patient will give evidence of resolution of these problems.

The researchers were able to identify specific criteria of improvement to measure the progress of the cardiac patient. Examples of such criteria were: the patient will gradually show less apprehension toward pain as he is given an understanding of the physiological process causing pain; the patient permits the nurse to perform necessary activities for him; the patient will tend to sleep during the day after major activities and during the entire night without medication.

Meltzer and Pinneo[25] at Presbyterian Hospital in Philadelphia sought to find the answer to this question: Can the modification of nursing practices result in the reduction in the death rate of cardiac patients? Attention was directed at lowering the fatality rate of coronary patients developing arrhythmias during the first 72-hour period of hospitalization. Intensive nursing care and observation by utilizing special monitoring systems to identify subtle changes in the patient's status might make it possible to take action during the precatastrophic period. Specific steps have been outlined for the nurse to follow once the catastrophe has occurred.

As a result of this study several lives have been saved owing to the professional nurse's being able to recognize signs early enough and to initiate countershock therapy within *a few seconds* of the detection of the arrhythmia. The researchers have developed tools to assess the patient's condition on admission and during hospitalization in order to predict patient behavior prior to the occurrence of the catastrophe.

Attempts to measure quality nursing by the nurse's performance have had limited use in measuring the effect of nursing care upon patient recovery. A small but significant study was conducted by Dumas,[26] in which she showed that clinical experiments in nursing practice are feasible and can be used to measure quality nursing. The aim of this research was to observe the effect of an experimental nursing process on the incidence of vomiting during recovery from anesthesia.

One experiment included the study of a sample of patients who were scheduled for surgery. Patients assigned to the experimental group were given nursing care by research nurses who used the experimental nursing process. This is a process directed toward helping the patient obtain a suitable psychological state for surgery. Specific steps are described in this process: (1) the nurse observes the patient's behavior and explores with him whether or not he is experiencing distress; (2) the nurse explores further to find out what is causing the distress and what is needed to relieve the distress; (3) an appropriate course of action is next undertaken to relieve the stress; and (4) the nurse follows through on her action(s) to see if the distress was relieved. This experimental nursing process was proved to be successful in reducing postoperative vomiting.

An important theoretical basis for this study is that emotional reactions of surgical patients to their illness and treatment have important consequences for their postoperative course. The study has demonstrated further that the relief of emotional distress is a part of the nurse's professional role.

A major problem in measuring quality nursing is the lack of instrumentation to measure it directly. Smith[27] at the University of Florida proposed that we measure nursing practice more indirectly than directly. Measurement of the nursing care of a "patient as a whole" may not be possible. Measurement of quality nursing might be made on the basis of the "scientific rightness" of our assessment of the patient's nursing problems and our management of them. It is proposed that ". . . we need a system—an organized framework wherein we can see plainly and definitely what is to be done and what we must do to accomplish it." It is proposed that the nursing problems that professional nurses are called upon to assess and manage daily might form the basis for evaluating quality nursing care. Quality nursing might be measured indirectly by examining the system or organization provided for dealing with these nursing problems. For example, the degree to which communications are systematized might be one of the most important criterion measures that can be used in assessing quality nursing practice.

Hegyvary and Haussmann[28,29] developed a methodology for monitoring the quality of nursing care which focuses on the nursing process and the actual delivery of nursing care. This research effort began in 1972 and later resulted in the development of a project designed to develop an improved methodology for monitoring the quality of care by:

- Synthesizing and incorporating methodologies available;
- Establishing a conceptual framework for nursing care, one that could accommodate both existing and new criteria;
- Designing an observation and scoring methodology using a set of criteria to maximize measurement efficiency; and
- Testing the methodology and refining criteria.

The basis of the quality monitoring methodology is a master list of 220 criteria applicable to medical, surgical, and pediatric nursing units. Not all are used with each patient.

The researchers pilot-tested the research in two hospitals to test the applicability, comprehensiveness, and reliability of criteria. Further intensive testing and analysis demonstrated the instrument to be reliable and valid. Nurse observers, once trained, can achieve reliability in their interpretation of evaluation criteria. The quality-monitoring methodology developed proved to be an important tool for nursing management in controlling nursing performance at a unit level. It was found that it is not enough to assess patient outcomes. Nursing management must know and understand both process and outcomes to be able to make decisions regarding quality of care.

This research effort also identified important problems to consider in developing criteria. These are: establishing and maintaining validity and reliability in quality monitoring; observers' general ability and willingness to interview patients; nurses' loyalty to hospital policies; poor quality of records; and writing criteria for specific populations.

The American Nurses' Association (ANA) has a long history in the involvement in efforts of quality assurance. A major effort beginning in 1974 resulted in a milestone document, *Guidelines for Review of Nursing Care at the Local Level*.[30] The guidelines, contained in the manual, had been developed as one part of the contract between ANA and the Department of Health, Education, and Welfare (DHEW). Mrs. Geraldine Ellis served as the DHEW Project Officer. The manual is intended to help registered nurses develop a system for evaluating the quality of nursing care.

Examples of guidelines suggested in developing outcome criteria are:

- Screening criterion is a crucial factor (outcome or process) that, if not met, may indicate a significant deficiency in nursing care. Screening criteria are used to survey a large number of cases to determine acceptable levels of patient outcomes.
- The outcome stated in the criterion must be possible to achieve.
- Each criterion should be a statement of one specific outcome representing its optimal achievement.
- In establishing criteria, select the most critical time for the measurement of the identified outcome for a particular population.
- A criterion must be appraisable and phrased in positive terms.
- Criteria are not static and will change as values and scientific knowledge change.

STEPS IN WRITING OUTCOME CRITERIA

- Choose a category.
- Identify the target population.
- Select the appropriate population variables.
- Select criteria subsets.
- Generate outcome criteria.
- Establish critical time of measurement.
- Establish the standard.
- Establish any exceptions to the criteria and standards.
- Document the sources for the criteria.
- Select screening criteria.

The development of outcome criteria in nursing is particularly significant as nurses become more involved in peer review mechanisms such as Professional Standards Review Organizations (PSROs) enacted by Congress in 1972 under P.L. 92–603. PSROs are modeled after the fundamental concept of peer review, which holds that health professionals rather than third party payors are the most appropriate individuals to evaluate the quality of services they deliver and that peer review should be done at the local level.

In 1974, Lang[31] developed a Model for Quality Assurance, which was later adapted for use by ANA/DHEW. The components of the model are:

- Clarification of values.
- Establishment of outcome, process and structure standards, and criteria of nursing care.
- Assessment of the degree of discrepancy between the standards and criteria and the current level of nursing practice.
- Selection and implementation of an alternative for changing nursing practice.
- Improvement of nursing practice.

The function of the Lang model is to provide a mechanism into which one may feed specific data. The model can accommodate a variety of practice situations.

The development of patient assessment approaches and related outcome criteria for long-term care patients started more than 25 years ago and culminated in the work of Densen, Jones, Flagle, Katz, and Danehy.[32] A dictionary of common definitions and single data base were significant contributions of this effort.

In 1974, DHEW launched a nationwide Long Term Care Facility Improvement Campaign.[33,34] A significant finding of this effort was that in order to improve the quality of care in nursing homes one must first assess the patient's/resident's needs for care, develop a plan of care with specific goals, and determine through outcome criteria if the goals have been met. DHEW has now developed, tested, and modified a systematic process for assessing health care. The process is referred to as Patient Appraisal and Care Evaluation (PACE). PACE can provide a single data source which is consistent and a current source of patient/resident data including demographic descriptors, impairments, functional status, services provided, etc. Specifically, PACE provides accessible and measurable data on appropriateness of care as well as outcome criteria for use by such groups as PSROs, JCAH, DHEW, state, and regional surveyors. The PACE system needs to be adpated for use in hospitals and in noninstitutional care settings such as home care, day care centers, hospices.

The identification of criterion measures of nursing practice poses many problems because of its complexity. Multiple studies will have to be undertaken before measures of quality nursing can be identified. Measurement of quality care will have to be both direct and indirect before a complete assessment of the effect(s) of nursing practice upon patient welfare can be made.

References

1. Genevieve R. Meyer, *Tenderness and Technique: Nursing Values in Transition*. Los Angeles, Institute of Industrial Relations, University of California, 1960, p. 13.
2. Miriam A. Safren and Alphonse Chapanis, "A Critical Incident Study of Hospital Medication Errors." *Hospitals, J.A.H.A.*, **34:**62, 64, May 1, 1960.
3. Claire Selltiz *et al.*, *Research Methods in Social Relations*. New York, Holt, Rinehart and Winston, 1962, p. 435.
4. Morris R. Cohen and Ernest Nagel, *An Introduction to Logic and Scientific Method*. New York, Harcourt, Brace and Co., 1934, pp. 289–290.
5. Helen Peak, "Problems of Objective Observation," Chapter 6 in Leon Festinger and Daniel Katz (eds.), *Research Methods in the Behavioral Sciences*. New York, The Dryden Press, 1953, p. 256.
6. Stuart Wright, "Turnover and Job Satisfaction," *Hospitals, J.A.H.A.*, **31:** 47–52, October 1, 1957.
7. Rena E. Boyle, *A Study of Student Nurse Perception of Patient Attitudes*. U.S. Public Health Service Publication No. 769. Washington, D.C., Government Printing Office, 1960.
8. Faye G. Abdellah and Eugene Levine, "Developing a Measure of Patient and Personnel Satisfaction with Nursing Care." *Nursing Res.*, **5:**100–108, February 1957.
9. Eileen G. Hasselmeyer, *Behavior Patterns of Premature Infants*. U.S. Public Health Service Publication No. 840. Washington, D.C., Government Printing Office, 1961.
10. Macolm W. Klein *et al.*, "Problems of Measuring Patient Care in the Outpatient Department." *J. Health and Human Behavior,* **2:**138–144, 1961.
11. W. Stephenson, *The Study of Behavior, Q-technique and Its Methodology*. Chicago, University of Chicago Press, 1953.
12. William G. Cochran, "Research Techniques in the Study of Human Beings." *Millbank Memorial Fund Quarterly*, **33:**125, April 1955.
13. Selltiz *et al., op. cit.*, pp. 196–197.
14. W. Allen Wallis and Harry V. Roberts, *Statistics: A New Approach*. New York, The Free Press of Glencoe, 1956, p. 133.

15. Wright, *op. cit.*

16. Jane Wilcox, "Observer Factors in the Measurement of Blood Pressure." *Nursing Res.,* **10:**4–17, winter 1961.

17. Joseph Wood Krutch, "Through Happiness with Slide Rule and Calipers." *The Saturday Review,* **XLVI:**14, November 2, 1963.

18. Mindel C. Sheps, "Approaches to the Quality of Hospital Care." *Publ. Health Rep.,* **70:**877–886, September 1955.

19. Faye G. Abdellah *et al., Patient-Centered Approaches to Nursing.* New York, Macmillan Publishing Co., Inc., 1960.

20. Frances Reiter and Marguerite E. Kakosh. *Quality of Nursing Care,* A Report of a Field Study to Establish Criteria 1950–1954 (P.H.S. Grant #RG 2734). Institute of Research and Studies in Nursing Education, Division of Nursing Education, Teachers College, Columbia University, 1963.

21. Reiter and Kakosh, *op. cit.*

22. Myrtle K. Aydelotte and Marie E. Tener, "An Investigation of the Relation Between Nursing Activity and Patient Welfare." Iowa City, State University of Iowa, Utilization Project, 1960.

23. J. Richard Simon, "Patient Activity as a Measure of Patient Welfare." State University of Iowa, October 1962 (P.H.S. Grant, GN 7610, unpublished).

24. Gladys Nite and Frank Willis, *The Coronary Patient: Hospital Care and Rehabilitation.* New York, Macmillan Publishing Co., Inc., 1964.

25. Lawrence E. Meltzer, Rose Pinneo, and J. R. Kitchell, *Intensive Coronary Care.* A Manual for Nurses. Philadelphia, The Charles Press, 1970.

26. Rhetaugh G. Dumas and Robert C. Leonard, "The Effect of Nursing on the Incidence of Post-operative Vomiting." *Nursing Res.,* **12:**12–15, winter 1963.

27. Dorothy M. Smith, "Myth and Method in Nursing Practice." *Am. J. Nursing,* **64:**68–72, February 1964.

28. Sue Thomas Hegyvary and R. K. Dieter Haussmann, "Monitoring Nursing Care Quality." *Journal of Nursing Administration,* **6:**9:3–9, November 1976.

29. R. K. Dieter Haussmann, Sue T. Hegyvary, and John F. Newman, *Monitoring Quality of Nursing Care.* Part II, Assessment and Study of Correlates. Bethesda, Md., DHEW Pub. No. (HRA) 76–77, July 1976.

30. American Nurses' Association, *Guidelines for Review of Nursing Care at the Local Level,* Rockville, Md., DHEW Contract HSA 105–74–207, September 1976.

31. Norma Lang, "A Model for Quality Assurance in Nursing." Unpublished doctoral dissertation, Marquette University, Milwaukee, Wis., May 1974.

32. Ellen W. Jones, *Patient Classification for Long-Term Care: User's Manual.* Rockville, Md., DHEW Pub. No. HRA 74–3107, December 1973.

33. DHEW, *Long-Term Care Facility Improvement Study.* Rockville, Md., DHEW Pub. No. (OS) 76–50021, July 1975.

34. Faye G. Abdellah, "Patient Assessment. Its Potential and Use." *American Health Care Association Journal,* **1:**3:69–80, November 1975.

Problems and Suggestions for Further Study

1. Describe five variables that could serve as either a dependent or independent variable in patient care research. What kinds of dependent variables could never conceivably serve as independent variables?

2. Study the 25 hypotheses listed on pp. 135–36. Describe how you would go about quantitatively measuring the dependent variables stated in these hypotheses. Do measuring instruments already exist to measure these variables, or will fresh ones have to be developed?

3. Review some periodicals containing reports of research in nursing and patient care (like *Nursing Research*) to obtain some examples of the use of nonquantified data in a study. What are some of the limitations in using nonquantified data in research? What are the benefits to be gained by the use of such data?

4. Read the article "Measurement" by Norman Campbell in *The World of Mathematics,* James R. Newman (ed.) (New York, Simon and Schuster, Inc., 1956, Vol. 3. pp. 1797–1813). What are the three rules the author gives for determining what properties (variables) are measurable? How does the author distinguish between fundamental and derived measurement?

5. Describe five types of nominal scales commonly used in nursing and patient care. Can you conceive of a way in which these scales can be converted into quantitative scales? How meaningful would such quantitative scales be?

6. Comment on the following statement by M. Sidman in his *Tactics of Scientific Research* (New York, Basic Books, Inc., 1960): "The best that we can be presumed to do is to determine that specific data have a low probability of belonging to Chance, and with some trepidation, we accept such data into the fold. If they do not belong to Chance, they belong to Science. Thus data are accepted into science by exclusion. They possess no positive virtues, only the negative one of being due to chance with a low level of confidence." (p. 43.) Is the author's definition of chance the same as the uncontrolled extraneous variables in a study? Are extraneous variables that are randomized really uncontrolled?

7. Develop a graphic rating scale for the following variables.
   a. Quality of performance of a nursing aide
   b. Cooperativeness of a patient
   c. Ability of the patient to verbalize his feelings
   d. The sleep behavior of an adult patient
   e. Degree of mobility of a patient
   f. The severity of a surgical operation

8. What are the essential differences between the graphic rating scale, the Thurstone-type scale, the Likert-type scale, and the Guttman scale? How would you rank these scales in the order of their usefulness to research in nursing and patient care?

9. The Q-sort technique has been widely used in research in nursing. Referring to the journal *Nursing Research,* locate a report of a study in which the Q-sort method has been used (several have been reported). Write a summary and critique of the use of the method in the reported study.

10. Perform the following experiment. Take the temperatures (orally) of a group of patients, say, a dozen or so. Have a few nurses independently read the same patient's thermometer and record the readings. In comparing the readings for the same patients do you find any variation? Next, take the same patient's temperature with two thermometers simultaneously. Do this for a number of patients. Do the readings always agree exactly?

11. Make the following scale conversions:
    a. 200°F. to the centigrade scale
    b. 25 pounds avoirdupois to the metric scale
    c. 34 centimeters to linear measure
    d. 44° centigrade to the Fahrenheit scale
    e. 8 quarts (liquid) to the metric scale
    f. 100 yards to the metric scale

12. Analyze the criterion measures used in the following studies:
    a. Mary A. Bochnak, Julina P. Rhymes, and Robert C. Leonard, "The Comparison of Two Types of Nursing Activity on the Relief of Pain," in Monograph No. 6 of papers presented in the clinical sessions of the 1962 American Nurses' Association Convention. New York, American Nurses' Association, 1962, pp. 5–11.
    b. Florence C. Austin, Ellen Donnelly Davis, and Judith Rubenstein Steward, "Characteristics of Psychiatric Patients Who Utilize Public Health Nursing Services." *Am. J. Pub. Health,* **54:**226–238, February 1964.
    c. Edith M. Lentz and Robert G. Michaels, "Comparisons Between Medical and Surgical Nurses." *Nursing Res.,* **8:**192–197, fall 1959.
    d. Leonard I. Pearlin and Morris Rosenberg, "Nurse-Patient Social Distance and the Structural Context of a Mental Hospital." *Am. Sociol. Rev.,* **27:**56–65, February 1962.
    e. Rosemary Rich and James K. Dent, "Patient Rating Scale." *Nursing Res.,* **11:**163–171, summer 1962.
    f. Marie E. Meyers, "The Effect of Types of Communication on Patients' Reactions to Stress." *Nursing Res.,* **13:**126–131, spring 1964.
    g. Robert A. Hoekelman, Harriet J. Kitzman, and Anne W. Zimmer "Pediatric Nurse Practitioners and Well Baby Care in a Small Rural Community," in *ANA Clinical Sessions,* 1972, pp. 103–113. New York, Appleton-Century-Crofts, 1973.

13. Write a critique of Joseph Wood Krutch's article, cited in this chapter, in *The Saturday Review* ("Through Happiness with Slide Rule and Calipers," November 2, 1963). Which of the points made by the author do you think are especially pertinent. To what extent, if any, has he overstated his case against measurement of subjective phenomena like happiness?

14. Read the article by Faye E. Spring and Herman Turk, "A Therapeutic Behavior Scale" (*Nursing Res.,* **11:**214–218, fall 1962). How do the authors employ the scalogram analysis in this study? How was reliability of the scale assessed? Do you think the scale developed could have applicability in other studies?

15. The following data are taken from a descriptive study reported in the *American Journal of Public Health* by Testoff and Levine on the characteristics of patients 65 years of age and over who received public health nursing services in their homes on April 30, 1963.

Number of patients 65 years of age and over receiving nursing care at home from public health agencies, on April 30, 1963.

Age	Number of Patients
Total All Ages	17,501
65–69	3,400
70–74	4,148
75–79	3,776
80–84	3,376
85–89	1,825
90–94	770
95–99	170
100 and over	36

    a. Convert the numbers into a percentage distribution.
    b. What is the modal age group? What is the median age?
    c. Would you say that this distribution is approximately a normal one? Is it symmetrical?
    d. How would the arithmetic mean be computed from such data? The standard deviation?

16. Clearly distinguish between a direct measure of a variable and an indirect measure. Are some measures more indirect than others? Describe some direct and indirect measures of patient care that could serve as criterion measures in research.

17. Carl G. Hempel in his *Fundamentals of Concept Formation in Empirical Science* (*International Encyclopedia of Unified Science*, Volume II, No. 7, Chicago, The University of Chicago Press, 1952), distinguishes between natural and artificial classifications in discussing (pp. 50–54) what have been called in this chapter, nominal scales. Which of the following classification scales are natural or artificial according to the author's definition?
Disease
Race
Occupation
Blood grouping (A, B, O, etc.)
Sex (male, female)
Nursing education program (baccalaureate, degree, associate degree, diploma)
Nursing units in a hospital (e.g., three east, four west, etc.)

18. On page 58 of his monograph, Hempel distinguishes between fundamental and derived measurement. Can you give some examples of derived measurement that are used in nursing and patient care? Cite some examples of fundamental measurement in these areas. How does the author distinguish between derived measurement by stipulation and derived measurement by law? (p. 70.)

19. Obtain a copy of the book by Charles M. Bonjean and others, *Sociological Measurement: An Inventory of Scales and Indices.* San Francisco, Chandler Publishing Co., 1967. Comment on the application of some of the scales described to nursing research. Also, see Gary M. Maranell, *Scaling: A Sourcebook.* Chicago, Aldine Publishing Co., 1974.

20. Read the article by Alex Barr and others, "A Review of the Various Methods of Measuring the Dependency of Patients on Nursing Staff." *Int. J. Nurs. Stud.,* **10:**195–208, August 1973. What are some of the measurement problems in developing an index of patients' dependency on nursing staff?

21. Read the article by Fabienne Fortin and Suzanne Kérouac, "Validation of Questionnaires on Physical Function." *Nursing Res.,* **26:**128–135, March-April, 1977. Is the CICCHETTI statistic a good method of testing reliability?

Additional Reading

A. Donabedian, "Evaluating the Quality of Medical Care." *Milbank Mem. Fund Q.,* **44:**166–206, July 1966, Part 2.

L. S. Rosenfeld, "Standards for Assessing Quality of Care." *Quality Assurance of Medical Care.* St. Louis, Regional Medical Programs Service, February 1973.

J. W. Taylor, "Measuring the Outcomes of Nursing Care." *Nurs. Clin. North Am.,* **9:**2:337–348, 1974.

M. J. Zimmer, "A Model for Evaluating Nursing Care." *Hospitals, J.A.H.A.,* **48:**5:91–95, 131, 1974.

D. Block, "Evaluation of Nursing Care in Terms of Process and Outcome: Issues in Research and Quality Assurance." *Nursing Res.,* **24:**256–263, 1975.

Chapter Eight

METHODS OF COLLECTING AND PROCESSING DATA

THIS CHAPTER will be concerned with three interrelated topics: first, the selection of study subjects from the target population; second, the means by which the data are obtained from the study subjects; and third, the ways in which data are processed and organized.

Decisions made concerning how the data will be gathered and processed are closely related to the other elements of the research process. Thus, if we have chosen for our study a highly controlled experimental type of research design, collection of data would most likely involve direct contact with the study subjects. On the other hand, if we selected a nonexperimental design, we can use indirect means of collecting the data such as by a mailed questionnaire.

If the variables can be quantitatively measured, we might need to use scientific measuring instruments requiring direct observation of the study subjects. Data on qualitative variables can often be gathered by indirect methods like self-administered tests or scales. Moreover, the ease with which the measurements can be made will influence the number of study subjects included in the research. If measurements are difficult and time-consuming to make, the number of study subjects may need to be restricted.

Each of the different methods of selecting study subjects and collecting data on the variables being measured has certain advantages and limitations. The choice of method for a particular study should be tailor-made to fit the requirements inherent in the nature of the research problem.

SELECTION OF THE STUDY SUBJECTS

The subjects included in a study are often human beings, but they can also be animals, plants, cells, or inanimate objects such as equipment, buildings, chemicals, plots of land, or even nonmaterial subjects such as words, constructs, processes, or procedures. The subject of a study is the person or thing from whom data are collected. In some studies the whole subject is the concern of the measurement—as, for example, determination of the level of wellness of a person. In other studies only a part of the subject is measured, as in a study of dental cavities among children. The definition of the variable being studied—in the first example, level of wellness, and in the second, condition of teeth—describes which aspect of the subject we are examining in the study.

Definition of the Target Population

The first step in selecting the study subjects is to define the *target population*. The target population consists of the total membership of a defined set of subjects (people, animals, plants, etc.) from whom the study subjects are selected and to whom the data from the study will be generalized. The target population must be defined as to the nature of the individual subjects composing it as well as its geographic and temporal scope. Thus, we may speak of the population of professional nurses in the United States who were licensed to practice in 1979. Or we may define the target population as all hospitals in the state of New York accepted for listing by the American Hospital Association in 1979.

Each individual nurse or each individual hospital that composes the target population is potentially a study subject in research. The individual members of the target population are called the *sampling units*. A study usually focuses on the measurement of particular variables relevant to the sampling units, as for example, the nurse staffing (variable) of general hospitals. Thus a population actually consists of all the measurements that could theoretically be made of the variables under study. Nevertheless, in this example the population would be conceived as consisting of hospitals, called the primary sampling units, not as the measurements of staffing in the hospitals. Similarly, if we are studying the effect of different brands of toothpaste on prevention of dental caries, the target population would ordinarily be defined in terms of individual people, not as measurements of teeth, and the primary sampling units would thus consist of whole people.

Theoretically, the same individual can be a member of many different target populations at the same time depending on how the scope of the population is defined as well as the types of variables being measured. For example, the nurse who was licensed to practice in 1979 could be a sampling unit in various geographically defined target populations of registered nurses. These populations could encompass the entire world, or be limited to the country she lives in, or her state, city, neighborhood, block, or even confined to her household. The same nurse could also be a sampling unit in target populations defined according to different characteristics, as, for example, populations of working mothers, people who voted in the last election, all alumnae of a certain school of nursing, residents of urbanized areas, or nurses who work in the field of public health.

Some writers make a distinction between the *target population* and the *sampled population*. The target population is considered to be the entire population to whom the findings of the study are held to be applicable while the sampled population is considered to be the aggregate of all the identifiable sampling units from whom the study subjects were actually drawn. In many studies these two populations are identical. However, if we select our study subjects from all nurses registered in the state of New York and make generalizations from the data for all nurses in the United States, the latter would be considered the target population and the former the sampled population.

In the following discussion the term target population is used interchangeably with the sampled population—as the population for whom the data can be statistically generalized. The concept of the "hypothetical universe" to be discussed shortly will be used to designate the notion of the broader population that exists beyond the sampled population.

A target population is thus a finite population, its boundaries fixed and described by time, geography, and the characteristics of the individual members composing it, as well as the nature of the variables being studied. The importance of precisely defining this population arises from the fact that in most research studies we aim to generalize to some larger population the findings we obtain from our study subjects. Thus, if we are testing the effect of providing increased nursing hours to psychiatric patients in one hospital, we would undoubtedly be interested in applying the data from our particular study subjects to psychiatric patients in other hospitals. Only through a widespread application of the findings will the time, effort, and money expended on the study be considered worthwhile. It is indeed a rare study that does not look toward generalization of its findings beyond the immediate study setting. Generalization of findings is considered to be an essential characteristic of meaningful research.

The boundaries of statistical generalization of research findings are fixed by the limits of the population from which the sample was drawn. In many studies, a population is not defined in advance. Instead a group of subjects is studied—say, all the freshman students in a particular school of nursing. In studies like these implicit generalizations of findings to some larger population are often made through the style in which the data are interpreted. The use of the present rather than the past tense in reporting the findings of such studies creates a sense of generality: "Students whose initial exposure to the nursing situation in a hospital is a traumatic one are more apt to withdraw from school before the end of the first year than those whose exposure is pleasant."

Even where a target population has been defined in advance and the study subjects carefully chosen from the population so as to be representative of it, generalizations often extend beyond the population limits, particularly those limits imposed by time. Research findings are frequently extended into the future, and in so doing the fact is often overlooked that a study has been conducted during a specific time period in the past. Since most situations are not static, the same findings might not be true for an indefinite time in the future.

Broad generalizations are frequently made from findings obtained in experimental research even though the study was conducted in a limited way as when subjects are brought into the experiment because of convenience—e.g., patients who happen to be in the hospital at the time. On the other hand, in nonexperimental studies the study subjects are more likely to be broadly representative of some larger population and they are frequently selected through scientific means. Sweeping generalizations of the findings of experiments are considered warranted because of the strict controls exerted over the extraneous variables. Perhaps such generalizations are possible when the subjects are inanimate and the variables are precisely and relevantly quantified. When the subjects are human beings and when the measuring instruments are not precise, the caution offered by McGinnis[1] should be borne in mind:

> There is no such thing as a completely general relationship which is independent of population, time, and space. The extent to which a relationship is constant among different populations is an empirical question which can be resolved only by examining different populations at different times in different places.

Studies in which findings are generalized beyond the boundaries of target populations, whether the target population is specified in advance or not, are essentially being generalized to a hypothetical universe. The notion of a hypothetical universe has been postulated to enable a researcher to extend his findings beyond the finite target population and provide them with more general applicability. As described by Hagood:[2]

> This superuniverse must be a universe from which our finite universe can be considered a random sample. It has been defined as an unlimited or infinite universe of all the possible finite universes that could have been produced at the instant of observation under the conditions obtaining. It is therefore only an imagined possibility and whether or not one wishes to utilize the concept is still at the discretion of the individual research worker.

It can be argued that the notion of a hypothetical universe is vague and somewhat contrived. General laws or principles can be established only by replications of studies in which findings are confirmed or reinforced from one study to the next. If repeated tests of the same hypothesis produce the same findings, the formulation of a general relationship has been strengthened. Multiclinic trials of drugs is an example of such repeated studies that can broaden the scope of generalizations. Before the Salk and

Sabin vaccines were released for general usage, their effectiveness in reducing the incidence of polio was tested and retested among numerous study groups.

The importance of carefully defining the target population in advance of a study is illustrated by the famous *Literary Digest* poll undertaken to predict the presidential election in 1936. The *Literary Digest* was a popular magazine during the 1930's, but it went out of business soon after erroneously predicting that Landon would defeat Roosevelt. The error in the survey arose from the way in which the sampling units were selected. Telephone directories and other specialized lists were used to obtain a listing of the names and addresses of persons to whom straw ballots were mailed. The target population for the poll was considered to be all voters in the United States although the sampling frame actually was restricted to owners of telephones, thus overrepresenting persons with high income.

The reason for the erroneous prediction was that income level was related to voting behavior in the 1936 election. In general, lower income persons voted for Roosevelt, higher income persons for Landon. Thus, the distorted interpretation of the poll was inevitable.

SAMPLING

After the target population for a study has been carefully defined, the study subjects can be selected. If the target population is small—that is, if it consists of a limited number of sampling units—all the sampling units may be taken into the research as study subjects. Thus, if we are studying the types of patients who receive home nursing care from public health agencies in the United States, and if the total number of primary sampling units (agencies) in this population is around 1,000, we might decide to include all of them in the study, particularly if our measurements can be made simply and quickly. If the number of sampling units is very large and the data difficult to obtain, the number selected for study will be fewer than the total number composing the target population.

The process of selecting a fraction of the sampling units of a target population for inclusion in a study is known as *sampling*. The set of sampling units chosen for the study is called the *sample*. Studies that include all members of the target population are sometimes known as 100 per cent samples. Summary measures—such as percentages, means, medians, percentiles, and standard deviations—that are computed from measurements obtained from a sample of the total population are called *statistics*. Summary measures based on all the sampling units in the target population are known as *parameters*. Statistics, therefore, are estimates of population parameters.

One important objective of sampling is to obtain a sample of study subjects that will be representative of the total population in terms of important organismic variables. Thus, if our target population consisted of patients who are receiving home nursing care, and if 40 per cent of the patients are males and 60 per cent are females, if 30 per cent are 65 years of age or over and 70 per cent under 65 years of age, and if sex and age were considered to be important organismic variables in relation to the hypothesis we are testing, our sample would be representative if the characteristics of the sampling units we selected approximated these percentages. A sample should be a replica in miniature of the total population. The extent to which our sample findings are different from what they would be if we had studied all the sampling units is known as *sampling error*.

History of Sampling

The process of selecting a sample of the total members of a population is a very ancient one. Thousands of years ago, Aristotle made some valid generalizations of the behavior of celestial bodies by observing just a few stars. The use of sampling among human populations became prevalent in England prior to the 1700's when estimates were made from small samples of the number of people composing the total population of cities. In the 1800's, stimulated by Bentham and his philosophy of utilitarianism, various health surveys were undertaken based on samples of the total population.[3]

The application of the mathematical theory of probability to sampling originated in the twentieth century, although probability theory was well established 200 years ago. A. L. Bowley, considered to be the father of scientific sampling, undertook a sampling study of the economic classes in England in 1912.[4] In 1927, L. H. C. Tippett[5] produced his table of random sampling numbers which facilitated the selection of probability samples. In the 1930's many descriptive surveys were undertaken in the fields of health, welfare, and social relations in which probability sampling was used. And in the 1950's and early 1960's, partly based on the extensive work on sampling done by the U.S. Bureau of the Census, several major texts were produced in the field,[6,7,8] one specifically directed to the sampling of hospitals.[9] Today the theory and practice of sampling are of major importance in the work of statisticians. Indeed, many applications of sampling in research require the specialized attention of sampling experts, since the quality of a sample can vitally affect the validity of the research findings.

Advantages of Sampling

The benefits of sampling, particularly where the target population is very large or difficult to reach, are numerous. Briefly, these benefits can be summarized as follows:

1. We must sample in studies where complete measurement of all members of the target population is not possible. Thus, if we wanted to test the effects of a drug in the treatment of patients with cancer, we could not practically include every patient who has cancer as study subjects, even if we had large amounts of time, money, and personnel to do the study, because the total number of sampling units is too large and too dispersed.

2. It is usually cheaper and quicker to measure a sample of study subjects than all the members of a target population. Sampling thus reduces the cost and time of doing research.

3. The gain in accuracy from inclusion of all members of a population is often not worth the time and expense required. Sometimes sample data can be almost as precise as data obtained from the total population. For example, it has been found in the decennial census of population that a sampling produces almost as precise data for some of the variables studied as does the complete enumeration.

4. In some studies the process of measurement can introduce spurious influences into the research. The Hawthorne effect, mentioned in Chapter 6, is the reaction of the study subjects to the study process itself, which can obscure or bias the effects of the independent variable we are actually testing. By keeping the number of study subjects as small as our need for precision of study results will permit, we can more easily control the Hawthorne effect as well as other psychological biases that can be introduced during the measuring process.

5. The number of study subjects should be kept as small as is feasibly possible when the independent variable could have unpleasant side effects on the study subjects. Trials of new drugs, especially when not all of the effects of the drug on the patient can be assessed in advance, are usually based on small samples. Any potentially dangerous phases of the study are usually restricted to animal subjects.

6. In studies involving nonhuman subjects, the measuring process sometimes destroys the sampling units. In such studies economics would dictate a limitation of sample size. For example, in the evaluation of alternative products—e.g., x-ray equipment produced by different manufacturers—we might have to break down the equipment to obtain certain measurements. To keep the cost of such tests from getting out of hand, the number of sampling units must be kept to a minimum.

Scientific Sampling

As has been stated, the aim of sampling is to obtain a group of study subjects that is a replica in miniature of the target population. The method of probability sampling has been developed to provide a measure of how good a replica of the population the sample is. Probability sampling, also called random sampling, is a method whereby each sampling unit in the target population has a known—greater than zero—probability of being selected in the sample. Moreover, in drawing a probability sample, neither the sampler nor the sampling unit has any deliberate influence over the inclusion of a specific sampling unit. In other words, the process of drawing a probability sample is a random one. This process is analogous to that of random assignment of study subjects to the various alternative groups of an experiment. Random sampling can be achieved in the same manner as random assignment. We can put the names or the numbers of each sampling unit on slips of paper, put the slips in a bowl, and then draw a number of slips at random which will compose the sample. More scientifically, we could assign numbers to each sampling unit and then select the sample members by choosing the numbers from a table of random numbers, as described in the method of randomization in Chapter 6.

Instead of drawing a probability sample we might deliberately select the sampling units according to certain criteria that we as subject-matter experts in the field know to be important. Thus, if the sampling units in a study of nurse staffing patterns consist of hospitals, we might stipulate which particular hospitals are to be included in the study because we are familiar with their characteristics and we feel that the hospitals chosen are typical of all hospitals in general.

Probability samples have two advantages over deliberately selected, nonrandom samples:

1. Statistical techniques can be applied to evaluate the precision of summary measures based on randomly selected samples. Thus, we can compute the *sampling error* of these statistics which tells us how good an estimate they are of the parameter values. In nonrandom samples we have no adequate way of estimating sampling error.

2. By random selection of sampling units we can help to avoid the possible unconscious selection of a biased sample. An example of a biased sample that was drawn nonrandomly is the Kinsey study on sexual behavior in females. The subjects for this study were invited through advertisements to enter the study voluntarily. Thus, the essence of randomness was missing. By volunteering, the subjects deliberately controlled who was to be included in the study. A woman who voluntarily provided details on such an intimate variable as sexual behavior was not likely to be representative of the total population of females. The findings in this study of high rates of premarital and extramarital sexual activity can be questioned as being applicable to all females.

Random selection of the sampling units does not guarantee that the sample will be representative or typical of the target population. It may well be possible to select a more typical sample by nonrandom selection.

But such gains in representativeness must be weighed against the inability to evaluate statistically the precision of summary measures obtained from nonrandom samples.

TYPES OF PROBABILITY SAMPLES

There are numerous methods by which a probability sample may be drawn. The ones most applicable to research in nursing and patient care will be briefly discussed.

Simple Random Samples

This is the most fundamental type of sampling design. In this design each sampling unit has an equal probability of being selected as the first member of the sample; after the first member is selected each of the remaining units in the population has an equal chance of being the second member of the sample, etc. Thus, if the target population consists of a total of 100 units, each sampling unit has a 1 per cent probability (chance) of being chosen as the first member in a sample of size 1, a 10 per cent chance in a sample of size 10, and so on. Most important, in a simple random sample each possible combination of the various sampling units has an equal chance of being chosen. Thus, in a sample of 10 units drawn from 100, each possible combination of 10 (and there are millions of them) is as equally likely to be selected as any other.

Selection of a simple random sample includes the following steps. First, we must define the target population. Then we must establish a complete listing, sometimes called a frame, of all the sampling units in the population. Such a listing might be in the form of a roster or a deck of index cards containing the names and addresses of all the people, hospitals, schools, or public health agencies composing the target population. Then, we decide how many sampling units we want to include in the sample. Determination of sample size is a rather technical matter often best handled by a professional statistician. His determination takes into consideration the following factors, many of which have been discussed in Chapter 6 in relation to the number of experimental subjects required in the alternative experimental groups.

1. *The amount of precision required in the statistics (summary measures) that are computed.* Precision essentially means how accurate we want to be in estimating the values of the parameters of the target population. The amount of precision needed in a study depends upon the nature of the research problem. If the findings of the study can affect the health of people, we would want a high degree of precision. If we can tolerate rough approximations of the values of the parameters, a smaller sample might suffice.

The basic formula for computing the sampling error of a sample estimate of a population parameter is as follows:

$$\text{Sampling error} = \frac{\substack{\text{Variability of the values of the measurements} \\ \text{among the sampling units}}}{\sqrt{\text{Size of sample}}}$$

This formula is applicable to estimates obtained from simple random samples. For other types of sample designs an elaboration of this formula is required. As can be seen, precision depends upon the ratio of the variability of the measurements among the individual sampling units to the square root of the number of sampling units included in the sample. Precision can, therefore, be increased either by reducing the variability among the sampling units, which can be accomplished by altering the method of selection of the sample from simple random sampling to other methods that will be discussed shortly, or by increasing the size of the sample. Because of the "square root" operation, however, doubling the sample size (with variability of the measurements held constant) will only increase the precision by the square root of two. (1.4), not by two. Quadrupling the sample will double the precision.

2. *The variability of the measurements among the sampling units we are studying.* The greater the variability of the values of the measurements, the larger the sample needed to attain a desired level of precision among the sampling units. If the measurements had little variability among the sampling units, it is obvious that a smaller number of sampling units would be required to make as precise an estimate of the population parameter than if variability were high. To illustrate, suppose we were interested in estimating the average number of hours of nursing care per patient per day in a target population consisting of five hospitals. If there were little variability among the sampling units, the data might look as follows:

Hospital	Average Hours per Patient per Day
1	4.6
2	4.1
3	4.5
4	4.9
5	4.8
Average	4.6

If we chose any one of these hospitals as our sample, we would have quite a precise estimate of the average hours per patient in all hospitals— 4.6—since none of the hospitals deviates by more than one-half hour from this average. However, if the individual values varied as widely as in the following target population, a sample of only one hospital could differ from the average as much as two hours.

Hospital	Average Hours per Patient per Day
1	4.6
2	1.8
3	3.7
4	5.9
5	4.3
Average	4.1

3. *Sensitivity of the measuring instruments.* Other things being equal, the more sensitive the instruments are that we use to measure our variables, the smaller is the sample required to detect significant differences among the study subjects being measured. For example, let us assume that our study involved the testing of the realtionship between alternative methods of training nursing aides, and our criterion measure was a rating scale of the proficiency of the aide. We would need a larger sample to detect significant differences among the study subjects if the scale consisted of only two broad qualitative categories than if it were a highly refined quantitative scale that could validly and reliably detect small but significant differences in proficiency.

4. *Amount of detailed descriptive data required.* In experimental studies the end product might simply be a test of statistical significance of the differences among the values of our summary measures for the alternative groups. In nonexperimental studies, where the time and expense involved per sampling unit in collecting the data usually are less than in an experiment, we are often interested in obtaining detailed descriptive data relevant to the research problem, even when the purpose of the study is primarily one of explanation. Such descriptive data might refer to the important organismic variables concerning our study subjects—their age, marital status, educational level, occupation, and so on. We may wish to cross-tabulate these variables against the dependent variable—that is, to simultaneously tabulate the summary measures by the organismic variables as well as the explanatory variables. To the extent that we desire detailed, meaningful cross-tabulations of the data, the size of the sample will have to be enlarged in order to provide sufficient data for the additional cells of the table. To illustrate: assume we are interested in assessing the relationship between the size of a public health agency (the independent variable with, say, four size groups according to case load) and the cost per visit to patients in home nursing care programs (dependent variable); the table showing this relationship would need only four cells—one for each

of the four size groups. If we were interested in seeing the effect of the control of the agency (official, nonofficial, combination) on this relationship, we would need a larger sample, since the table showing this relationship would now have 12 cells:

	Control of Agency		
Case Load of Agency	*Official*	*Nonofficial*	*Combination*
Less than 50 patients			
50–99 patients			
100–199			
More than 200 patients			

Another reason for enlarging the sample size is to be able to detect rarely occurring events. For example, the effectiveness of the vaccines to combat polio was measured in terms of the reduction in the incidence of paralytic polio. Since this type of polio rarely occurs, even among un-vaccinated populations—only a few cases are reported each year—it was necessary to include a very large number of individuals in the study in order to detect any significant reduction in this rare event after vaccination.

5. *Number of sample units in the target population.* When the target population is small, a smaller number of sampling units can serve to provide precise statistics than if the target population is very large—assuming, of course, relatively equivalent variability among the sampling units of the different-sized populations. Data from a sample of 100 would very precisely measure the parameters of a target population consisting of 100 units—in fact there would be no sampling error. This same-sized sample would produce less precise data if the target population consisted of 1,000 units, and even less precise data if it contained 100,000 units.

6. *Practical limitations.* Size of sample is often restricted by such practical limitations as time and money available to collect the data. Such criteria as precision of sample estimates and the detail desired in the results must be balanced against the availability of resources. The aim of sample design is to secure an efficient sample, one that produces the most information at the lowest possible cost per sampling unit.

Selecting a Simple Random Sample When size of sample has been determined, the next step is to actually select the sampling units from the target population. The previously described table of random numbers provides the best selection procedure. If we desired to choose a sample of 100 patients' records from files containing 50,000 records, each having a unique five-digit identification number, we would open the table of random numbers at random and copy out 100 five-digit numbers, beginning randomly at any place in the table, and continuing up and down the columns or across the rows of figures until we obtained our 100 numbers. The patient records bearing these numbers would compose our sample.

The simple random sample has perhaps more applicability in research in nursing and patient care than other types of sampling, particularly in studies involving the selection of a sample of patients, personnel, students, or records from within an institution or a limited geographic area. In studies like these the target population consists of a relatively small, fairly homogeneous number of sampling units, so that the simple random sample is a very adequate sampling method. For large, heterogeneous target populations, other sampling methods are generally more efficient than the simple, unrestricted type. However, even in the more elaborate sample designs, which essentially involve grouping the sampling units in terms of certain criteria prior to selection of the units, simple random sampling is often employed for the actual selection.

Systematic Sampling

When the sampling units are arranged in some order, such as names on a list or by geographic location, it is sometimes simpler to select the sample in a systematic way: every tenth name on the list, the patients in the odd-numbered rooms, every fifth house on a block, every tenth baby born in the hospital. The random element in such a sampling method is provided by the random start. That is, if a list contains 1,000 names and we wish to select 100 for our sample, we would select every tenth name, but we would start by selecting our first name by chance and then take every tenth name after that. Thus, if the first randomly selected name were the seventh on the list, the next sample subject would be the seventeenth name, the next would be the twenty-seventh, and so on.

A variation of the systematic sampling technique is the work sampling method advocated by the U.S. Public Health Service's Division of Nursing.[10] In this method, after a random start, the activities of nursing personnel are observed every 15 minutes and classified in terms of such variables as the area of the activity (patient care, housekeeping, maintenance of environment) and skill level of the activity (head nurse, staff nurse, aide, clerk, and so on). This systematic sampling of activities is in contrast to the simple random sampling advocated by work sampling theorists in other fields.[11] Tests of the two sampling approaches indicate that both provide approximately the same precision.

Systematic sampling has two limitations. One is the fact that the sampling error formula for such samples is difficult, if not impossible, to derive. This would hinder the computation of the sampling error of any statistics computed from such samples. Another is the danger that the

order in which the sampling units are arranged on a list, or their geographical arrangement, or, as in the case of work sampling, their time
ordering, would be systematically related to some extraneous variable,
which if unknown to the researcher might result in the selection of a
biased sample. In other words, the use of a systematic sample assumes
that the order in which the units are arranged is essentially random in relation to the variables being studied. But this assumption may not always
be correct. We might find, for example, that the patients located in the
odd-numbered (or even-numbered) rooms had certain special characteristics. Such rooms, because of the peculiarities of construction of the hospital, might be higher-priced, and the patients in them in the higher income
brackets. Consequently our sample, like the *Literary Digest* poll, would
be overweighted with wealthier people. Or in the systematic time sampling
there may be a cyclical pattern of activities in the work of the nurses we
observe: certain activities begin precisely every 15 minutes. If our observation schedule coincides with these cycles, it would give us a distorted
picture of the total range of activities performed by the personnel. In systematic sampling, then, we must be sure that there is randomness in the
arrangement of the sampling units in the population. This can be done by
taking a number of random starts, not just one.

Stratified Random Samples

In this type of sample the target population is subdivided into homogeneous subpopulations. Then a simple random sample, or a systematic
sample, or some other type of sample is selected from each subpopulation.
Thus, if we wished to select for study 200 patients out of a total target
population of 5,000, we might first subdivide the 5,000 sampling units in
terms of certain important organismic variables—say, the age and sex of
the patients. If we established four groups for age and two for sex there
would be eight cells, called strata. From each stratum we would take a
certain proportion of sampling units to provide us with a total of 100. The
proportion of sampling units selected from each stratum for the sample is
identical with the proportion of sampling units in each stratum in the
population. This can be illustrated in Table 8-1.

For the same-sized sample, stratification generally increases the precision of summary measures above that obtained by simple random
sampling. This is achieved by making the various strata from which the
samples are drawn as homogeneous as possible. Such homogeneity tends
to reduce the value of the numerator in the formula used to compute the
sampling error—the variation of the individual measurements among the
sampling units—for each stratum. This results in a reduction of the
sampling error for all strata combined.

Essentially, stratification is a process of sampling from subdivisions of

TABLE 8-1

A Stratified Sample
(Proportions in per cent are in parentheses)

Age	Population Total	Sex Male	Sex Female	Sample Total	Sex Male	Sex Female
Total	50,000 (100)	20,000 (40)	30,000 (60)	200 (100)	80 (40)	120 (60)
Under 21	5,000 (10)	4,000 (8)	1,000 (2)	20 (10)	16 (8)	4 (2)
21–44	15,000 (30)	3,000 (6)	12,000 (24)	60 (30)	12 (6)	48 (24)
45–64	10,000 (20)	5,000 (10)	5,000 (10)	40 (20)	20 (10)	20 (10)
65 and over	20,000 (40)	8,000 (16)	12,000 (24)	80 (40)	32 (16)	48 (24)

the target population. The most common procedure is to select the number of sampling units from each stratum proportionately, as in Table 8-1 since this simplifies the computations. However, this is not a necessary feature of this type of sample design. A disproportionate number of sampling units could be selected from each stratum. For example, a stratum that consists of only a few sampling units may represent an important group regardless of its small numbers. Thus, when all nonfederal, short-term hospitals in the United States are stratified by size, one would find only approximately twelve hospitals with more than 1,000 beds. Such a stratum may be sampled in its entirety, even though it represents only a tiny fraction of all sampling units—five hospitals compose less than 1 per cent of all general hospitals in the United States. Disproportionate sampling would require the adjustment of any summary measures that are computed from such samples by weighting each stratum according to its relative contribution to the value of the summary measure for all strata combined.

A technical procedure known as *optimum allocation* can be used to determine the best possible allocation of the sampling units into strata. This procedure can tell us what is the most efficient size sample for each stratum, balancing precision obtained against cost per sampling unit.

For many sampling situations encountered in research in nursing and patient care, a simple random sample will suffice. The next most frequently used design would be stratified random sampling with proportionate allocation. Disproportionate allocation would be the least frequently used of the three designs. The gain in precision may not always be worth the additional complexities in selecting the sample and in determining the sampling error of estimates obtained by the latter design. Its use would generally be limited to those research situations where a significant enhancement of the precision of estimates can be obtained.

Cluster Sampling

In large-scale descriptive studies involving target populations with geographically dispersed sampling units, it is often necessary to use cluster sampling. Suppose, for example, that our research problem required that we obtain certain measurements on hospitalized psychiatric patients by visiting each sample hospital. Our basic sampling unit is the patient. But since we do not have a list of such patients, we must select our sample in terms of some other identifiable sampling unit, such as the hospital in which they are located. Moreover, since the more than 500 psychiatric hospitals in the United States are geographically well distributed, it would be very costly and time-consuming to select the sample of patients from a list even if one were available, because we might find our sample patients scattered far and wide. Thus our procedure would be, first to select a random sample of hospitals (our clusters of patients). Then we would either include all the patients in the selected hospitals as the subjects for our research, or we would subsample by randomly selecting only a proportion of the patients in each hospital. This sample design involving more than one stage of sampling is called a multistage sample. The hospital or whatever entity serves as the unit that is selected first is called the primary sampling unit. The patients are the secondary or second-stage sampling units.

Multistage sampling can have numerous stages. The primary sampling unit might be a hospital. The second stage could be a random sampling of various nursing units in each hospital, and the third stage could be a sampling of patients on whom the actual measurements are made for the research.

Multistage sampling is applicable where the target population can be grouped according to some formal or informal organizational or structural entity. In cluster sampling, the cluster, or primary sampling unit, might represent a hospital, as in the previous example, or a school, a state, a city, a neighborhood, a block within a neighborhood, a house, an association, a family, an agency, a work team, and so on. An advantage of this type of sampling is that it is usually possible to obtain a greater amount of data at a lower cost than with other methods. In the example of the psychiatric patients, it is obvious that it would be cheaper to collect data from 100 patients all located in one hospital than from one patient in each of 100 hospitals.

Also, cluster sampling is often the only kind of sample design that can feasibly be employed in many research situations. If there are no lists available identifying the basic sampling units in a target population—as, for example, in a study of part-time nurses who work in public health agencies—we can only reach the individual members of the target population through the group to which they belong. Cluster sampling is an especially good approach to uncovering data that cannot be obtained in any other way. In epidemiological studies cluster sampling can be most helpful. If we wished to determine the prevalence of certain diseases among people living in a community, we could select our sample so that our primary sampling unit would be a block of the different streets in the community, the second stage of sampling would be a house on a block, and the third and final stage a resident of a house. The U.S. Public Health Service has frequently used such designs in studies of the prevalence of illnesses among the population of the United States.[12,13]

There are several disadvantages to cluster sampling. One is the fact that for the same-sized sample it will usually yield less precise data than other sample designs, such as stratified random sampling. Another is the greater complexity in determining the sampling error of estimates based on cluster sampling. Such error formulas need to take account of the fact that the individual sampling units being measured were not selected independently. Therefore, they may not be independent of each other in relation to relevant environmental variables that could influence the variables being measured. In the example of the sample of patients in psychiatric hospitals, all patients in a particular hospital have been exposed to a similar set of environmental variables. These variables may well be different from those to which patients in other hospitals are exposed. Thus, if we measure two patients from the same hospital to determine the kind of nursing they receive, the measurements are correlated, since both patients would be likely to receive similar kinds of care. If we measure two patients who have been independently and randomly selected from different hospitals, the measurements are not correlated. The latter sample is more apt to be "representative" of the total target population than is the cluster sample.

The effect of clustering thus must be taken into account in determining the precision of summary measures computed from cluster samples. As Kish[14] points out, the formula for a simple random sample is used to compute sampling error in many studies when in fact the sample was based on a cluster design. The wrong formula would result in an incorrect determination of the sampling error.

The researcher generally finds it economical and convenient to use for his sampling units existing clusters (blocks, cities, counties, work groups, school classes, etc.). These clusters usually exist as ecological, perhaps geographical units, and sometimes as "psychological groups" as well. The individuals in these units tend to resemble each other—there is usually some homogeneity of characteristics, of attitudes, of behavior—but homogeneity is generally not complete. It may be due to common selective factors, or to joint exposure to the same effects, or to mutual influence (interaction), or to some combination of these three causes. Because of this homogeneity, the use of these clusters for sampling units has definite consequences: it destroys the independence of the characteristics of the sample elements. The correspondence with the "well-mixed urn," inherent in the assumption of independence, is neglected; and formulas that depend on that assumption fail to apply.

As has been indicated, cluster sampling has not been widely employed in research in nursing and patient care, since most studies have involved geographically limited target populations, and lists identifying the sampling units have been readily available. One example of a cluster sample was in a study of the relationship between hours of nursing care available and the satisfaction of patients and personnel with the care provided.[15] Here the primary sampling unit was a hospital, and a total of 60 were randomly selected for inclusion in the study. The sampling was actually done at one stage only, as all patients and personnel in the hospitals selected were included in the study. In another study of hospitals conducted by the Bureau of Hospital Administration at the University of Michigan, described in the monograph *Probability Sampling of Hospitals and Patients*,[16] the technique of *controlled selection* was used to select a sample of hospitals in Michigan. The hospitals served as clusters for a study of the characteristics of a sample of patients discharged from the hospitals.

Mixed Sampling Designs

Combinations of the major types of sampling techniques can be employed to maximize economy and efficiency in data collection. Thus, stratification and clustering could be combined into a single design. In a study of nursing students, we might first stratify all the schools of professional nursing by size of student body and type of program. Then we would select a sample of schools from each strata as the primary sampling units. A sample of students from each school could be selected as the second-stage sample.

Sequential Sampling

In the sample designs discussed thus far, the number of sampling units to be included in the study is fixed in advance of the data collection. Such designs are sometimes called "fixed sample plans." In the sequential design the sampling units are taken into the study sequentially, and the number to be included in the study is not fixed in advance. That is, we start with a sample of one and measure it. Then we select another sampling unit, measure it, combine it with the first, and obtain a summary measure for the two. Then we select another unit, measure it, and so on. The sampling is stopped when the summary measure for the cumulated sampling units reveals that we are within the sampling error range that has been established prior to the initiation of the sampling process. The process of deciding when to terminate the sampling is known as the "stopping rules."

Sequential sampling has proved to be very useful in testing hypotheses. It has been used to experimentally test the effects of drugs on patients.[17, 18] In such studies it has been found that the sampling is always terminated at a level below the number of sampling units that would have been included in a fixed-sample-size design. Sequential sampling is, therefore, an economical sampling method.

However it does have its limitations. Among these is the impracticality of using such a design in testing hypotheses where there is a large time lag between the application of the independent variable and the measurement of the effects produced in the dependent variable. Since the decision to either terminate or continue the sampling depends on the sequential measurement of each sampling unit, the progress of the study would be ground to a halt if it took a few months for an effect on the study subjects to appear.

Another limitation is the narrow focus of studies based on sequential sampling. A sequential sample is geared to providing information on a specific and limited set of variables—the variables formulated in the hypothesis. Many studies of patient care are more broadly conceived than a specific test of a hypothesis concerned only with "what happens to dependent variable Y when we make a certain change in independent variable X?" The small-sized sample generally required by the sequential approach to test such narrow hypotheses would be inadequate to investigate the multivariable, complex research problems so frequently encountered in the field of patient care. Even though a fixed-sample-size design may overshoot the number of sampling units actually needed in a study, it will yield more information concerning the variables being measured and is, therefore, not a wasteful design.

TYPES OF NONPROBABILITY SAMPLES

Many studies are conducted with subjects that have not been chosen by truly random sampling methods. This does not mean that such studies are bad or that their data are inaccurate. The main limitation of the use of data obtained through such samples is the difficulty of generalizing them to a larger target population. Basically, nonprobability samples are not samples at all but could be regarded as complete populations from which no *statistical* generalizations to larger populations can be made.

There are various kinds of nonprobability samples. All are popular because they are usually cheaper and more convenient to employ than probability samples. In some types of nonprobability samples a target population is specified in advance of the sample selection, but the sampling units are not selected randomly. In other types the target population is defined ex post facto—that is, after the data have been collected and analyzed and the characteristics of the sampling units have been fully investigated. In still other types of nonprobability samples a certain element of randomness may be said to be present in the selection of the sampling units included in the study in that the selection is not done purposively but by chance or accident. A few of the more common types of nonprobability samples will be described.

Purposive Samples   Many samples are of the kind where the researcher deliberately selects the sampling units that are to be included in the study because he feels that they are representative of the target population. Such handpicked samples, also known as judgment samples, are widely used in research in nursing and patient care. Thus, if we are interested in studying the differences between a "good" school of nursing and a "bad" school or a "well-run" health agency and an "inefficient" one, we might rely on the judgment of knowledgeable people to select the actual institutions. Also, if we are conducting a study involving patients we might select Mr. X, Mr. Y, Mr. Z, and so on, because we are sure they have typical or average characteristics that would make them very representative subjects for our research. In other studies we might select the most typical day to observe the patients in the hospital or to test the students or to interview the personnel.

The danger in the use of such purposive samples is that there is no way of measuring the precision of the estimates. Also, unconscious bias may exert an influence, so that we choose Mr. X, not because he is the typical patient we think he is, but because he is cooperative and we are sure he will be a good study subject. Moreover, the most typical day might not be typical at all, but a quiet day without any problems when it would be convenient to do a study.

Convenience Samples   Another common type of nonprobability sample is the kind where we select for study the patients who happen to be in the hospital at a certain time, or the patients who will be receiving home nursing care on the day when the agency has a large staff making home visits, or the students who happen to be receiving their field experience in psychiatric nursing, or the first 50 visitors who come to the hospital that afternoon, and so on. It is true that there is an element of randomness in the entry of such subjects into the study. The subject has not been purposively selected as in the previously discussed sample. But a convenience sample is not a true random sample, since the subjects have not been selected out of some larger population in which all members of the population had some stated chance—greater than zero—of being selected.

Quota Samples This, too, is essentially a convenience sample, but it has controls to prevent overloading the sample with subjects having certain characteristics, as in a sample of patients with too many males or too many younger patients. The controls are established by determining the distribution of the members of the target population according to certain significant variables. These distributions serve as limits or quotas for the number of subjects with these characteristics to be taken into the study. Thus, by using the data in Table 8-1, the selection of a quota sample of 200 patients from a population of 50,000 can be established in terms of the age and sex of the patients. The quota would be 16 males under 21 years of age, 4 females under 21, 12 males between 21 and 44, 48 females between 21 and 44, and so on. The appropriate number of patients with these characteristics would then be selected as they conveniently could be found, rather than through random selection. This design thus resembles stratified sampling with the omission of randomization.

In another type of quota sample, used frequently in market research, the quotas are not established in accordance with the proportionate distribution in a target population. Instead the data collector is told to interview a group of subjects well-distributed according to sex, marital status, income level, and so on. The interviewer selects his cases by seeing that they are dispersed more or less evenly among the different strata.

Quota samples have an element of chance or accident in the selection of a particular subject for inclusion in the study. However, we cannot be sure that bias has not entered into the selection process. In quota sampling the tendency to choose the most convenient or the most cooperative subject can result in a distorted sample.

Volunteers Samples composed of volunteers can be thought of as the reverse of judgment samples. In judgment samples, the sampler handpicks the sampling units. In voluntary samples, the individuals being sampled do the selecting by deciding whether they will enter the study or not. The previously mentioned Kinsey study of females is an example of a sample composed of volunteers. Also, studies in which questionnaires are mailed to a random sample of a target population and where only a fraction of those who are mailed the questionnaires respond represent a voluntary not a random sample. The danger in the use of volunteers as sampling units is that they may not be representative of the target population in terms of the variables being measured, making it difficult to draw unbiased generalizations from the sample to the target population.

Random sampling, if strictly adhered to, is a disciplined and quite difficult approach to the selection of study subjects from a target population. Once an individual has been selected for inclusion in the study by the method of random sampling, he must enter the study regardless of his lack of cooperativeness or the inconvenience in collecting the data. If a household is selected for interviewing we would have to keep calling until we find someone at home regardless of the expense involved. In actual practice, however, many studies using random sampling allow a certain amount of nonresponse or provide for a substitute sampling unit for an uncooperative individual. Nevertheless random sampling is a more time-consuming and more expensive method of selecting study subjects from a target population than is nonprobability sampling. However, it can yield more valid data than other sampling methods.

METHODS OF COLLECTING DATA

The ways by which data on the variables being studied can be collected are outlined as follows:

  I. Use of existing data
 II. Use of the observer to collect the data
    a. Nonparticipant observer: use of quantitative scales
    b. Nonparticipant observer: use of qualitative scales
    c. Participant observer
    d. Interviewing
III. Self-recording collection of data
    a. Factual questionnaires
    b. Psychological and sociological pencil and paper instruments
    c. Mechanical instruments
IV. Combined methods

Existing Data

Existing data play a role in all types of research. In retrospective and in some prospective nonexperimental studies, existing data may provide all of the needed data for the study. In experimental studies, existing data may provide a background for the new data that are collected and assist in the analysis and interpretation of the findings of the experiment.

Existing data can be found in two forms, raw and tabulated. In its raw form there are such basic documents as patients' records, personnel folders, birth, death, and other vital records, licensure forms, applications of various kinds, financial records. Such records are originally designed as administrative documents, not as research instruments. However, it is often possible to prepare statistical tabulations from them that can serve as meaningful, valid, and reliable data for a study. Thus, from existing patients' hospital records, in a study described in Chapter 13, it was possible to tabulate the number of patients discharged from the hospitals who were in each of the major diagnostic categories. Such data were then used to assess the variety of clinical experiences the hospital could provide to nursing students.[19] In another study, personnel folders of all the members of the nursing department were used to provide an analysis of the stability of the work force.[20] Another study used the Kardex to obtain data on the work load of the nursing department.[21]

Data that are already tabulated can be used either as supplementary data or as the major source of data in a research study. Data produced by such governmental organizations as the Bureau of the Census, the Public Health Service, and the Bureau of Labor Statistics can serve many other purposes in addition to those for which they were primarily designed. Such a report as that by Lerner and Anderson[22] largely consists of an analysis of data from agencies like these.

In the field of nursing and patient care there are a variety of useful source documents that can provide data for a study. These include the Public Health Service's *Health Manpower Sourcebook* series, the American Hospital Association's Annual Guide Issues, and the American Nurses' Association's *Facts About Nursing*.

A major limitation to the use of existing data is that the definitions of the variables for which data are available may not correspond to the definitions of the study in which they are to be used. If we were to use as a criterion measure of the effectiveness of a public health program a tabulation from existing records of the number of deaths from different diseases, we may not have a valid measure, since the death rate may not be a function of how well a program is executed, particularly on a short-run basis. What would be needed in a study like this would be a more sensitive and responsive measure of effectiveness.

A second drawback to the use of existing data is the difficulty in evaluating its quality. Tabulated data, particularly if published, have a very authoritative appearance. However, even published data sometimes possess certain limitations. They may be incomplete or they may contain errors of one kind or another, or possess some other deficiency that could destroy their usefulness as research data. Such deficiencies are often unknown to the potential user of the data, since they are usually not advertised. It is therefore advisable to be cautious in the use of secondary data and to maintain at all times a skeptical attitude regarding their quality.

Use of an Observer to Collect the Data

In many studies, particularly of the prospective type, the requirements are such that the data collection has to be tailor-made for the study. Data available from existing sources are either nonapplicable, or not sufficiently reliable or not complete enough for studies like these. One of the most widely used methods of collecting new data is through the use of an observer. There are several means by which an observer obtains the required data.

Nonparticipant Observer: Use of Quantitative Scales In Chapter 7 discussion of the measurement process mentioned various types of quantitative scales that could be used to make measurements of the variables included in a study. These scales are usually incorporated into mechanical instruments such as weight scales, thermometers, or clocks to provide a precise and sensitive source of research data. The observer using mechanical instruments serves as the recorder of the data by applying the instruments to the study subjects and reading them. If the observer is well-trained, a high level of precision can be achieved in the use of quantitative scales, since subjective judgment in making the readings is kept to a minimum.

Nonparticipant Observer: Use of Qualitative Scales The use of an observer to obtain data on qualitatively scaled variables permits the observer to exert more judgment than in the use of quantitative scales. As a nonparticipant in the events being observed, the observer stands outside of the phenomena being measured and as objectively as possible records the required data. The recording may be in the form of a direct scaling of what is observed. For example, the observer could rate the performance of nursing personnel on a graphic rating scale with categories ranging from "high proficiency" to "low proficiency." Or she could classify patients on a scale according to their nursing needs. Instead of a direct scaling, the recording could be in the form of a narrative description of what transpires, or entries on a checklist, or a questionnaire type of form —material that will later be classified in terms of a nominal or ordinal type of scale.

Many examples of the use of this method of observation can be cited from research in nursing and patient care. In the assessment of the activities of nursing personnel by work sampling, the observer either makes a narrative recording of what she sees or directly classifies the activities into a nominal scale. In another approach to the study of the work of nurses, a watch is used to quantitatively measure how long it takes to perform different types of activities as well as to nominally classify the activity.

The use of an observer to gather data on qualitative variables requires a high level of control to insure the reliability of the observations, because the observer employs considerable judgment in making decisions about the categorization of the phenomena she is observing. It has been said that nurses make very precise observers, since they have been trained to assess the behavior of patients. This may well be true, but there is often a big difference between the kinds of observations made for the purpose of patient care and those required in research. Research observations are often concerned not with signs and symptoms presented by patients but rather with very subtle and intangible phenomena that are detected through the application of unstructured data-collecting instruments. A high level of skill is required on the part of the observer to insure the relevance and precision of such observations.

The worthwhileness of data collected by an observer on qualitative variables will depend not only on how well-trained the observer is, but on the clarity, meaningfulness, and sensitivity of the scale employed to measure the variables, the definitions of the categories included in the scale, and the format of the instrument used to gather the data. In making unstructured observations, the observer has maximum freedom to record what she sees, since the instrument used to collect the data is essentially a blank piece of paper. Here the burden of classifying and scaling the data is placed upon the editor of the data, who must be provided with definitive rules to guide his work. In more highly structured observations, the observer must fit the observations into predetermined categories. This procedure relieves the editor of much of the burden of classifying and scaling the observations, but it requires the observer to have a thorough understanding of the scale being used.

Participant Observer   One limitation to the use of the nonparticipant observer is the possibility of introducing psychological bias by the presence of the observer—the familiar Hawthorne effect. In observing people at work, for example, those being observed may work harder, or at least may behave differently from normal. One way of eliminating the possibility of observer bias is to disguise the observer by having her blend into the situation being observed. Maximum blending is obtained when the observer becomes a participant of the situation being observed.

The use of the participant observer is very popular in sociological research. The term "sociometry" has been applied to measurement of the social interactions among a group of people. A participant observer may be a member of the group, collecting the required data while taking part in the activity. The observer could assess the attractions and repulsions among the group's members by plotting their interactions on a device called a sociogram. This device has been used to analyze leadership exerted at meetings and conferences by recording who talks to whom, who initiates topics, and so on.

Nonsociological evaluations can also be the subject of participant observation. Thus, in evaluating the service provided in a hospital the observer can be disguised as a patient, rating not only the services she receives but all activities that come within her purview. A question can be raised as to the ethics of such a procedure, since it can be called "spying."

It would appear that for much of the research in nursing and patient care, the participant observer technique would have value if a dual observer (another outside observer) could be involved in the process to corroborate the participant observer's observations. A closed-circuit television screen or a one-way viewing screen can be most helpful.

A major principle of nonparticipant observation is for the observer never to intrude into the situation being observed. This may be difficult to do for a nurse observer who sees something being done that she regards as harmful to a patient.

Interviewing In the process of interviewing, the observer gathers her data by verbal questioning of the study subjects to elicit data on the variables being studied. The format of the interviews can vary from the highly structured kind where the interviewer actually reads the questions to the study subject and records the answers, to the highly unstructured interview where only a general framework is provided for the content of the questions and the interviewer is given much leeway in framing the actual questions and in the extent of coverage of the material. The unstructured interview permits greater probing into the responses of the subjects to verify meaning and to obtain data with depth and breadth. However, the highly structured interview also usually allows the interviewer to probe in order to clarify and broaden responses. One advantage of the structured interview is the greater ease with which the data can be processed. Another is that the observer does not need to be too highly skilled in the interviewing process. To obtain valid data in an unstructured interview, the interviewer must be well trained.

Direct Collection of the Data

In direct collection of the data the observer is eliminated and the study subjects themselves supply the material needed for the research. This can be in the form of a rating on a qualitative scale, a reading on a quantitative scale, a narrative description, or responses to a checklist, test, or questionnaire.

By eliminating the observer three important benefits are achieved. First the cost of collecting the data can be reduced. In studies where large amounts of observation are required, such costs can be quite high. The savings obtained by elimination of the observer can be used to increase the *size* of the sample for the study to provide greater coverage.

Second, elimination of the observer removes a source of possible bias from the study—observer error. However, this may well be offset by the introduction of a new source of bias—response error. Without an observer trained to interpret the meaning of the information being sought, the respondent can frequently misinterpret the items on the instrument he is responding to, thus reducing the precision of the data.

Third, with self-recording techniques it is possible to guarantee the study subject that his responses will be kept anonymous. When a study deals with sensitive or highly personal data this may be an important advantage.

A major disadvantage of the self-recording method of data collection, as compared to the use of an observer, is the lesser degree to which depth of response can be obtained. This can be a particularly serious disadvantage if the research problem is a thorny one and the variables studied are highly complex. An observer asking questions in an interview can probe into the meaning of a response. This cannot be easily done when the subject is responding to questions on a standardized form.

Also there are many variables of importance to research in nursing and patient care that can be studied only through the use of an observer. For example, if we are interested in studying the flow of some ongoing process or activity, such as the provision of nursing care, we would usually employ an observer to record the observations. Such substitutes as recording by a motion picture or television camera would be much more costly if done on a large scale. Moreover, such instruments do not entirely eliminate the observer, but only make the process of observation an indirect one.

Three of the ways in which data can be collected directly from the study subjects without the need for an observer are by the use of factual questionnaires, psychological and sociological tests and scales, and mechanical instruments.

Factual Questionnaires   Perhaps the single most widely used instrument for data collection, particularly in nonexperimental studies, is the factual questionnaire. These often consist of a battery of questions aimed at eliciting data on demographically oriented organismic variables such as age, marital status, occupation, educational level, size of family, or on economic variables such as possessions owned, salary earned, expenditures made, as well as on variables concerned with behavioral characteristics such as kinds of books read, hobbies pursued, hours of work performed, television programs watched, jobs held. Included also are variables that describe preferences—Who is your best friend? What is your most liked food? Who is your favorite political candidate? Factual questionnaires also deal with specific events—When were you last ill? Where did you purchase your car? How many times did you visit a dentist last year? How long did you spend on different activities on your job last week?

Responses to many kinds of factual questions are readily amenable to validation. If a study subject claims she is 29 years of age, an independent check is available on the accuracy of the data—the respondent's birth certificate. If a respondent states that her favorite television program is the evening news, corroboration may be possible by checking with family members, friends, or fellow workers.

Although a low response error is expected in factual questionnaires, such is not always the case.[23] A major source of error in responses to factual questions, particularly questions relating to past events, is faulty memory. Bell and Palmer reported a study[24] in which the identical factual questions were presented to the same respondents one week to ten days apart. There was an amazing lack of agreement in the responses to some of the variables.

Variable	*Per Cent of Agreement in Response*
Race	99.9
Marital status	98.2
Number of persons in household	85.3
Occupation	78.1
Age	68.5
School grade completed	55.8
Length of service in present job	40.0

For many factual questions, standardized wordings are available that can be used from one study to the next. One of the virtues of standardized items is that the comparability of data from different studies is insured.

Factual questionnaires can serve as useful criterion measures for a research study. Since they contain questions related to concrete, observable behavior, it is possible to use such questions to measure the effects of the independent variable. If, for example, the independent variable represents different kinds of treatment given to patients while they are hospitalized, a factual questionnaire can be used in a longitudinal follow-up study of the patients to determine what their health history is after discharge.

Factual questionnaires are perhaps the simplest type of data-collecting instrument to administer. Many factual questions are self-evident and require little interpretation. Assuming no major lapses in memory on the part of the respondent or a conscious determination on his part to distort a reply, the precision of such questions is rather high. Questionnaires of this type can be distributed through the mails, enabling wide coverage at low cost. With appropriate controls over return of the questionnaires, such as follow-ups to delinquent respondents, a high response rate should be obtained, thus keeping the bias of a "voluntary" sample to a minimum.

Factual questionnaires are generally easy to process. The response categories for qualitative variables can be framed in such a way as to make the questionnaire "self-coding," so to speak. A "self-coded" questionnaire is one in which the respondent replies to the items by checking the appropriate category of response. In the tabulation of the questionnaires the number of checks are counted to obtain the total frequency for the different classes of each question. A questionnaire is not self-coded if it requires open-ended, narrative responses to qualitative variables. These have to be coded after they are returned, a process of categorizing the responses into the various classes. One type of open-ended factual instrument is the so-called diary method. Here the study subject makes a continuous narrative recording of events, impressions, or findings concerning the variables under study. These narrative data are then coded and tabulated. Some structure could be incorporated into the diary method by including questions or checklists to which the study subjects regularly respond.

Psychological and Sociological Pencil and Paper Instruments   Many of these instruments have been mentioned in the previous chapter in the discussion of measurement of variables. These instruments measure such variables as personality, intelligence, interest, motivation, attitudes, and perception. They are called "pencil and paper" instruments because the study subjects respond by writing a narrative statement or making a check mark, or some other similar type of response. For a few psychological variables mechanical instruments can provide an indirect measure, but these are not commonly used. As an example, anxiety might be measured in terms of blood pressure level, loudness of heartbeat, or amount of moisture on the skin.

Instruments to collect data on some psychological and sociological variables could be administered in the same way as factual questionnaires. Graphic rating scales as well as other types of sociological scales could be distributed by mail to the study subjects. However, many psychological tests need to be highly controlled in their administration and require the presence of a member of the research project when they are being filled out by the study subjects. This is necessary because many of these instruments have to be regulated as to the time permitted for reply by the study subject. Also, there is need to insure the fact that the respondent receives no assistance while he is replying to the instrument and that he is free from distractions and interruptions. For economy, study subjects are often assembled and the test administered on a group rather than an individual basis. Some tests require that an observer be assigned to one study subject during the entire course of the administration of the instrument, acting as an interviewer or nonparticipant observer. In such a situation, the instrument cannot be classified as a self-recording one, but rather as one that employs an observer-recorder.

Psychological and sociological instruments are of two broad types— those that are direct and highly structured, and those that are less direct and unstructured. The latter are called nondirective or projective techniques and include such methods as the Rorschach test and thematic apperception test. These usually require a high degree of skill for proper administration and interpretation. Many instruments like these are available for use as a means of collecting the data for a study. To develop one especially for a study could be a formidable undertaking. However, this should not discourage the use of such instruments, since they can provide valuable criterion measures in studies of nursing and of patient care.

Mechanical Instruments   Many instruments are now available that can provide quantitative measurements on a self-recording basis. For example, certain types of thermometers can be attached to a patient to provide a continuous reading of his temperature. A variety of devices known as electronic patient monitoring apparatus are available as tools for diagnosis and therapy. They can also be used as instruments for research. Such instruments are useful in that the observer is eliminated, thus removing one possible source of bias, and quantitative measurements are provided of a highly precise and sensitive nature. A question remains as to the validity of such measurements. As was discussed in the previous chapter, a measurement can be very precise and sensitive, but it might not be valid because the variable being measured is not relevant to the research problem. Validity is the overriding consideration in the determination of the adequacy of a criterion measure in a research study.

An interesting example of a mechanical instrument used to obtain data without an observer is the equipment used in measurement of the size of the audience of television programs. This equipment is a monitoring device called an audimeter that is attached to the television receivers of sample viewers. When the viewer turns on his receiver the monitoring device records the station to which he is tuned and the amount of time the set is in use. These recordings are collected routinely and the data tabulated to provide ratings of the size of the audiences for different programs.

One difficulty in the use of such devices is the lack of control over the data-collecting process. This is somewhat analogous to permitting a subject to take an intelligence test home and work on it at his leisure. The lack of validity of such audience measurement was underscored during a congressional investigation of TV ratings. One of the sample viewers was found to have a very high rate of viewing, much higher than would be expected of people with similar socioeconomic characteristics. Closer investigation revealed that this viewer owned a dog. When she left the house for an extended period of time, she would turn the set on to keep the dog company. The monitoring device was indeed making precise recordings of the amount of time the set was in use, but the data did not portray a valid audience for the programs to which it was tuned.

Combined Methods

Many studies employ not just a single method of data collection but a combination of methods. In experiments that test the effects of drugs on patients, data on the criterion measure are usually collected by an observer. Data on important organismic variables related to the patient are obtained through factual questionnaires, interviews, and existing records.

Sometimes two or more different methods of data collection are employed to gather data on the same variable. The separate approaches are used to reinforce the findings or as a means of elaborating the amount of information gathered on the explanatory variables. Thus a factual questionnaire may be filled out by the study subjects. Later an interviewer will repeat some of the questions to the study subjects to corroborate the replies as well as to obtain more interpretative depth for these replies.

Another combined approach, also used to enhance the precision of the data, is to give a factual questionnaire to a study subject while an interviewer stands by to assist the subject in clarifying the meaning of any questions that the subject does not fully comprehend.

How to Select a Method of Data Collection for a Study

The choice of methods to use in a study for collecting the data will depend on consideration of a number of elements:

The research problem
The design of the study—experimental or nonexperimental, prospective or retrospective
The variables being studied—how they are defined, how they are measured
The sampling units to be included—their type, number, location
The amount of time available in which to complete the study
The amount of resources available to do the study

Often the nature of the variables will dictate the method to be used for data collection. A variable that can be measured quantitatively may require the use of mechanical apparatus. This will necessitate the employment of observers to read the instruments. Variables that are essentially factual can be measured with questionnaires, while psychological and sociological measurements are usually in the form of pencil and paper tests, rating scales, questionnaires, or a projective design. Data to be collected longitudinally on phenomena that are ongoing will require the use of observers or mechanical monitoring systems, such as the electronic devices now widely found in health agencies.

Highly controlled experimental studies usually require direct observation of the phenomena being studied. Nonexperimental studies, particularly where the subjects are widely dispersed geographically, often collect data with instruments that are distributed through the mails.

Where the measurements required are complex, difficult to make, and need considerable interpretation, the use of an observer to collect the data from the study subjects will be a greater necessity than where the variables are well-defined, specific, unidimensional, and easy to measure.

Importance of a Pretest

The adequacy of a data-collecting instrument can best be assessed by pretesting it before it is applied to the subjects in the actual study. The pretest should be done on subjects representative of the actual study subjects. Sufficient time should be allowed for the pretest to fully analyze the results so as to make all necessary changes in the data-collecting procedures.

A pretest can be used to validate the measures of the variables being studied by correlating them with outside criteria. It can also be used to check the reliability of the data-collecting instruments by such means as comparing responses to alternative ways of constructing the items relating to the same variable, by test-retest, and by comparison of independent observations of the same phenomena. The pretest also provides a "dry run" of the total administration of the data collecting as well as the tabulating phases of the research. It goes without saying that validity and reliability of the data-collecting instruments and procedures should be established by the pretest. The actual data collection phase should not begin until this has been achieved.

Criteria for Evaluating Data-Collecting Instruments

The criteria for evaluating data-collecting instruments are the same as those for assessing the quality of the measurement of variables:

Validity—Does the data-collecting instrument yield data that are relevant to the problem being investigated?

Reliability—Are the data that are collected precise? Would two independent observers observing the same phenomena record comparable data?

Would two independent interviewers asking the same questions elicit similar responses from the same subject?

Will identical responses to the same factual questionnaire be obtained if given to the same subject at short-spaced intervals?

Will the subject respond to the same test or scale consistently on a retest?

Sensitivity—Are the scales for different variables on which data are being collected of sufficient sensitivity to be discriminating and selective? Can they detect significant differences among the study subjects?

Meaningfulness—What is the substantive significance of the differences found among the subjects from whom data are collected? What practical importance do the data possess?

Enhancing Precision in Data Collection

The precision of the data that are collected is influenced by various sources of error. Many of these sources have been discussed in the previous chapter. Fortunately some errors that occur in data collection are random rather than systematic and as such can cancel each other out. This would tend to be truer as the number of study subjects on whom data are being collected increases. An error arising from a subject who mistakenly checks her field of practice on a factual questionnaire as hospital nursing when it really is private duty nursing may well be offset by another respondent checking private duty nursing when it should be hospital nursing.

However, some errors are systematic in nature. Such errors can harm the precision of the data. Many studies have shown that a variable such as age is consistently underestimated, particularly by women. Also, there is a tendency to round off data reported for certain variables such as age. The U.S. Bureau of the Census finds, for example, in its decennial census, that there are more persons reported at ages such as 20, 25, 30, 35, etc., than at the in-between years.

Questions such as age can be independently verified by asking for the same information in two ways on a questionnaire. Thus, an early question might be: How old are you? A later one might ask: What is the date of your birth? Underestimation or rounding off is likely to be picked up by the response to the latter question, since it is more difficult for the subject to either round off or underestimate his birth date than his age.

Systematic errors are troublesome when the criterion measure is to be assessed in terms of the absolute units of the scale of measurement. It is of less serious consequence if we are interested only in relative comparisons or trends. As Deming[25] remarked:

When trends or proportions rather than absolute numbers are to be considered no harm is done if the figures to be compared are all in error by the same percentage. Moreover, in some problems an error of 100 percent or even more will not affect the decision one way or another.

For example, if our study is concerned with measuring the effects of teaching on the weight reduction of diabetic patients, we might be interested simply in the fact that the experimental group weighed less than the control group at the end of the study. If there was a systematic bias in the weight scales that underestimated the weights of the study subjects by about 5 per cent on the average, the comparison would be unaffected by the error. If the average weight for both groups was the same at the beginning of the study, and if at the end of the study the control group averaged 150 pounds and the experimental group weighed 140 pounds, we still can make a valid interpretation of the data—weight loss was related to patient teaching—even though the true final weights were 160 pounds for the control group and 150 pounds for the experimental group.

Collection of data by observers can be fraught with both random errors, which hopefully will cancel themselves out, and systematic errors, which are more likely to reduce precision. A poorly trained observer can consistently make the same mistake in reading a mechanical instrument or in applying a rating scale to the events she is observing. Psychological bias, too, can systematically distort the data collected by an observer. In a study where the criterion measure is a rating of the quality of patient care, an observer, if she is a nurse herself, might unconsciously substitute her own system of values as well as her own prejudices for the definitions of the scale categories established in the study.

The major sources of error in a study that can reduce the precision of the data can be summarized as follows:

Sampling Error This error has been defined as the ratio of the variation of the values of the measurements among the sampling units of a target population to the square root of the number of sampling units in the sample. This is the most important kind of error in data collection that is actually measurable, since precise, mathematical formulas are available to assess it. Of course, such errors should only be computed where the sampling units were randomly selected from some larger target population. If nonrandom sampling is used, or if the whole target population is studied, sampling error should not be computed.

Sampling error is computed in terms of the summary measures that we derive from our sample of measurements. Each summary measure has its own sampling error formula. In statistical textbooks, these are called *standard errors*. The formula for the standard error of the mean in a simple random sample is identical with the one stated above. The numerator of the formula is the standard deviation of the values of the measurements among the sampling units of a target population. Since in most studies we do not know the standard deviation of the values of measurements for all sampling units in a target population, but only for those units actually in the sample, we use the standard deviation of the sample measurements in the computation of the standard error as the "best" estimate of the population standard deviation.

To illustrate the computation of the standard error of the mean, we can use the data presented in the last chapter on the blood pressure measurement for a sample of 15 patients. For the Group A patients we found a mean of 133 and a standard deviation of 16. The standard error of the mean is therefore:

$$\frac{16}{\sqrt{15}} = \frac{16}{3.9} = 4.1$$

The standard error of a summary measure like the mean is interpreted in the same way as a standard deviation of the values of the individual measurements among the sampling units. A standard error of a summary measure is, conceptually, the standard deviation of all the values of the summary measures that can be computed from successive samples drawn from the same target population. Thus, if our target population consisted of, say, 100 patients (a very small target population indeed), we could sequentially draw samples of 15 patients, compute the mean blood pressure for each sample, and return the 15 patients to the target population. Each sample of 15 would be randomly drawn from the population of 100 patients so that the same patients could appear over and over again in the different samples that are selected. However, each sample is likely to be a different set from every other sample set. Consider the fact that although as many as 14 of the sampling units may be the very same patients that composed another sample that was selected, the fifteenth may be an entirely new patient in the sample set. In fact, the number of different samples that could be drawn is astronomical. This is obvious if you consider the number of different bridge hands that can be drawn from a deck of 52 playing cards—over 600 billion different combinations of 13 cards can be selected. In mathematical terms the number of different samples that can be drawn from a population is: $\binom{n}{r}$, where $n =$ the total number of different sampling units in the population and $r =$ the number of sampling units in the sample. This is the well-known combination theorem that gives us the total number of combinations of n total units selected r at a time. Mathematically, $\binom{n}{r}$, which can also be stated as nCr, is equal to:

$$\frac{n!}{r!\,(n-r)!}$$

The exclamation point $!$ designates the mathematical operation called "factorial," which means that the number preceding the factorial is multiplied by all the positive integers preceding it. Thus 15! would be equal to $15 \times 14 \times 13 \times 12 \times 11 \times 10 \times 9 \times 8 \times 7 \times 6 \times 5 \times 4 \times 3 \times 2 \times 1$.

Substituting our values we find that the number of different samples of 15 patients that can be selected from a target population of 100 patients by simple random sampling is:

$$\frac{100!}{15!\,85!} = 25{,}333{,}846 \times 10^{10}$$

After drawing successive samples of 15 patients and computing the mean blood pressure for each sample, if we plotted the values of these means for all samples, we would find that they would form a normal curve, even if the actual blood pressures of the 100 patients in the target population did not. The mean of this distribution of means—called a sampling distribution—would be equal to the population mean, the mean for the 100 different blood pressures. The standard deviation of this sampling distribution is called the *standard error of the mean* and its value is estimated by the standard error of our sample mean. We can therefore interpret the value of a standard error in the same way as a standard deviation: ± 1 standard error would include 68 per cent of the values of all the mean blood pressures that could be selected from the $25{,}333{,}846 \times 10^{10}$ means in the sampling distribution; ± 2 standard errors would include 95 per cent of all the means; and so on.

The standard error of a sample statistic thus provides us with an estimate of the range within which the population parameter can be found at a stated level of probability. This range is called *confidence interval,* and the level of probability is called the *confidence coefficient.* Since our sample of 15 patients had a mean of 133 and a standard error of 4.1, we estimate, with a confidence coefficient of 95 per cent, that the interval 124.8 to 141.2 embraces the true population mean: $133 \pm 2(4.1)$.

The size of the confidence interval around a summary measure is the measure of the sampling error of the statistic computed from the sample. It provides a measure of the precision of the statistic as an estimate of the value of the population parameter. For other types of summary measures the measure of the sampling error is analogous to that of the standard error of the mean. Sampling errors can be computed for data obtained from qualitative scales as well as from quantitative ones. As has been described previously, summary measures of the frequencies in each of the qualitative scale categories (e.g., the number of males, the number of females; or the number of patients who died, the number who recovered) are known as rates or proportions. For a simple random sample, the standard error of a proportion is the square root of the ratio of the proportion multiplied by its complement (1 minus the proportion) to the number of sampling units in the sample. The numerator in this case, although it seems far removed from the numerator of the standard error of the mean, is quite analogous to it, since it is also a measure of the variability of the measurements among the sampling units of the target population.

To illustrate the computation of a standard error of a percentage, assume we took a random sample of 25 patients and wanted to estimate the percentage of patients in the target population who needed intensive care. If among our sample of 25 patients 10 per cent needed intensive care, our estimate of the population percentage would be 10 per cent ± 12, a confidence interval of 0 to 22 per cent with a level of confidence of 95 per cent, since the standard error of our sampling percentage is:

$$\sqrt{\frac{(.10)\,(.90)}{25}} = .06 \text{ or } 6\%$$

Observer Error   This type of error has been described as being either random or systematic. Random errors occurring more or less accidentally and with no particular pattern may offset each other, particularly when the number of measurements made is very large. Systematic errors, arising from such causes as inadequate training or psychological biases, can damage the precision of the data. One way of assessing the extent of observer error is to have two observers independently measure the same phenomenon and then compare the results obtained by each.

Response Error   Such error may also arise either randomly or systematically. It is more apt to be present where self-recording methods of data are employed and there is no observer to check the accuracy or completeness of responses. One type of response error is nonresponse. In mailed questionnaires some of the subjects selected for study may fail to cooperate and not reply. Those who do reply may not provide an adequate sample of the target population.

The various kinds of response errors can be controlled by making the instruments used as unambiguous and self-explanatory as possible and by making the aims of the study clearly known to the respondents. Also, the importance of submitting complete and accurate replies should be stressed.

Processing Errors This type of error should be under the complete control of the researcher. It should, therefore, be kept to a minimum. With the ready availability of highly accurate mechanical and electronic data-processing equipment there is little reason why any significant amount of error should occur during this phase of the research process. One possible source of processing errors in the translation of open-ended responses into categories in order to obtain the frequency of occurrence of the different categories. However, if the categories composing the scales for the variables are clearly defined there should be little difficulty in keeping the data free of errors during this stage of data processing.

Processing Data by Machine

The main steps in transforming the data from their raw state to a finished product include the following: editing the raw material; coding, scoring, and scaling the data; summarizing the data into statistical tables. These steps assume that the data are to be processed by either mechanical or electronic equipment. In small studies, which involve few variables and a handful of study subjects, it would not be advantageous to process the data mechanically or electronically. Whenever possible, machine processing should be used, as it is more precise, quicker, and less burdensome, and can also yield a greater amount of information per dollar spent on data processing. Moreover, the data can be permanently stored on cards or magnetic tape for re-use in the future if desired. A brief description of the major steps in data processing using punched cards as input follows:

1. *Edit the Raw Material* This usually involves an examination to see that all the questions have been answered and to evaluate the reliability of the responses. If reliability questions are included—asking a person's age in two different ways—these can be compared.

2. *Code, Score, and Scale the Data* If machine processing is to be used, it is necessary to transform data on qualitative variables into numerical codes that can be entered into the punched cards that will be used to tabulate the data. If a questionnaire or checklist contains no open-ended items or if the responses are in terms of a number (How many years of schooling do you have?), the instrument is said to be "self-coded" and after editing is completed can be turned over for card punching. Where responses are in narrative form, the material has to be coded. This operation not only assigns a scale category for the response, but also prepares it for the card-punching operation.

When psychological tests are used, the responses have to be scored. It is advantageous in the use of such tests in research to employ a device like "mark-sensing" in which the subject indicates his reply on a specially prepared answer sheet that can be fed directly into an optical scan machine for scoring. This process is similar to that of self-coding in the use of questionnaires and checklists. Projective tests in the psychological area present their own special problems. The scoring of these often has to be done by specially trained personnel. Sociological instruments may also have to be scaled if they are not of the self-scaling type, as are the graphic rating scales.

3. *Punch the Data into Cards* Card punching of data for research is done by specially trained personnel. Often the researcher has to contract for services like these, since only large research organizations have personnel trained in the use of such equipment and have the necessary equipment available. Sometimes card-punching and computing equipment and the staff to operate them are maintained by the institution in which the research is being done, and it may be possible for the research staff to make use of it. Many large hospitals have such equipment for their administrative and financial record-keeping.

Card punching consists of transferring the coded data from the basic document on which it was collected—a questionnaire, a checklist, an observer's record, a diary, or an interviewer's schedule. The punched cards serve as the input to the mechanical or electronic equipment that will be used for tabulating the data. If certain types of electronic data-processing equipment are used, the input might be magnetic tape rather than cards. One type of equipment used by the U.S. Bureau of the Census, known as FOSDIC, directly transfers raw data from the basic document into magnetic tape.

4. *Tabulate the Data* The end product of descriptive studies is the computation of summary measures for the data that have been collected and the preparation of statistical tables that portray the data in summary form in terms of the variables that have been studied. If the data are based on samples, confidence intervals are computed for the various statistics.

In explanatory studies a procedure known as testing the significance of the data is performed. This procedure, to be discussed in the following chapter, is analogous to the computation of confidence intervals for sample estimates. It essentially tests whether there is any statistical significance in the differences between the values of the criterion measures for the alternative groups that have been studied.

Mechanical data-processing equipment can summarize data into tables, but the actual computation of the summary measures—means, medians, rates, standard deviations—and their confidence intervals, as well as the tests of significance concerning these measures, ordinarily has to be done with desk calculators. In many studies this is a manageable chore. However, in studies that involve a large number of summary measures or employ more complicated tests of significance, the use of electronic computers is the most efficient way of processing the data. Computers, which are essentially giant desk calculators of a highly sophisticated kind, can accomplish huge tasks. As described by Rand:[26]

A Cambridge couple . . . have begun studying crime and juvenile delinquency by computer analysis of figures they have been collecting since the nineteen-thirties. Someone else has calculated word frequencies in twelve of the Federalist Papers as a means of assigning their authorship to either Madison or Hamilton; Madison was declared the winner. And last winter a visiting psychologist did a computer study of a nine-session psychotherapy undertaken by a psychiatrist several years ago and recorded by him verbatim in book form. In this study, the text was fed into a machine programmed to count various word usages of the patient and the psychiatrist throughout the nine sessions— and also to calculate changes in the frequency of these usages as the sessions progressed . . . the psychologist's work is typical of much that is being done in Cambridge today—by historians, anthropologists, public health experts, and many others. With the computer's help, they are paying profound attention to small, specific details that may mean little singly but when plotted in a big way are expected to reveal larger, less tangible truths.

Computers can be used not only to process great masses of data and to perform mathematical operations quickly, but also to solve problems in a manner analogous to the research process. One such technique, known as "simulation," is a method of programming a computer—a term signifying a process of telling the computer what to do—to imitate a real-life situation in terms of an abstract mathematical model. The purpose of the model is to find out what might happen if certain variables included in the model were altered. Computer simulation has been used widely in the military field by specialists in operations research to test out alternative courses of action in defense and warfare situations. In the field of patient care, Flagle[27] directed a simulation of the flow of patients into a hospital as a means of determining the optimum allocation of beds in the Progressive Patient Care type of hospital organization.

An electronic computer can thus be a most valuable aid to research, as a tool for processing data as well as a problem-solving instrument. For many studies, however, the amount of data collected might not warrant the expense involved in employing electronic computers. It is difficult to set forth generally applicable guidelines for determining when to consider the use of electronic computers in a study. However, it would be advantageous to consider their use in any study with reasonably large data requirements.

Processing Data by Hand

The steps in hand processing of the data are analogous to the use of machines. Briefly the steps are:

1. *Edit the Raw Data*   Review the data contained in the data-collecting instruments—questionnaires, checklists, observers, records, tests, scales, interviewers' records—for completeness and accuracy.

2. *Tally the Data on Worksheets*   Worksheets are a means of bringing together in one place the data collected on all the study subjects. For each variable studied, the frequency with which each scale value was reported for the individual subjects can be recorded by means of tally mark as follows:

Male	⫫⫫	⫫⫫	⫫⫫	/	
Female	⫫⫫	⫫⫫	⫫⫫	⫫⫫	///

Worksheets are so arranged as to permit the cross-tabulation of variables —the simultaneous tallying of the scale values of two or more variables for each individual:

	Improved	*Not Improved*
Male	⫫⫫ ⫫⫫ //	⫫⫫
Female	⫫⫫ ⫫⫫ ⫫⫫ /	⫫⫫ //

3. *Tabulate the Data*   This involves converting the tally marks to actual numbers, computing summary measures, preparing summary tabulations of the data, and if required by the study, computing confidence intervals for sample estimates. In explanatory studies this step frequently includes performing tests of statistical significance. For these activities a desk calculator is usually employed.

Preparing Summary Measures and Tabulations of the Data

In the previous chapter the main summary measures have been discussed:

For qualitative data: rates, ratios, percentages
For quantitative data:
  Measures of central tendency: mean, median, mode
  Measures of variation: range, standard deviation

In addition to these, other types of summary measures can be computed. The decision concerning which to compute should be based on the nature of the variables studied—qualitative variables require one type while quantitative variables require another type. The types of summary measures computed also depend on the nature of the distribution of the values of the measurements in the population—highly skewed distributions, for example, are better summarized by the median than the mean.

The end product in processing data is usually the preparation of statistical tables. Such tables can take many different forms, but all essentially contain the same basic ingredients. The preparation of statistical tables begins with the design of the outline of the table, called dummy or skeleton tables. In all studies it is highly advisable that such skeleton tables be prepared before any data are actually collected, since they can be of great assistance in clarifying the variables being studied and in directing and focusing the analysis of the data. This in turn clarifies the focus of the total study.

Table 8-2 contains a skeleton outline of a table which can be called an "explanatory table." Explanatory tables show the data for a dependent variable—in this case the average percentage of patients reporting dissatisfaction with length of time spent waiting for nursing service—in relationship to an independent variable. In Table 8-2 there are actually two independent variables: age of the patients and size of the room accommodations. Explanatory tables, thus, present data concerning the relationship among the variables studied. By contrast "descriptive tables" often present data for only one variable at a time:

Number of Patients by Size of Room Accommodations

Size of Room	Number of Patients
All room accommodations	227
Private	20
Two beds	94
3–6 beds	60
7 or more beds	53

Or, if data in descriptive tables are shown for two variables they are usually not related in terms of being dependent and independent.

The major components of an explanatory table containing two independent and one dependent variable are:

1. *Title*—Describes the data contained in the table—the variables for whom the data are presented, the study subjects, where the data were collected, and the time period to which they refer.

2. *Headnote*—Contains further information pertaining to the table as a whole that would be unwieldy if placed in the title. Headnotes are used infrequently.

3. *Stub*—Contains the scale categories for one of the independent variables. If there is more than one independent variable, the main variable is usually shown in the stub.

TABLE 8-2

A Skeleton Layout of a Statistical Table

Average percentage of patients* reporting dissatisfaction with length of time spent waiting for nursing services, by age of patient and size of room accommodation, 60 general hospitals, 1956. } (1) **Title**

(Percentages denote the percentage of the total number of patients in each age and accommodation group who reported dissatisfaction with length of time spent waiting for nursing services.) } (2) **Headnote**

(6) **Column**

(4) **Box Head**

Age of Patients	All room Accommodations (Average)	Number of Beds in Room			
		Private	2 beds	3–6 beds	7 or more beds
All ages (average)					
Under 20 years	(7) Cell				
20–29					
30–39					
40–49					
50–59					
60 and over					

(8) **Body**

(5) **Line**

(3) **Stub**

*Nonobstetrical patients.} (9) **Footnote**

Source: Questionnaires to patients in 60 general hospitals. For a complete report of the study see Faye G. Abdellah and Eugene Levine, *Effect of Nurse Staffing on Satisfactions with Nursing Care,* American Hospital Association, Monograph No. 4., 1958. } (10) **Source**

4. *Box Head*—Contains the scale categories for the second independent variable. If there is only one independent variable, it is shown in the stub and the box head is not used.

5. *Line*—Shows the data on the dependent variable for one scale category of the independent variable contained in the stub according to the scale categories of the independent variable contained in the box head.

6. *Column*—Shows the data on the dependent variable for one scale category of the independent variable contained in the box head according to the scale categories of the independent variable contained in the stub.

7. *Cell*—The intersection of a scale category of one variable with a scale category of the other variable.

8. *Body*—The aggregate of all the cells in the table.

9. *Footnote*—Provides additional information for a specific part of the table, if needed.

10. *Source*—Describes where the data came from.

Summary

The data collection phase of the research process involves the making of four important decisions:

1. The target population must be defined. This definition sets the boundaries of generalization of the data.

2. The method of selecting the individual sampling units from the target population must be determined. Scientific (probability) sampling, which involves the selection of the sampling units by a random process, is the most desirable selection method. It can summarize the selection of a biased sample, and it enables the assessment of the precision of the summary measures computed from the sample data. Some types of probability sampling include simple random sampling, systematic sampling with a random start, stratified random sampling, cluster sampling, and sequential sampling. Nonprobability sampling includes purposive samples, convenience samples, quota sampling, and the use of volunteers.

3. The method of collecting the data must be determined. The three major ways of collecting the data include the use of existing data, use of an observer to collect the data, and self-recording collection of data.

4. The way in which the data are to be processed must be decided. The two main processing methods include machine processing and processing the data by hand. For many studies some form of machine processing should prove to be the most advantageous method. The use of electronic data processing should be explored in the planning stage of a study.

The following chapter will discuss the phases of a research project that follow the processing of the data. These phases include analyzing and interpreting the data and reporting the findings.

References

1. Robert McGinnis, "Randomization and Inference in Sociological Research." *Am. Sociol. Rev.,* **23**:412, August 1958.

2. Margaret J. Hagood and Daniel O. Price, *Statistics for Sociologists,* rev. ed. New York, Henry Holt and Co., 1952, Chap. 16.

3. Sidney and Beatrice Webb, *Methods of Social Study.* London, Longmans, Green and Co., Ltd., 1932.

4. Frederick F. Stephan, "History of the Uses of Modern Sampling Procedures." *J. Am. Statistical A.,* **43**:12–39, March 1948.

5. L. H. C. Tippett, *Random Sampling Numbers.* Cambridge, Cambridge University Press, 1927.

6. M. H. Hansen, W. H. Hurwitz, and W. G. Madow, *Sample Survey Methods and Theory,* Vol. 1. New York, John Wiley and Sons, Inc., 1953.

7. W. E. Deming, *Some Theory of Sampling.* New York, John Wiley and Sons, Inc., 1950.

8. W. G. Cochran, *Sampling Techniques.* New York, John Wiley and Sons, Inc., 1977.

9. Irene Hess, Donald C. Riedel, and Thomas B. Fitzpatrick, *Probability Sampling of Hospitals and Patients.* Bureau of Hospital Administration, Research Series No. 1. Ann Arbor, University of Michigan, 1975.

10. Faye G. Abdellah and Eugene Levine, "Work Sampling Applied to the Study of Nursing Personnel." *Nursing Res.,* **3**:11–16, June 1954.

11. C. L. Brisley, "How You Can Put Work Sampling to Work." *Factory Management and Maintenance,* **110**:84–89, July 1952.

12. Theodore D. Woolsey, *Sampling Methods for a Small Household Survey.* U.S. Public Health Service Monograph No. 40. Washington, D.C., Government Printing Office, 1956.

13. Staff of the U.S. National Health Survey and the Bureau of Census, *The Statistical Design of the Health Household-Interview Survey.* U.S. Public Health Service Publication, No. 584-A2. Washington, D.C., Government Printing Office, 1958.

14. Leslie Kish, "Confidence Intervals for Clustered Samples." *Am. Sociol. Rev.,* **22**:154, April 1957.

15. Faye G. Abdellah and Eugene Levine, *Effect of Nurse Staffing on Satisfactions with Nursing Care.* Hospital Monograph Series No. 4. Chicago, American Hospital Association, 1958.

16. Hess *et al., op. cit.*

17. Peter Armitage, *Sequential Medical Trials.* New York, John Wiley, and Sons, Inc., 1975.

18. E. J. Anscombe, "Sequential Medical Trials." *J. Am. Statistical A.,* **58**:365–383, June 1963.

19. Faye G. Abdellah and Eugene Levine, *Appraising the Clinical Resources in Small Hospitals*. U.S. Public Health Service Monograph No. 24. Washington, D.C., Government Printing Office, 1954.

20. Eugene Levine, "Turnover Among Nursing Personnel in General Hospitals." *Hospitals, J.A.H.A.*, **31**:50–53, 138, 140, September 1, 1957.

21. Marion J. Wright, *Improvement of Patient Care*. New York, G. P. Putnam's Sons, 1954.

22. Monroe Lerner and Odin W. Anderson, *Health Progress in the United States*. Chicago, University of Chicago Press, 1963.

23. Deming, *op. cit.*

24. Gladys L. Palmer, "Factors in Variability of Response in Enumerative Studies." *J. Am. Statistical A.*, **38**:148–152, 1943.

25. Deming, *op. cit.*, p. 24.

26. Christopher Rand, "Center of a New World." *The New Yorker Magazine*, April 1964, pp. 58, 60.

27. Charles D. Flagle, "How to Allocate Progressive Patient Care Beds," Chapter 6, in Lewis E. Weeks and John H. Griffith (eds.), *Progressive Patient Care: An Anthology*. Ann Arbor, University of Michigan, 1964, pp. 47–57.

Problems and Suggestions for Further Study

1. Define the target populations for the hypotheses listed on pp. 135–36. For which of these target populations would listings of the sample units be readily available? Discuss the pros and cons of defining the target population as broadly or as narrowly as possible.

2. Read the article by Morris J. Slonim, "Sampling in a Nutshell" (*J. Am. Statistical A.*, **52**:143–161, June 1957). Discuss the following statement by the author, "In addition, many who insist that the only accurate way is to make a complete count, overlook the fact that often there are many sources of error in the basic data and that a 100 per cent count can be highly erroneous, as well as nearly impossible to achieve." (See pp. 146–147 in Slonim article.)

3. It has been said in this chapter that the same person is simultaneously the member of many different conceivable target populations that could be defined for a study. Can you list at least five different target populations of which you are a member that could be the populations for a study (e.g., a target population of voters, a particular occupational group, the alumni of a school, etc.)? Is it possible for one individual to participate in more than one study at the same time?

4. Suppose we wanted to experimentally test the effects of a nursing procedure on patients who are hospitalized with a certain type of illness, say, a chronic disease. If we selected our patients from only one hospital would we be able to generalize our findings to other hospitals? If we included two hospitals would we be in a better position to generalize findings? What about a dozen or two dozen hospitals?

5. In agricultural experiments a plot of land is subdivided into smaller plots, each representing a different sampling unit. Is it possible to take a human being and treat him similarly? Could we, for example, in testing out various sunburn preventatives apply a different preventative to various parts of a person's body, expose him to the sun, and determine which does the best job in preventing sunburn? Would each part of the body represent a different sampling unit? What are the limitations of such a design?

6. Discuss the sampling designs employed in the following studies. Which of the studies employed probability sampling? How would you classify the nonprobability samples?

   a. Dorothy E. Reese and Stanley Siegel, "Educational Preparation of Nurses Employed in Non-federal Hospitals." *Hosp. Mgmt.*, **89**:108–112, April 1960.

   b. Sharon Ringholtz and Miriam Morris, "A Test of Some Assumptions About Rooming-In." *Nursing Res.*, **10**:196–199, fall 1961.

   c. Janice E. Mickey, "Findings of Study of Extra-Hospital Nursing Needs." *Am. J. Pub. Health*, **53**:1047–1057, July 1963.

   d. John S. Hathaway *et al.*, "The Role of the Nurse in a University Health Service." *Nursing Outlook*, **10**:533–537, August 1962.

   e. Margaret L. Schell and Peter J. Korstad, "Work Sampling Study Shows Division of Labor Time." *Hospitals, J.A.H.A.*, **38**:99–102, January 16, 1964.

   f. Irene S. Palmer, "Surgical Intervention and Social Class." *Nursing Sc.*, **2**:15–37, February 1964.

   g. Louis E. Davis, George M. Parks, and Samuel R. Wickel, Jr., "A Sampling Technique for Estimating Linen Supply." *Hospitals, J.A.H.A.* **37**:118, 120, 122, 123, 141, March 16, 1963.

7. On pages 10 and 11 of their *Probability Sampling of Hospitals and Patients* (Bureau of Hospital Administration, Research Series No. 1, Ann Arbor, University of Michigan, 1975), the authors (Hess, Riedel, Fitzpatrick) describe a method of selecting a simple random sample of patients admitted to a hospital during a period of a year. Since some patients may be admitted more than once to the same hospital during the course of a year, what technique do the authors propose to obtain a sample of different persons?

8. How would you classify the following types of samples that are selected for a study? Discuss their adequacy as sample designs.

   a. After a random start, select every fifth patient who visits the outpatient department during the week.

   b. Select all the home visits made by the public health nurses to patients whose last names begin with an odd letter (i.e., A, C, E, G, I . . . etc.).

   c. Select all patients admitted to the hospital on Tuesdays and Thursdays during a three-month period.

   d. Select at random 6 diploma nursing schools out of 35 located in a state. For the study population choose at random the first-year class in two of the schools, the second-year class from two of the remaining four schools, and the third-year class from the remaining two schools.

   e. Obtain a copy of the classified telephone directory (yellow pages) for a dozen large cities. Select every twentieth name listed under "Nurses."

   f. Obtain the latest copy of *State Approved Schools of Practical Nursing* (published by the National League for Nursing, 10 Columbus Circle, New York). Number the schools consecutively, beginning with 1. Choose 25 schools for a sample by selecting the numbers from a table of random numbers.

g. Choose a sample of medication orders by putting a copy of all medication orders written during a month into a box, mixing up the slips (as in a lottery), and selecting 100 slips at random.

9. Why does the design of a sample have to consider the other phases of the research process—e.g., definition and measurement of variables, types of data-collecting methods used, methods for analyzing the data? What are some of the pitfalls in designing a sample for a study without considering other phases of the research process?

10. Read the article by Abdellah and Levine in *Nursing Research* (**3**:11–16, June 1954), "Work Sampling Applied to the Study of Nursing Personnel." How would you go about designing a study to demonstrate that systematic work sampling is as reliable as random work sampling? What is the basic sampling unit in a work sampling study?

11. Define the following:
    a. Random start
    b. Confidence level
    c. Level of significance
    d. Self-coding
    e. Pencil and paper instrument
    f. Parameter
    g. Response error
    h. Standard error

12. Read the article, "On the Use of Sampling in the Field of Public Health" (*Am. J. Pub. Health*, **44**:719–740, June 1954). What are some of the guidelines offered in the article as to when to enlist expert assistance in the design of a sampling plan? Discuss the disadvantages of sampling that are presented in the article, and indicate at least three situations in which sampling is inappropriate or will offer no advantages over study of the whole target population.

13. Obtain a recent edition of *Facts About Nursing* (published by the American Nurses' Association, Kansas City, Missouri). Examine some of the data contained in this book. Discuss three studies that could be made that would be based wholly or in part on these data, assuming, of course, that previous editions of *Facts* could be used for the study. (Example: a study to answer the question: Have the salaries of public health nurses kept pace with the rise in the cost of living over the past 15 years?)

14. Design a factual questionnaire containing 8–12 items to gather data on one of the following topics:
    a. To what extent do professional nurses marry physicians?
    b. The characteristics of patients in private psychiatric hospitals.
    c. Staffing patterns in operating rooms of short-term general hospitals.
    d. The family characteristics of patients receiving home nursing care from public health agencies.
    e. A comparison of reasons for turnover of nursing personnel employed by nongovernment hospitals and government hospitals.
    f. The amount of information patients possess about their illnesses.

g. How do directors of nursing service evaluate recent graduates of collegiate programs in nursing?

h. The work patterns of private duty nurses.

15. Describe what methods you would use to collect the data needed to test the hypotheses listed on pp. 135–36. What are some of the ways in which the costs of collecting the data for these studies could be kept as low as possible?

16. Comment on the following statement by Hyman in his *Survey Design and Analysis* (New York, The Free Press of Glencoe, 1955, p. 28), "There is the realization that the standardization of inquiry in large scale survey research, while making for efficiency and necessary to insure comparability among field workers, at the same time may impose some artificiality on the phenomenon studied, particularly when the analyst does his planning away from the live events."

17. Discuss the following statement by Walter I. Wardwell and Claus B. Bahnson ("Problems Encountered in Behavioral Science Research in Epidemiological Studies," *Am. J. Pub. Health,* **54**:972–981, June 1964): "A very great advantage of home interviewing is that the patient's home and often also his family can be observed as well as the patient's behavior in relation to them. In his natural habitat, as it were, a different quality of information may be obtained about the patient than would be possible in the more standardized and possibly threatening environment of the hospital or examination clinic" (p. 979). Are there any disadvantages in obtaining research data by interviewing the patient in his home? What are the advantages of conducting an interview study of institutionalized patients?

18. How could you go about deciding whether an electronic computer would serve a useful purpose in a research project you are planning. (Note: Some comparative information on computers available on a rental or purchase basis is contained in an article entitled "Layman's Guide to Computers," *Business Week,* September 1960. Although many changes have occurred in the computer field since 1960, much of the information in this article is still relevant and would be helpful in answering a question like this.)

19. Computers are used for a variety of purposes including the statistical processing of data. Discuss the various applications of computers and indicate how these could be helpful in conducting research. In answering this question the following book could be helpful: Charles A. Myers, *Computers in Knowledge-Based Fields.* Cambridge, Mass., MIT Press, 1970.

Chapter Nine

ANALYSIS AND INTERPRETATION
OF RESEARCH FINDINGS

MOST RESEARCHERS are concerned with drawing inferences from sample data about populations. The two main purposes of statistical inference are to test statistical hypotheses and to estimate population parameters. In testing statistical hypotheses we are testing, on information obtained from a random sample, some preconceived notion that we have concerning the population from which our data are a sample. Statistical estimation deals with estimating the values of parameters from observations in a random sample.

A single value, which is in a sense the best single guess as to the value of the parameter being estimated, is called a point estimate. Examples of point estimates are measures of central tendency and rates. However, the point estimate does not provide a measure of the degree of confidence we may place in the estimate. The sampling error serves as a measure of the precision of the estimate. This precision is expressed in terms of the confidence interval.

In essence the fundamental purpose of statistical analysis of data is to determine the amount of sampling error in the data. In random sampling the sampling error arises from having randomly selected one set of sampling units out of the many different sets that could have been selected. As was shown in the previous chapter the number of different samples of size 15 out of a target population of 100 is $\dfrac{100!}{15! \quad 85!}$.

In random assignment of subjects to alternative groups in an experiment the sampling error arises from having randomly allocated the subjects to certain groups from the many different groups that could have been formed out of the total number of subjects in the study. The number of different groups (samples) of study subjects that could be formed by randomly assigning 30 subjects to two equal-sized groups is $\dfrac{30!}{15! \quad 15!}$, a huge number indeed.

In descriptive studies the sampling error is computed as a measure of the precision of the estimate obtained from the sample. This is done by computing confidence intervals around the sample estimates of the population parameters. The interpretation of the confidence interval is as follows: If we draw repeated samples of size *n,* and if for each of these samples we estimate the population parameter and its corresponding confidence interval, which is a random variable, then we may expect a certain percentage of these intervals, called the level of confidence, to include the population parameter. Thus, in the example of blood pressure measures, introduced in Chapter 7, the mean blood pressure for Group A patients was 133, and the sampling error (standard error) of the mean was computed to be 4.1. At a level of confidence of 95 per cent the mean blood pressure for the population was estimated to lie within the range of 124.8 to 141.2. The mean blood pressure for Group B patients was 144, and with a standard error of 10.3 the 95 per cent confidence interval is 123.4 to 164.6. Because the variability of the measurements among the Group B patients is considerably higher than for Group A— the standard deviation for Group B is 40 compared with 16 for Group A—the estimate of the population mean for Group A is more precise than for Group B.

In explanatory studies the aim is to evaluate whether the values of the summary measures obtained for the alternative groups are different. Such an evaluation is done through a technique known as a *test of significance.* Basically, the purpose of the test is to see whether the summary measures being compared, after making allowances for sampling error, could be independent estimates of the same population parameter.

TESTS OF SIGNIFICANCE FOR QUANTITATIVE VARIABLES

Variables that are measurable in terms of either interval or ratio scales are called quantitative variables. Such variables have a continuous numerical distribution and when used as criterion measures are capable of providing refined distinctions among the subjects being measured. In explanatory studies the aim is to assess the relationship between the independent variable, whose different levels or versions are represented by the different groups of study subjects, and the dependent variable, which is measured by the criterion measure. When the criterion measure possesses a numerical scale, summary measures such as a mean and standard deviation are computed for the values of the measurements of the individuals composing the groups. The test of significance is aimed at evaluating the differences in the values of the summary measures for the groups to see to what extent they could have arisen by random sampling. In comparing two means, the *t*-test is usually employed. In comparing more than two means, as in studies having more than two study groups or where more than one independent variable is being tested at the same time, the technique of *analysis of variance* is the most widely used method.

Test of Significance of the Difference Between Two Means

In a test of the significance of the difference between the mean blood pressure readings for Group A patients of 133 and Group B of 144, the question being answered is: considering the sampling error for these means, what is the probability that they could have come from the same population? That is, are the patients in the two groups actually samples from the same population? For Group A patients the interval within which the population mean could be estimated to lie with 95 per cent confidence is 124.8 to 141.2 and for Group B the interval is 123.4 to 164.6. The interval for B encompasses that for A, giving rise to the belief that the two sample estimates could have come from the same population. In other words, the difference between the means of the two samples, 133 and 144, may well be due to sampling error and not to the independent variable being tested.

Sampling error could have been generated in these data in two ways. In a nonexperimental explanatory study of the relationship between the variables quality of nursing care provided and blood pressure levels of the patients, we could have selected a random sample of 15 patients from one hospital known to provide high-quality care, called Group A, and another random sample of 15, called Group B, from a hospital known to provide lower-quality care. Or, in an experimental study we could have taken 30 patients, randomly assigned them to two groups, the A patients receiving high-quality nursing care (lots of reassurance, emotional support, T.L.C., etc.) and the B patients receiving minimal care. Then, after both groups have been suitably exposed to the independent variable we could measure their blood pressures. The hypothesis to be tested would be concerned with the relationship between quality of care and patients' blood pressure.

Instead of comparing the confidence intervals for the summary measures for the two groups, the usual procedure is to apply a test of significance of the difference in the values of the summary measures. For a comparison of two means computed from small samples the test is called a *t*-test. This test is based on Student's *t* distribution rather than the normal distribution that was discussed in Chapter 7. The *t*-test is in the form of the following ratio:

$$t = \frac{\text{Difference in sample means minus difference in population means*}}{\text{Standard error of the difference in sample means}}$$

* In most applications of this test the difference in population means is hypothesized as being zero (null hypothesis), therefore, in the following discussion this term will be omitted from the formula.

The denominator of this ratio, the standard error of the difference between two sample means, is directly analogous to the standard error of a sample mean. As has been discussed, the standard error of a sample mean is the standard deviation of a sampling distribution of means—the distribution of the values of all the means that could be calculated from repeated samplings of a specified number of sampling units from the target population. The standard error of the difference between sample means is the standard deviation of a sampling distribution of differences between means—the distribution of the values of all *differences* between means that could be calculated from repeated samplings of a specified number of sampling units from two populations. And if the two population means have the same value—in essence, the two populations are the same population with respect to their mean values—the mean of the sampling distribution of differences between means would be equal to zero. Such a sampling distribution, with a mean equal to zero and a standard deviation equal to the standard error of the difference between two means, is the statistical model underlying tests of differences between two sample summary measures.

The standard error of the difference between two sample means is calculated from the following formula:

$$s_p \sqrt{\frac{1}{n_1} + \frac{1}{n_2}}$$

Where: s_p = a weighted average of the two sample
          standard deviations
n_1 = size of first sample
n_2 = size of second sample

Note that the denominator of the t-test is in terms of standard error units. Thus, the t ratio converts the numerator of the ratio—the difference in sample means—into standard error units. In interpreting the t ratio value, the size of sample upon which it is based must be considered. For example: in samples of size 5, ± 2.6 standard errors include 95 per cent of all the values, and in samples of size 30 ± 2.0 standard errors will include 95 per cent of the values. Thus if our ratio exceeds 2.0—that is, the difference between the sample means is larger than twice the value of the standard error of the difference between the means—it has exceeded the 5 per cent level of significance. In other words, the difference that we have found in the values of the summary measures for the alternative groups would occur less than 5 times out of 100 in repeated random samplings. Since such an occurrence is rare, we say that the difference between the sample measures is significantly greater than zero.

The normal distribution can be used to evaluate the differences between sample means where the samples are large, consisting of more than 30 sampling units; in smaller-sized samples the t distribution is used. From the properties of a normal distribution, we have seen that approximately $\pm$ 2 standard errors includes 95 per cent of all the values in a distribution. Tests based on the normal distribution are called by some T-tests and by others the K-test or Z-test. This test is identical with that of t, having the ratio:

$$T = \frac{\text{Difference in sample means}}{\text{Standard error of the difference in sample means}}$$

The 5 per cent level has been traditionally accepted as a suitable level of significance for many studies, although other levels could be chosen. The 1 per cent level—that of finding a difference in the sample summary measures that, in a sample of size 30, would be nearly three times larger than the value of the standard error of the difference between the sample measures—signifies that such a difference could occur by chance only 1 time in 100. This is a more stringent significance level than the 5 per cent level because larger differences are required between the sample statistics before they are considered to be significantly greater than the value that could be attributable to random sampling error.

The levels of significance of the values of the t ratio for various-sized samples are as follows:

Size of Sample	Level of Significance	
t-test	*5 per cent*	*1 per cent*
5	2.57	4.03
10	2.23	3.17
15	2.13	2.95
20	2.09	2.84
25	2.06	2.79
30	2.04	2.75
T-test	1.96	2.58

Applying the t-test to the data on the difference between the mean blood pressures for Groups A and B, we find that the value of this difference is $144 - 133 = 11$. The standard error of this difference, determined from the formula just provided, is 11.1, $(30.5 \sqrt{\frac{1}{15} + \frac{1}{15}})$, since Group A's standard deviation is 16 and Group B's is 40, and as both have sample sizes of 15 the weighted average of the two sample standard deviations (s_p) is 30.5. The t ratio value is, therefore, $11/11.1$ or 1, which is well below the 5 per cent level and thus not considered statistically significant. This confirms the conclusions from the comparison of the confidence intervals for the means of the two groups where it was found that the interval for Group A fell within the interval for Group B. The conclusion is that both means come from the same population, and are therefore not considered significantly different. In terms of the hypothesis being tested we can say that there is no relationship between quality of nursing care and blood pressure levels of patients.

Analysis of Variance

Many explanatory studies are directed toward a comparison of the values of quantitative criterion measures for more than two groups. Instead of comparing the mean blood pressures for Groups A and B, more than two groups could have been set up in the experiment, each representing a different scale value of the independent variable, quality of nursing care. Moreover, many studies are concerned with the analysis of the effects of multiple independent variables, as in the previously discussed factorial design. The method of statistical analysis of such data is called the *analysis of variance*. Originally conceived by the late R. A. Fisher and his co-workers, this is a powerful statistical tool for analyzing multiple comparisons. It is intimately related to the design of experiments and is the analytical method for treating data obtained from such designs as the *latin square* and the *factorial design*.

The computational procedure for the analysis of variance is contained in most texts on statistical methodology. This procedure is a rather straightforward and ingenious one. It consists in its simplest application of computing two kinds of variances (the square of the standard deviation): the variance of the measurements within each of the alternative groups and the variance among the means of the alternative groups. The first measure of variation is called the "within-group" variation whereas the second is the "among-group" variation. The within-group variation should reflect only the effects of chance—as a consequence of randomization—since theoretically all subjects within a group have been treated identically. The among-group variation, in addition to being influenced by chance, should also reflect the effects of the independent variable being tested. The test of significance is called the *F*-test (for R. A. Fisher) and is the ratio:

$$\frac{\text{Variance among groups}}{\text{Variance within groups}}$$

If there were no difference in the measurements among the groups, except for chance variation attributable to randomization, the value of the numerator of the *F* ratio would be similar to that of the denominator. To the extent that the means of the groups differ significantly from each other, the numerator would tend to be larger than the denominator and the value of the ratio would increase. Tables are available by which the level of significance of the value of the *F* ratio can be assessed. Thus, the *F*-test is analogous to the *t*-test. It provides the relative frequency (5 times out of 100, 1 time out of 100, etc.) of obtaining a value as large as that computed from the ratio by random sampling (randomization). The higher the value of the *F* ratio for specified-size samples, the greater the probability that the means being compared are really different from each other.

The analysis of variance is an important technique because it provides more information in factorial experiments than just a test of the significance of differences among the means of the groups. It also yields an assessment of the effects of combinations of the variables included in the study, known as the interactions.

Regression Techniques

The simplest type of statistical model underlying hypotheses that express a relationship between independent and dependent variables is called the general linear hypothesis. In its most basic expression it possesses the formula $Y = a + (b) X$, which states that Y, the dependent variable, is a function of X, the independent variable. In this equation a is called the *intercept* and (b) the *slope of the line*. The equation states that whenever X is changed Y also changes. In studies of independent and dependent variables that are both measurable in terms of quantitative scales, if we had a sufficiently large number of sampling units, it would be possible to fit a regression equation to the data that would precisely express the relationship between the two variables. The test of significance of the relationship between the variables would be based on an evaluation of the slope of the line that is fitted to the data, called the *regression coefficient*. That is to say, if two variables are positively related, the line fitted to the data—assuming that the relationship is linear, e.g., in the form of a straight line—should look as follows when plotted on a chart:

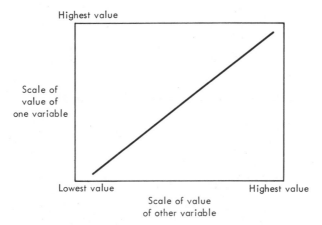

Fig. 9-1. **Positive relationship between two variables.**

Or, if the variables had a negative relationship the chart would appear as follows:

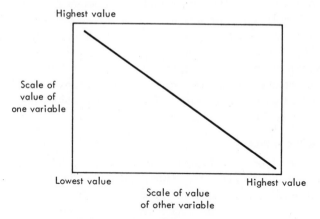

Fig. 9-2. **Negative relationship between two variables.**

If there were no relationship between the variables, the slope of the line would be zero and the chart would appear as follows:

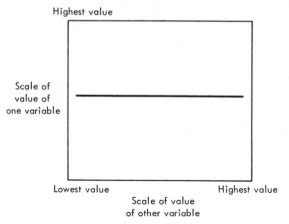

Fig. 9-3. **No relationship between two variables.**

The test of significance would be:

$$t = \frac{\text{Slope of the regression equation for sample data} \quad \text{minus} \quad \text{Slope of the regression equation for the population*}}{\text{Standard error of the slope}}$$

Regression analysis can be extended to include more than one independent variable. Known as multiple regression, the contribution (weight)

* Assumed to be zero (null hypothesis).

of the values of each of the independent variables toward the value of the dependent variable can be assessed. Such an approach is analogous to a factorial design in which the data are analyzed by the method of analysis of variance.

An example of the use of multiple regression analysis in a study in nursing is reported in *Effect of Nurse Staffing on Satisfactions with Nursing Care*.[1] In this study, the dependent variable was a measure of the unfulfilled needs for nursing services as perceived by patients and personnel in 60 general hospitals. Four independent variables were included in the regression equation: total hours of nursing care provided per day, hours of professional nursing per day, size of hospital, and ownership of hospital. The equation for the regression analysis was:

$$Y = u + b_1X_1 + b_2X_2 + b_3X_3 + b_4X_4 + e$$

Where: Y = satisfaction with care
X_1, X_2, X_3, X_4 = independent variables
b_1, b_2, b_3, b_4 = weights of independent variables
u = general mean
e = random error (due to random sampling)

Computationally the values of the b's were estimated by a mathematical procedure known as the method of least squares. The statistical significance of each of the four factors in terms of their contribution to the value of Y was determined by the analysis of variance technique.

Correlation Techniques A technique related to regression analysis is that of *correlation*. In some applications of statistical methods, particularly in the field of educational statistics, it is one of the most widely used techniques. In the correlation method a coefficient of correlation, called r, is computed. This coefficient varies between -1 and $+1$, and its value is a measure of the degree of association between the variables studied. The closer the computed value of the r is to $+1$ or -1, the higher is the degree of relationship between the variables studied.

The coefficient of correlation is a summary measure, not a test of significance. For quantitative variables the coefficient of correlation is computed by a technique known as the product-moment method, which is essentially the ratio of two standard deviations. The numerator of the ratio is the standard deviation of the values of the dependent variable *calculated* from the regression equation, and the denominator is the standard deviation of the *actual* values of the dependent variable that were obtained from the sample.

For qualitative variables, the coefficient of correlation can be estimated by a variety of techniques. One technique, known as *Yule's coefficient of association*, is applicable to data concerning two variables, each of which has only two scale values. To illustrate, Safford and Schlotfeldt[2] conducted a study a number of years ago in a general hospital to test the relationship between the number of patients assigned to a nursing team consisting of one registered and two practical nurses and the ratings of the quality of care provided by the team. The independent variable is the number of patients assigned to the team. In this comparison two groupings were used: 13 and 19 patients. The dependent variable is the rating of the care by patients and personnel. Here also, two groupings were used: "excellent" and "all other." The number of ratings in each category were as follows:

Number of Patients Assigned to Team	Rating of Care		
	Excellent	All Other	Total
13	51	39	90
19	38	55	93
Total	89	94	183

Yule's coefficient of association has the following formula:

$$A = \frac{ad - bc}{ad + bc}$$

A is equivalent to r, the coefficient of correlation, and also varies between ± 1. The letters in the formula represent the four cells in the table:

		Rating of Care	
		Excellent	All Other
Number of patients	13	a	b
assigned to team	19	c	d

It is obvious that if all the frequencies fall into the a and d cells and none in b and c or, conversely, all fall in b and c and none in a and d, there would be extremely high correlation between the variables and the value of A would be $+1$ or -1.

The value of A for the study of the work load of a nursing team and the rating of the care provided by the team is computed to be *.31*. Since a perfect correlation is designated by $+1$ or -1, and complete lack of correlation by zero, these variables can be interpreted to be mildly related.

TESTS OF SIGNIFICANCE FOR QUALITATIVE VARIABLES

Much of the data gathered in research in nursing and patient care are concerned with qualitative variables—those whose scales of measurement are either nominal or ordinal. Such scales yield counts of the frequency with which each scale value is recorded for the sampling units included in the study. When the dependent variable of an explanatory study is measured in terms of such a scale, tests like the ones just described—the difference between two means and the analysis of variance—cannot be used. However, other tests can be applied to the data to determine the probability (level of significance) that the differences observed in the criterion measures among the groups being compared could have arisen from random sampling. In one of these tests we can evaluate the differences in the percentage of subjects in certain classes of the criterion measure, similar to the test of the difference between means. For example, the percentage of subjects in the experimental group who recovered after treatment can be compared with the percentage recovered in the control group. Such a test can use as its model the t or normal distributions previously described to evaluate the level of statistical significance of the difference in proportions. In another test, we can compare the actual numerical frequencies in each of the scale categories for the study groups and evaluate their differences by use of a test known as *chi-square*.

Tests of Significance for Proportions

Many qualitative variables—those possessing nominal or ordinal scales —are often summarized into relative frequencies, called rates, such as the percentage of total number of study subjects possessing each value of the scale. If the variable has only two values—sometimes called an all-or-nothing variable—and there are two groups being compared, a direct test can be made of the statistical significance of the difference between the percentages for the two groups. This test is analogous to the test of the difference between two means. The t ratio for small samples is computed from the following formula:

$$t = \frac{\text{Difference in sample percentages}}{\text{Standard error of the difference in sample percentages}}$$

The formula for the standard error of the difference between two percentages is:

$$\sqrt{\frac{P(1-P)}{n_1} + \frac{P(1-P)}{n_2}}$$

Where: $P = \dfrac{n_1 p_1 + n_2 p_2}{n_1 + n_2}$, a weighted mean of the two sample percentages, n_1 = size of first sample and n_2 = size of second sample. (For computational purposes the figures are expressed as proportions not percentages: e.g., 50 per cent = .50).

To illustrate, assume that instead of recording *quantitative* blood pressure measurements on the two samples of 15 patients each, we had simply recorded whether the patient's blood pressure was high or normal according to a qualitative scale. These data could be tabulated as follows:

	High Blood Pressure		Normal Blood Pressure		Total	
	Number	Per Cent	Number	Per Cent	Number	Per Cent
Group A	7	47	8	53	15	100
Group B	13	87	2	13	15	100
Total	20	67	10	33	30	100

The t ratio would be:

$$t = \frac{(.87 - .47)}{\sqrt{\frac{(.67)(.33)}{15} + \frac{(.67)(.33)}{15}}} = \frac{.40}{.1715} = 2.3$$

Thus, $t = 2.3$. This value exceeds the 5 per cent level of significance but is below the 1 per cent level. Since the sample size is small, the t rather than the normal distribution is used. In large-sized samples, the T-test, based on the normal distribution, would be used to assess the difference between two percentages.

Chi-square Test

When the qualitative variable being studied has more than two categories, the chi-square test can be applied to analyze the significance of differences among the groups being compared. The chi-square test is applied directly to the actual frequencies in the various categories of the variables and not to the percentages. In a sense chi-square is an extension of the test of the significance of the difference between two percentages (or any other type of relative frequency) and is similar to the extension of the test of significance of differences between two means to differences among more than two means by the analysis of variance.

The chi-square test of significance is analogous to the t- or F-tests in that it is computed from a test ratio. The value provided by the computation of this ratio is a measure of the probability of obtaining the value by random sampling. The higher the value of chi-square for specified-size samples, the greater the probability that the frequencies for the different groups being compared are really different from each other and not just the result of random sampling.

The computation of chi-square requires the determination of theoretical frequencies for each of the cells in the table, subtracting each theoretical frequency from the actual frequency in each cell, squaring this difference, dividing by the theoretical frequency for the cell, and then summing up all the quotients. The formula for chi-square is thus:

$$\text{The sum for all cells of the table of:} \left(\frac{\text{The squared difference between sample and theoretical frequencies for a cell}}{\text{The theoretical frequency for the cell}} \right)$$

Chi-square can be applied to data in which the scale has only two classes—the all-or-nothing variety. Although such data can also be analyzed by a test of significance of the difference between two percentages, the chi-square test is often used because of the ease in computing it. The level of significance of a chi-square test of such data would be identical with a *t*-test applied to the differences between the percentages.

Using the data on blood pressure readings for the two groups of patients, we can calculate the chi-square value and compare it with the previously computed *t*-test of the difference between the two percentages. The results of the two tests should be identical.

As has been indicated the frequencies in each of the cells are as follows:

	High Blood Pressure	Normal Blood Pressure	Total
Group A	7	8	15
Group B	13	2	15
Total	20	10	30

Theoretically, the chi-square test does not work well in studies where the frequencies in any of the cells are less than 10. However, for illustrative purposes the test will be applied to the data anyway.

The first step is to calculate the theoretical frequencies for each of the cells. These are computed by determining what the frequencies in each cell would be if there were no difference in the distribution of blood pressure readings for the patients in the two study groups. If this were the case the number of patients in Groups A and B with normal and high blood pressures would be equivalent to the distribution of all 30 patients—two-thirds (20/30) in the high blood pressure group and one-third (10/30) in the normal group.

Thus, the theoretical frequencies—those denoting how many patients would be in each cell of the table if the two groups were actually one sample of 30 patients from the same target population—are as follows:

	High Blood Pressure	Normal Blood Pressure	Total
Group A	10	5	15
Group B	10	5	15
Total	20	10	30

Each sample frequency is then subtracted from each theoretical frequency, the difference squared, and the result divided by the theoretical frequency. All of the quotients would be totaled, providing the value of chi-square.

For the blood pressure data, a correction factor known as *Yate's correction for continuity* should, theoretically, be applied. This correction is applied to data being tested by chi-square where the scale of classification for each variable has only two discrete values, known as a 2 by 2 table, and where the expected frequencies are small. The correction, which involves reducing the absolute value of each difference between the actual and theoretical frequencies by one-half prior to squaring, is fully described in an article by Allison.[3]

For simplification, Yate's correction will not be applied to the blood pressure data. The computed value of chi-square is thus:

$$\frac{(7-10)^2}{10} + \frac{(8-5)^2}{5} + \frac{(13-10)^2}{10} + \frac{(2-5)^2}{5} = 5.4$$

To determine the level of significance of the computed value of chi-square we refer to the distribution of chi-square values. This distribution, as is the case for the normal t and F distributions, can be found in tabled form in the appendices of most statistical texts. The table shows, for different levels of *degrees of freedom,* the relative frequency (probability) of obtaining the value of chi-square by random sampling as high as that computed for the data.

The value of chi-square for various degrees of freedom at the 5 and 1 per cent levels of significance are as follows:

	Level of Significance	
Degrees of Freedom	*5 Per Cent*	*1 Per Cent*
1	3.8	6.6
2	6.0	9.2
3	7.8	11.3
4	9.5	13.3
5	11.1	15.1
10	18.3	23.2
15	25.0	30.6
20	31.4	37.6
25	37.6	44.3
30	43.8	50.9

The degrees of freedom for the data in the above example are found by multiplying the number of scale values of one variable (the number of columns in the table) minus one by the number of scale values of the other variable (the number of rows in the table) minus one. For the blood pressure data there are two scale values for blood pressure and two for the groups representing different qualities of nursing care. The degrees of freedom, therefore, are: $(2 - 1) \times (2 - 1) = 1$. Thus, with one degree of freedom the value of chi-square of 5.4 exceeds the 5 per cent level of significance, which is 3.8, but is below the 1 per cent level, which is 6.6. This means that such a value of chi-square could be obtained by chance in less than 5 but more than one samplings out of 100. We would thus say that the relationship between quality of nursing care and the blood pressure of patients is significant at the 5 per cent level. This conclusion is identical with that found when the test of the difference between the two percentages was used.

Short-cut Method of Calculation   A short-cut method is available for the calculation of chi-square for data in tables with two columns and two rows, the so-called 2×2 table just discussed. The formula for this short-cut is:

$$\frac{N\,(ad - bc)^2}{(a + b)(c + d)(a + c)(b + d)}$$

Where N = total number of subjects in the study and a, b, c, d, the various cells in the fourfold table: $\dfrac{a\mid b}{c \mid d}$

Applying the short-cut method to the blood pressure data we compute the following value of chi-square:

$$\text{chi-square} = \frac{30(14 - 104)^2}{(15)(15)(20)(10)}$$

$$= \frac{30(90)^2}{(15)(15)(20)(10)}$$

$$= \frac{243,000}{45,000} = 5.4$$

This is a value identical with that obtained by the long method.

Chi-square for Other than 2×2 Tables   To illustrate how the chi-square value would be computed from data containing variables having more than two scale categories we can assume the following study. Suppose we randomly assign 200 undergraduate nursing students to two groups, one in which the course in nursing arts is taught by conventional methods, and one in which programmed instruction is used.

At the end of the course we give an achievement exam to the students which grades them into three categories: low, medium, and high achievement. We then apply a chi-square test to the data to see if there is any relationship between teaching method and achievement score. The data are as follows:

Computation of Chi-Square for a 2 × 3 Table

	Actual Frequencies Score on Final Exam				Theoretical Frequencies Score on Final Exam			
Teaching Method	Low	Medium	High	Total	Low	Medium	High	Total
Programmed instruction	a30	b 50	c20	100	a20	b 65	c15	100
Conventional instruction	d10	e 80	f10	100	d20	e 65	f15	100
	40	130	30	200	40	130	30	200

Cell	Actual Frequencies	Theoretical Frequencies	Difference	Difference Squared	Chi-Square Ratio
a	30	20	+10	100	100/20 = 5.000
b	50	65	−15	225	225/65 = 3.462
c	20	15	+5	25	25/15 = 1.667
d	10	20	−10	100	100/20 = 5.000
e	80	65	+15	225	225/65 = 3.464
f	10	15	− 5	25	25/15 = 1.667

Chi-square = 20.260 or 20.3

The degrees of freedom for these data are 2: $(3 - 1$ columns $\times$ $2 - 1$ rows). Since the calculated chi-square value, 20.3, is considerably larger than 6.0, the chi-square value at the 5 per cent level with 2 degrees of freedom, we can say that there are significant differences among the two groups in terms of the achievement scores of the students on the final exams. In other words a value of chi-square of 20.3 can be expected to occur by chance alone considerably fewer times than 5 out of 100 samples —in fact fewer than 1 out of 1,000.

Distribution-free Methods

With the exception of the chi-square test, all statistical tests thus far discussed have two features in common. First, they make an assumption about the form of the underlying distribution of the measurements in the target population—i.e., the values of measurements are normally distributed, or, that at least, the distribution is approximately symmetrical and has a single peak. Second, they focus upon testing hypotheses about *parameters* of the underlying distribution, as in testing the significance of differences in sample means or percentages.

For data where little is known about the underlying distribution of the measurements of the variable being studied, or where the distribution is not of the type required by the test of significance, certain tests can be employed that are valid regardless of the character of the distribution of the measurements in the target population. The only assumptions that have to be met are that the samples were selected randomly and that the measurements made of the sampling units are independent of each other. Such tests of significance are called distribution-free or *nonparametric* tests in contrast to tests based on the normal, t, or F distributions, which are called *parametric* tests. A chi-square test is essentially a nonparametric test since its application is not restricted to variables whose measurements are normally distributed nor is it used to test or estimate means or standard deviations of these measurements, but rather is applied to qualitative variables, where the measurements are in the form of frequency counts for the different categories of a qualitative scale.

Nonparametric tests possess several useful features. First, they may provide the only way of testing the statistical significance of frequency data obtained through nominal or ordinal scales. However, by converting the actual frequencies into relative frequencies, it is possible to apply a parametric test to the data such as the t-test of the difference between two proportions. Converting frequencies into rates essentially transforms the data for the groups of study subjects as a whole from a qualitative to a quantitative scale.

For example, when we calculate the percentage of patients in a sample who have recovered from an illness, the basic qualitative scale may contain only two classes: recovered, died. By computing the rate of recovery we have substituted for this very discrete scale a continuous numerical scale ranging from 0 to 100 which represents the degree to which patients, considered as a group, recover from their illnesses. Our sample percentage is an estimate of the population percentage of patients expected to recover from the illness. If we took a large number of samples, the values of the percentages computed from each sample should approximate the normal distribution, and the value of the standard deviation of the sampling distribution is estimated by the standard error of a sample percentage.

Second, nonparametric methods are generally quicker and easier to compute than parametric techniques. A method like the analysis of variance can involve a great deal of computational work requiring the use of elaborate data-processing equipment. On the other hand, some nonparametric tests do not even require a desk calculator. Nonparametric techniques can be applied to quantitative data as short-cut substitutes for parametric techniques. For example, a nonparametric analysis of variance test is available that is quicker to compute than the parametric test, although, of course, it is considerably less sensitive.

Third, most nonparametric tests provide an exact statement of the probability of obtaining the test results for the sample irrespective of the shape of the distribution of the values of the measurements in the target population, i.e., these values do not have to be distributed normally.

A major limitation of nonparametric tests of significance is that they can be very wasteful of information. This is particularly true if a nonparametric test is employed as a substitute for a parametric test. The parametric test would have yielded a more sensitive and discriminating test of the data. To illustrate this we can apply the nonparametric test known as a *sign test* to evaluate the effect of an independent variable on a criterion measure. Assume that twenty newly born normal infants were paired according to a number of important characteristics, as birth weight, sex, race, etc. One of the pair is randomly assigned at birth to the experimental group, which receives a newly developed feeding formula while its mate is assigned to the control group and receives the usual formula. At the time of discharge the weights of the two groups are compared. Since the weights are quantitative measurements, the mean weight for each group can be computed and a t-test applied to assess parametrically the significance of the difference in weights between the two groups.

In the nonparametric sign test, only the fact that the experimental infants' weight is higher (plus sign), or lower (minus sign), than his control is considered, not the extent to which the actual weights for the pair differ. The significance of the difference between the groups is evaluated by determining the probability of obtaining that many plus signs by chance alone. Suppose the data collected in this experiment were as follows:

Infant Pair No.	Weight at Discharge (in grams)		Sign
	Infants Fed Enriched Formula	*Infants Fed Regular Formula*	
1	3,682	3,143	+
2	2,970	3,012	−
3	3,422	2,815	+
4	4,082	3,677	+
5	4,312	3,785	+
6	3,075	2,633	+
7	3,857	3,059	+
8	4,490	3,990	+
9	3,951	3,344	+
10	3,222	3,240	−

If the study showed that for 8 of the paired infants, the experimental members weighed more at discharge than their control while in 2 pairs the reverse was true, the probability of getting such a result is the same as the probability of obtaining 8 or more heads in 10 tosses of a coin, where the chance of getting either a head or tail in one toss is ½. This probability is found by the following formula:

$$P = (nCr)\, p^{n-r} \cdot q^r$$

Where n = total number of coins tossed (total number of pairs of infants)
r = number of heads (number of plus signs)
p = probability of obtaining a tail (minus sign)
q = probability of obtaining a head (plus sign)

for eight heads

$$_{10}C_8 \left(\frac{1}{2}\right)^2 \cdot \left(\frac{1}{2}\right)^8 = \frac{10!}{8!\,2!} \cdot \left(\frac{1}{2}\right)^{10} = \frac{45}{1024}$$

for nine heads

$$_{10}C_9 \left(\frac{1}{2}\right)^1 \cdot \left(\frac{1}{2}\right)^9 = \frac{10!}{9!\,1!} \cdot \left(\frac{1}{2}\right)^{10} = \frac{10}{1024}$$

for ten heads

$$_{10}C_{10} \left(\frac{1}{2}\right)^0 \cdot \left(\frac{1}{2}\right)^{10} = \frac{10!}{10!\,0!} \cdot \left(\frac{1}{2}\right)^{10} = \frac{1}{1024}$$

Thus

$$P = \frac{45}{1024} + \frac{10}{1024} + \frac{1}{1024} = \frac{56}{1024} = .054$$

According to this statistical model if we tossed 10 coins many times and did nothing to the coins to influence the greater occurrence of either a head or tail, we would expect that 8 or more heads would appear purely by chance alone in our random tossing (random sampling) slightly more than 5 times out of each 100 tossings of the ten coins.

In terms of our experimental data, this means that, by chance alone, we would expect that in a little more than 5 out of 100 samplings we would obtain at least 8 plus signs in 10 comparisons. Since this is greater than the 5 per cent level, which we have selected as our level of significance, we say that there is no relationship between type of feeding and weight gain. Even though they were fed the enriched formula the performance of the experimental infants was not any better than what could be expected by chance alone.

However, if we look at the actual weights we can see that the infants fed the enriched formula did reach a substantially higher weight level than those fed a conventional formula. For several of the pairs the infant fed the enriched formula weighed several hundred grams more than his control who was fed a regular diet. In pair number 7 the difference was nearly 800 grams, or over a pound and a half. In the two pairs where weights of the control infants were higher than the experimental infants—numbers 2 and 10—the difference was slight, less than 50 grams in both instances.

The mean weights for the two groups are:

Experimental group	3,706	grams
Control group	3,270	grams

When a t-test is applied to these means in a test of the significance of the difference between means, the result is highly significant. The t ratio value is 2.88, which means that such a difference could occur by chance alone only 1 time in 100 samplings.

These data illustrate the loss of information that results from the application of a nonparametric test to data that could be validly analyzed by a parametric method like the t-test of the difference between two means. The nonparametric sign test in this example took highly refined quantitatively scaled data—the actual weights of the infants—and converted them into a crude ordinal scale consisting of only two categories: more than $(+)$ and less than $(-)$. As a result there was a great reduction in the sensitivity of the statistical test and differences in the weights of the infants in the two groups was found to be nonsignificant. The only advantage in the use of the nonparametric test is that it provides a short-cut in the computation, a slight advantage when compared to the great loss of sensitivity.

Nonparametric tests have their most useful application when the data cannot be treated by a parametric test. Another widely used nonparametric technique often employed just for this purpose is the *rank correlation* method. This technique is analogous to the product-moment coefficient of correlation computed from numerically scaled data. The rank correlation coefficient has the following formula:

$$r_s = 1 - \frac{6(\text{sum of the squared differences in the ranking of the subject on the two variables})}{n(n + 1)(n - 1)}$$

Where n = number of subjects being ranked

To illustrate: Assume we randomly selected 10 freshman students in a school of nursing and ranked them from highest to lowest, 1 to 10, in terms of two ordinally scaled variables: (1) their intelligence level as determined from scores on preadmission tests, and (2) the degree of interest they showed in their educational program. The rankings are as follows:

Student No.	Intelligence Level	Interest in Educational Program	Difference	Difference Squared
1	1	1	0	0
2	5	4	1	1
3	3	5	−2	4
4	7	3	4	16
5	9	2	7	49
6	8	10	−2	4
7	2	8	−6	36
8	4	7	−3	9
9	6	6	0	0
10	10	9	1	1
			Total	120

$$r_s = 1 - \frac{6 \times 120}{10 \times 11 \times 9} = 0.27$$

Since perfect correlation between the two variables would result in a value of +1 if the variables were positively associated and −1 if they were negatively associated, while 0 would indicate no association at all, a value of 0.27 indicates a slight association.

It is possible to determine the probability of obtaining such a value of r_s by chance alone by reference to tables showing the level of significance of the values of r_s for different numbers of subjects:

	Level of Significance	
Size of Sample	5 Per Cent	1 Per Cent
5	0.90	1.00
10	0.56	0.75
20	0.38	0.53
30	0.31	0.43

From these figures it can be seen that a value of r_s of 0.27 with 10 subjects can be expected to occur by chance more frequently than 5 times in 100, since the 5 per cent level value is 0.56. Even if the sample had included as many as 30 subjects such a value of r_s could not have exceeded the 5 per cent level.

Nonparametric tests of significance are sometimes called *order statistics*. Many of these tests essentially treat data in terms of ordinal rankings or comparisons, as in the rank correlation and the sign test techniques, as well as in other nonparametric methods such as the runs test, median test, and the so-called Mann-Whitney U test. Thus, the designation, order statistics, is an apt description of their method as well as their purpose— to see whether the ordering of the data follows a random pattern or not.

THE MEANING OF STATISTICAL SIGNIFICANCE

As has been indicated, statistical tests of significance, whether they are parametric or nonparametric, are applied to the analysis of research data where measurements of either quantitative or qualitative variables have been made of the study subjects who have been selected for study through a random process. Randomization can enter into a research study in several ways. In nonexperimental studies the subjects may be randomly drawn from some larger target population. In an experimental study the subjects not only may have been drawn randomly from some larger population but are also randomly assigned to the alternative groups in the experiment.

The function of the test of significance is to test whether two or more groups being compared in terms of some summary measure—a mean, a standard deviation, a percentage, or nonparametrically in terms of their rank order on a qualitative scale—could be considered to have come from the same target population or not—i.e., are they essentially two independent samples from the same population? In a nonexperimental study the target population could be all general hospitals in the United States. We could group the hospitals into two subpopulations by the amounts of nursing care they provide, high and low, which would serve as the independent variable. We could then draw random samples of hospitals from the two groups. For our dependent variable we could measure the quality of care the patients receive, say, in terms of some valid quantitative criterion measure. We would then test the significance of the difference in the values of the summary measures for the two groups of patients. If, at the level of significance we have chosen, let us say, the 5 per cent level, we find that the difference is not statistically significant—the difference would occur more frequently than 5 times in 100 repeated samplings—we say that the hospitals belong to the same population in terms of the variable "quality of care provided." In other words, the distinguishing characteristic of the two subpopulations—the different amounts of care received by patients—is not significantly related to the dependent variable that was measured.

In an experimental study, patients could be randomly assigned to two groups, analogous to the subpopulations in the nonexperimental study—in one group higher amounts of nursing care would be provided to the patients than in the other group. Here the subpopulations are actually formed by the experimenter, whereas in the nonexperimental approach they have been formed outside of the study and beyond his control. If the test of significance shows that the difference in the values of the summary measures is not significant, we can say that the two groups are samples from the same population. If the difference in the values of the summary measures is statistically significant, we say that the groups represent different populations and that quality of care *is* related to the amount of care provided.

A test of significance, then, is basically a test of the extent to which random sampling error is the explanation for the difference in the summary measures we computed for the sample subjects in our alternative groups. At the level of significance we have chosen, if sampling error explains all of the difference observed in the summary measures, we say that the difference is not significant and there is no relationship between the dependent variable and the variable that distinguishes the alternative groups. If sampling error does not explain all of the difference, we say that the summary measures are significantly different from each other and there is a relationship between the dependent variable and the variable distinguishing the alternative groups.

If the study subjects have not been randomly selected from the target population or randomly assigned to the alternative groups, or both, a test of statistical significance should not be applied to the summary measures obtained for the subjects. In such cases any differences in the values of the summary measures could not be attributed to random sampling error. To apply a test of significance to such data, which is an evaluation of the extent to which the difference observed exceeds the amount attributable to random sampling, is not only inappropriate, but meaningless.

The Null Hypothesis

In explanatory studies that employ tests of statistical significance to evaluate a difference in the values of summary measures for the alternative groups studied, the hypothesis that is being tested is that the population difference is really zero and any difference we find in the sample values is due to the fact that we sampled. Thus, the null hypothesis says that the alternative groups can be considered as independent samples from the same population and their summary measures are independent estimates of the same population parameter. To the extent that the difference in sample summary measures does not exceed the value that we have established in our test of the significance as attributable to random sampling error, we accept the null hypothesis as being true.

When we sample we expect to obtain results that are not exactly the same as if we had studied the entire population. The smaller the sample, the greater is the possible deviation between the sample value and the actual population value. Conversely, the larger the sample the smaller the sampling error would be. If we had a 100 per cent sample—that is, if we had studied all the sampling units in the population—the sampling error would be zero, and the value of our sample statistic would be equal to the value of our population parameter.

As has been stated before, the basic model for most tests of significance is the following ratio:

$$\frac{\text{Difference in values of sample summary measures}\;\textbf{minus}\;\text{Difference in values of population summary measures}}{\begin{array}{c}\text{Standard error (sampling error) of the difference in}\\\text{the values of sample summary measures}\end{array}}$$

The hypothesis for a study describes the expected differences in the values of the population summary measures for the alternative groups being compared. The way of stating the hypothesis for a statistical test of significance is in the form of a *null hypothesis*—that there is no difference in the values of the population measures for the alternative groups being compared. Examples of null hypotheses are:

There is no relationship between smoking and lung cancer.
The amount of nursing care provided is not related to the quality of care provided.
A graduate of diploma program in nursing is just as proficient as a graduate of collegiate program.
There is no difference in the amount of nursing care required by patients in different age groups.
Nurses do not have any greater job mobility than members of other occupational groups.

Because a hypothesis is stated in the null form does not mean that the researcher actually expects that his data will support it. Generally, just the opposite is true; the researcher expects that in the real world the alternative to the null hypothesis will be found to be true—that smoking *is* related to lung cancer, that higher amounts of nursing care *will improve* the quality of care, and so on.

The use of the null form in stating hypotheses is dictated by the nature of statistical tests of significance. In a statistical test we are evaluating the extent to which the difference we have actually measured in the sample deviates from the difference that could be expected due to chance, as a result of random sampling.

When our study is based on a sample, we are uncertain about the real state of affairs in the total population. We can only estimate it based on data from our sample subjects. In testing hypotheses in explanatory studies, we are estimating from our sample data whether there is a relationship between the variables studied or not. Since the data are based on only sample evidence, which may not correspond with the true state of affairs, there is the possibility that the sample could yield a result different from what would be found if we studied the total population. In other words, because our sample can differ significantly from the population as a whole, we might find that a relationship exists between the variables studied in the sample when in fact such a relationship does not hold for the entire population. Our level of significance tells us the probability of such an occurrence. By setting this level at a relatively rare frequency—5 times out of 100, or even less—such an erroneous interpretation becomes relatively unlikely to occur.

When the difference between the groups studied is statistically significant, we reject the null hypothesis and accept the alternative hypothesis— that there *is* a relationship between the independent and dependent variables studied. By rejecting the null hypothesis we have not *proved* that the alternative hypothesis is true with absolute certainty, just as when we accept it we have not proved that the null hypothesis is true with absolute certainty. We have only demonstrated that our difference exceeds or falls below the value that, with a certain relative frequency, called the level of significance, could be attributable to chance. If our difference can occur by chance fewer times than our level of significance, we are willing to accept the alternative hypothesis, knowing full well that there is a small possibility it may not be true.

Although the null hypothesis is meant to denote a hypothesis of zero difference between the summary measures, a more meaningful approach might be to test the differences obtained for the study groups against some value greater than zero that is considered to be the minimum value of no importance. For example, if we are testing the effects of an educational program on weight reduction, we might establish our null difference not as zero but say as 10 pounds, if this were considered to be the minimum weight loss of any practical importance. An average weight loss of less than 10 pounds would be considered as not being significant. Our statistical test of significance would be:

$$\frac{\text{Difference in values of sample summary measures } \textbf{minus } 10}{\substack{\text{Standard error (sampling error) of the} \\ \text{difference in the values of sample measures}}}$$

Thus, "null" really should mean a difference of no particular importance, not just a zero difference.

Alternative Hypothesis

The alternative hypothesis is that form of statement of the hypothesis that represents the expectation of the researcher. A researcher embarking on a study often expects, or at least is hopeful, that the independent variable he is manipulating is really related to the dependent variable he is measuring. If he were certain that the variables were unrelated, he would most likely not undertake the research.

The alternative hypothesis to the null hypothesis may be either implicit or explicit. In many studies, the alternative hypothesis needs no explicit statement, since it is so obvious as to be self-evident. In others it may be necessary to clearly spell out the alternative hypothesis, since it can be formulated in various ways. Broadly speaking, alternative hypotheses can state that:

1. The independent variable will have some effect, either positive or negative, on the dependent variable.
2. The independent variable will have a positive effect on the dependent variable.
3. The independent variable will have a negative effect on the dependent variable.

Thus, if we are studying the effect of a nursing procedure on a patient, we might be interested in any statistically significant effect produced, whether it be a positive or a negative one. Or we may only be interested in whether we can produce a positive effect—a negative effect would be interpreted as if the independent variable had produced no effect at all and would lead to an acceptance of the null hypothesis.

In assessing the effects of testing drugs on patients we would only accept the drug as being effective (reject the null hypothesis) if we could produce a positive effect on the patients. However, we would also be interested in any significant negative results, since this could well have important implications for further development of therapy. Therefore, although in many nursing and patient care studies we are fundamentally interested in seeing whether the effect we are producing by the manipulation of our independent variable is a positive one, we are also interested in negative effects. We are interested, then, in any effect produced.

Studies with alternative hypotheses that are directed toward any effect, regardless of direction, employ what is called two-sided or two-tailed tests of significance. Studies that are interested only in either a positive or a negative effect employ a one-sided or one-tailed test.

The examples previously shown in this chapter were all two-tailed tests. We did not care whether sample A's summary measure was higher than sample B's, or vice versa, but only that there was some difference between the two sample values. If we were interested only in a one-sided alternative—that is, we would consider our difference as statistically significant only if A were higher than B and not if B were higher than A—we actually would achieve a greater level of significance for the same difference in the values of the summary measures than for the two-sided alternative. In other words, for the same data we can reject the null hypothesis and thereby accept the alternative hypothesis with lower values of t when a one-tailed test is used. To illustrate, if our level of significance is 5 per cent we will reject the null hypothesis and accept the alternative hypothesis if our t ratios for various-sized samples are as follows:

Size of Sample	Two-tailed Test	One-tailed Test
5	2.57	2.02
10	2.23	1.81
15	2.13	1.75
20	2.09	1.72

Level of Significance

As has been indicated a test of significance provides us with an evaluation of the extent to which our sample data depart from what would be expected if only chance factors are affecting the data. Thus, for example, in the t ratio we divide our sample difference by the measure of random sampling error. The probability of getting such a t ratio value in repeated random sampling by chance alone is called the level of significance. Customarily, the .05 (5 per cent) level of significance is employed, particularly in sociological and psychological research. This means that 5 times out of 100 such a difference in the summary measures found in the study can be attributable to chance factors arising as a result of random sampling. It should be noted that there is nothing magical about the

.05 level. Other levels can be used in research. The .01 (1 per cent) level is a more stringent one, because the chances of finding a difference in the summary measures attributable to random sampling rather than to the independent variable being studied is one in a hundred, an even rarer occurrence.

If we want to be more certain that our results are not just accidental, due to having selected an atypical sample from the target population, we would choose a more stringent level of significance. If our study is concerned with matters of vital importance to the health and welfare of human beings, or if decisions based on the study would involve great expense, we might want to be surer in rejecting the null hypothesis and accepting the alternative that our results were not accidental, and therefore we would select a .01 or even .001 level of significance. If we were less concerned about rejecting the null hypothesis when it were really true, we might select a less stringent level: .05 or even .10, and in some instances, .20.

The level of significance actually tells us the risk of rejecting the null hypothesis and accepting the alternative hypothesis when in fact the null hypothesis is true. This risk is called the Type I error in applying tests of significance. Assuming sample size is not changed, the risk of committing a Type I error can be reduced by using a more stringent level of significance, say, .01 instead of .05. However, reducing the risk of Type I error increases the risk of a Type II error. The Type II error is incurred when we accept the null hypothesis and reject the alternative hypothesis when the alternative hypothesis is true.

There is an inverse relationship between the two types of errors, since if we decrease the probability that one will occur, we increase the probability that the other will occur. If we change our level of significance from 5 to 1 per cent, we will reject the null hypothesis falsely only 1 time in 100 rather than 5 times in 100. However, by so doing we will increase the probability of rejecting the alternative hypothesis falsely.

For many studies the danger of a Type I error may be more serious than that of a Type II. If we are testing the effects of a drug on a patient, we might want to be sure that these effects really exceeded what would be expected to occur purely by chance before we marketed the drug.

Thus we might select a .01 or .001 level of significance, even though we would be more likely to attribute real effects of the drug to chance and thus conceal its true value. In other words we would make the level of significance more stringent, say, .01 instead of .05, in order to decrease the Type I error if the findings of our study can result in life or death of a patient and we want to be very sure that the differences we have observed are not accidental, but real. We would accept a higher level of significance, .05 instead of .01, if we were not so concerned with the consequences of falsely accepting the alternative hypothesis and wanted to decrease the chance of masking any real differences in the data.

Each study must balance the risks in committing Type I and II errors. Usually a compromise is made which serves to optimize the balance between the two errors. In reaching this balance the *power* of the test is evaluated. The power of a test can be defined as the probability of rejecting the null hypothesis when it is actually false. The power is determined by the following formula:

1 minus probability of Type II error

The probability of committing a Type II error can be assessed by the computation of the power curve for the test, also known as the power function. By reducing the probability of committing a Type II error the power of the test is increased.

The power of a test is actually a measure of the sensitivity of the test—the extent to which it uncovers real differences among the groups that were studied. Power can be increased in several ways. First, it can be increased by employing the most powerful test of significance that the characteristics of the data will permit—an analysis of variance, for example, is more powerful than a nonparametric test. Second, the use of one-tailed tests, when warranted by the nature of the hypothesis being tested, will provide a more powerful test than a two-tailed one. Finally, the power of the test can be increased by enlarging the size of the sample, although unlike the other approaches to the increase of power, this can significantly add to the cost, time, and effort required to do the study.

Use of Prior Probabilities

In recent years, some research has begun to employ what is known as "Bayesian inference" in the analysis and interpretation of statistical tests of significance. Traditional tests of significance, known as the Neyman-Pearson approach, are those in which the null hypothesis is formulated, the alternative hypothesis is explicitly or implicitly stated, and the level of significance established *in advance* of the actual data collection and kept fixed during the course of the study. This procedure is very objective. The tests of significance that are employed make no use of prior knowledge gained from previous studies. In the Bayesian approach, so named because it derives from and employs Bayes' probability theorem, the use of prior knowledge is employed in the test of significance. In this sense it is a subjective approach to significance testing. As described by Mosteller and others,[4] the Bayesian approach involves the following:

An experimenter might assign probabilities that are in some way proportional to the "intensity of belief" he has in the various hypotheses. (Another investigator might assign quite different probabilities.) An experiment is performed, with the aim of discovering evidence to modify these prior probabilities. Such evidence may even assign such low posterior probabilities to some of the hypotheses as to eliminate them from further consideration. . . .

Each new experiment can begin with *a priori* probabilities of the remaining hypotheses proportional to the *a posteriori* probabilities that resulted from the previous experiments. In this way, scientific evidence accumulates and modifies our beliefs, weakening our intensity of belief in some hypotheses, strengthening it in others.

ERRORS COMMITTED IN THE USE AND INTERPRETATION OF TESTS OF STATISTICAL SIGNIFICANCE

Much concern in recent years has been expressed over the misuses of statistical tests of significance in research studies.[5-9] One of the main criticisms has been that the use of tests of significance have become a sort of ritualism in research. They are applied indiscriminately to data, often as window dressing to give a veneer of scientific authority to the study. To avoid the mistaken use of tests of significance a clear understanding should be had of their purpose. Pure and simple, they are a means of testing whether the data the researcher has gathered through a random process of some kind vary from what would be expected if the influences on the data were solely chance influences. In other words, a test of significance, like the determination of a confidence interval for a sampling estimate of a population parameter, is essentially a measure of sample error around the estimate. For example, in a t-test of the difference between two sample means, the sample estimate is the value of the difference between the means. The standard error of this difference is a measure of its sampling error and can serve as the value of the confidence interval around the estimate. The t ratio measures the probability that a confidence interval around the sample estimate of the difference will include the value of the hypothesized population difference. With the null hypothesis the population difference is hypothesized to be zero.

The misuses of tests of significance are numerous. The following are the most common ones:

1. *Inapplicability of tests of significance.* Not every study employs randomization either in the selection of study subjects from the target population or in the assignment of subjects to the alternative groups being compared. Therefore, such studies do not involve sampling, but actually encompass a total target population. For such studies the use of tests of significance are inappropriate, since the data do not contain random sampling error. Of course, such data may contain other types of error, but these are not measurable by confidence intervals or significance tests.

The notion of a "hypothetical universe" has been advanced to provide a rationale for the use of significance tests in studies in which random sampling has not been employed. The rationale of a "hypothetical universe" is that every finite target population is in reality a subpopulation from some superpopulation. Therefore data from such a subpopulation is a sample and, like a random sample, is subject to sampling error. Thus, if we conduct a study in one school of nursing, it can be considered to be a sample from the superpopulation of all nursing schools. Although this may well be true, the tests of significance and the formulas for calculating confidence intervals have been derived from models in which random sampling is an important, fundamental assumption. And in a study in which a school of nursing has been selected because of convenience and not by random methods, we do not have by any stretch of the imagination a *random* sample as technically defined. Consequently, we cannot apply conventional statistical tests to our data.

A clear distinction should be made between statistical and nonstatistical generalizations. A statistical generalization derives from the computation of a test of significance or a confidence interval. Thus, we may say, "One hundred patients' records were selected randomly from the 10,000 records in the files of the agency to evaluate the completeness and usability of the information contained in the records. From these sample records we estimate that in 16 to 24 per cent of all the agency's patients' records the information is of poor quality."

A nonstatistical generalization does not derive from significance tests or confidence intervals but from the researcher's own interpretation of the data he has collected. The quality of this interpretation will depend on many things, including his expert knowledge of the subject matter to which the data pertain as well as his ability to logically fathom the meaning of the data he has gathered. When the data have been collected through a random process of some kind, both types of generalizations can be made. The statistical generalization is concerned with assessing the degree to which random error has influenced the data. The nonstatistical generalization is concerned with interpreting what the data mean, how they have contributed to the fund of accumulated knowledge in the field, and how they can be applied.

If the data collection has not involved a random process, only the latter type of generalization need be made, since the former would be superfluous and not add anything meaningful to an understanding of the data. And it is often this latter type of generalization that is the most important one for a study, particularly where the data are not amenable to treatment by statistical analysis, as in nonquantified data.

2. *Significance and causal relationships.* In explanatory studies in which the relationship between the independent and dependent variables is assessed, a finding that is statistically significant is sometimes taken to

mean that the dependent variable is *causally* related to the independent variable. This certainly is not the case. Significance of a statistical relationship among variables does not prove causation. As has been indicated in the discussion of research design, causal relationships are extremely difficult to establish, particularly in studies concerned with human beings, because the interconnection between a cause and an effect is often very complex, having many intervening variables. In highly controlled experimental research, we can hope to come closer to causal relationships than in nonexperimental studies. In the latter, the most we can often aim for is to demonstrate a clearly defined, stable association between the variables which can be useful for predictive purposes, even though it may not provide us with a basic explanation of the phenomena studied.

The ability to establish cause and effect relationships is thus a function of the design of the research and is influenced by the degree to which intervening, extraneous variables can be kept under control. A test of significance in no way assesses this ability. However, to the extent that we define our variables precisely and meaningfully, sharpen up our measuring instruments, employ designs that will sort out and control extraneous variables, and minimize the psychological biases that can distort our data, the greater will be the likelihood that we will find statistically significant differences in the measures we compare as well as produce findings that will be substantively significant.

3. *A finding of statistical significance is no indication of the quality of a study.* The fact that a statistical analysis reveals that our findings are statistically significant does not put a stamp of approval on the quality of the total study design. A poor study can produce statistically significant findings, whereas a well-designed study may turn up nonsignificant results. Sometimes the poor quality of a study design is obscured, perhaps intentionally, in the reporting of results by the inclusion of page after page of esoteric mathematics. The mathematics prove nothing but serve as a convenient smokescreen for the inadequacies of the study design. Some of the most significant—meaning *substantively* significant—research findings have been completely free of any mathematical manipulations.

It should be borne in mind that the determination of sampling error through the calculation of a standard error measures only one type of error. Actually this is not error in the common usage of the term—a mistake, something done wrong. The "error" of sampling is basically the consequence of the variability of the sampling units in the target population and the fact that we happened to select only a small number of these units to serve as our study subjects. If we included the whole population in the study, or if there was no variability among the subjects, this source of error would be eliminated. But we do not want to include the whole population because that would usually be too expensive if not impossible to achieve. Moreover, in everything that is measured there is variability among sampling units. Therefore, in research we must contend with sampling error.

Nonsampling errors are often caused by mistakes—mistakes in defining the problem or in the measuring instruments or in the data collection procedures or in the handling of the data after collection, or in interpreting the meaning of the data, or in providing sufficient control over extraneous factors. These errors are not assessed by tests of significance or by confidence intervals.

4. *Use of the wrong tests of significance.* In the discussion of the various types of random sampling methods it was pointed out that each method employs a different mathematical formula for the calculation of sampling error. Thus, the standard error of a mean for a sample that has been selected by the cluster method has a more complicated formula than that for means based on a simple random sample, since the intercorrelations among the sampling units within a cluster need to be considered. Quite often the simple random sampling standard error formula is used indiscriminately, regardless of the nature of the sampling method employed.

Moreover, each of the various tests of significance, particularly parametric tests, require that the data meet certain assumptions before the test can be applied. For example, in addition to the requirements that the measurements be obtained through a random process and that they be independent of each other (i.e., that the value of the measurement for sampling unit A should not be influenced by the value of the measurement for B), the analysis of variance test has certain other requirements. These include that the distribution of the values of the measurements in the population from which the sampling units were randomly selected be reasonably normal, that the scale underlying the measurements be a continuous one, and that the effects attributable to the independent variable(s) being tested be additive. Frequently, tests of significance are employed for data that deviate widely from the assumptions underlying the tests. Nonparametric tests can provide a safeguard against this problem, although they may have a serious drawback in the large amount of information that is lost and decreased sensitivity that results from the use of such tests.

5. *Fishing for statistical significance.* Quite often the researcher may apply a rash of statistical tests of significance to his data after they have been tabulated. Every summary measure is compared in *t*-tests with every other summary measure. New summary measures are often computed and tested by regrouping the scale values of the criterion measure. Thus, tests of significance are applied on an ex post facto basis to differences in the values of summary measures even though no hypotheses concerning these comparisons were stated prior to the data collection.

With such wholesale significance testing, sooner or later t ratio values are going to be found that exceed the 5 or even 1 per cent level of significance, when maybe no significance should really be attached to the differences. As has been indicated, significance levels actually state the risk of rejecting the null hypothesis when it is in fact true—the Type I error. If we were to run one hundred significance tests based on the same data—as in dividing our sample into smaller samples, computing the means of the measures for the subsamples, and running tests of significance on differences in the means—we would expect to commit the Type I error about 5 times in 100 tests at the .05 level of significance.

Hypotheses that are formulated retrospectively, particularly if they are suggested by the data that have been collected to test the hypotheses originally stated for the study, cannot be legitimately tested by traditional tests of significance. The Bayesian approach, with its use of prior information and the notion of "intensity of belief" the researcher has in various hypotheses about the subject he is investigating, may appear as a modification of this rule. However, prior knowledge in this approach is used as a basis for formulation of the hypotheses to guide the collection of new data, not to suggest a new hypothesis to be tested by the data from which this knowledge was gained.

6. *Impermanence of statistically significant results*. The fact that a test of significance has shown the data to be statistically significant does not mean that the research problem we have explored has been settled for all time. The finding of statistical significance today does not mean that we will find significance if we repeated the study a year from now or even next month. Particularly when the research is concerned with a complex set of variables that are operating in a fluid population, we cannot be sure how far into the future we can project the results of our statistical significance tests. Many findings, even those that are highly significant, may be transitory in nature. A finding that the team organization for providing nursing care yields a significantly higher quality of nursing care, even if based on a large, representative, and randomly selected sample, might only hold true for a limited time period. The many variables impinging on the model for this relationship are undergoing continual change—the education of the team members is changing, the characteristics of patient care are being modified, attitudes toward care on the part of the patients are changing, new facilities and new methods of patient care are being introduced, to name just a few of the dynamic ingredients in this situation.

The extent of statistical generalization is limited by the boundaries of the target population. One dimension of this boundary is the time period in which the population exists. Any generalization beyond this time period will require a nonstatistical generalization, and the scope of the generalization will depend on the researcher's assessment of the stability of the total situation with which his research is concerned.

Since one study will not answer a question for all time, the need for replication of studies cannot be stressed too strongly. By replication the stability of previous findings can be assessed. If these findings are confirmed by a series of studies, we are then justified in treating them as possessing some of the attributes of a principle or law.

7. *The level of significance does not necessarily denote the strength of a relationship.* In testing hypotheses concerning the relationship between independent and dependent variables the fact that the test indicates significance well beyond the level chosen—say, at the .0001 level—does not necessarily indicate a stronger relationship than if the level turned out to be .01. For example, assume that our independent variable involved a comparison of two newly employed groups of public health nurses: those who had taken a course in public health nursing as part of their basic undergraduate educational program and those who had not. The dependent variable is a measure of the ability of a nurse to adjust to a work situation in the field of public health nursing the first six months after graduation. If in a comparison of the values of the summary measures of the dependent variable for the two groups, the difference is found to be well beyond the level of significance adopted for the study—5 per cent—we should not jump to the conclusion that the variables are very strongly related—more strongly than if a lower level of significance were obtained.

We need to bear in mind that the level of significance of the difference we find is influenced not only by the effects of the independent variable but also by the homogeneity of the sampling units composing the population and by the research design we have used, which in essence is an artifact. We need to consider that such elements of the research design as the sensitivity of the measuring instruments employed, the control exerted over the extraneous variables, and the size of the sample, to name just a few, can be greatly influenced by the researcher. For example, for a given difference in the values of the summary measures for the groups studied and a stated amount of variability of the values among the population, the significance of the findings can be increased by enlarging the size of the sample. This would not necessarily indicate a stronger relationship among the variables, but rather a more precise estimate of the true difference among the groups being compared.

8. *The use of a statistical significance test is not a guarantee of a good study.* Many studies, excellently designed and concerned with important research problems, do not employ tests of significance. This may be because the data do not warrant the use of tests—random sampling was not involved, or the study was concerned largely with nonquantitative data. The absence of tests of significance does not depreciate the findings of a study, just as the use of such tests does not necessarily raise the quality of a study. Very often the key interpretation of study results is made from analysis of the tabulations of the data. Such interpretation of

statistical tables, to be discussed shortly, can bring out the real meaning of the data.

Statistical analysis through significance testing should be placed in a proper perspective. It is essentially a technique for evaluating the influence of sampling error and should not be regarded as the final step in determining what the data really mean. We should not try to make these tests perform interpretative functions, which they were not created to do.

9. *Insufficient time for significance to be revealed.* In some studies the time lag between the application of the independent variable and measurement of the effect in the dependent variable may be too short. As a result we do not observe any significant difference in the values of the summary measures for the groups being compared. If we had waited a longer period of time—enough time for the "treatment to take," so to speak—significance might well have been obtained in the results. Thus, in order to avoid the possible commitment of a Type II error—accepting the hypothesis of no difference when it is really false—the study should allow for a sufficient period of time to elapse before measurement of the dependent variable is made.

One of the factors in a study situation that might militate against obtaining short-run results in a study is resistance to change. Wallis and Roberts[10] give the following example:

A restaurant attempted to evaluate the effect on its cigarette business of changing from sales by cashier to sales by a coin-operated vending machine. The number of packages sold during the first month of machine sales was 51 per cent less than during the last month of cashier sales. As a basis of comparison sales for the same two months in two comparable restaurants were used. These showed decreases of 15 per cent and 3 per cent, respectively. As a result of this comparison, it was concluded that the "installation of the cigarette vending machine was detrimental to sales."

Perhaps if cigarette sales were measured a year later when customers had a chance to adjust to the change in the method of vending, the volume would have risen to a level at least as high as it was prior to the change.

10. *Overuse of the null hypothesis.* Many studies employ the null hypothesis as the model for the test of significance almost by rote. From a practical standpoint, in some research areas a hypothesized zero difference has no real meaning, and some positive value should be used instead. In other studies any difference, no matter how small, is important. If, for example, we are testing the effect of a drug on weight reduction, we might be interested only in differences between our experimental and control groups that significantly exceed a certain amount, say, a minimum of 10 to 20 pounds, before we accept a decision that the drug is effective. We would not just be interested in the fact that the difference was greater than

zero. If, on the other hand, we are testing a drug in terms of its ability to reverse an incurable illness, we might use any amount greater than a zero difference as our standard of acceptance of the drug, since even one life saved would be a significant contribution.

11. *Confusion of statistical significance with practical significance.* One of the most common misuses of statistical significance is to confuse it with practical significance. As discussed previously, a finding of statistical significance may in fact have little or no substantive meaning, particularly if it is based on the null hypothesis. Consider the fact that if our sample is large enough, even small differences not much greater than zero would be statistically significant regardless of how unimportant these differences might be. Moreover, artificial refinements in our measuring scale, such as dividing our intervals into small segments, as in reading patients' temperatures to one-hundredth of a degree, can yield statistically significant findings that would be somewhat meaningless. We must constantly remind ourselves that statistical significance means that the difference we observed among our sample subjects could only rarely have occurred by chance as a result of random sampling. It does not tell us anything about the practical importance of this difference.

The substantive significance of a finding can only be assessed by the researcher's evaluation of its meaning within the subject matter framework of the area of the research. In applied research this may be a pragmatic evaluation in terms of dollars and cents. If our study showed that raising salaries of the nursing staff by 10 per cent resulted in a 10 per cent reduction in turnover, the significance of this reduction can be appraised in a "balance sheet" type of analysis that weighs the cost of the salary increase against the monetary savings achieved by a turnover reduction as well as any nonmonetary gains such as higher morale and improved quality of performance.

In many studies, where the criterion measure cannot be correlated with some external pragmatic standard such as lives saved, improvement in services, or lowered costs, the practical significance of the findings is more difficult to assess. If our criterion measure is a subjective rating scale of some kind, how can we evaluate a statistically significant difference between an average rating of say, "excellent" and "very good," or "very satisfactory" and "satisfactory"? But even objective numerical measurement does not guarantee practical significance. How, for example, do we interpret the practical importance of changes in blood pressure which although small might be statistically significant?

Until we can demonstrate that such statistically significant findings also have substantive significance, our interpretation of the data is limited. This would hold true for basic as well as so-called applied research, even though the basic research is not concerned with the immediate application of findings. Application of results may well be the long-range objective of basic studies. The findings of one basic study often serve to formulate the problem and hypothesis for another study. Each study, through the substantive contribution of its findings, provides a further step in the progression toward a meaningful real-life contribution of the total research effort.

The significance of findings is dependent upon the quality of the measurement of the variables in the study. This quality is assessed by the criteria of validity, reliability, sensitivity, and meaningfulness. To the extent that the process of measurement in a study meets these criteria, the likelihood is increased that the findings will be not only statistically significant but substantively significant as well.

INTERPRETING DATA IN STATISTICAL TABLES

Perhaps the most useful approach to the interpretation of the statistical findings of a study is through organization of the data into statistical tables. Such organization helps to focus attention on the practical meaning of the data in two important ways. First, since a table is a summarization of the data, the researcher must often regroup his measurements into scale categories, called class intervals, that possess substantive meaning. Thus, if an independent variable included in the study is the age of a patient, recorded in actual years, the regrouping into class intervals will help to focus attention on the uses to which the data might be put. If the data are to serve in planning health programs for the elderly patient, perhaps two groupings will suffice: 65 years of age and over, under 65 years. Or if the study were concerned with health problems in each age group, a more refined grouping will be employed, such as under 1 year of age, 1–5, 6–20, 21–44, 45–64, 65 and over.

Second, the process of organizing data in tables enables the researcher to assess the relationship between the variables studied. Not only can the simple relationship between an independent and a dependent variable be studied, but the combined effects of several independent variables on the criterion measure can be assessed.

How the relationship between variables can be assessed through tabulation of the data is illustrated by the following study. A health department desired to evaluate the factors influencing people to become vaccinated against poliomyelitis. A total of over 600 people were interviewed to find out why they did or did not obtain immunization against polio.

The most basic tabulation of data from a study is called a *univariate distribution*. Such a tabulation presents the data for only one variable at a time. For the immunization study a univariate distribution of the criterion variable—the extent of vaccine acceptance among the respondents —is presented in Table 9-1.

TABLE 9-1

Percentage of Study Subjects Immunized Against Poliomyelitis

Total	Nontakers	Injections Only	Oral Only	Both Vaccines
100%	19	20	14	47

Source: A. L. Johnson, C. D. Jenkins, R. Patrick, and J. T. Northcutt, Jr., *Epidemiology of Polio Vaccine.* Florida State Board of Health, Monograph No. 3, 1962, p. 35.

This table simply shows in percentage form the distribution of respondents according to one variable—their acceptance of the vaccine. The interpretation of the data is that nearly half of the respondents took both types of vaccine and less than one in five took neither type.

In Table 9-2 another variable is introduced into the analysis: the educational level of the respondents. Such a table is called a *bivariate distribution.* In this table, vaccine acceptance can be considered as the dependent variable—the criterion measure of the success of the polio immunization program—while educational level can be considered as an independent variable—a variable that may help explain the vaccine acceptance behavior of the respondents. As is seen in the table there is a direct relationship between the two variables: as educational level increases, so does acceptance of the vaccine. This suggests that the content of the program that was used to induce people to seek vaccination may have been pitched above the understanding level of people with lesser educational attainment. The table demonstrates how the introduction of additional variables can provide meaningful insight into the behavior of the dependent variable.

Tables that contain more than two variables can be called *multivariate*

TABLE 9-2

**Percentage of Study Subjects Immunized Against Poliomyelitis
by Educational Level**

Educational Level	Number of Respondents	Total	Non-takers	Injections Only	Oral Only	Both Vaccines
All levels	624	100%	19	20	14	47
Less than eight grades	42	100%	52	7	24	17
Grade school graduate	43	100%	42	12	18	28
Some high school	133	100%	25	25	13	37
High school graduate	228	100%	16	21	15	48
Some college	128	100%	6	19	9	66
College graduate	50	100%	2	24	6	68

Source: as for Table 9-1.

distributions; an example of such a table is Table 9-3 in the following section.

HOW TO INTERPRET A STATISTICAL TABLE

The various elements of a statistical table were discussed in the previous chapter. These elements provide the framework for the data incorporated in the table. There are many approaches to the interpretation of data contained in a table. Some persons direct their attention first to the body of the table and make a quick, overall evaluation of the data it contains. Others take a more leisurely approach, reading the title first, then the boxhead, stub, source, and even footnotes before actually studying the data. The following is a suggested step-by-step guide for interpreting the data in a statistical table, which, if followed in the sequence presented, should help the reader to derive the maximum amount of interpretative information from the table.

The steps in interpreting a table will be presented in the form of guide questions. The usefulness of these questions will be illustrated by applying them to a table containing some findings from a study in which the relationship between the amount of nursing care provided and patient and

TABLE 9-3

Average Percentage of Patients* Reporting Dissatisfaction with Length of Time Spent Waiting for Nursing Services, by Age of Patients and Size of Room Accommodation (60 general hospitals, 1956)

(Percentages denote the percentages of the total number of patients in each age and accommodation group who reported dissatisfaction with length of time spent waiting for nursing services)

Age of Patients	Number of Beds in Room				
	All Room Accommodations, Average	*Private*	*2 Beds*	*3–6 Beds*	*7 or More Beds*
All ages average	*9.8*	*8.8*	*9.2*	*9.9*	*12.0*
Under 20 years	14.9	12.8	13.0	12.9	18.8
20–29	12.5	14.1	12.1	12.3	12.7
30–39	9.9	9.0	8.2	10.2	8.1
40–49	9.3	9.0	8.2	9.5	9.3
50–59	8.0	7.1	8.7	7.7	8.6
60 and over	8.1	7.2	8.1	8.9	7.4

* Nonobstetrical patients.

Source: Questionnaires to patients in 60 general hospitals. For a complete report of the study see Faye G. Abdellah and Eugene Levine, *Effect of Nurse Staffing on Satisfactions with Nursing Care.* American Hospital Association, Monograph No. 4 (1958), 88 pp.

personnel satisfaction with the care was explored. Discussed in greater detail in Chapter 14 of this book, the design for this study was a non-experimental one. A sample of 60 general hospitals was selected according to the average daily amounts of nursing care provided to their patients: high, medium, and low. The dependent variable, satisfaction with care, was assessed by checklists in which the patients and personnel in the sample hospitals reported omissions in nursing services. Table 9-3 is a by-product of this study. For this table a subscore of the dependent variable was computed indicating dissatisfaction with the length of time spent waiting for services. This variable is analyzed in relation to two independent variables—the age of the patients and the size of their room accommodations.

Table 9-3, then, is a multivariate distribution. In such a table not only can the relationship between each independent variable and the dependent variable be assessed, but the interactions between the independent variables can also be evaluated.

The guide questions for interpreting data in a table are:

1. What does the title of the table and other explanatory material tell us?
2. How were the data obtained?
3. What is being measured?
4. How much variation is there in the grand totals or averages for each variable?
5. How much variation is there within each of the scale values (classes) of the variables?
6. How are the variables related to each other?
7. Do the data reveal any unusual pattern?
8. What can be concluded from the interpretation of the data?

1. *What does the title of the table and other explanatory material tell us?* The title indicates that the purpose of the study is an attempt to determine whether age of patients or the size of their accommodations or a combination of the two variables is related to patients' dissatisfaction with nursing services in general hospitals. The data are classified according to two variables, age of patient and size of room accommodations. There is a third variable in the table. This is the dissatisfaction of patients with nursing services. Age of patients and room size are the independent variables. Dissatisfaction is the dependent variable. The table portrays the relationship between the independent variables, age of patient and size of his room accommodation, and the criterion measure, dissatisfaction with nursing service. The data were collected in 60 general hospitals, thus being a sample. The adequacy and scope of the sample can only be assessed by reference to the complete study. The headnote spells out specifically what

the percentages in the table represent. The footnote limits the data to non-obstetrical patients.

2. *How were the data obtained?* The source tells us the data were collected by questionnaires filled out by patients. The data have come from an original source and not a secondary one.

3. *What is being measured?* The sampling unit in the study is a patient. Measurements have been made on three variables concerning each patient. The size of his room, his age, and his dissatisfaction with waiting for services. The table shows how these variables are related to each other.

4. *How much variation is there in the grand totals or averages for each variable?* There are two sets of overall averages in the table, one for each of the independent variables. These are the figures in the first column of the table under "All Room Accommodations, Average" and on the first line "All ages, average."

The figures on the line "All ages, average" indicate that as size of room increases, dissatisfaction with nursing services also increases. The per cent of patients dissatisfied with nursing services in rooms with seven or more beds is nearly 50 per cent greater than the per cent dissatisfied in private rooms.

The figures in the column "All Room Accommodations, Average" show the following pattern: As age increases, per cent of patients dissatisfied with nursing services decreases. The range of difference among the age groups is greater than for room size. The percentage of patients under 20 years of age dissatisfied with nursing services is nearly twice as high as the percentage of patients 50 years of age and over. This suggests age is more closely related to dissatisfaction than is size of room accommodation.

5. *How much variation is there within each of the scale values (classes) of the variables?* Data in each of the room size groups follow the same pattern as the overall average. In each of the different room accommodation groups, as age of patients increases, dissatisfaction decreases. The greatest variation is in the group "7 or More Beds," where the range is from 18.8 per cent in the youngest group to 7.4 per cent in the oldest.

The data behave differently for the age variable. Only in the youngest age groups is there an increase in dissatisfaction as room size increases, while among older patients there is no relationship at all between amount of dissatisfaction and room size.

6. *How are the variables related to each other?* The age of a patient has a considerably stronger relationship to dissatisfaction than size of room accommodation. While the average for all patients combined shows a rise in dissatisfaction as room size increases, only the youngest age group reveals this same pattern. Apparently, the pattern found in the youngest age group has a strong influence on the average for all ages combined.

7. *Do the data reveal any unusual pattern?* Why does the average for

all patients combined show increasing dissatisfaction in waiting for nursing services as room size increases, when this pattern does not hold true for any age group except the youngest? The key to the answer to this question lies in Table 9-4, which gives the actual number of patients participating in the study for each cell of the table. As can be seen from the table the largest proportion of younger patients are in the larger rooms, while the largest proportion of older patients are in private and semiprivate rooms. Since younger patients are more dissatisfied with nursing services than older patients regardless of room accommodation, the average percentages are weighted by the number of patients in the different age groups who are in the various room size groups. Since there are more younger patients in larger rooms, and more older patients in smaller rooms, and since younger patients are more dissatisfied than older patients, the average for all patients combined shows an increasing dissatisfaction as room size increases. If considered only by itself, this average is thus misleading, since it is distorted by the underlying disproportionate age distribution of patients in the different-sized rooms.

8. *What can be concluded from the interpretation of the data?* There is a strong relationship between the age of a patient and his dissatisfaction with time spent waiting for nursing services. As age increases, dissatisfaction decreases. Except for the youngest patients, there is no relationship between size of room accommodation and dissatisfaction with nursing services. Patients under 20 years in large rooms are more dissatisfied than patients under 20 in private rooms. The greatest range of dissatisfaction,

TABLE 9-4

Total Number of Patients* in 60 General Hospitals Study, by Age of Patients and Size of Room Accommodations (1956)

| Age of Patients | All Room Accommodations, Total | Number of Beds in Room | | | |
		Private	2 Bed	3–6 Beds	7 or More Beds
All ages, total	7,024	1,330	2,425	2,408	861
Under 20 years	720	63	162	249	246
20–29	846	107	285	315	139
30–39	1,057	159	364	411	123
40–49	1,264	255	481	412	116
50–59	1,333	285	498	430	120
60 and over	1,804	461	635	591	117

* Nonobstetrical patients.
Source: See Table 9-3.

according to age, is in the largest room accommodations. Patients under 20 are nearly two and a half times more dissatisfied with the amount of time they have to wait for nursing services than patients who are 60 years of age and over.

SOME PITFALLS IN INTERPRETING DATA IN TABLES

There are a number of pitfalls that can be encountered in interpreting a table like the one just discussed. If these are not avoided, the interpretation of the data can be spurious. If a spurious interpretation of data is used to guide action it can lead to costly wastes of effort, time, and money. A few of the major pitfalls will be discussed using the table just presented as an illustration.

1. *Misinterpretation of cause and effect.* Because a table reveals that the variables are related to each other does not by any means establish the fact that they are causally related. Particularly in nonexperimental studies, where many of the important extraneous variables may not be controlled, relationships between two variables shown in a table may actually reflect the influence of an extraneous variable. This point is demonstrated by the fact that the relationship between room size and patient satisfaction actually reflects the influence of patients' ages. When age is held constant, no important relationship can be seen between room size and satisfaction.

2. *Failure to consider variability around the measures of central tendency.* The figures shown in each cell of a table are summary measures around which may exist considerable variation of the individual values upon which they are based. The extent to which a summary measure, such as a mean, is a good descriptive measure of the individual values depends on how great the variation is. Thus, in interpreting data the fact that some summary measures may describe the individual values better than other summary measures should be kept in mind in evaluating differences between the values in different cells of the table. For example, suppose we had two samples, each consisting of five hospitals, for which the average percentage of patients reporting dissatisfaction with length of time spent in waiting for nursing services is computed as follows:

	Sample 1	Sample 2
	11.0	5.0
	11.0	7.0
	12.0	14.0
	13.0	14.0
	13.0	15.0
Mean	12.0	11.0

In sample 1 the individual values fall within a narrow range, whereas in sample 2 the values are highly variable. If we only examined the means it would appear that the hospitals in sample 2 had better satisfaction scores than those in sample 1. However, in sample 2 the scores of three of the hospitals indicate higher dissatisfaction than any of the hospitals in sample 1. This raises the question as to whether for a comparison of the two samples of hospitals the mean is a good summary measure of the average satisfaction level.

3. *Failure to account for the possibility of noncomparability of the groups included in the table.* In nonexperimental studies the comparison groups are usually not equalized by a process of random assignment. Therefore, it is possible that the groups could differ in certain important characteristics that could affect the values of the criterion measures being compared. One such characteristic is the fact that for some of the very young patients, where highest dissatisfaction levels were found, it may have been the parent who responded to the checklist rather than the patient, since the protocols for the study permitted this. In some cases, enough to influence the data significantly, the parents may have been more apt to be impatient with the length of time it took for a nursing service to be provided than the patients would be themselves.

4. *Limitations of data due to possible inadequacies of measuring instruments.* In interpreting data in tables a skeptical attitude should be maintained concerning the quality of the measuring instruments employed, particularly their reliability and validity. This is particularly true in data such as those in these tables. The instrument used to collect these data was developed especially for the study and at the time of the study had not undergone extensive use, although it received multiple pretests to check its validity and reliability.

5. *Limitations of sample size in making generalizations.* Before any generalizations of the data could be made beyond the study setting, the method of selection of the sample as well as its size must be considered. In interpreting the data the following questions should be raised. Were the hospitals selected from a larger target population? If so, how was this population defined? Were the sample hospitals chosen randomly so that confidence intervals could be computed for the summary measure? What kind of sample is this—if it is not a simple random sample, is it a cluster sample? If so, what formulas should be used in computing the sampling error? How many hospitals were included in the sample, and how many patients in each of the hospitals submitted checklists?

Answers to many questions like these are not usually available just from inspection of a table. They can only be obtained by referring to the complete report of the study. If the data are to be definitively interpreted this would need to be done.

6. *In interpreting a statistical table it is important to consider all possible limitations of the data.* In addition to the limitations already mentioned—spurious relationships, possible weaknesses in the measurement process, lack of comparability of study groups, small size of sample, and its method of selection—all other limitations of the data should be weighed. These include the possible transient nature of the relationships found among the variables in the study. What was found in this study would have to be corroborated by other studies to demonstrate stability and permanence of the findings.

7. *The substantive meaning of the data needs to be assessed.* Finally, the data need to be evaluated in the light of what substantive meaning they possess. Are the data merely an interesting academic exercise, or do they offer any constructive suggestions, advice, or guidelines for pursuing a course of action in the real world?

COMMUNICATION OF RESEARCH FINDINGS

Unless research findings are communicated, they cannot benefit mankind nor improve the environment in which man lives. The research investigator has an obligation to publish his research so that he can share his knowledge with the world and subject his findings to testing by others. Some researchers view publication as only a scholarly achievement and do not feel obligated to publish. In instances where this occurs one can only wonder if the researcher fears exposure of inconsequential research and sanction by his colleagues. Some researchers, on the other hand, are perfectionists and never feel that their manuscripts are ready for publication. This attitude only delays the sharing of new knowledge that might be valuable to other researchers.

Many universities have now adopted the philosophy of "publish or perish." The intent here is to use one criterion—namely, publication—as a means of assessing the individual's readiness for promotion within the academic hierarchy. This pressure has sometimes led to premature publication of inconsequential research. The following pages present some guidelines that the investigator might find helpful in thinking through the steps in preparing a manuscript for publication, as well as providing suggestions as to what to look for in scientific papers that have been published.

Initial Planning for Publication

The way in which research findings are communicated is dependent upon how the original proposal was prepared. The type of thinking that has gone on initially is often reflected in the final report. Therefore, it is often helpful to consider how the research findings are to be communicated early in the research process.

Brockington[11] refers to the formative stage of writing as reflective thinking. Its quality is based upon the clarity with which the research question is posed. If it is stated ambiguously the entire report is apt to reflect this confusion. Discussion of the research question with experts in the field will further help to crystallize the problem.

Various steps in the research process have been considered previously. These need to be thought of within a framework of preparing the final report. Following is a checklist that might help to summarize important points.

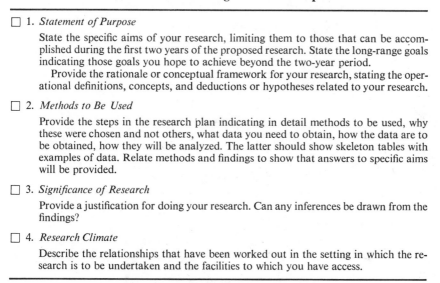

Checklist for Planning a Research Report

☐ 1. *Statement of Purpose*

State the specific aims of your research, limiting them to those that can be accomplished during the first two years of the proposed research. State the long-range goals indicating those goals you hope to achieve beyond the two-year period.

Provide the rationale or conceptual framework for your research, stating the operational definitions, concepts, and deductions or hypotheses related to your research.

☐ 2. *Methods to Be Used*

Provide the steps in the research plan indicating in detail methods to be used, why these were chosen and not others, what data you need to obtain, how the data are to be obtained, how they will be analyzed. The latter should show skeleton tables with examples of data. Relate methods and findings to show that answers to specific aims will be provided.

☐ 3. *Significance of Research*

Provide a justification for doing your research. Can any inferences be drawn from the findings?

☐ 4. *Research Climate*

Describe the relationships that have been worked out in the setting in which the research is to be undertaken and the facilities to which you have access.

Preparation of the Final Report

An aid in preparing the final report is the development of a skeleton outline specifying chapter titles, subheadings, table outlines, with examples of kinds of data you hope to find. This is more than a mental exercise and can save many months of pursuing an approach that does not answer the research question.

The selection of the title of the report should be given considerable thought. It should be stated concisely and communicate the central theme of the research. Following is a sample table of contents.

Sample Table of Contents*

* Based upon material prepared by Dorothy Sutherland for a Nursing Research Conference, Columbia Union College, Takoma Park, Maryland, November 1961.

List of Appendix Tables

1. A scxc cxcx cxcxc cxc.	xx
2. The vxczv vxvzuxvz vxv.	xx
3. Etc.	xx

Sample Arrangement of the Research Paper

1. Title page: title of project, author's name, date, location, and other pertinent identifying information.
2. Preface or foreword containing acknowledgments.
3. Table of contents:

> Chapter or other subheadings
> List of tables
> List of illustrations
> Bibliography
> Appendix

Tables and graphs should be so clearly presented that they are self-explanatory: this means that headings and captions to figures and graphs must be complete.

4. Introduction:

> Should be included in the first section of the text. (Separate introduction not recommended. To many "forewords" slow down pace of getting into the substance of the report.) Note special limitations of report here. Mention special techniques employed in gathering and handling of material. Define terms used if unusual or "coined" for purposes of the study.

5. The text:

> Repeat title at top of first page, centered.

Number pages consecutively.

Begin each new section of the report on a new page.

6. Bibliography:

List on separate page, with self-heading.

Continue pagination of report.

7. Appendix:

Material not legitimately a part of the text itself, but helpful to the reader; e.g., some tables, sample questionnaire forms, complete transcripts of documents or other reference materials, etc.

8. Index:

An index can be an invaluable aid to the reader and should be included in a research report that is published as a monograph or book. Its value rests in the appropriateness of the classification of concepts that it uses.

Reviewing a Research Report

Hillway[12] cites four main purposes that a review of a research report should accomplish. First, the main thesis of the report should be stated. Were the research aims initially stated achieved? Were hypotheses formulated? Was there an original contribution to knowledge? Second, there should be a clear analysis and assessment of the data presented. What controls were identified and used? Third, has the author presented his ideas logically in understandable terms? Fourth, does the review contain a critique of the work presented in terms of its contribution to its field of knowledge?

Suggested Checklist for Reviewing a Research Report

---

1. Does the report clearly state the purpose of the study?
2. Is the methodology adequately described?
   (a) Did the investigator use the method cited in his proposal, and if not, does his report explain his reason for deviating?
   (b) Are the instruments fully explained and (when appropriate) included as figures in the text or as exhibits in an appendix?
3. Have raw data (source tables) been placed in an appendix? Are summary tables integrated into appropriate places in the text? Are the tables understandable? Does the text merely restate content of tables, or does it interpret and point out significant relationships?
4. Does the report plainly summarize the findings? Does it contain the investigator's conclusions? Interpretation of results?
5. Do the findings, as reported, suggest need for further research or recommendations for application of the new knowledge discovered (if the content is applied research)?
6. Does the report adequately credit all sources and resources tapped during the study? Are there an acceptable bibliography and index?
7. Was the report difficult to read? Did the language obscure the content and value of the research? Were you interested in the study, regardless of the manner in which the report was written, despite its style?
8. Does the report convey that the research was useful or important, even though the subject investigated might have been a small one? Or, conversely, is it so verbose that it suggests the entire investigation was "much ado about nothing"?
9. Is the report interesting?
10. Do you know what the investigator accomplished?
11. If human subjects are involved, have they been informed of their rights? Have appropriate steps been taken to protect the subjects?

The importance of communicating research findings cannot be over-emphasized. To be meaningful, research must be communicated. The writer has a responsibility of predigesting his material into clear, concise writing. It is not uncommon to find that a researcher has submitted a voluminous, unedited document to be published. Many of these reports are actually working papers from which the researcher has failed to extract the relevant material.

It is helpful to focus the report upon a central theme to provide continuity from chapter to chapter. Be sure to indicate the significance of your research and questions that still remain unanswered. Above all, write enthusiastically to express rather than impress. There is no substitute for simplicity and clarity in writing.

Selected Standard Abbreviations

anon., anonymous
bull., bulletin
ca. or c., (*circa*): about, approximately
c., copyright
cf. ante, (*confer-ante*): compare above
cf. post, (*confer-post*): compare below
chap(s). or ch., chapter(s)
col(s)., column(s)
ed., editor, edition, edited
ed. cit., edition cited; where specific reference is being made to one edition that has already been noted in the documentation
e.g., (*exempli gratia*): for example
et al., (*et alii*), (*et alibi*): and others, and elsewhere
et seq., (*et sequens*): and the following
fig(s)., figure(s)
ibid., (*ibidem*): in the same place. When two or more successive footnotes refer to the same work, use *ibid.* instead of repeating reference. If different pages are referred to, pagination reference must be shown
id., idem: the same
i.e., (*id est*): that is
loc. cit., (*loco citato*): in the place cited
o.p., out of print
op. cit., (*opere citato*): in the work cited. If reference has been made to a work and new reference is to be made without intervening references to other works, ibid. may be used; if intervening reference has been made to different works, op. cit. must be used. The name of the author must precede.
q.v., (*quad vide*): which see
rev., revised
sic: thus; indicates an error of which you are aware, especially in matter
tr., trans., translator, translated, translation
vid. or vide: see, refer to
V. or Vol(s)., volume(s)

Summary

This chapter has been largely devoted to a discussion of the meaning of statistical tests of significance and their role in research in nursing and patient care. It has been stressed that tests of significance should be applied only where the research has involved randomization in the process of data collection, by either random sampling of the study subjects from the target population, random assignment of the study subjects to the alternative groups, or both.

A test of statistical significance measures the extent to which the observed difference in the values of the summary measures of the dependent variable for the alternative groups studied exceeds the sampling error of the difference. The level of the significance of the observed difference, therefore, is the relative frequency of obtaining such a difference by chance alone in repeated random samplings from the target population.

Various misuses of statistical tests of significance have been discussed. One is the frequent confusion of statistical significance with the practical importance of the findings. It should be kept in mind that a statistically significant result may not have any substantive significance. Conversely, an important result may not turn out to be statistically significant if the sample size employed in the study was too small.

Another misuse of tests of statistical significance is the wholesale application of such tests retrospectively, after the data have been collected. The only hypotheses that can be validly tested for statistical significance are those formulated *prior* to data collection.

Some guidelines for interpreting data in statistical tables have been provided in this chapter. A thoughtful and painstaking interpretation of tabulated data can bring to light the real meaning of the findings of a study. In interpreting data the limitations of the study should be constantly kept in the forefront.

The final step in the research process is to communicate the findings. Implementation of the study results, confirmation of the results through replicated studies, and advancement of the accumulated knowledge in the field cannot take place until research findings are clearly and comprehensively communicated.

References

1. Faye G. Abdellah and Eugene Levine, *Effect of Nurse Staffing on Satisfactions with Nursing Care.* Hospital Monograph Series No. 4. Chicago, The American Hospital Association, 1958.
2. Beverly J. Safford and Rozella M. Schlotfeldt, "Nursing Service Staffing and Quality of Nursing Care." *Nursing Res., 9:*149–154, summer 1960.
3. Harry E. Allison, "Computational Forms for Chi-Square." *Am. Statistician,* **18:**17–18, February 1964.
4. Frederick Mosteller, Robert E. K. Rourke, George B. Thomas, Jr., *Probability with Statistical Applications.* Reading, Mass., Addison-Wesley Publishing Co., Inc., 1961, p. 146.

5. Hanan C. Selvin, "A Critique of Tests of Significance in Survey Research." *Am. Sociol. Rev.*, **22:**519–527, October 1957.
6. Robert McGinnis, "Randomization and Inference in Sociological Research." *Am. Sociol. Rev.*, **23:**408–414, August 1958.
7. Leslie Kish, "Some Statistical Problems in Research Design." *Am. Sociol. Rev.*, **24:**328–338, June 1959.
8. Patricia L. Kendall, "Methodological Appendix," in Robert K. Merton, George G. Reader, and Patricia L. Kendall (eds.), *The Student Physician.* Cambridge, Harvard University Press, 1957.
9. Herman Wold, "Causal Inference from Observational Data." *J. Royal Statistical Soc.* (A), **119:**28–61, January 1956.
10. W. Allen Wallis and Harry V. Roberts, *Statistics: A New Approach.* New York, The Free Press of Glencoe, 1956, p. 133.
11. Fraser Brockington, "Preparation of a Research Proposal and Preparation of the Final Report," in Margaret G. Arnstein and Ellen Broe (eds.), *International Conference on the Planning of Nursing Studies.* London, International Council of Nurses, 1956, pp. 44–50.
12. Tyrus Hillway, *Introduction to Research.* Boston, Houghton Mifflin Co., 1956, pp. 261–262.

Problems and Suggestions for Further Study

1. Comment on the following remarks by R. A. Fisher in his *The Design of Experiments* (London, Oliver and Boyd, 1953 ed., p. 16).
   ". . . it should be noted that the null hypothesis is never proved or established, but is possibly disproved in the course of experimentation. Every experiment may be said to exist only in order to give the facts a chance of disproving the null hypothesis."
2. Discuss the use of tests of statistical significance in the following studies:
   a. David J. Fox *et al.*, "Freshman Characteristics and Expectations Related to Anticipated Satisfaction from Attending Nursing School." *Nursing Forum,* **2:**49–59, No. 3, 1963.
   b. George K. Tokuhata, "Familial Factors in Human Lung Cancer and Smoking." *Am. J. Pub. Health,* **54:**24–32, January 1964.
   c. Betty L. Cuthbert, "Sex Knowledge of a Class of Student Nurses." *Nursing Res.,* **10:**145–150, summer 1961.
   d. Jane Wilcox, "Observer Factors in the Measurement of Blood Pressure." *Nursing Res.,* **10:**4–17, winter 1961.
   e. Dorothea M. Lenarz and Norris D. Vestre, "The Effect of a Course in Psychiatric Nursing on Insight Test Scores of Nursing Students." *J. Psychiat. Nursing,* **2:**137–141, March–April 1964.
   f. Evelyn Crumpton and Eileen P. Rogers, "Some Effects of Team Nursing on a Psychiatric Ward." *Nursing Res.,* **12:**181–182, summer 1963.
   g. Judith T. Shuval, "Perceived Role Components of Nursing in Israel." *Am. Sociol. Rev.,* **28:**37–46, February 1963.
   h. Margaret W. Linn, Lee Gurel and Bernard S. Linn, "Patient Outcome as a Measure of Quality of Nursing Home Care." *Am. J. Pub. Health,* **67:**344–77, April 1977.
   i. Marlene Kramer and others, "Extra-Tactile Stimulation of the Premature Infant." *Nursing Res.,* **24:**324–334, September–October, 1975.

j. S. E. M. O'Brien and K. A. Stoll, "Attitudes of Medical and Nursing Staff Towards Self-Poisoning Patients in a London Hospital. *Int. J. Nurs. Stud.,* **14**:29–35, 1977.

3. For each of the following tests of significance describe a study in which the test would be used:
   a. A *T*-test of the difference between two percentages
   b. A chi-square test
   c. A sign test
   d. A *t*-test of the slope of a regression equation
   e. An *F*-test

4. Why do you think the chi-square test is so popular in research on human beings as a test of significance of the data? What are the advantages in the use of this test? What are the disadvantages? Why is chi-square a more widely applicable test than the analysis of variance? But why is the analysis of variance a more powerful test than chi-square?

5. What is the relationship between regression analysis and the analysis of variance? Are the two techniques identical in that they are concerned with the relationship between dependent and independent variables? How are they different? How does regression analysis differ from correlation analysis?

6. Read the article by Hanan C. Selvin, "A Critique of Tests of Significance in Survey Research," (*Am. Sociol. Rev.,* **22**:519–527, October 1957). Do you agree with the author's conclusions that "Statistical tests are unsatisfactory in nonexperimental research for two fundamental reasons. It is almost impossible to design studies that meet the conditions for using the tests, and the situations in which the tests are employed make it difficult to draw correct inferences" (p. 527). Also read the reply to this article by Leslie Kish, "Some Statistical Problems in Research Design." (*Am. Sociol. Rev.,* **24**:328–338, June 1959). Comment on this author's statement that "Selvin's logic and advice should lead not only to the rejection of statistical tests; it should lead one to refrain altogether from using survey results for the purposes of finding explanatory variables. In this sense, not only tests of significance, but any comparisons, any specific inquiry based on surveys, any scientific inquiry other than an 'ideal' experiment, is inapplicable. That advice is most unrealistic" (p. 331).

7. Discuss the comparative advantages and disadvantages of parametric and nonparametric tests of significance. Are there any assumptions at all that have to be met concerning the data before nonparametric tests can be applied? Why are nonparametric tests useful in research on nursing and patient care? Explain why there is a loss of information when a nonparametric test is used in place of a parametric test. Discuss the statement by Wallis and Roberts in their *Statistics: A New Approach* (New York, The Free Press of Glencoe, 1956) that "Not all non-parametric tests are quick and easy, by any means, even though most quick and easy methods are non-parametric" (p. 592).

8. Read Chapter 2 in R. A. Fisher's *The Design of Experiments* (London, Oliver and Boyd, 1953 ed., pp. 11–25), "The Principles of Experimentation Illustrated by a Psycho-Physical Experiment." What are some of the ways indicated by Fisher that the sensitivity of the experiment can be increased? How can the practical significance of the results of such an experiment be assessed?

9. Does all explanatory research require that the data be evaluated by tests of significance? What other ways are there of evaluating data in addition to tests of significance? What really does a test of significance do? Why, in looking at the process of research in its entirety as it is currently being applied to problems in nursing and patient care, might the process of applying tests of significance to the research data be of minor importance?

10. Comment on the following statement by Selltiz and others in *Research Methods in Social Relations* (New York, Holt, Rinehart and Winston, rev. ed., 1962). "If we want to make causal inferences—that is, to say that one variable or event has led to another—we must meet assumptions over and above those required for establishing the existence of a relationship" (p. 422). What are these assumptions?

11. This chapter has focused primarily on guidelines for analyzing and interpreting quantitative data in research. Can any guidelines be established for analyzing nonquantitative data? Is it possible to make a scientific interpretation of nonquantified data?

12. Comment on the following remarks by Robert S. Morison in his article, "Gradualness, Gradualness, Gradualness" (*Am. Psychologist,* **15:**187–197, March 1960). "It can be demonstrated that medicine, most notably in the case of the infectious diseases, has made astonishing progress by adopting an oversimplified view of causality. Perhaps it was simply lucky to grow up in an unsophisticated era when no one took David Hume's billiard balls very seriously, questioned the validity of the inductive method, or reflected on the proposition that everything is probably related to everything else in some multivariable system with lots of feedback. Maybe the explanation lies in the fact that most medical men have been relatively simple minded souls anxious to do something to help mankind" (p. 193). Are these same comments also applicable to research in nursing? Explain.

13. Discuss the following statement by Neyman in his article, "Statistics— Servant of All Sciences" (*Science,* 401–406, September 2, 1955). "The development of modern science is marked by a pronounced tendency toward indeterminism. A somewhat brutal description of this tendency may be stated as follows. In relation to some phenomena, instead of trying to establish a (deterministic) functional relationship between a variable y, and some other variables x_1, x_2, . . . x_n, we try to build a (stochastic or probabilistic) model of these phenomena predicting frequencies with which, in specified conditions, the same variable y will assume all of its possible values" (p. 401). Is Neyman's distinction between a deterministic, functional relationship and a stochastic or probabilistic model the same as the distinction drawn earlier between a mathematical and a statistical model?

14. Evaluate the manner in which the data were interpreted in the following reported studies. Do you feel the authors provided sufficient data in their reports to enable the reader to verify the author's interpretation?
   a. Fred Davis and Virginia L. Olesen, "Initiation into a Woman's Profession: Identity Problems in the Status Transition of Coed to Student Nurse." *Sociometry,* **26:**89–101, March 1963.
   b. Joyce D. Sloane, "Bladder Atonia After Vaginal Delivery." *Nursing Res.,* **8:**26–32, winter 1959.
   c. Jack P. Gibbs, "Rates of Mental Hospitalization: A Study of Societal Reaction to Deviant Behavior." *Am. Sociol. Rev.,* **27:**782–792, December 1962.

    d. Peter Kong-Ming New and Gladys Nite, "Staffing and Interaction." *Nursing Outlook,* **8:**396–400, July 1960.

    e. Daniel Horn, "Behavioral Aspects of Cigarette Smoking." *J. Chronic Dis.,* **16:**383–395, May 1963.

    f. Leo G. Reeder, Don H. Zimmerman, and Eleanor B. Sheldon, "Improving Nursing Home Administration: A Report of an Experiment in Education." *J. Health and Human Behavior,* **4:**29–36, spring 1963.

    g. Beverly J. Volicer and Mary Wynne Bohannon, "A Hospital Stress Rating Scale." *Nursing Res.,* **24:**352–359, September–October 1975.

    h. John A. Ward and John M. Griffin, "Improving Instruction Through Computer-Graded Examinations." *Nursing Outlook,* **25:**524–529, August 1977.

15. Read Chapter 14, "Probability and Induction," in Morris R. Cohen and Ernest Nagel, *An Introduction to Logic and Scientific Method* (New York, Harcourt, Brace and Co., 1934, pp. 273–288). How do the authors define inductive reasoning? Discuss the author's remarks that "an inductive argument, while it does not, in the strictest sense, demonstrate a universal proposition, may prove it to be the best evidenced of all suggested hypotheses" (p. 284).

16. Discuss the distinction between the following terms:
    a. Practical significance of research findings and statistical significance of the findings
    b. One-tailed and two-tailed tests of statistical significance
    c. The Neyman-Pearson method of statistical inference and Bayesian inference
    d. Analysis of data and interpretation of findings
    e. Random sampling and random assignment
    f. Level of significance and confidence level
    g. Statistics and parameters
    h. Correlation and regression
    i. Type I and Type II errors.

17. Obtain a copy of the latest edition of *Facts About Nursing* published by the American Nurses' Association (Kansas City, Missouri). Select five tables and apply the guidelines for interpreting data in tables contained in this chapter. Write a brief interpretation of the data they contain.

18. Read the following work as an example of a major research report in nursing:
Doris Schwartz, Barbara Henley, and Leonard Zeitz, *The Elderly Ambulatory Patient: Nursing and Psycho-social Needs.* New York, Macmillan Publishing Co., Inc., 1964.
Prepare a paper commenting on the way in which the authors handled the analysis and interpretation of the data. What are some of the ways in which the authors make it possible for others to replicate this study? In other research reports that you have read, have you found that it would be possible to replicate the study from the information given in the report?

19. Discuss the following statement by E. J. G. Pitman, "Statistics and Science," (*Journal of the American Statistical Association,* **52:**322–330, September 1957), "The scientist with ideas frames his hypotheses and wishes to test them. He would be happy if he could devise a test which would decide with certainty whether a hypothesis is true or not. When he cannot do this, he must use a test which has only a certain probability of giving the right answer" (p. 323).

20. Read Chapter 7, "Some Fundamental Problems and Limitations to Study by Experimental Designs" in F. Stuart Chapin, *Experimental Designs in Sociological Research* (New York, Harper and Row, 1947, pp. 165–190). What are the various definitions of "probability" that are given by the author in this chapter? Explain what the author means in stating that probability tests (tests of significance) serve only as an "empirical safety device, and not to provide the basis for extensive generalizations" (p. 185).

21. Read the article "Study Shows How Computerization Affects Nursing Activities in ICU," by Samuel H. Talbert and Alvaro E. Pertuz in *Hospitals, Journal of the American Hospital Association*, 51:79–84, September 1, 1977. Study the table on page 81. Can you tell what test of significance was used from either the table or the text? What practical significance can be placed on the statistical significance that was found in the study?

22. Read the report *Delphi Survey of Clinical Nursing Research Priorities*. Western Interstate Commission for Higher Education. Boulder, Colorado, The Commission, August 1974. Does the absence of tests of significance of the data detract from the report? Applying the *Checklist for Reviewing a Research Report* write a review of this report.

Chapter Ten

RESEARCH TACTICS

THE FIVE PRECEDING CHAPTERS have been concerned with the technical side of conducting a research project. In addition to the technical aspects, every researcher is also confronted with certain administrative problems in attempting to pursue his study as efficiently and expeditiously as possible. This chapter will briefly touch on some of the more important of these problems. The decisions a researcher makes in solving them can be called research tactics or strategy.

The major administrative problems in pursuing a study include those related to securing and maintaining adequate resources to conduct the study. These resources include staffing for the research, facilities in which to conduct the research, study subjects from whom the data are collected, and financial support for the conduct of the research.

Research as an Organized Activity

It is rare today for a research project to be conducted by a lone investigator. In many areas of research the solo researcher, toiling long hours in his laboratory, performing all of the tasks required by the research, perhaps with only the help of a research assistant, has disappeared. This does not mean that much useful research cannot be pursued individually. Research conducted for a doctoral dissertation is an example of research still being undertaken as a solo effort, although some dissertation topics might better be accomplished as a group activity. In the nursing and patient care areas a number of very important research problems are sufficiently delimited to be conducted by a single investigator with assistance from others when needed in the more routine aspects of data collection and processing. Many valuable contributions have been made toward the advancement of knowledge in nursing in small, modestly financed studies, pursued by a lone researcher.

However, many of the research problems in the area of patient care are too complex to be approached through a small study. When a research project requires the attention of more than one full-time professional person and a supporting staff of technical and clerical workers, it is called group or team research. If the professional persons are members of different speciality fields—as, for example a nurse researcher and a psychologist —the research effort is called interdisciplinary research. Some interdisciplinary research projects involve specialists from a large variety of professional fields.

Considerable criticism has been directed at interdisciplinary research. It is said that the total research effort can become, when pursued by a team, too fragmented, and this can result in a deterioration in the level of interest among members of the research team and a failure to reach the objectives of the research. On the other hand, the benefits of team research include greater efficiency in the pursuit of a study as well as the capability it provides to investigate broad, complicated problems.

When a research project becomes large enough to require a team of workers, the administrative problems of securing adequate resources and maintaining the cohesiveness and productivity of the group are multiplied. Very large projects needing a large research staff are essentially autonomous organizational entities, often managed by an administrative staff and a project director who devotes much of his time to administrative problems rather than to the technical problems of the research. Such large-scale research efforts often become institutionalized, pursuing an organized program of research studies and engaging in more than one study at the same time.

There is some question as to whether research should be pursued as a full-time, specialized activity or whether it should be combined with other functions. Some advocate that teaching and research should be combined, either in a pattern whereby the two functions are carried on simultaneously or as consecutive activities. Among the various patterns are the faculty members who engage in research in the summer and teach during the rest of the year. Then, there is the administrator who carries out a research study in his spare time.

Although there is indeed great value in combining the functions of teaching and research, many research problems require the continuing full-time attention of members of a team. In fact, if an organization whose primary objective is that of teaching or service desires to pursue research on a fairly large scale it is essential that this function be conducted by a specialized unit. This is essential not only to provide sufficient resources for the research effort but to create a proper climate for the careful, unhurried pursuit of the study free from the possible disturbing influences of the workaday world. In a service agency, research should be separated from the agency's primary objective in order to avoid the biases that could affect the research and distort the findings when the two activities are intermixed.

SECURING ADEQUATE STAFF FOR THE RESEARCH

When a research project becomes too large for one investigator to manage by himself, he must enlist the services of other workers. These may be either professional staff, such as biologists and social scientists, industrial and systems engineers, statisticians and mathematicians, or supportive personnel, such as statistical clerks, electronic data-processing technicians, interviewers, and typists. These personnel can be employed on either a full- or part-time basis, depending on the requirements of the study. One type of part-time professional research staff member is the consultant, generally a specialist in some specific aspect of the research problem who can be called upon when needed. Consultants can play a most valuable role in a research project, particularly in many of the more technical phases for which it would be impractical to employ a full-time team member. Such methodological problems as development of the measuring instruments, selection of the sampling units, and processing of the data can often be satisfactorily solved by a consultant.

Another device for obtaining services for a research project other than hiring a full-time staff is to contract with specialized service agencies for certain requirements of the study. For example, if the data for the study are to be collected by mailed questionnaires from a large number of sampling units, the total mailing procedure can be handled by organizations whose primary function is that of addressing and mailing correspondence. Also, there are available, even in the smallest community, agencies devoted to the processing of statistical data. Such agencies usually maintain data-processing equipment of all kinds and have electronic computers available if they are needed.

In team research, one person is designated as the principal investigator. He has the major responsibility for the administration of the research. The principal investigator is generally the individual who originated the study, developed the initial research plan, is mainly responsible for its execution, and may write the final report. In large projects the principal investigator may devote all of his time to administrative problems associated with the research, leaving the supervision of the technical aspects to a project director or research associate.

In order to determine the staffing requirements for a research project it is necessary that the research plan be fairly well developed so that the demands for personnel can be assessed. Development of the research plan should not be the sole responsibility of the principal investigator and/or the project director but should involve other members of the team. A research plan should include a staffing budget in addition to a financial budget to carry out the study. This can be formulated on the basis of an assessment of the staff requirements for each phase of the study. Heaviest requirements will often arise during the data-collecting phase of the study. This is particularly true when the data are to be collected by direct observation or interviewing involving multiple observers.

It is highly advisable that all professional personnel who are to be involved in the study, even those on a part-time or consultative basis, be given an opportunity to become familiar with and offer suggestions about the research plan before it is finalized and any data are collected. Early involvement of all members of the research team not only can lead to constructive suggestions for the improvement of the total research design, but can serve to promote a sense of participation among the members of the research team and stimulate a coordinated effort toward the accomplishment of the research aims.

The value of early participation in the development of the research plan by all team members is frequently illustrated by reference to the role of a statistician in a study. Statisticians are often called in after the data have been collected and are asked to make sense out of them. If a statistician is involved before the data are collected, he can frequently offer constructive advice on the entire process of data collection and analysis as well on the total research design. If these suggestions are implemented before the data are actually gathered, they can significantly improve the quality of the research.

A useful device in executing a research plan is to set up an advisory committee consisting of persons who are not full-time members of the research team. The committee can include consultants to the project, persons in administrative positions in the service agency where the study is done, or faculty members if the study is being pursued within a university setting; they can provide overall guidance for the project and can serve as a sounding board to clarify objectives, concepts, and approaches.

Motivation of Research Team

During the execution of the study the principal investigator and/or project director must concern himself with ways of motivating and stimulating the members of the team toward the attainment of the objectives of the research. Ways of keeping the interest of the team high, of overcoming the frustrations and disappointments that can accompany any research effort, must be sought. Some phases of nearly all research projects can be repetitious and dull. It is essential, particularly in the data-collecting stage, for the project director to see that the members of the team are sufficiently motivated to sustain them over the less exciting but essential phases of the study's execution.

Turnover in any organized enterprise can be deleterious, but in a research project it can be especially harmful. Since the reliability of the data that have been collected depends to some extent on minimizing errors through the appropriate training of investigators, losses of personnel through attrition can slow the project down because of the need to see that replacements for personnel who have left are sufficiently oriented to the research methods employed in the study. Also, the introduction of a new person into the process of data collection increases the risk that unconscious psychological bias will be introduced into the study. For this reason the morale of the members of the research team must be kept as high as possible. One of the ways in which this can be achieved is to keep the research team informed about the objectives of the research and about progress made in achievement of these objectives. Opportunity should be provided for the team members to participate in discussions concerning the progress of the research, changes in its design occurring during the course of the study, and accomplishments that have been achieved.

The end product of many studies is a written report, hopefully one that is published. A boost to the morale of members of the research team is appropriate recognition of their contributions in the final report. If possible, they should participate in the actual writing of the report with due credit, of course, for authorship. Members of the research team should be strongly encouraged to publish separately whenever they can report on a selected aspect of the research for which they had special responsibility. Publication should be planned for at all stages. It is particularly important for researchers to publish their studies in scientific and professional periodicals where their peers can challenge their research findings.

A useful device for keeping all members of the research team fully informed of the progress of the study, as well as providing material that can serve as the foundation for the final report, is the preparation of periodic progress notes in the form of working papers during the execution of the study. These should be more than just a "news item" type of informational release and should contain preliminary analysis of the data, discussions of problem areas encountered in implementing the research design, elaborations of the conceptual model underlying the research. Such reports, or working papers, can serve as stimulants for discussion and for critical examination and refinement of the entire research effort. They can also be useful as historical documents concerning the development and progress of the research and as sources of ideas and guidance in the development of further research.

Acquiring staff for a research team is only one phase of the problem of administering a research project. And it may not be the most important phase. Keeping the team intact after the research has been launched is a persistent administrative problem. The success in accomplishing this is dependent on the ability to motivate the members of the team toward fulfillment of the research aims. This can be done by keeping interest high, encouraging the participation of team members in decisions that are

made, keeping the research goals always in sight of all team members, and
offering appropriate incentives to maintain a high quality of performance.

THE NURSE AS A RESEARCHER

An emerging role of the nurse as a researcher has highlighted some of
the problems as well as the successes in carrying out this role.

The authors would like to present two underlying assumptions before
discussing the conflicting elements affecting the role of the nurse as a researcher. These are:

1. The raison d'être for nurses doing research is to improve nursing
   practice.
2. Research in nursing is primarily interdisciplinary rather than multidisciplinary. Interdisciplinary research is usually considered group
   research in which the individual scientist may use the methods and
   theories of two or more disciplines and may become a specialist in a
   newly recognized discipline.[1] In multidisciplinary research scientists
   from several disciplines work relatively independently.[2]

Almost all of nursing research carried out since 1950, which marked
the period when research in nursing came to be recognized, has been interdisciplinary. In the early days it was the social scientist, sometimes the
physician, who assumed the key role of principal investigator. Therefore, it
is not surprising that the problems emerging in relation to achieving effective interdisciplinary research are those centered upon the social scientist
and the nurse.

The Russell Sage Foundation has pioneered in introducing the social
scientist into situations where he or she would work with other disciplines.
It is from the foundation's many years of experience in trying to achieve
collaboration between the social scientist and the health disciplines that
we can better understand the problems involved.[3]

The social scientists reported to the foundation the following ways of
attaining effective communication and collaboration:[4]

1. Achieving an optimal initial orientation and realistic level of expectation
2. Achieving maximum assimilation of "professional subcultural
   values" such as ideologies, technologies, and language
3. Making certain that the organizational structure in which the social
   scientist has to work permits him to fit into an appropriate position
4. Specific understanding and clarification of the roles involved in collaborative research
5. Improving the "interpersonal skills" of the participants.

Following the above guidelines does not assure effective collaboration, but achieving some of these objectives is essential. Orientation efforts probably will have to be continuous. A systematic effort on the part of both disciplines to assimilate a working knowledge of the other's field is crucial. The foundation suggests a very practical way in which the latter can be achieved—namely, making it possible for the social scientist and key professional staff involved to exchange courses for which they are responsible for teaching.

The introduction of the social scientist as part of the nursing faculty in a few schools of nursing has followed a hazardous and frustrating course for both the social scientists and the nurse. Lack of specific clarification of the roles of the professional practitioner and the social scientist has been a major deterrent. The scientist, at home in an academic setting, finds his freedom hampered in a quasi-militaristic setting of a school of nursing or hospital. Maintaining this freedom is essential if the scientist is to continue to be creative and productive.

There have been repeated situations in which the social scientist has been employed by a school of nursing or department of nursing in which he or she has survived in the situation for about one year before being sacrificed. This has occurred so frequently that the social scientist employed on the nursing faculty is referred to as the "sacrificial lamb." This unusual phenomenon raises several questions: Are nurses masochistic? Because the social scientist is a change agent, would he find survival difficult in any situation for the first three years?

Much can be learned from those situations where the "sacrificial lamb" phenomenon has occurred. The social scientist who is employed full time in the department of nursing without a dual appointment in his own discipline, or a specific time allotted to spend with his discipline, is apt to survive for the shortest period of time. Universities that have invited social scientists and nurse researchers as visiting professors have made good use of such "change agents" and have successfully prepared their faculty to utilize them when they become a part of the faculty. The importance of having the social scientist maintain one foot in his own discipline and one foot in the adopted profession cannot be overly stressed.

The nursing profession has adopted a feverish pace in carrying out its research endeavors. This, too, contributes to the shortening of the period of survival for the "change agent," for he is caught up in this haste and is pressured to produce. The social scientist, new in his role as collaborator, finds little, if any, time to familiarize himself with the new profession. It is estimated that it takes approximately three years for a social scientist to become thoroughly familiar with the profession with which he has chosen to collaborate.

Strong administrative backing and support as well as a climate conducive to research have also contributed to a longer survival period. A built-in safety valve, such as permitting the social scientist to return to his discipline periodically, was also found to be crucial. This might be achieved by initially planning to have the social scientist spend part of his time in his discipline—teaching, consulting, and/or doing research. Without this mechanism, within as little time as one year the social scientist might find it impossible to withdraw intellectually and emotionally from the situation.

Another survival feature noted was the social scientist's awareness of what strategy is essential if one is to survive—i.e., knowledge of where to avoid existing cross factions that might block any attempt at communication. Prior knowledge of the adopted profession and the health field in general can help to avoid errors of communication and the lack of identity of problems crucial to nursing. The same problems of survival will be faced by the nurse scientist, for she, too, must maintain identity, with her profession as she prepares herself in a related discipline.

The Russell Sage Foundation sums up the problem succinctly by stating that as long as professional practitioners and social scientists find themselves in interactive situations, hopefully there will be mutual learning of viewpoints if not acceptance of viewpoints.[5]

The nurse as a researcher faces many struggles similar to the social scientist's. Maintaining one's identity was recognized by Malone[6] when she joined a group of social scientists. As other nurse researchers, she had to face the constant struggle of whether to identify with her profession or with social scientists. The choice at times can be a lonely one, for her research training and associations teach her to observe from a scientific point of view, which might ostracize her from her own group. She is faced with two alternatives—either withdrawal from nursing or redefining the concepts of nursing.[7]

Major barriers to collaborative effort often find their basis in the ways in which research is perceived by the practitioner and the scientist. Research as perceived by the practitioner and the scientist may be summarized as follows:

Practitioner	Scientist
Clinical Nurse Specialist or Nurse Practitioner	Social, Physical, or Biological Scientist (This may be a Nurse Scientist)
1. Problems selected for study are operational, requiring immediate solution and have practical application.	1. Problem selected for study may or may not have immediate relevance to the real world. (Research is both basic and applied.)

Practitioner	*Scientist*
Clinical Nurse Specialist *or* *Nurse Practitioner*	*Social, Physical, or Biological* *Scientist (This may be a* *Nurse Scientist)*
2. Conceptualization of research is empirical and pragmatic.	2. Theoretical framework for research stems from literature, previous research, and basic postulates.
3. A practical plan of action is outlined.	3. Operational definitions are spelled out and hypotheses formulated.
4. Methods are selected and adopted from other fields rather than developing new methods.	4. Methods may need to be developed. Other disciplines may provide models and methods.
5. She observes the consequences of her action in light of the total program goals.	5. Criteria to evaluate the results of the project, particularly those dependent variables that are observable, are determined.
6. Analysis of the results is often based on subjective judgments.	6. The research design is set up in a way to permit an objective analysis of the data as they are obtained. This would permit modification or changing of the hypothesis(es). (Serendipity.)

7. Weighs the results of action as they affect individual patients or groups of patients.
    Is slow to initiate change and may not do so if the patient(s) is not ready to accept the change.
	7. Evaluation is based on criteria which are checked consistently for their validity and reliability.
	    The theoretical framework provides the source to which the results of the experiment are directed.

8. Results of actions are limited to one situation and cannot be generalized.	8. Inferences can be drawn from the findings that can be related to other situations.
9. She uses the results of action to add to her experience to resolve similar problems.	9. New hypotheses are identified for future study.
10. Results of action are communicated immediately to permit solution of the problem. Experiences may be reported in professional journals as descriptive reports of one situation.	10. Research findings are reported to a body of scientists and practitioners through scientific and professional journals, papers, and conferences.

As nurses become increasingly oriented to the basic science disciplines and are able to direct their own research projects, is is hoped that collaborative research can be achieved to a much greater extent.

SECURING FACILITIES TO CONDUCT THE RESEARCH

Obtaining a site in which to conduct the research is particularly important in experimental research. Experimental design requires that the setting in which the research is conducted be highly controlled. Often, a specially devised setting is employed, such as an experimental unit or a laboratory. These might be specially constructed facilities containing equipment and layout tailor-made for the research. In experimental studies the problem of securing facilities is usually greater than in research conducted in a natural or in a partially controlled setting. In studies conducted in natural settings, however, there may not be a clear separation between the research setting and the actual work situation. As a consequence, a problem often encountered is interference with the work being performed. Thus, if our study requires that we observe the actual delivery of infants on an obstetrical unit in a hospital, we must make sure that the process of observation will not disturb the functioning of the delivery room.

Where the data are to be collected by indirect means, such as by a questionnaire, the interference problem is less obvious to the researcher but can raise havoc in an institution or agency when multiple questionnaires are received. It is the responsibility of the researcher, or the adviser of graduate students, to clear with the institution before questionnaires are sent out. Researchers and student advisers must assume greater responsibility in screening all questionnaires.

A research unit that is part of an operating agency, such as a school, public health department, or a hospital, has fewer problems in securing a setting for the research than does an independent research agency that may have to depend on the cooperation of others for the site in which to conduct the research. Experimental studies involving radical modifications of existing facilities require detailed planning. Securing facilities for non-experimental research is largely a matter of having office space for the members of the team and facilities where the data can be processed.

OBTAINING COOPERATION OF RESEARCH SUBJECTS

As nurse investigators seek to develop and refine scientific knowledge and theory in nursing through clinical investigations, increasing emphasis is being placed upon the protection of research subjects.

Nurse practitioners involved in data collection for other investigators are equally involved and must be concerned about the protection of human subjects, particularly when the outcomes are not known.

The American Nurses' Association as part of the activity of the ANA Commission on Nursing Research has developed a very useful document for human rights guidelines for nurses in clinical and other research.*

* American Nurses' Association. *Human Rights Guidelines for Nurses in Clinical and Other Research.* ANA Publication No. D-465M, July 1975.

It is suggested that:

- All proposals, investigative instruments, protocols, and techniques to be used need to be specified and discussed with the prospective subject and other workers who are expected to participate.
- Safeguards be developed to make sure that no unanticipated physical, psychological, or social disadvantage accrues to subjects either during the investigation or as a result of the dissemination of findings.
- Protection of the subjects' anonymity be assured.
- Protection of the confidentiality of information when not under control of the investigator.
- Consent to participate in research or clinical activities be obtained from the prospective subject. Such consent is expected to cover an explanation of the study, the procedures to be followed, their purposes, a description of physical risk or discomfort, any invasion of privacy, any threat to dignity and the methods used to protect anonymity and insure confidentiality.

The Privacy Act (Public Law 93–579) effective on September 27, 1975, states that its primary purpose is to provide safeguards for individuals against invasions of personal privacy. The Act requires federal agencies and federal contractors to:

- Permit individuals to determine what records pertaining to them the agency collects, maintains, uses, or disseminates;
- Permit individuals to prevent records pertaining to them obtained for a particular purpose from being used or made available for another purpose without their consent;
- Permit individuals to gain access to information pertaining to them in federal agency records, to have a copy made of their records, and to correct or amend their records;
- Collect, maintain, use, or disseminate records of identifiable personal information in a manner that assures that such action is for a necessary and lawful purpose, that the information is current and accurate for its intended use, and that adequate safeguards are provided to prevent misuse of information;
- Be subject to civil suit for damages which occur as a result of willful or intentional actions that violate any individual's rights under the Act.

In addition, subsection (i) of section 3 of the Act states that employees of an agency maintaining a system of records shall be subject to criminal penalties for willful or intentional actions which violate any individual's rights under the Act.

Comprehensive guidelines for ethical standards have also been issued by the American Psychological Association.*

Research subjects may take a variety of forms. If the subjects are inanimate objects, as in a study of the cost of different types of disposable syringes, or animals, as in a study of the effect of sensory deprivation on monkeys, the problems are few in obtaining the cooperation of subjects. Where human beings are the study subjects, problems of cooperation might be formidable, particularly where the research may involve some unpleasantness for the subjects.

An important requisite in obtaining the cooperation of human research subjects is to explain fully the purpose of the study and to impress the subject with the importance of his participation in it. Sometimes an inducement, such as a promise to make the report of the study available to the subject, will help to obtain cooperation. Or where the study requires a large expenditure of time, perhaps an incentive as tangible as providing the subject with a free physical examination, free drugs, or services, or even the payment of money may help to offset any unpleasantness or bother to which he is exposed. In any event, written permission from the patient to participate as a study subject is a *must*.

In studies involving cluster sampling, in which random samples are drawn at several stages—say, first a sample of schools is drawn, then a sample of students—the cooperation of two groups must be obtained. Random sampling, even at one stage, presents special problems. Theoretically each unit selected for study by the random process must be included in the study. Failure to secure cooperation of a sampling unit that has been selected can bias the results of the study. In studies using mailed questionnaires such bias is called the error of nonresponse. To reduce this error various techniques can be employed, including sending follow-up questionnaires to those not returning the original and including a strong appeal for cooperation.

In prospective longitudinal studies where contact with study subjects often extends over a lengthy period of time, the problem of maintaining the cooperation of the subjects throughout the course of the study can be formidable. Attrition from such a study can seriously harm its validity. In developing the plan for a longitudinal study, safeguards must be provided to keep attrition of subjects to a minimum.

One way of increasing the likelihood that the cooperation of study subjects will be secured and maintained is to assure the confidentiality of the data that are collected. This is particularly important where the study deals with matters of a rather personal nature. Assurance that the data

* Ad hoc Committee on Ethical Standards in Psychological Research. *Ethical Principles in the Conduct of Research with Human Participants,* Washington, D.C., American Psychological Association, Inc., 1973, 104 pp.

collected from the subject will be kept strictly anonymous and that they will be used only for research purposes will help to alleviate any fears the subjects may have in this regard.

SEEKING FINANCIAL SUPPORT FOR RESEARCH

"Grantsmanship" is something that is learned empirically. Few researchers have this skill. The following discussion is intended to provide some guidelines for researchers in developing research proposals for which financial support might be sought. The administrator of a university, hospital, or health agency has an important role to play if the research is to be conducted successfully by these institutions. The responsibilities of the administrator and researcher in conducting research will be discussed first.

Responsibilities of Universities and Health Agencies in Conducting Research

What are the responsibilities of universities and health agencies in conducting research? It is generally agreed that the goals of a university are teaching, research, and service. Teaching hospitals can be said to have similar goals. State universities, particularly land grant institutions, and hospitals must of necessity give more attention to service.

Many universities lack the organizational structure to facilitate interdisciplinary research. Existing departmental barriers inhibit rather than facilitate interdisciplinary research.[8] In an attempt to solve this problem, universities have set up centers, institutes, and laboratories that provide a research climate where interdisciplinary research might be conducted.

In nursing, as well as in other fields of knowledge, the quality and volume of research can have a direct influence upon the caliber of education provided by the university. If the research being conducted is pedestrian, the quality of teaching can suffer. There must be a balance between research and teaching. The dean, director, or department head of the school must decide how much and what kind of research can be conducted within the school of nursing as well as in the clinical divisions of the hospital or health agencies associated with it. Too often administrators force research upon members of their staff who have no training or talent for it.[9] Hopefully, how much research and what kind, as well as the need for interdisciplinary research, can be determined by the dean, the faculty, and appropriate representatives of other departments (including hospital and nursing service administration) prior to initiating specific research projects.

Many difficulties encountered in conducting research often stem from the way in which the institution administers its research grants program.

Price[10] has provided some guidelines which should help those responsible for administering such a program.

1. No research grant or contract should be secured and then assigned to someone to carry out who has not been involved in the research design.

2. The university or health agency concerned should support and encourage principal investigators to apply for and secure financing for their research projects.

3. Whenever possible, graduate and undergraduate students should be involved in the research program.

4. A research contingency fund should be set up by the institution to handle research expenses not chargeable elsewhere. Such expenses include support for time to develop a research proposal, travel to institutions conducting related research, and for conducting small pilot studies.

5. Research activities that utilize space of the university or health agency should administer funds through that agency.

6. The institution administering the research should have prior publication and patent rights. Any royalties resulting should be shared by the institution and the investigator.

7. Salary supplements and consultant fees for those within the university or health agency should be prohibited. Those participating in research activities should be permitted to do so only on a released time basis.

8. Membership on the graduate faculty should include active participation in a research program that would justify a reduced teaching load.

9. Research proposals in departments of arts and sciences that relate to a particular profession such as nursing or public health should be reviewed by the professional school in that university or one within the immediate vicinity. Likewise, proposals developed in professional schools that utilize the research tools and/or resources of university departments should be reviewed by the chairman of the department. Some universities have found it helpful to set up specific procedures regarding clearance of research proposals before they are submitted for support.

10. The principal investigator should be a member of the university faculty or institution receiving the grant. This permits the administrator of the institution to achieve a proper balance between research and teaching and/or research and service.

11. To deal with the complex problems of grants management some institutions, particularly universities, have employed a grants management officer. A scientist administrator would be an ideal person for this position. The grants associate program at the National Institutes of Health provides a 12-month training program for this type of person.

Preparing a Research Proposal in Applying for Financial Support

In the preparation and review of research proposals it is wise to give equal consideration to the substantive and methodological aspects of the study as well as to the administrative problems in carrying it out. The scientific substance of the plan is the responsibility of those who will execute it. The principal investigator should be given every opportunity to maintain his scientific freedom in carrying out his research objectives. However, once the plan has been approved and receives financial support, the investigator should be allowed to make only those changes in methodology, approach, or other aspects of the project that would expedite achievement of the research objectives already stated.

When support is requested for a project from an outside agency it becomes all the more important for the institution in which the research is initiated to carry out its own preliminary review process before the application is submitted. Use of an internal advisory committee, previously discussed, can be useful for this purpose.

The large amounts of federal funds being expended for medical research have brought about an external control by panels representing the special interests of particular fields of science. These panels review research proposals submitted for grant support and pass on their scientific merits and worthiness to receive financial backing. For example, the U.S. Public Health Service has fifty study sections responsible for providing the scientific evaluation of a proposal. These study sections are made up of multidisciplinary health professionals and consumers.

The following pages contain a suggested outline* of a research proposal that might be used in applying for financial support to undertake a research project. Although the immediate purpose of such a proposal is to convince the money-granting authority of the merits of the project and secure their financial backing, it can serve as the plan for study and be used to guide its execution. A proposal contains not only a description of the design of the research, it also provides a financial budget and a staffing plan that can be most useful in administering the project efficiently and economically.

Part I

1. *Research Plan*

    A. Research Objectives
       State your research objectives in terms of your immediate aims (those to be accomplished the first two years) and your long-range goals.
       Present the rationale for your research, giving particular attention to the theoretical basis for your research.

    B. Research Design
       Provide a statement of the nature of your proposed research—i.e., is it descriptive (experimental or nonexperimental), explanatory (experimental or nonexperimental), methodological, or a combination of these.
       Describe your research plan, detailing the steps in your methodology, relating each step to the specific aims stated under A. If you are testing hypotheses, state these

* Adapted from U.S. Public Health Service Research Grant Application.

concisely, providing operational definitions and relating the hypotheses to concepts that led you to make these deductions.

Specify what data you need to collect, relating it to the research question(s) posed, and how the data are to be collected, tabulated, and analyzed. Whenever possible provide examples of data to be collected, sample work sheets, and skeleton table outlines. If the research is experimental in nature, show how you propose to control for any biases—e.g., observer bias, contamination between control and experimental groups.

C. Significance of the Proposed Research

Relate the significance of the research to the rationale. What will the research contribute—e.g., new knowledge (specify), a new theory, a new method or approach? Does the research design permit inferences to be drawn from the data?

D. Research Climate

Present a concise statement of the personnel resources and facilities available to carry out your work. State what steps have been taken to assure close working relationships with administration, the school of nursing, nursing and medical services, and, if appropriate, the community agency.

2. *Supporting Data*

A. Previous Work Done on the Project

State any previous work that you and/or members of your research team have completed that would have bearing on the present research.

B. Related Research

Select approximately five references that show related work in this area or indicate significant developments that have a bearing upon your proposed research.

Part II

Biographical Sketches

Provide a curriculum vitae for each key member of the research team.

Part III

Budget (for first 12 months of project)

1. Personnel........................ Category Total $_____

List all professional (these should be named), technical, secretarial personnel on the research team, even if salary is not requested. For professional staff, indicate per cent of work effort on the project as averaged out over the year. For other staff, state the number of hours per week on the project. Separate out any deductions for social security, retirement, etc., and state as a separate amount for each member of the research team. On a separate page state the functions of key members of the research team.	Hours per week	Per cent time on project	Funds requested	
			Institution	Outside sources

2. Consultants...................... Category Total $_____

If needed, list consultants to the project. These should be named and their contribution indicated. Include fees, travel and per diem costs.

3. Equipment...................... Category Total $_____

List all large items of equipment separately. Small items may be grouped. Indicate which items are available at the institution and which ones will have to be purchased. Equipment items should be grouped into scientific equipment (e.g., tape recorder) and other equipment (e.g., desk, etc.).

4. Supplies........................ Category Total $_____

List major items, such as tapes, office supplies, etc. Separate materials for scientific purposes (e.g., animals), from other supplies.

5. Travel.......................... Category Total $_____

Travel of the research team to related projects, professional meetings and patient travel costs essential to the project are examples.

6. Patient Costs.................... Category Total $_____

It may be necessary to cover the hospitalization costs for patients for study purposes. (The institution should be able to supply average per diem costs for patients to help you arrive at an estimate.)

7. Alteration and Renovation......... Category Total $_____

Any proposed changes should be detailed with justification. (Granting agencies usually set ceilings for this category).

8. Publication..................... Category Total $_____

Specify any publication costs, reprints, etc.

9. Other Costs..................... Category Total $_____

Machine tabulation, rental, and maintenance costs are examples that might be specified.

10. Indirect Costs................... Category Total $_____

Each institution or agency usually has a set indirect cost allowance. This amount usually goes to the institution to help to defray the costs of building maintenance, rent, etc. The amount of indirect cost allowance may vary from 50 to 100 per cent.

11. Total, All Categories.............. Category Total $_____

This should represent the total costs for the *first* 12 months of the project.

Budget Estimate for Total Years of Project

Category	1st year	2nd year	3rd year	4th year	5th year
1. Personnel					
2. Consultants					
3. Equipment					
4. Supplies					
5. Travel					
6. Patient Costs					
7. Alteration and renovation					
8. Publication					
9. Other costs					
10. Indirect costs					
11. All Categories Total					

Guidelines for Setting up Budget Determinations

Professional Salaries Persons employed by the university, institution, or health agency full-time should be reimbursed from grant funds only on a released time basis. If a person is part-time or wishes to work on a research project during his vacation, compensation from grant funds should be at the same rate as for full-time employment.

Consultants who are not employed by the institution may be reimbursed from grant funds in an amount sufficient to cover honoraria, per diem, and travel if necessary.

An institutional policy should be established regarding the way in which time and effort should be reported on a research project. Most institutions now use an ex post facto time and effort estimate report to be completed on a quarterly basis, within one month following the end of the quarter concerned. The professional staff on the project should report an average amount of time and effort spent on the research project during each quarterly period. (In most instances it is easiest to base this estimate on a forty-hour week.) All other staff should use hours per week as a way of reporting time on the project.

Equipment Institutions will want to develop a clear policy regarding the use and purchase of equipment. It is helpful to have an institutional official determine that there is no other equipment available or suitable for the intended use. He should also approve the purchase of each item of equipment that has been fully justified by the investigator.

Travel This category more than any other seems to create many problems. Many of these could be avoided if the institution has developed specific policies regarding domestic and foreign travel. It is often highly desirable for members of the research team to visit related research projects and to attend professional meetings. However, when one institution has multiple research projects it becomes necessary to set up a mechanism to review the travel needs of each investigator, to control attendance at meetings, and to evaluate the pertinence of the travel to that project being supported. The record should show that an institutional official has approved the travel. A "hard" and "soft" money travel policy should be avoided.

Transfer of funds from one category to another should be permissible with the exception of "equipment" and "travel," which should be fixed and require permission from the institution and/or granting agency before funds are added to these categories.

Reducing the Costs of a Research Project

Research can be a costly activity. Competent research workers have highly developed and often hard-to-find skills. They should be paid at a level commensurate with their skills. The collection of data can incur sizable expenses and is often the largest single cost item. This is particularly true where direct collection is employed, involving observers or interviewers.

It has been estimated that the cost per sampling unit for various methods of data collection are as follows:*

Mailed questionnaire	$ 2.00 to $ 10.00
Interview	10.00 to 100.00
Direct observation	10.00 to 150.00

There are several ways in which the costs of collecting data for a research project can be controlled. Briefly, these are:

1. *Use of existing data.* For some research projects it may be possible to use data originally gathered for some other purpose. Care must be taken, however, that the data meet the specifications for the research in which they are to be applied—that the definitions of the variables parallel those in the study and the data are sufficiently reliable and valid.

---

* Includes costs of developing and printing the forms, selecting the sample, mailing costs (questionnaires), travel costs (interview, direct observation), and salaries of interviewers and observers. The figures are based on a questionnaire of average length, 15–20 items; an interview of an hour's duration; direct observation totaling about an hour per sampling unit but perhaps fragmented into a series of observations of small duration. Higher costs reflect need to travel sizable distances to conduct interviews or to make observations, the use of expensive equipment, or the need to employ highly skilled personnel to collect the data—e.g., physicians to make physical examinations of the subjects.

2. *Use of sampling.* Among the numerous advantages of sampling is the lowering of the costs of collecting data. When the cost per sampling unit for data collection is very high, the size of the sample should be kept to the minimum number that will yield the level of precision desired for the study.

3. *Use of volunteers.* In some research situations it may be possible to use volunteer assistance in the collection of the data. For example, if we are conducting our study in a hospital, it may be possible to enlist the help of the hospital's volunteer organization in collecting the data, particularly where special skills are not required for this task. A training period for those collecting data must be planned for and carried out prior to the data collection phase.

Economies can also be introduced into the data-processing phase of the study. The use of mechanical equipment in tabulating the data can often reduce processing costs below what they would be if the hand method were employed, particularly when the equipment is available in the school, hospital, or other agency where the research is being conducted.

SOME MAJOR DETERRENTS TO RESEARCH

Insufficient time and funds are cited by researchers as the main deterrents to the research effort.[11] To counteract this there is an attempt now in many universities to establish research career award positions to provide sustaining support for investigators who are solely dependent upon research grant funds for support but who have a distinguished record in the research field. Appointing researchers to faculty positions with tenure also helps to provide the researcher with some security regarding his future assignments.

Another deterrent is lack of information on important areas of research. Researchers have expressed a need for the following information:

1. Sources of financial support
2. Current research
3. Research personnel and consultants in the field
4. New innovations in equipment and techniques
5. Resources available on the campus or in the community

Another major deterrent to research is the lack of clarity with which a researcher prepares his protocol. In a study conducted by the National Institutes of Health, it was found that over half (58 per cent) of the research proposals were disapproved because of weaknesses in the statement of the problem[12]—for example, the proposed problem was scientifically premature and based on unsound hypotheses. In 73 per cent of the applications disapproved, it was felt that the proposed research would not yield any useful data; and in 55 per cent the research team did not give evidence of sufficient competencies to carry out the research.

Summary

A scientifically sound research plan does not guarantee that the research itself will be successfully executed. The plan has to be soundly managed, and this includes securing and maintaining adequate resources for the conduct of the research. Among the resources for a research project are personnel, money, a site to conduct the research, and study subjects from whom the data will be collected.

Administering a research project is similar to the management of any organized enterprise. Its quality can be improved by the use of such techniques as a financial and personnel budget, incentives for staff productivity, and the use of labor-saving devices.

References

1. Daniel Howland, "Engineering in Interdisciplinary Research," *J. Engineering Education,* **52:**664–670, June 1962.
2. *Ibid.,* p. 665.
3. Russell Sage Foundation, *Annual Report 1959–1960.* Russell Sage Foundation, New York.
4. *Ibid.,* pp. 8–9.
5. *Ibid.,* p. 16.
6. Warren G. Bennis, Norman H. Berkowitz, Mary F. Malone, and Malcolm W. Klein, *The Role of the Nurse in the Outpatient Department.* New York, American Nurses' Foundation, Inc., 1961, pp. 86–88.
7. Mary F. Malone, "Research as Viewed by Researcher and Practitioner." *Nursing Forum,* **1:**43, spring 1962.
8. William R. Willard, "The Present Status and Future Development of Community Health Research—A Critique: From the Viewpoint of Educational Institutions." *Ann. New York Acad. Sc.,* **107:**776, May 22, 1963.
9. Charles V. Kidd, "The Effect of Research Emphasis on Research Itself." *Research and Medical Education,* **37:**100, December 1962.
10. Daniel O. Price, *University Research Administration Policies.* Atlanta, Georgia, Southern Regional Educational Board, 1962, pp. 4–14.
11. Southern Regional Educational Board, *Mental Health Research in the South on the Threshold of the 60*'s. Atlanta, SREB, August 1960, pp. 19–21.
12. Ernest M. Allen. "Why Are Research Grant Applications Disapproved?" *Science,* **132:**1532–1534, November 25, 1960.

Problems and Suggestions for Further Study

1. Make an analysis of university, hospital, or health agency policies regarding the use of grant funds for travel, equipment, and the use of consultants. Develop proposed policies that your institution might consider regarding these categories.

2. Prepare a budget page for a three-year research project relating it to the stated specific aims of your research. Develop a time schedule for your proposed research indicating which phases of the research will be covered.

3. What are some guidelines for determining when the services of a consultant are needed? How would you go about obtaining the services of a consultant for a research project?

4. Read the article by D. Mainland, "The Clinical Trial—Some Difficulties and Suggestions" (*J. Chronic Dis.,* **11:**484–496, May 1960). Comment on the quotation from Bradford Hill in this article that "Every departure from the design of the experiment lowers its efficiency to some extent; too many departures may wholly nullify it."

5. Refer to the article by King and Spector, "Ethical and Legal Aspects of Survey Research" (*Am. Psychologist,* **18:**204–208, 1963). Discuss the question raised by the authors, "Can the survey research turn information against the respondent that the respondent has voluntarily offered?"

6. In Chapter 6 of his book, *An Introduction to Scientific Research* (New York, McGraw-Hill Book Co., 1952), E. Bright Wilson discusses some of the practical problems in executing a research study. Explain some of the "search" principles provided by the author in this chapter. Comment on his statement, "When Sherlock Holmes mystified his friend Dr. Watson by his amazing deductions, he was utilizing to the fullest degree the data available to him—the muddy boot, the ash of a cigar, the torn ticket. This is a practice which is also basic in the highest forms of scientific research" (p. 148).

7. George Bush and Lowell Hattery in their *Scientific Research, Its Administration and Organization* (Washington, American University Press, 1950) give some principles of administration applicable to research, and in the same authors' *Teamwork in Research* (Washington, American University Press, 1953) they offer some guidelines for motivating the research team. Which of these principles and guidelines are pertinent to research in nursing and patient care? See also, Editorial, "University Responsibility." *Science,* **140:**861, May 24, 1963.

8. Indicate some of the practical problems that might be encountered in undertaking research on the following problems:
   a. The "real" reasons why student nurses drop out of school
   b. What is the best way of teaching family members of patients in home care programs when there are difficulties in communication (language barriers, illiteracy, etc.)?
   c. The role of the nursing aide in the care of emotionally disturbed patients in the short-term general hospital
   d. Developing a tool to measure the quality of performance of the staff nurse in a public health agency
   e. Is private duty nursing no longer necessary?

  f. The use of television in monitoring patients

  g. What is the independent role of the professional nurse in patient care?

  h. How can errors in the provision of patient care be controlled?

9. What are some of the benefits to be gained from the use of an advisory committee for a research study? Are there any problems that can arise from the use of such committees? What are some ways in which advisory committees can be utilized most effectively?

10. From an administrative standpoint how might the following situations that can arise in executing a research project be dealt with?

  a. A hospital administrator refuses to participate in a study even though his institution was selected in the random sample drawn for the study.

  b. During the processing of the data it is discovered that the original estimate for the cost of data processing was much too low. There is no money available in the budget to pay for the increased costs.

  c. In a study that involves the direct observation of nursing personnel as they perform their tasks during the regular workday it appears that the personnel are not behaving naturally. Aware of being observed, they have altered their normal routines and are performing atypically.

  d. A key research assistant has been offered a higher paying, more responsible position during the data-collecting phase of the study. If he leaves, the study will suffer a serious setback.

  e. The research project was the joint effort of several investigators. Each contributed equally to its development and execution. Questions concerning who shall write the report, how shall credit be assigned, who is the senior author have arisen.

  f. In collecting data on hospitalized patients by direct interviewing of the patients, the researcher notices a number of instances of poor practice in the provision of care to the patients. The interviewer does not know whether to communicate this to the nursing service administrator or not.

11. Read Chapter 2, "Who Should Do Research," in Hans Selye *From Dream to Discovery: On Being a Scientist* (New York, Arno, 1975). Comment on the following statement by the author:

> We have become accustomed to thinking that while religions are built on faith, and poetry on dreams, the prime prerequisite for research is pure intellect. Yet, the basic researcher must also be able to dream and have faith in his own dreams. To make a great dream come true, the first requirement is a great capacity to dream; the second is persistence—continued faith in the dream. Pure intellect is largely a quality of the middle-class mind. The lowliest hooligan and the greatest creator in any field of human endeavor are driven by imponderable instincts and emotions, especially by an unreasoned desire for, and faith in, success. Scientific research —the most purely intellectual creative effort of which man is capable— represents no exception in this respect. The initial impulse and the strength to persevere both feed on emotion; intellect is merely a powerful weapon that faith uses to attain its goal.

12. Describe a study involving patients in which you must collect clinical data directly from the patients. Specify the procedures to be followed, their purposes, describe any physical risk or discomfort, any invasion of privacy, and how you propose to handle the data to assure anonymity.

3

CASE STUDIES OF RESEARCH

The following chapters will present detailed discussions of various studies that have been conducted in the field of nursing. These studies will be presented within a typology of research that groups the studies according to two characteristics: their broad purpose and their design. Chapter 11 will explain this typology, and the following three chapters will contain extended discussions of selected research projects, which will be grouped according to their placement in the typology for research in nursing.

The purpose of Part III of this book is twofold. First, the presentation of a typology for research will serve to identify concretely the similarities as well as the distinguishing dissimilarities—of purpose, setting, methodology etc.—of many studies that have been conducted in the area of nursing. The typology can serve as an aid to future researchers in clarifying the purpose of their research, in selecting methodology, and perhaps most important of all, in determining where in the many ramifications of research being conducted in a particular area, the findings of a research project contribute to a further understanding of the area studied. Moreover, such a typology could suggest areas for future research.

Second, a purpose of presenting analyses of completed research is to provide the reader with some deeper insight into the way the researcher went about conducting his study. By seeing the problems faced by researchers and the ways in which they were resolved, future researchers might obtain useful leads in the conduct of their own projects.

The material presented as case studies is essentially the same as that which appeared in the first edition of this book. Although many studies have appeared in the nursing field since 1965 it was the decision of the authors to keep this material intact rather than update it. Although taken from an earlier era in nursing research the studies are still very useful as examples. Moreover, they cover a period when a very rich variety of studies were undertaken. Too, in some instances the studies presented are out-of-print, or difficult to retrieve, so that this collection serves as a useful reference source.

To update this collection, at the end of each chapter an update note is presented that provides references to more recent study collections. These easily obtainable sources can supplement the case studies presented herein.

Chapter Eleven

A TYPOLOGY FOR NURSING RESEARCH

THERE are many ways to classify research. Chapter 3 of this book presented one possible categorization which consists of numerous dimensions. One of these dimensions can be called the reason for doing research. Two broad reasons were delineated:

Basic or pure research—to establish fundamental theories, facts, and/or statements of relationships among facts, in an area of knowledge, which are *not* intended for immediate use in a real-life situation. Basic research is useful in advancing scientific knowledge and in furthering research.

Applied research—to obtain facts and/or identify relationships among facts which are intended to be used in a real-life situation, specifically to:
1. Solve a problem
2. Make a decision
3. Develop a program, procedure, process or product
4. Evaluate a program, procedure, process, or product

Basic research is regarded as "pure research" conducted in some remote laboratory or experimental unit, uncontaminated by any real-world considerations. In a similar vein, basic research is often regarded as theoretical and abstract in nature, far-removed from any concrete, lifelike substantive matters. By these considerations most studies conducted in nursing would be categorized as applied research, since they deal with the solution of practical problems. They are often also conducted in naturalistic settings.

The delineation of basic and applied research can often lead to sterile arguments. The test of the usefulness of such a distinction should be a pragmatic one: What purpose does it serve?

For one thing, this distinction, more than any other dimension of the typology, influences expectations concerning how the findings of the research will be used. If the research is basic, the findings can be expected to augment the intellectual storehouse of the field with which it is concerned. The augmentation may be in the form of descriptive facts, or there may be statements of relationships that the study found to be true.

One example of the former is: "The study revealed that 90 per cent of the nurses employed part-time in hospitals were married." An example of the latter is: "As the hierarchy of nursing service organization is ascended, greater deviation is found between the incumbent's conception of what her job ideally should be and what the demands of her job actually are."

If the research were "applied," the findings would be expected to have applicability to the field in which it was done and to be capable of influencing human behavior. Thus, one example of the findings of an applied study might be: "The number of medication errors was nearly twice as high on the surgical ward as on the medical ward." Another example is: "Fewer nursing visits are required to be made to the patients in their homes when the family members receive orientation by the nurse on the care of the patients after discharge from the hospital." It is difficult to see how a finding that most part-time nurses are married or that nurses in supervisory positions view their jobs with some disillusionment could influence behavior except in an indirect way. This influence would certainly be less direct in its impact on behavior than a finding that instructing family members can reduce the need for nursing visits or that more medication errors occur on surgical units than on medical units.

However, in much of the research in nursing that has already been done or that might be done in the near future, the distinction between applied and basic research, in terms of the use to which the findings may be put, can often be quite blurred. In the natural sciences rather sharp distinctions exist between research conducted purely for the advancement of knowledge and research for the purpose of producing practical results. By contrast, research on human beings often produces a mixture of results that add to knowledge and/or might influence human behavior in a practical way.

The distinction between "applied" and "basic" research in nursing not only influences the expectations concerning the use to which the research findings can be put—the final stage of research—but also influences the very early stages of research—the formulation of the problem. The intermediate steps of the research process differ little whether the research is basic or applied. This statement may appear to contradict popular belief that basic research is more tightly controlled, more "scientific," more experimental in design than applied research. Although it is probably true that a higher proportion of studies categorized as basic research have used tightly controlled experimental designs as compared to applied studies, there is no reason why such designs should be restricted only to basic research. The main differences between basic and applied research lie in the applicability of the findings to practical matters and in the formulation of the problem.

The way in which the researcher formulates his problem is influenced by the use to which the findings are put. To maximize the usefulness of basic research the research problem should be so formulated as to be referable to the mainstream of developments in knowledge and theory in the area being studied. To maximize the usefulness of applied research the problem should be so formulated as to provide widespread generalization of results beyond the research setting and subjects. A finding concerning anxiety states among leukemic children can be said to have fulfilled the reason for doing basic research if it can be integrated with existing knowledge of patient care and contribute to a general advancement of knowledge in the field. A finding that the use of intensive care nursing units reduces mortality of patients with cardiac arrest can be said to have accomplished the goal of applied research if the finding can be put to use beyond the hospital where the research was conducted. Therefore, in formulating a research problem it is important to conceptualize how the findings might contribute to knowledge and theory, as in basic research, or how they will be used in other situations, as in applied research.

As has been indicated, the distinction between basic and applied research in the field of nursing may not be of much value to either the user or doer of research because the two purposes are often intermixed in studies involving human beings. It would seem that for nursing the most useful classification would be one that would distinguish between the *specific aims* of the research and the *methodology* that was employed in conducting it. In Chapter 3 two aims of research were discussed: to discover new facts, called *descriptive* research, and to discover relationships among facts, called *explanatory* research. To these can be added a third aim of research: to develop methods, tools, products, or procedures for conducting further research or for use in practice. This can be called *methodological* research.

Also in Chapter 3, two broad types of methodology were delineated: the *experimental* method, in which the research is conducted under highly controlled conditions, and the *nonexperimental* method, in which the research is conducted under largely uncontrolled conditions. To this classification can be added a third category, called the partial experimental method, in which the study has features of both experimental and nonexperimental research design.

The remainder of this chapter will discuss this typology of research. An attempt will be made to show how it can be useful to the researcher as well as to the consumer of research. The following chapters will analyze completed studies in nursing in terms of their placement within this typology.

AIMS OF RESEARCH

In discussing the distinction between basic and applied research we have delineated two broad purposes in undertaking research: to add to knowledge (basic) or to influence behavior (applied). Research purposes can be viewed in a more specific way: to develop a tool, method, product or procedure for research or for practice (methodological); to discover new facts (descriptive); or to discover relationships among facts (explanatory). Often these three specific aims are incorporated within a single research study. Thus, *Studies in Social Psychology in World War II*,[1] a series of studies of American soldiers in World War II, made important methodological contributions to the theory of scaling and questionnaire construction, produced a considerable amount of interesting descriptive data on the social and psychological characteristics of the participants of World War II, and uncovered a number of valuable explanatory relationships concerning behavior patterns of the study participants. Similarly, Hasselmeyer's study[2] of the effects of a diaper roll support on premature infants produced several new tools of value to nurse practitioners, including a weight chart for recording weight gain of premature infants.[3] The study also yielded masses of statistical data on the behavior of premature infants during their first 40 days of life and provided the results of tests concerning the hypothesis of a relationship between diaper roll support and infant behavior.

The classification of studies by the "basic-applied" dichotomy can be superimposed on the classification by specific aim. Thus, we can add to knowledge by developing new methodology, producing new facts, or discovering relationships among facts. Similarly, we can influence behavior by accomplishing any or all of these purposes of research.

Methodological Research

To some the development of a tool, method, product, or procedure is not research in the strictest sense. Sometimes a distinction is made between research and development, the former referring to the descriptive or explanatory studies that are conducted as a prelude to the actual development of the tool or product. If the tool being developed is to be used in collecting data in a research study, such as a measuring instrument of some kind like a scale or a test, there is usually no question as to the appropriateness of labeling this activity as research. In fact, Greenberg[4] goes so far as to classify the development or refinement of measuring tools as pure or basic research.

In research in nursing, two main types of methodological research can be identified: (1) that which develops tools for research methodology and (2) that which develops tools for nursing administration, practice, or education. In terms of total volume produced, the second type has far outnumbered the research tools. This probably reflects the demand in nursing for discovering new and improved ways of providing patient care.

Very often, tools that were originally developed for administrative or educational purposes find their way into use as research methodologies.

Thus, as will be discussed in detail in the following chapter, instruments that have been developed to measure the needs of patients for nursing services were primarily intended to be used as administrative tools to assist nursing administration in the prediction of nurse staffing requirements. However, several studies have used these same instruments to gather research data—as, for example, the research at Johns Hopkins Hospital to determine optimum nurse staffing patterns.[5] Conversely, some instruments that were originally developed to be used as methodology for research have later been adopted as administrative tools. The methodology developed by Abdellah and Levine[6] to measure the extent of unfulfilled needs for nursing care, also discussed in the following chapter, was intended for use in a study of the relationship between amount of nursing care available and patient satisfaction. This same methodology has been used as an administrative tool for the appraisal of the adequacy of nursing care provided to patients.[7]

Few research projects in the nursing field have been conducted for the sole purpose of developing research methodology. Much of the methodology has been developed as an adjunct of a descriptive or explanatory study. This methodology has often been tailor-made for the studies in which they were developed and cannot be readily adapted for use in other research. Little work has been done to develop new methodologies for nursing studies that could be widely used. A considerable share of the methodology that has been used in research in nursing was developed in other fields and for other purposes than that to which they were put in the nursing studies. Psychological instruments like the Edwards personal preference schedule, the thematic apperception test, and the Strong vocational interest inventory are just a few of the instruments used in nursing studies. Methodology developed in the behavioral sciences such as the Q-sort, critical incident technique, and scalogram analysis have been applied to the construction of questionnaire items containing nursing content.

The absence of research methodology especially developed for research in nursing can be explained by the highly technical nature of this work. In the physical sciences, instrumentation is often the full-time activity of specialists trained in this field. In the social sciences, too, research methodology is frequently developed by specialists called psychometricians or sociometricians. As more and more of such specially trained personnel become interested in research in nursing, the output of specialized methodologies for studies in nursing should increase. In the meanwhile, most purely methodological research in the nursing field will probably be concerned with the development of methods and tools for nursing administration, practice, and education.

However, there is another area of methodology developing in nursing that has received increasing attention as a distinct research activity. This is the area of theory and model development. Researchers in nursing have borrowed not only their instrumentation for data collection from the social and physical sciences, but their theories as well. Examples of theories that have been applied in studies in nursing include small groups, sensory deprivation, cybernetics, learning, motivation, and personality.

Recently, attempts have been made to develop theories and models that are unique to the nursing field. Some of these have been discussed previously in Chapter 4. The purpose for developing such theories has been twofold: to serve as the basis for research or to promote the improvement of nursing practice. Often, these theories and models have had to be extended beyond the area of nursing in order to provide a meaningful frame of reference. Thus, Howland's hospital system model,[8] which has possible uses in both research and practice, is a broadly conceived formulation that encompasses many components of the hospital system in addition to that of nursing.

Methodological research differs from other types of research in two important ways. First, it usually does not include all of the stages of research design as discussed in Chapter 5. Thus, if the purpose of the methodological research is to develop a new theory or a model, the stage of research where data are collected may never be reached, thereby eliminating many steps in the research process. Moreover, even if quantification is involved in methodological research, as in the development of a research tool, it may not be necessary to become as deeply involved in such statistical problems as sampling, randomization, and data analysis as is often necessary in descriptive and explanatory research.

Second, it is held by some that to engage successfully in methodological research requires a more creative and ingenious approach than do other forms of research. Since some products of methodological research can be viewed as inventions—whether it be a theory, a tool, or a new procedure for doing something—this viewpoint may have some validity. There is no question that a considerable amount of the effort expended by the researcher in methodological research is intellectual—thinking through the problem and developing ideas—whereas in descriptive and explanatory research much of the effort centers around actual collection and analysis of the data, activities which may not be of a comparable intellectual level. However, all research presents intellectual challenges at every stage of the research process. The degree to which one type of research might be more of an intellectual challenge than another essentially depends on the nature of the problem being studied.

Descriptive Research

In this type of research the primary aim is to discover new facts—i.e., to provide a factual, descriptive picture of the situation. To some, descriptive research is considered to be pedestrian because it does not offer the intellectual challenges of inventing a new theory, method, or procedure as in methodological research, or of discovering causative or predictive relationships as in explanatory research. It is probably true that some descriptive research often commences from a meager theoretical base and ends with a superficial analytical treatment of the data. Also, the largest share of the effort in descriptive research is devoted to the routine data-collection phases rather than to the more thought-provoking stages of research.

This is not to deprecate descriptive research as being less important than other types of research. Other research may not be able to proceed until descriptive studies shed light on the variables in the situation. Often, descriptive studies provide the basis for undertaking explanatory research. In many areas this has been the usual mode of progression—from a broad descriptive study that uncovers problem areas to explanatory research that investigates the possible causes of the problem. Much of the research into the causes of diseases was first stimulated by the descriptive data showing a rise in the number of cases of the disease—as, for example, the rise in lung cancer among men.

Descriptive studies that are undertaken solely to throw some light on an area or to generate hypotheses for later investigation in an explanatory study are sometimes called *exploratory* studies. Such studies are never considered as final products, but rather as one step in a total research program that might eventually yield explanatory inferences.

Fortunately, sufficient descriptive data exist in some areas, making it unnecessary to engage in preliminary exploratory research to obtain the needed data. Thus, if one were to embark on a study of the differences between survival rates of hospitalized patients with cardiac arrest who are cared for in intensive care units as compared with patients cared for in conventional hospital nursing units, sufficient descriptive data already exist on the main explanatory variables—survival rates of hospitalized patients with cardiac arrest and type of nursing units—so that an exploratory descriptive phase would not be needed. However, if a comparative study were to be made of alternative systems of recording and transmitting patient data (electronic data processing versus peripheral punch cards), a descriptive study might have to be made of current practices regarding patient data so that the comparative study could be designed along realistic, meaningful lines.

As was discussed in the case of methodological studies, a single study frequently combines descriptive and explanatory purposes. Indeed, most explanatory studies include a descriptive phase. This phase is sometimes treated as an independent entity in reporting the results of the study. Moreover, explanatory findings are themselves new facts and can be considered as "descriptive" research. To illustrate, Bredenberg[9] in 1951 published the results of a study in which she investigated differences between the team plan for nursing care and the traditional case method of patient assignment. Her basic hypothesis was that the team method of patient care assignment would lead to an improvement in the quality as well as quantity of patient care. A one-group before-and-after design was used, in which the same personnel employed two different methods of assignment during consecutive periods of time. The alternative methods were evaluated by numerous criterion measures, including number of trips to central supply room, average minutes of overtime per day, average minutes per day spent on clerical work, and amount of nursing care actually received by patients. Results of the study appeared to indicate that the team plan improved both quality and quantity of nursing care.

In addition to this explanatory finding, a considerable amount of descriptive facts was provided by the study. These included data showing the distribution of time spent by personnel on various kinds of nursing and nonnursing activities. Finally, the explanatory findings that showed that the team method of assignment led to improved patient care also had certain descriptive aspects such as an indication of the number of hours of professional nursing care per patient per day (2.0 hours) and the proportion of nonprofessional to professional nursing personnel composing the nursing team (1:2) that maximized the quality of patient care.

Frequently, studies that are largely oriented toward the development of methodology yield valuable descriptive data. Thus, in attempting to develop measures of patient welfare, Aydelotte[10] collected much descriptive data on physiological responses of patients. Also Boyle[11] obtained a considerable amount of descriptive facts concerning nursing students and the patients they cared for while she was attempting to construct a method for assessing students' perceptions of the needs of patients.

Although descriptive studies may not present as formidable an intellectual challenge as do methodological and explanatory studies, they occupy an important place in the total research spectrum. In nursing, descriptive research has yielded important data for program planning and for decision making. It has also provided the basis for undertaking explanatory research. Some of the outcomes of descriptive studies as well as discussion of their methodology will be presented in Chapter 13.

Explanatory Research

To some the only true research is the kind that seeks answers to questions concerned with "why does something happen?" or "what would happen if . . . ?" Studies directed to such questions are called explanatory studies. Their purpose is to offer an explanation for the occurrence of certain phenomena. Essentially, explanatory studies are concerned with relationships among two or more variables. As was discussed in Chapter 5, explanatory studies are basically concerned with testing whether a stated hypothesis is true or false, the hypothesis being a statement of the expected relationship between two or more variables. Thus, the statement that "chronically ill patients are happier being cared for in their homes than in a hospital" is an example of a hypothesis that could precipitate an explanatory research study in which the relationship between two variables might be tested: type of facility in which care is provided and level of happiness of patients receiving care.

Not all explanatory studies are based on such clearly defined hypotheses. In fact some may not contain explicit statements of any hypotheses at all. An illustration of the first type of study is one in which the purpose is to determine the optimum staffing pattern for, say, a nursing unit consisting largely of patients with neurological disorders. If this is an area where little descriptive data exists, it may be difficult to set up in advance the alternative staffing patterns that could be tested in an experimental type of research design. In other words, such a study might not have a clearly defined independent variable. Thus, it would not be possible to state a prior hypothesis that staffing pattern A is more effective than staffing pattern B. This study might have to proceed on a trial and error basis. First one kind of pattern would have to be tried and evaluated, then another, and so on, until the most effective one is found. Of course, in this kind of design each trial of a different staffing pattern would have to be carefully controlled so that differences between the various patterns that are studied could be clearly described in order that the findings could be generalized beyond the experimental setting.

Other studies, instead of being based on a single, explicit hypothesis may be addressed to a large number of questions. An example of this is a study that seeks to discover whether a school health program should be under control of a public health or an educational agency. Here the independent variable is clearly defined—type of agency administering the school health program. But the dependent variable—the measure by which the more appropriate of the two types of agencies is determined—is not so clearly or easily defined. It is possible to conceive of dozens of criteria by which to evaluate the independent variable, including quality of service (which can itself be broken down into many specific factors), financial factors, political considerations, community acceptance, efficiency of personnel use. In addition to the difficulty of developing this research problem so that it includes concise and manageable hypotheses, there exists the further complication that many of these criterion measures are highly interrelated, making it rather meaningless to treat each one as a separate and distinct hypothesis.

Generally, it is possible to formulate hypotheses for every explanatory study, since, by definition, the researcher is seeking answers to questions concerning the relationship among variables. The existence of the relationship can be postulated as a tentative and speculative explanation which is then tested in the research itself. For the studies just discussed it would be possible to state the following tentative hypotheses: in the first study as, "The type of nurse staffing pattern employed can influence the effectiveness of the care of neurological patients," and in the second study: "There is a difference in the quality of school health nursing services when they are administered by the board of education as compared with the health department." Although vague, the hypotheses would at least serve the purpose of imposing a unifying framework for the research.

Causal Explanation Explanatory studies can take many forms. In its most basic and, for some, its most important role, explanatory research is employed to find out why something happens—to discover the causes of events.

Why do some children develop cerebral palsy?
Why do nursing students withdraw from school?
What is the reason that heart attacks are more common among males than females?
Why are nurses spending less time on direct patient care?
Can home care programs lower the cost of providing health care?
Does authoritarian leadership in nursing cause high turnover among nursing personnel?

As was discussed earlier, except in simple, uncluttered situations, it is often very difficult to draw a clear and straight line between cause and effect in areas involving human beings. This is so because one variable alone usually does not represent the total cause. Often many independent variables affect the results observed in the dependent variable. Moreover, in many situations the independent variables, rather than being causative variables, are really correlated variables. That is to say, both the independent and dependent variables are affected by some other more fundamental independent variable. Thus, a relationship may be found between age of nursing student and rate of withdrawal from school—older students may drop out at a higher rate than younger ones. But this does not necessarily mean that younger students are intellectually superior to older ones. It may well be that marriage, which is more likely to occur with older students, is the important factor in the attrition differential.

Predictive Studies In addition to investigating causes, explanatory studies seek to make predictions: What will happen if something is done? Studies concerned with seeking causal relationships are also predictive, since if the cause of an event is isolated it is then possible to predict the occurrence of the event in the future on the basis of the occurrence of the cause. Thus, if research indicates that prematurity is caused by the occurrence of a certain illness in the mother during pregnancy, say, measles, then it would be possible to predict whether the mother will give birth prematurely on the basis of her health history during pregnancy.

But not all predictive studies are based on causal relationships. Some, perhaps the majority, are based on correlated variables that are not necessarily causally related. If we know that when A occurs B is also likely to occur, we can predict B from the occurrence of A, or vice versa, without A being causally related to B. Therefore, if a study finds that patients with diabetes who are given formal instruction about their illness are more likely to keep their illness under control than patients who do not receive such instruction, it does not matter if it is the actual transmission of factual knowledge that influences the diabetic's behavior in a positive way or some other factor associated with the teaching process. The other factor—the psychological act of imparting a feeling of reassurance, security, and support to the patient, which could well be accomplished in other ways than through the process of teaching the patient—may be the actual causative factor. If we know we can influence (predict) the desired behavior by teaching the patient, then we can employ this means to accomplish our ends even in the absence of a direct causal relationship.

Another illustration: if it is found that maternal mortality is higher among primigravidas who are in older age groups, the public health nurse could be alerted to take precautionary measures for patients over 35 years of age who are pregnant for the first time. This should be done even though it is not age per se or even a variable related to the aging process that causes the higher mortality, but rather some other unknown factor. In other words, we do not have to know what causes something to take action to influence that "something." The exact mechanism by which poliomyelitis is transmitted is still not fully known, although vaccines have been perfected for preventing the disease.

Studies of causal relationships are essentially diagnostic and are concerned with questions of "why does something happen?" Predictive studies focus on questions of "what happens if . . . ?" If we can predict the occurrence of certain phenomena, we may also be able to control it. Thus predictive research provides a very powerful tool for influencing and directing behavior. If we learn from a study of the nursing care of hypertensive patients that patients who receive nursing care through the team method of assignment show a better prognosis than patients cared for by conventional methods of patient assignment, we can favorably influence the course of the hypertensive patient's progress by promoting the team plan of organization. If we discover in a study of recruitment to nursing than an appeal emphasizing the intellectual aspects of nursing attracts a higher caliber student who is less apt to drop out of school, we then have a powerful means of raising both the quality and quantity of students produced by the schools.

Predictive studies are particularly popular in the educational field where much of the work in developing predictive instruments, such as tests, scales, inventories, and profiles, has been done. These tools have been used to assist in the selection and placement of students. They have also been used to measure an individual's aptitude—for learning, for developing a mechanical or other type of skill, and for getting along well with other people. The field of personnel management makes wide use of such predictive devices also for the purposes of selection and placement of people. And in the health field, increasing attention is being given to predicting the chances of falling prey to certain illnesses. In nursing, methods to forecast patients' needs for nursing care are receiving considerable attention (see Chpater 12).

Evaluative Studies　Explanatory research serves yet a third function. Not only can we discover predictive and causal relationships through this form of research, but we can evaluate the effect of alternative courses of action. That is to say, we can test whether one way of doing something is better than another (or, in retrospect, was better). Here, the way of doing something—the independent variable—can be a method, procedure, product, program, system, or some behavior of an individual or group. Evaluation of the independent variable is made in terms of a criterion variable that measures its performance effectiveness. Much of the research in nursing and patient care is of this kind. In fact many studies in these areas include the term "evaluation" in their title:

An Evaluation of Three Methods of Treatment of Patients with Personality Disorders
A Comparative Evaluation of Hospital Beds
Evaluation of Group Counseling for Nursing Students
Evaluation of an Experimental Nursing Curriculum
An Evaluation of Different Methods of Interviewing Patients for Case-Finding Purposes
An Evaluation of Faculty Research Potential

Perhaps more than any other type of research, evaluative studies deserve the label "applied research." By definition, the problem areas of evaluative studies are drawn directly from real life and their findings have very practical consequences. Often, evaluative studies have meager theoretical foundations, and their findings contribute little to the advancement of scientific knowledge. One reason for this is the fact that such studies often arise from a pressing, felt need to solve an immediate problem and not as part of a long-range, integrated research program. Examples of such studies are abundant in every area of activity. In medicine there are the clinical trials of drugs; in government there are studies to evaluate the effects of policies and programs; and in business there is market research on consumer preferences for goods produced.

For nursing, evaluative studies offer a wide range of fruitful possibilities. At the direct patient care level, to illustrate just a few of these possibilities, there can be studies of alternative ways of performing physical care for patients, providing staffing patterns for patient care, teaching patients, assessing patients' requirements for nursing care, achieving continuity of care, recording and communicating patient care data, providing emotional and other supportive care, planning for comprehensive patient care. At the nursing administration level there can be studies of different methods of recruiting and selecting personnel, assigning personnel to patient care, organizing patient care units, providing leadership to nursing staff, establishing personnel policies, evaluating nursing performance, providing in-service education, enhancing utilization of personnel, influencing levels of job satisfaction, promoting employment stability, and establishing effective communication channels. At the nursing education level there can be studies of alternative ways of recruiting and selecting students, using instructional time, utilizing some of the newer teaching methods such as television and programmed instruction, evaluating teacher and student performance, determining appropriateness of curriculum content, preventing student withdrawals, improving faculty competencies, and recruiting and retaining an adequate teaching staff.

These topics represent broad areas in which evaluative research might be done. Any one of the areas can be narrowed down into a very specific research problem. For example, an evaluation of different methods of achieving continuity of patient care could be directed toward patients with particular illnesses or in particular age groups or in certain geographic areas. Or the study could be concerned with a particular organizational system of patient care such as Progressive Patient Care. Or it can focus on the staffing and personnel aspects of continuity of care. Finally, such a study could be slanted toward either the economic, psychological, sociological, administrative, or medical care aspects of achieving continuity of patient care.

Evaluative studies are closely related to the decision-making process. In decision making, a set of alternative courses of action are weighed in terms of their possible consequences. The decision is made when one of the alternatives is selected as the course of action to pursue. In evaluative studies alternative ways of doing something are tested in a research design. On the basis of the research findings, one of the alternatives is selected as being the most desirable.

In the real world most decisions are taken without benefit of formalized research. Decisions are usually based on previous experience or on already collected factual data or on some other available evidence. As has been pointed out in Chapters 3 and 5, when there is paucity of evidence available concerning which of the alternatives to select, and only when the decision involves large amounts of money, or has a close relation to the health and welfare of people, or arises frequently, is evaluative research actually undertaken.

Not all evaluative research is prospective. That is to say, not all such studies are concerned with testing alternatives and applying findings to some future action program. Some evaluative studies are retrospective, to see what has been done, to evaluate how well it has been done, and to attempt to discover reasons for any shortcomings. A clear example of such studies—although they are often not identified as research—are quality control procedures employed in the inspection of manufactured products. By a method of random sampling, a fraction of each batch of the product —say, a drug—is selected for testing as it is completed. If the product does not meet the test criteria, the entire batch is rejected, and the manufacturing procedure is carefully scrutinized to uncover the reasons why the product failed to meet standards of quality.

In nursing, a type of retrospective evaluative study that is widely used, and one that in some aspects resembles quality control methods, is the study of activities of nursing personnel. Called by various designations— time studies, function studies, utilization studies, work sampling studies (described in detail in the following chapter)—their purpose is to assess the amount of time nursing personnel devote to various categories of work activities. Certain statistical tabulations are prepared that provide an indication of whether time is being properly utilized. One of these shows the percentage of time nursing personnel spend on clerical activities. If this percentage is exceptionally high, attempts are made to find out why this is so in order to rectify the situation. Here, as in quality control of manufactured products, data that are essentially retrospective play a valuable role in improving future courses of action.

From this discussion of the three major aims of research—to develop methodology, to discover new facts (descriptive), to discover relationships among facts (evaluative)—it should be clear that few studies fall purely into one of these three areas. Methodological studies frequently generate descriptive facts and sometimes even provide explanatory data. Descriptive data, even if not the intention of the researcher who obtained them, are sometimes used for explanatory purposes. And, of course, every explanatory study also produces descriptive facts. As in all classification schemes, it is not possible to construct categories that have the properties of water-tight compartments. The value of this trichotomy is to describe the three main areas of research and to provide a means of at least grossly classifying studies in terms of their major emphasis.

CLASSIFICATION BY RESEARCH DESIGN

In Chapter 6, the two major types of research design were discussed in detail: the experimental and the nonexperimental. In that discussion, the experimental design was described as the classical research design, usually conducted in a specially constructed research setting, called a laboratory, experimental unit, or test unit, in which all the major elements of the study were under the control of the researcher. An experiment was called a prospective study. The independent variable is applied to the study subjects and the effects observed in terms of the dependent variable. By contrast, a nonexperimental study—also called a survey, a field study, or an investigation—is usually conducted in a natural setting, which, in patient care research, can be a hospital, a ward, an outpatient department, a physician's office, a classroom, or the patient's home. Moreover, in nonexperimental research some elements of the study are not under the control of the researcher. In some nonexperimental studies the application of the independent variable has preceded the initiation of the study itself and, thus, is beyond the control of the researcher. Therefore, this type of explanatory research can be labeled retrospective.

In between these two extremes a third type of research design can be identified which has some elements of both. This type can be called partially experimental. An example of such a study design is one in which experimental changes are made in a natural setting. Conversely a laboratory study in which changes are allowed to occur without the influence of the experimenter would also be an example of a partially controlled experimental design. The former type of study has the advantage of avoiding the artificiality that often attaches itself to experiments conducted in laboratories or specially devised experimental units. Avoidance of artificiality is important in patient care research where much of the virtue of a study stems from the ability to generalize its findings to a larger population. Similarly, the partially experimental study seems to have the worst features of the two types of research design—the artificiality of an experimental environment and the absence of complete controls over the study found in nonexperimental research. However, for some kinds of research problems this type of design may be useful. For example, in sociological studies of the proces of communication it may be desirable to place the study subjects in a controlled environment but to allow the transfer of information among the study subjects to proceed without interference.

The classification of studies by research design affords another dimension by which both completed and contemplated research can be assessed. To obtain a perspective on the role of the three types of research design in studies in nursing and patient care, the following discussion is provided.

Experimental Design

Just as some people consider explanatory research that is concerned with discovering causal relationships as the only true form of research, so do some feel that experimental design is the only valid research design. In combination—experimental explanatory research—is an extremely powerful tool, the scientific method par excellence, which has made it possible for researchers to make substantial contributions to the advancement of scientific knowledge.

As has been reiterated numerous times in this book, the experimental method has certain limitations as a research design when applied to human populations. The difficulty in manipulating human beings and the restricted scope of generalization of experimental findings are two of these limitations. Nevertheless, if research in nursing is going to further the advancement of scientific knowledge, more experimental studies will have to be undertaken.

Until now, few studies in nursing can be categorized as being truly experimental. This is quite in contrast to such related fields as medicine, physiology, and biology where a considerable amount of research activity has been experimental in nature. Of course, much of this research is conducted in laboratories with animals as the experimental subjects.

Animal research should not be completely ruled out in patient care research. After all, a considerable amount of research in the field of human psychology was conducted with animals as subjects, and the knowledge gained from studies was transferred to human beings. Some thought is now being given to the place of animal research in nursing. Among the possibilities for the use of animals are studies that emphasize psychological or physiological concepts. For example, studies concerned with measures of patient welfare or with analysis of nurse-patient relationships could conceivably profit by first observing responses in animals.

Experimental research in nursing and patient care, however, does not have to be restricted to animal subjects. It is possible to conduct meaningful experiments with humans, particularly where they are members of an institutionalized population. Thus, patients in hospitals, especially long-term patients such as psychiatric, chronic, or convalescent patients, are likely subjects for an experiment. They could be placed on an experimental unit without causing a drastic disturbance to their normal routines. Students in schools are also convenient experimental subjects, and in fields like education, psychology, and sociology, they have participated in numerous experimental studies. Some would call such subjects as patients or students a captive audience. Difficulty arises in generalizing results of studies that use specialized subjects to broader population groups.

If an experiment is of sufficiently short duration, and if the manipulation of the experimental variables does not have unpleasant consequences for the subjects, it is quite possible to draw experimental subjects from a broadly representative target population. Many research problems in the areas of nursing and patient care can conceivably lend themselves to experiments having these attributes. For example, studies of alternative ways of performing certain types of nursing procedures would not necessarily need to involve subjects for very lengthy periods of time, nor would they be placed in a situation that might endanger their health or well-being.

Nonexperimental Design

Studies conducted nonexperimentally can take a variety of forms. At one end, furthest removed from the very direct participation in the data-collecting phase by both researcher and study subject that is so characteristic of experimental studies, are studies that are based on data originally collected by others. The purposes of collecting the data in the first place might be quite remote from the study in which they are being used. In research based on existing data, the entire data-collecting phase of research is largely eliminated, and most emphasis is placed on problem formulation, review of the literature, and data analysis. A good example of such a study is reported in the article "Psychosocial Aspects of Cigarette Smoking."[12] Here the researcher extensively reviewed the literature in his field and summarized all the pertinent data that had been reported in studies of what motivates people to smoke. Through a careful analysis and synthesis of these data the author was able to develop his own interpretation of the reasons why people smoke. Similarly, in the area of patient care research, it is possible to pursue a research question on the basis of existing data from other studies or from source documents, such as patients' records, nurses' notes, Kardex systems, personnel forms, and other administrative documents.

Thus the use of existing data for nonexperimental research purposes can take several forms: the use of research findings by others to develop a new interpretation, the use of data compiled in statistical reports (e.g., Census Bureau Reports, *Facts About Nursing,* Reports of the National Center for Health Statistics), and the use of source documents that are part of administrative record-keeping systems such as patients' or personnel records.

A second type of nonexperimental research does involve the collection of new data from study subjects. But unlike experimental research, where there is direct, personal contact between researcher and research subjects, this design collects data through such impersonal means as questionnaires, tests, or some other type of data-collecting instrument. Because of the relative ease with which new data can be collected in this type of study design, it has been the most widely used method of conducting research in studies involving human populations.

A third type of nonexperimental design does involve the direct collection of data from study participants. This is done either through the method of observation or by interview. Since a nonexperimental study is frequently conducted in the natural setting, direct collection of data can involve considerable travel to contact the study subjects if, for example, they are to be visited in their homes. Or the study may involve some disruption of normal organizational routines, as when data are collected from persons in hospitals, schools, or other types of institutions. However, for certain types of studies, particularly where the data to be collected are too complicated, subtle, or sensitive, or for some other reason not easily obtainable by an impersonal instrument like a questionnaire, direct collection is the most desirable way to obtain the needed data.

Because of the great variety of approaches to the conduct of nonexperimental research and the ease with which many studies using this type of design can be carried out, it is a very popular design for research in nursing and patient care. However, its limitations must be recognized. Foremost among these is the great difficulty, if not impossibility, of deriving cause and effect relationships through such studies. As previous discussions of research design have shown, nonexperimental research is weak on control of extraneous variables. The effects of these variables on the explanatory variables can be confounded to such an extent as to lead to the drawing of spurious relationships when a nonexperimental design is used. The advantage of this type of research lies in the relative ease with which data can be collected and the possibility of extending the research to large study populations. When the fact that this type of research is often conducted in a natural setting is also considered, there is no question that it can provide greater applicability of findings than does the more narrowly restricted experimental study.

Partially Experimental Design

Two important aspects of research designs—adequate control over research variables and wide representation of study subjects and settings—can sometimes be achieved by incorporating features of the experimental and nonexperimental types of design. In such a design there may be experimental manipulation of the independent variable, but not complete control over the extraneous variables, because the factor of randomization is not strictly, if at all, adhered to. Such studies are usually labeled as incomplete experiments, since the researcher may not recognize that some crucial elements of the true experimental design are missing.

Another feature of the partial experiment is the fact that it is generally conducted in a natural setting rather than in a specially devised experimental unit or laboratory. The use of a natural setting does not automatically disqualify a research project from acquiring the status of a complete experiment. However, the use of such settings makes the achievement of all the essential controls that are necessary in a complete experiment difficult, if not impossible, to attain.

An example of a partially experimental study in nursing will be briefly described to show how it differs from a full experiment. The example is the study of the team plan of patient assignment that was discussed earlier in this chapter.[13] In this study the team plan was initiated at different times on various units of a hospital, and data were collected concerning activities of the personnel composing the team on a "before" and "after" basis. That is to say, the activities of the personnel were measured before the team plan was put into effect and again after they were organized according to the team concept. Analysis was made of changes in activities of personnel. The significant changes that occurred in the criterion measures, such as a decrease in time spent on clerical activities, were ascribed to the team method of organization.

Although the study director called her design experimental, it is obvious that it cannot qualify as a full-blown experiment. First of all, the researcher did not have complete control over the experimental variables. The independent variable studied was type of patient assignment, and it had two alternatives: team plan and case method. The researcher had only partial control over this variable. She devised the composition of the team organization and actually assigned the study subjects to this type of organization. However, the other alternative—the case method type of organization—pre-existed the "experiment." Its composition as well as the assignment of personnel to it were quite beyond the control of the researcher. Thus, the comparison of the "before" and "after" activities of the nursing personnel was subject to several important extraneous variables, making it difficult to ascribe all changes to the team plan of organization. Foremost among these is the "Hawthorne effect" (see Chapter 6). Since the experimental change that was introduced—the team plan—involved the same personnel, we do not know whether the changes in performance are attributable to the new type of organization or to the process of change itself, with the sense of participation in an interesting experiment that was generated and the undoubtedly stimulating effect that it had on personnel to alter their performance in a positive way. Of course, this type of spuriousness is possible in any one-group before-after research design where the same study subjects receive the various alternatives of the independent variable. Only the double-blind approach offers a solution to the problem, but it is very difficult to achieve in designs where the subjects are used as their own control.

Another extraneous variable that could have been present in this study was the condition of the patients. We do not know too much about the patients from the report of this study, but it is quite possible that the needs of the patients may have changed significantly from one study period to the next. Consequently, the changes in the activities of the personnel that were measured may have been related to a shift in the level of patients' requirements for nursing services rather than the change from the case method of patient assignment to the team plan.

If a study like this were to be conducted as a truly, complete experiment there would have to be tighter controls over the extraneous variables. This could be accomplished through randomization, in which the patients as well as the personnel would be randomly assigned to the two types of organization of nursing care—team and case methods. But, of course, truly scientific randomization is sometimes difficult to achieve. This is particularly so where radical administrative changes have to be made, such as shifting patients from one unit to another or altering their pattern of care.

Although partial experiments may be deficient in the degree to which all relevant extraneous variables are controlled, they do have certain real advantages as a research design. In evaluative studies where a new method or a product is to be tested, the completely nonexperimental approach cannot be applied, since existing uses of the method or product, of course, cannot be found. The decision to conduct a full or a partial experiment must consider the extent to which the study subjects can be experimentally interfered with and controlled. If a partial experiment is selected as the research design, full recognition of the limitations of this design will enhance the validity of the data analysis.

Just as research aims can be classified into three broad categories— methodological, descriptive, explanatory—so can research design be divided into the three categories—experimental, partially experimental, and nonexperimental. These two categorizations can be cross-classified so that a research study can be classified by both characteristics at the same time. This cross-classification provides a total of nine cells into which a research study could be placed. But this does not exhaust all possible dimensions for categorizing research in nursing and patient care. Another can be called the content of a research project. The following section will provide a brief discussion of this dimension.

CLASSIFICATION BY RESEARCH CONTENT

Research content signifies the subject matter of a study. What does it deal with? In their thorough review of completed research in nursing, Simmons and Henderson[11] have identified the following areas:

A. Historical, Philosophical, and Cultural Studies
B. Occupational Orientation and Career Dynamics
C. Specialties in Nursing by Occupational Categories
D. Nursing Organizations and Organizations Including Nursing
E. Administration of Nursing Services in Hospitals, Clinics, Public Health and Other Agencies
F. Nursing Care
G. Patients' Reactions and Adjustments to Identifiable Variables Related to Their Illnesses
H. Interaction Patterns Between Nurse, Patient, Patients' Families, Other Nurses, Physicians, and Other Members of the Health Team
I. Education for Nursing
J. Conducting Research—Facilities, Personnel, Support and Method

These categories can be regrouped into three broader content areas: nursing practice, nursing education, and nursing administration.

Nursing practice relates to studies concerned with the actual provision of care to patients, whether this be direct, as in the giving of an intravenous infusion, or indirect, as in preparing nurses' notes. In administrative terminology, nursing practice includes those activities occurring at the operational level of an organization. The range of subject matter available for studies of nursing practice is enormous and can include industrial engineering studies of equipment and supplies as well as sociological studies of interpersonal relationships among members of the nursing team. Such studies can be very broadly conceived—as, for example, a study of the total system of providing nursing care to patients—or they can be limited to a very narrow area such as a study of one nursing procedure. Studies concerned with nursing practice can have the greatest impact on patient care, since they are concerned with matters that have direct and immediate consequences on patients. For these reasons, there has been a rise in the number of studies performed in this area, which reflects the increasing concern with the need to achieve patient-centered nursing care.

Studies of nursing education represent perhaps the earliest type of research in nursing. Even today the number of such studies in progress is very large. Nursing education research includes a broad range of topical areas: recruitment and selection of students, development of curriculum, faculty preparation, design of schools, financing of education, evaluation of student performance, and so on. Included, too, are the areas of in-service and continuing education. In one respect, research in nursing education faces fewer difficulties than studies of nursing practice. Since many problems in nursing education are common to other fields of education, it is possible to borrow theory, methodology, and findings from these fields for studies in nursing. An elaborate variety of tests, measures, data, principles, and theories is available for use by the researcher in education. By contrast, the researcher in nursing practice is working in a relatively underdeveloped area. ·

Nursing administration can be defined as the specialized work of maintaining the nursing organization in operation,[15] as contrasted with the actual physical work of the organization, which is nursing practice. Historically, nursing administration developed much later than nursing education as a field of knowledge as well as a specialized occupational category, having in fact been for many years a kind of subspecialty of nursing education. In nursing administration the range of research problems is also very broad, with boundaries limited only by the span of imagination of the researcher. Among possible topics for research projects are personnel policies, organizational patterns, styles of leadership, job mobility, recruitment and retention of staff, morale and job satisfaction, evaluation of performance, and relationships with individuals and groups outside of the nursing department. Administrative research can call upon a host of skills from a variety of disciplines, including social psychology, cultural anthropology, economics, political science, systems and industrial engineering, and law.

These three broad content areas of research in nursing do, of course, overlap. How, for example, does one classify a study of administrative problems in the field of nursing education, as administrative or educational? Or how would a study of alternative methods of patient teaching be classified, as an educational or a nursing practice study?

It was stated at the outset of this chapter that there were several purposes in presenting a typology of research in nursing. First, to point out to consumers of research in a simple and systematic way the dimensions of the whole area of research in nursing. Second, to assist researchers in defining their research problems and to suggest new areas for research. Third, to provide a means for delineating differences and similarities in purpose, method, and content of completed research in order to enhance the usefulness of research findings. To fulfill these three purposes it is not essential that the typology possess precisely and rigidly defined categories. This would be impossible to attain. The aim is for the categories to be sufficiently discriminating to permit a clear-cut classification in the majority of uses to which it is put. Thus, we have described a typology of research in nursing and patient care that has three broad dimensions—research aims, design, and content. No doubt other dimensions could be developed. For example, studies could be categorized according to the size of their budgets (small, medium, or large) or kinds of research subjects (patients, students, personnel), kinds of research settings (hospital, public health clinic, patient's home), and so on. These latter characteristics are of lesser importance than the three discussed in this chapter.

To recapitulate and summarize the discussion contained in the preceding pages, the following typology is presented. This typology is a modification of that presented at the conclusion of Chapter 3.

A Typology of Research in Nursing

I. *Research aims*

  A. Methodological research
    1. To develop research methodology
    2. To develop tools for nursing administration or education
    3. To develop theories and models

  B. Descriptive research
    1. To discover new facts
    2. To gather exploratory data as a prelude for further research

  C. Explanatory research
    1. To discover causal relationships
    2. To make predictions
    3. To evaluate a program, method, procedure, product, system, or individual or group behavior

II. *Research design*
  A. Experimental design
  B. Partially experimental design
  C. Nonexperimental design

III. *Research content*
  A. Nursing practice
  B. Nursing education
  C. Nursing administration

The following three chapters will present a detailed discussion of some major research studies undertaken in the fields of nursing and patient care. These studies are presented as examples of various kinds of research —methodological, descriptive, and explanatory—in the various major content areas. Studies having the three major types of research design will be discussed. Some alternative design decisions that could have been taken in these studies will be examined. An assessment will be made of any limitations in the findings of some of these studies, as well as existing gaps in knowledge that might be filled by future research.

We can conclude this chapter by examining Figure 11-1, which attempts to show graphically the volume of research that has been completed in nursing according to the major areas of the typology. From this graph it can be seen that the preponderance of studies have been nonexperimental and descriptive. The graph points up a need for more explanatory research conducted experimentally, since these are the studies that can enrich and advance the scientific basis of any field of knowledge.

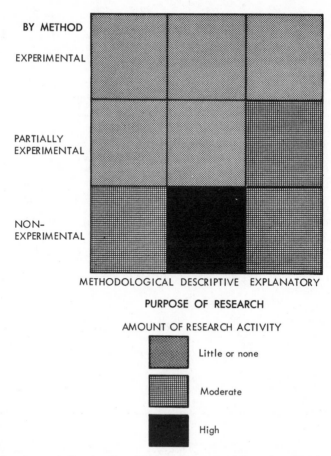

Fig. 11-1. Amount of research activity in nursing according to method and purpose.

References

1. See particularly Samuel A. Stouffer *et al., Measurement and Prediction: Studies in Social Psychology in World War II,* Volume IV. Princeton, Princeton University Press, 1950.
2. Eileen G. Hasselmeyer, *Behavior Patterns of Premature Infants.* U.S. Public Health Service Publication No. 840. Washington, D.C., Government Printing Office, 1961.
3. Eileen G. Hasselmeyer, Joseph de la Puente, Evelyn C. Lundeen, and Mary Morrison, "A Weight Chart for Premature Infants." *Nursing Res.,* **12:**222–231, fall 1963.
4. Bernard G. Greenberg, "The Philosophy and Methods of Research," in *Report on Nursing Research Conference,* Harriet H. Werley (ed.). Washington, D.C., Walter Reed Army Institute of Research, 1962, p. 51.

5. Robert J. Connor *et al.,* "Effective Use of Nursing Resources, a Research Report." *Hospitals, J.A.H.A.,* **35:**30–39, May 1, 1961.
6. Faye G. Abdellah and Eugene Levine, "Developing a Measure of Patient and Personnel Satisfaction with Nursing Care." *Nursing Res.,* **3:**100–108, February 1957.
7. Faye G. Abdellah and Eugene Levine, *Patients and Personnel Speak.* U.S. Public Health Service Publication No. 527, 2nd ed. Washington, D.C., Government Printing Office, 1964.
8. Daniel Howland, "A Hospital System Model." *Nursing Res.,* **12:**232–236, fall 1963.
9. Viola Bredenberg, *Nursing Service Research: Experimental Studies with the Nursing Service Team.* Philadelphia, J. B. Lippincott, 1951.
10. Myrtle K. Aydelotte and Marie E. Tener, "An Investigation of the Relation Between Nursing Activity and Patient Welfare." Iowa City, State University of Iowa, Utilization Project, 1960.
11. Rena E. Boyle, *A Study of Student Nurse Perception of Patient Attitudes.* U.S. Public Health Service Publication No. 769. Washington, D.C., Government Printing Office, 1960.
12. M. Powell Lawton, "Psychological Aspects of Cigarette Smoking." *J. Health and Human Behavior,* **3:**163–170, fall 1962.
13. Bredenberg, *op. cit.*
14. Leo W. Simmons and Virginia Henderson, *Nursing Research: A Survey and Assessment.* New York, Appleton-Century-Crofts, 1964, pp. 71–72.
15. Chester Barnard, *Organization and Management.* Cambridge, Harvard University Press, 1956.

Problems and Suggestions for Further Study

1. What are the values, if any, in making a distinction between basic and applied research? Does applied research always need to be preceded by basic research? Which type of research can potentially make the greater contribution to the advancement of knowledge?
2. Give five examples of research topics that could serve to initiate basic research studies in nursing. Apply the guidelines given in Chapter 5 to determine whether it would be worthwhile to pursue these topics as formal research.
3. How does Herbert Simon define the decision-making process in his *Administrative Behavior* (New York, Macmillan Publishing Co., Inc., 1957)? How is the decision-making process similar to the research process? How are they different? How can research contribute to the making of correct decisions?
4. Discuss why an exploratory or pilot study should adhere to the principles of good research design. Should an exploratory study always precede a definitive explanatory study? What is the difference between an exploratory study and a pretest? Why is it necessary for a pretest to be carefully designed?
5. One of the most comprehensive discussions of nonexperimental research (surveys) is contained in Herbert Hyman, *Survey Design and Analysis*

(New York, The Free Press of Glencoe, 1955, 425 pp.). In Chapter 9 of this book (pp. 350–363), the author distinguishes four types of explanatory surveys: the hypothesis-verifying survey designed to verify some hypothesis relevant to some larger body of theory, the diagnostic survey to explore some novel problem, the evaluative survey designed as a test of the practical value of some action program, and the programmatic survey designed to test the most effective application of a future action program. How does this classification differ from the one proposed in this chapter?

6. Cite some illustrations of descriptive research that might be useful to undertake in your area of interest. Which of the following would you think should be categorized as descriptive and which as explanatory research just from a knowledge of their titles:
   a. A study of licensing laws for professional nurses in the United States
   b. An experimental study of different methods of training nursing aides
   c. A history of the Canadian Nurses Association, 1920–1950
   d. The relation between neonate crying and length of labor
   e. The functions of a school nurse in a rural area
   f. Variations in respiration rate of patients with high temperatures
   g. An exploratory study of the nursing needs of patients with ophthalmic disorders
   h. A survey of nursing in India
   i. A quantitative analysis of the costs of attrition from schools of nursing
   j. A case study of pediatric patients in psychiatric hospitals
   k. The relationship between quality of nursing supervision and the adequacy of patient care provided

7. What are the limitations to the use of existing data in a study? What are some of the techniques that could be employed to make existing data more useful in a study? (Example: we can communicate with the supplier of the data to get further clarification of the data.)

8. Read the article by Walter Johnson, "Longitudinal Study of Family Adjustment to Myocardial Infarction," (*Nursing Res.,* **12**:242–247, fall 1963). What was one of the major problems faced by this researcher in conducting a longitudinal study? For what kinds of research problems are longitudinal studies especially useful? Could this study have been conducted retrospectively?

9. Is it possible for a completely uncontrolled nonexperimental study to discover causal relationships among the variables it investigates? What are the conditions for establishing cause and effect relationships among variables?

10. Apply the typology presented in this chapter to the following studies. In addition to determining the aims, design, and content of these studies, would you categorize them as basic or applied research?
    a. Sam Shapiro and Marilyn M. Einhorn, "Changes in Rates of Visiting Nurse Services in the Health Insurance Plan." *Am. J. Pub. Health,* **54:** 417–430, March 1964
    b. Leila Whiting and Joseph F. Whiting, "Finding the Core of Hospital Nursing." *Am. J. Nursing,* **62**:80–83, August 1962
    c. Rhetaugh G. Dumas and Robert C. Leonard, "The Effect of Nursing on the Incidence of Postoperative Vomiting." *Nursing Res.,* **12**:12–15, winter 1963

d. Helen M. Williamson, William E. Edmonston and John A. Stern, "Use of the EPPS for Identifying Personal Role Attributes Desirable in Nursing." *J. Health and Human Behavior,* **4:**266–275, winter 1963

e. Hazel A. Carpenter and Ralph Simon, "The Effect of Several Methods of Training on Long Term, Incontinent, Behaviorally Regressed Hospitalized Psychiatric Patients." *Nursing Res.,* **9:**17–22, winter 1960

g. Sr. Paula A. Larson, "Nurse Perceptions of Patient Characteristics." *Nursing Res.,* **26:**416–421, November–December 1977.

h. Bonnie Bullough, "The Measurement of Alienation as It Relates to Family Planning Behavior." In Marjorie V. Batey (ed.), *Communicating Nursing Research,* Vol. 8. Boulder Col., Western Interstate Commission for Higher Education, pp. 41–52, March 1977.

Update Note

Typologies of nursing research, different from the one presented in this book, are most plentiful. For example, Susan D. Taylor in "Bibliography on Nursing, 1950–1974." *Nursing Res.,* 24:207–225, May–June, 1975, classified over 1,000 items on nursing research appearing in the literature from 1950–1974. Another classification of nursing research is found in the article by Susan R. Gortner and Helen Nahm, "An Overview of Nursing Research in the United States." *Nursing Res.,* **26:**10–33, January–February, 1977.

Chapter Twelve

METHODOLOGICAL STUDIES

IN THE PREVIOUS CHAPTER, methodological research was described as that type of research whose aim it is to develop a new tool, method, procedure, product, program, research instrument, theory, or model. The uses to which methodological studies are put are varied. For example, a methodological study might produce a research instrument for use in other studies, or it might produce a new procedure for use in nursing practice. Or, in *basic* methodological research, the intended use might be to advance knowledge without necessarily being geared to a practical application.

As has been indicated, the development of methodology is often the work of specialists who devote full time to this pursuit. In nursing, few individuals have concerned themselves exclusively with methodological research. There are two reasons for this situation. First of all, there has been much adaptation in nursing, in both research and practice, of methodology developed in other fields. Moreover, many of the methods and procedures used in the provision of nursing care to patients have been developed outside of formal research settings, largely on the basis of common sense or through trial and error.

Second, few research efforts in nursing have been undertaken solely to develop new methodology. Usually, methodological developments have been part of comprehensive research projects that have also included descriptive or explanatory research, or both.

In this chapter some of the major methodological studies that have been undertaken in the field of nursing will be discussed. These studies have been selected for analysis because they represent examples of attempts to develop new methodology specifically for the field of nursing and are not transplantions of methodology from another field. Also, many of these studies exemplify research whose major or only purpose was to develop methodology, not as a by-product of some other purpose.

From a design standpoint all methodological studies to be discussed are essentially nonexperimental. Most were developed from data gathered in nonexperimental settings. This by no means represents a serious limitation of these studies. On the contrary, since most methodological studies are intended for practical uses it is essential that they be influenced by realistic considerations. Also, many of the control mechanisms that are essential to good research design, such as those aimed at enhancing the validity and reliability of the data, are of less concern in methodological studies, since actual collection and analysis of data are not the major aims. An important criterion for evaluating methodological research is a pragmatic one: How well does the product of such research work in actual practice?

ADMINISTRATIVE METHODS

Problems in the administration of nursing care are many and varied. Perhaps overshadowing all others are those dealing with personnel. These include assessing the needs for personnel, assigning personnel to meet these needs, evaluating the performance of personnel, assessing personnel utilization, and measuring personnel turnover. The emphasis on problems of nurse staffing is readily understandable. For many years needs for nursing personnel have exceeded the supply. Whether this imbalance is due to an actual numerical shortage of people or to the inefficient use of resources has been the subject of considerable speculation and study in recent years.[1] But regardless of its cause, the chronic personnel shortage has led to the initiation of some methodological studies for the purpose of attempting to make better use of scarce personnel resources.

The methodologies that have been produced thus far in the area of administration in nursing have by no means exhausted the subject. Many other administrative areas besides staffing and utilization of personnel await the development of tools, procedures, and methods. These areas include communication, budgeting, and appraising total organizational performance.

PATIENT CLASSIFICATION METHODS

If any particular area of research on methodology development can be singled out as receiving the most attention in nursing and patient care, the development of patient classification methods is such an area. Work on this type of methodology extends back many years and today occupies the attention of a considerable number of research workers.

Why has patient classification occupied such a prominent place in the field of methodology development? A number of reasons can be offered as possible explanations. First of all, although not exclusively applicable to inpatient care, patient classification systems do have certain uses in the inpatient area that are more readily apparent than in other fields. Institutionalized patient care represents the largest consumer of nursing skills. Since one important use of patient classification systems is in planning the assignment of nurse staffing, it is understandable that the demand for such a tool would be high in this area. However, this is not to say that the use of patient classification systems is restricted to inpatient care. The concept of "levels of wellness" represents a type of classification scheme that could be applied to all types of patient care settings.

Second, the worthwhileness of patient classification systems can be assessed in terms of dollars and cents. One stated aim of patient classification methodology is to match nurse staffing to patient requirements. Achievement of this aim should result in a savings of personnel costs by preventing overstaffing. For cost-conscious administrators this is a very appealing aspect of the methodology.

Third, more than any other methodology in the area of nursing administration, patient classification represents a methodological approach tailor-made to the field of nursing. Such techniques as audits, performance evaluations, cost accounting, and work sampling have their counterparts in other disciplines or, in fact, have been adapted from these disciplines. Because of its distinctive and authentic nursing flavor, much interest has been engendered in pursuing the development of patient classification and patient needs methodology.

Specifically, what are patient classification methods and to what uses can they be put? Essentially, patient classification methods are devices by which a patient's needs for nursing services can be assessed. This assessment can serve in determining the amount of nursing care he will require during some stated future time period, generally the next 24 hours, as well as the category of personnel (R.N., practical nurse, nursing aide) who should provide the required care.

Some classification schemes purport to provide only a general assessment of a patient's nursing needs without giving an actual numerical estimate of the amount of care required, while others supposedly provide a precise quantitative assessment of the time requirements of the patient for nursing care. Similarly, some of the methods claim to give only a limited picture of the patient's needs, say for the succeeding 12 to 24 hours, while others seek to provide an assessment extending over the entire period of hospitalization. Also, some of the classification methods are directed toward a certain segment of patients' needs—physical care or needs for instruction or emotional support—whereas other methodologies range over the entire spectrum of patients' requirements for services.

Of the greatest interest from the standpoint of research methodology are the differences in the design of the patient classification methods.

Basically, there are two general ways of designing such instruments. In one of these ways, which can be called "prototype evaluation," several mutually exclusive and exhaustive patient classification categories are established. These are graded in terms of an ordinal scale in which the categories represent greater or lesser requirements for nursing care. Each category is fully described in terms of the characteristics of the typical patient in that category. The methodology is applied by comparing the actual characteristics of a patient being classified with those described by the prototypes for the various categories. The patient is classified into that category in which his characteristics match the prototype characteristics most closely.

The other type of patient classification design can be called "factor evaluation." Here, instead of making a total evaluation of the patient's needs for nursing services, specific elements of care are delineated and the patient is rated on each of the elements. Ratings on individual elements are combined to provide an overall rating which determines the patient's classification according to an ordinal scale of needs for nursing care that contains a limited number of discrete categories. The scale, in fact, can be the same as that employed in the "prototype evaluation." Thus, the end product of the two types of evaluations is essentially the same. The difference lies in the method of rating. In one case (prototype evaluation) the patient is rated on a number of characteristics simultaneously, and in the other (factor evaluation) the characteristics are evaluated one by one.

Patient classification is, therefore, a scaling scheme in which the underlying continuum can be conceptualized as expressing a quantitative statement of a patient's requirements for nursing services. These range from no requirements at all, a condition of maximum self-help ability, to the other extreme representing total requirements for nursing services, a condition of minimum self-help ability. This scale can be thought of as falling within a still broader scale that expresses a person's level of wellness. In such a scale his/her needs for nursing services would commence at the point at which wellness has deteriorated to such a point that the person seeks medical attention. He or she, in short, has become a patient. At this point the patient may no longer be capable of providing all his individual needs and may require the assistance of another person. This other person could be a member of the family, if the individual is cared for at home. But if the family member cannot provide the needed assistance, the services of trained nursing personnel must be sought, either in the home or in an institutionalized setting such as a hospital, nursing home, or some other facility. Figure 12-1 shows graphically how the two scales are related to each other.

Patient classification scales have numerous uses. Briefly these include:

1. To determine staffing needs and to efficiently allocate staff to the various subdivisions (nursing units) of the institution
2. To provide a basis for developing a comprehensive plan of care for each patient
3. To provide a basis for determining the most effective facilities in which to provide patient care
4. To assist in the determination of equipment and supply needs
5. To serve as an instrument for gathering data for research purposes.

The development of patient classification systems extends back many centuries. When hospitals first became formally established, patients began to be grouped according to certain similarities, mainly by diagnosis, sex, and the broad age groups of adult and pediatric patients. Thus, some hospitals became specialized in the care of certain types of patients—psychiatric, tuberculosis, orthopedic—and the largest group of all, the general hospital, cared for patients with a variety of short-term illnesses. Within each type of hospital there was a further subdivision by the sex of patients and, particularly in the general hospital, by broad illness groupings—medical, surgical, obstetrical, and so on. As far as the nursing requirements of the patients were concerned, each of the nursing units contained patients with heterogeneous needs. Only in recovery rooms was there a grouping of patients with similar nursing requirements.

But such groupings are not completely without historical precedents. For many years the Japanese have been applying a system of grouping hospitalized patients according to their needs. Moreover, Florence Nightingale, among her many other innovations, placed the most acutely ill

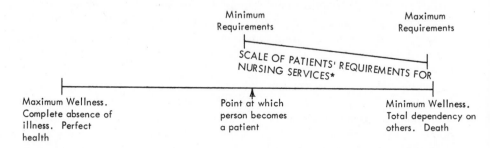

WELLNESS   SCALE

Fig. 12-1. A patient classification scale in relation to a level of wellness scale.

* *Note:* The relationship between "wellness" and "requirements for nursing services" is not a perfect one. A patient with minimum wellness may not necessarily have maximum requirements for nursing services and vice versa. Thus, a terminal cancer patient (low level of wellness) may have fewer needs for nursing services than an otherwise healthy patient with a fractured leg (moderate level of wellness). In general, however, the two scales are correlated with each other.

patients in a ward nearest the nurse's desk and the least ill patients furthest from the desk. And, today, the Progressive Patient Care concept of hospital organization is based upon grouping patients according to their common medical and nursing needs.

National League of Nursing Education System

One of the earliest attempts to develop a systematic method of assessing patients needs for nursing care was reported in 1947 in *A Study of Pediatric Nursing* published by the National League of Nursing Education.*[2] This classification system, designed for the care of pediatric patients, is an example of a factor evaluation in which a patient is rated on four factors: degree of illness, extent of activity, number and complexity of treatments and procedures, and nature of adjustment. As seen in Table 12-1, each factor can be rated in terms of a three-point scale of intensity. A profile can be drawn for each patient showing the degree to which he possesses each of the four factors (see Figure 12-2).

Some attempt was made in this study to relate the amount of nursing time required to the classification of the patient, but this was done in gross terms only and did not provide a sensitive tool for determining staffing

TABLE 12-1

National League of Nursing Education Method for Classifying Nursing Care Requirements of Hospitalized Children

Factors Affecting the Amount of Nursing Care Required by Children (Cutting across all of the factors is that of age)

1. Degree of illness
   a. Acute or critical illness
   b. Moderate illness or beginning to convalesce
   c. Long-term illness or convalescent

2. Extent of activity
   a. Bed care. May have definite restrictions. Usually able to do little for self
   b. Bed care. Ambulatory to a limited degree. Able to help self with care
   c. Limited bed care. Ambulatory to a large degree. Gives much of own care

3. Number and complexity of treatments and procedures
   a. Many and/or complex treatments and procedures
   b. Few and simple treatments and procedures
   c. Occasional or no treatments and procedures

4. Nature of adjustment
   a. Behavior problem or marked difficulty in adjustment
   b. Moderate difficulty in adjustment
   c. Little or no evident difficulty in adjustment

Source: National League of Nursing Education. *A Study of Pediatric Nursing.* New York, National League of Nursing Education, 1947, p. 98.
* Now the National League for Nursing.

	Degree of illness	Extent of activity	Number and complexity of treatments and procedures	Nature of adjustment
I	Acute or critical illness	Bed care. May have definite re- strictions. Usually able to do little for self	Many and/or complex treat- ments and procedures	Behavior problem or marked diffi- culty in ad- justment
II	Moderate illness be- ginning to convalesce	Bed care. Ambulatory to a limited de- gree. Able to help self with care	Few and simple treatments and procedures	Moderate dif- ficulty in ad- justment
III	Long-term illness or convalescent	Limited bed care. Ambu- latory to a large degree. Gives much of own care	Occasional or no treatments and procedures	Little or no evident diffi- culty in ad- justment

Fig. 12-2. Profiles showing four different types of children in terms of their degree of illness, extent of activity, number and complexity of treatments and procedures, and nature of adjustment. Note lines A, B, C, and Y represent profiles of four differ- ent patients. (*Courtesy* National League for Nursing. *A Study of Pediatric Nursing.* New York, National League of Nursing Education, 1947, p. 98.)

requirements. However, compared to earlier attempts to determine nursing needs of patients[3, 4] the pediatric study took a significant step forward in deriving a scaling of these needs.

In 1948, the National League of Nursing Education published the re- sults of the use of this patient rating method in a study of nurse staffing patterns known as *A Study of Nursing Service in One Children's and Twenty-One General Hospitals.*[5, 6] The rating method was employed as a guide in assigning nursing aides to care for patients. The method increased the number of factors affecting the nursing needs of patients by adding to the four used in the pediatric study, a fifth one—teaching and rehabilitative needs.

It is interesting to note that the development of a patient classification methodology following the National League of Nursing Education studies pursued a somewhat different path. Instead of rating the specific factors that could influence a patient's requirements for nursing services, the prototype evaluation system was employed in which, as has already been mentioned, the patient's characteristics were matched to a category of nursing care requirements that most closely described these characteristics. Later developments of this methodology also attempted to define more precisely the actual nursing requirements—timewise—of patients in the different categories.

Harper Hospital Method

In the early 1950's Marion Wright directed a study at Harper Hospital in Detroit which was concerned with increasing the efficiency of the provision of nursing care.[7] A battery of studies was conducted, including assessment of the satisfaction of patients with their care, work sampling of activities of nursing personnel, and measurement of work load. In the latter study the number of medications, treatments, and diagnostic procedures provided to each patient during a 24-hour period was counted. These counts were related to the intensity of illness of the patient as determined by the three-point degree of illness scale developed by the National League of Nursing Education in its studies (1947).

Patients in four hospitals in the Detroit area were classified according to the National League of Nursing Education scale. The following percentage distribution of patient days was found in these hospitals:

Illness Category	Hospital			
	Harper	*Grace*	*Cottage*	*Hackley*
Acutely ill	20	8	11	16
Moderately ill	19	25	48	58
Mildly ill	61	67	41	26

Army Method of Patient Classification

A major step forward in the development of patient classification methodology occurred in 1951 when the Army Medical Service began a study at Walter Reed Army Hospital in Washington, D.C., directed toward the determination of a system for classifying patients' needs for nursing services.[8] On the basis of this study, a scale was developed containing nine categories of patient classification. Further research in 1951–1952 at Valley Forge Army Hospital led to the reduction of the scale to eight categories for classifying patients. Also, studies of the time required to provide nursing service to patients in each of the eight categories were carried out so that the patient classification could provide a quantitative measure of nursing requirements.

In 1953, the development of this patient classification scale reached its final stage in a study at Fort Belvoir Hospital, Virginia. It was determined that four critical factors influenced the classification of patients by their nursing requirements. These are: nursing procedural requirements, physical restriction, instructional needs, and emotional needs. Based on these factors, the eight-category scale was reduced to four categories. Further study during 1954–1955 at Brooke Army Hospital led to the acceptance of the four-category scale as the method for patient classification in Army hospitals.

As finally developed, the Army method of patient classification—a prototype evaluation system—has served as a model for much of the subsequent work in this area. Shown in Table 12-2, this method of classification is applied by determining which of the four categories most closely describes the nursing requirements of the patient being rated. When all patients are rated (the head nurse of the unit is generally the rater in all systems of patient classification) an estimate of the nursing requirements is computed by multiplying the number of patients in each category by the average hours of nursing care required for patients in each category. Average hours of care are determined by time studies that relate the amount of nursing care received by the patient to his classification.

TABLE 12-2

Army Method of Patient Classification

Category A: A patient who requires *intensive* nursing care—i.e., one who may be helpless, hypoactive or hyperactive, and/or requires frequent treatments, observation, and/or instruction. This patient may or may not be able to perform acts of self-care but has a great many nursing care needs.

Category B: A patient who requires *moderate* nursing care—i.e., one who is able to perform some or all acts of self-care but requires daily treatments, observation and/or instruction. This patient may require bed baths and assistance with feeding.

Category C: A patient who requires *minimal* nursing and supervision by nursing service personnel—i.e., one who can perform all acts of self-care but requires observation, instruction, and/or occasional treatments.

Category D: A convalescent patient who requires *supportive* nursing or clinic facilities. This includes all patients who would ordinarily be placed in a holding detachment, but for some special reason have been assigned to units staffed by nursing service personnel. Examples: female military personnel for whom no holding detachment facilities are available; male officers and their dependents; other military personnel who in the opinion of the medical officers require observation not possible in the holding detachment.

In a study done in eight military hospitals in which the Army classification method was applied to over 5,000 patients, the following distribution was found:

Patient Category	Per Cent of Patients
A. Intensive care	17
B. Moderate care	27
C. Minimal care	36
D. Supportive care	20

It should be noted that this patient population is not representative of patients in all hospitals, since it consists largely of young males. However, the fact that this methodology was developed in a nonrepresentative population does not necessarily detract from its usefulness. There are other, perhaps more serious, limitations to its use. One of these is the strong orientation of the categorization toward the physical care of patients. Largely omitted are nursing requirements in the areas of psychological needs of patients, teaching, and observation. Another limitation, as in all scales of this type, is the possible lack of sensitivity of the instrument due to the use of such subjective, nonoperationally defined terms as, "frequent," "great many," "some," "moderate," "minimal," etc.

Still another shortcoming of this method, as well as of all methodologies that have fixed prototypes or a limited set of factors, is that it may not be sufficiently inclusive of all the needs of a patient that could influence his nursing requirements. In other words, what is lacking is the concept underlying the "level of wellness" scale. Moreover, there is the question of how far into the future data gathered by this method can be projected. It is obvious that the more restrictive such a scale is in terms of the range of patients' needs it includes, the shorter is the time period in which the data can be projected.

Nevertheless, with all its limitations, the Army method of patient classification represented a significant step forward in the systematic development of such a method through the process of research.

Division of Hospitals Classification Method

At the time the Army was conducting its research on a method for classifying patients according to their nursing requirements, the Division of Hospitals of the U.S. Public Health Service was also attempting to develop such a method for use in its own hospitals. The four-category classification scale that was finally developed is shown in Table 12-3. It is similar to the Army method except that it includes more of the non-physical nursing requirements of patients. Also the prototype descriptions are phrased in more operational terminology. This scale is extensively

TABLE 12-3

Division of Hospitals, U.S.P.H.S., Method of Patient Classification

Minimal Care

A patient whose nursing care needs are almost entirely met by routine collective ward activities. For example, a patient:

1. Requiring minimal or no physical care
2. Who is ambulatory without assistance
3. Requiring infrequent medications and/or treatments
4. Who is not undergoing special tests, research studies, or therapy that demand other than routine nursing service
5. With no psychological problem demanding other than routine nursing service

Partial Care

A patient who needs some nursing care, supervision, or assistance except for his own personal hygiene. For example, a patient:

1. Requiring a moderate amount of physical care (little other than A.M. or P.M. care)
2. Who needs little assistance to be up part of the day
3. Requiring moderately frequent medications and/or treatments
4. Who is undergoing occasional or limited special tests, research studies, or therapy that demand other than routine nursing service
5. With no unusual psychological problems demanding more than a minimal amount of nursing service

Full Care

A patient who has most of his activities initiated, performed and/or supervised by nursing personnel, or who is confined to bed for the major portion of the 24-hour period. For example, a patient:

1. Requiring a major amount of physical bedside care
2. Unable to help himself, or can help himself only to a limited degree, but not requiring the equivalent of special nursing service
3. Requiring frequent or relatively complex medicines and/or treatments
4. Who is undergoing frequent or complex special tests, research studies or other studies, or therapy that demand other than routine nursing service
5. With periodic or moderately severe mental disturbance demanding a moderate amount of nursing service

Complex Care

A patient whose nursing care becomes so intricate or time-consuming as to require the equivalent of special duty nursing service. For example, a patient:

1. Requiring time-consuming nursing activities, such as isolation precaution, multiple treatments occurring simultaneously, or such frequent treatments as to require constant nursing service attention
2. Who is physically or mechanically so handicapped as to seriously interfere with his ability to cooperate normally
3. Who is irrational or suffering from an extreme mental disturbance

used in Public Health Service Hospitals and has been quite useful in determining staffing assignments.

Office of Defense Mobilization Method

In 1955 Mrs. Helen G. Tibbitts, on assignment with the Office of Defense Mobilization, reoriented the patient classification methodology from a prototype evaluation to a factor evaluation. Six factors were delineated: observation, emotional support, medication and/or treatments, assistance with hygiene, tests, and teaching. Each patient included in the study was rated on each of these factors, according to a four-point scale of intensity of need. These ratings were then combined into four classification categories which corresponded very closely to the previously discussed prototype evaluation (see Table 12-4).

In studies conducted in 14 hospitals in Tennessee and 11 hospitals in Michigan by the Division of Nursing Resources staff, U.S. Public Health Service, in which this method was used to classify patients, the following distributions were found:

	Per Cent of Patients	
Patient Category	*Tennessee*	*Michigan*
1. Intensive care	13	22
2. Moderately intensive care	31	37
3. Minimal care	45	33
4. Equivalent to outpatient department care	11	8

It is interesting to compare these figures based on a civilian population with the Army data on 5,000 patients. Both sets of data show the clustering of patients in the middle two categories, with only about one-quarter to one-third of the patients in the two extreme classes.

The advantages of this method over the prototype methods are several. First, by having the rater focus on specific factors and rating them separately and independently, greater objectivity is obtained in the rating. The tendency to be influenced disproportionately by one factor when rating several factors simultaneously and nonindependently as in the prototype evaluation—known as the halo effect—is more likely to be reduced by this approach. Moreover, this method includes a larger number of factors in the evaluation of patients needs than does the Army method. This enhances its value as a tool for the planning of nursing care and also extends the range of time for which a patient's classification could be relevant.

Division of Nursing Resources Classification Method

A refinement of the Office of Defense Mobilization patient classification method was developed in 1957 as part of a project on comprehensive patient care under the direction of the Division of Nursing Resources (now Division of Nursing), U.S. Public Health Service. The comprehensive patient care project attempted to advance the classification of patients beyond the purpose of determining staffing requirements.

The project was concerned with assessing ways to enhance the utilization of personnel, to improve the process of communication within the nursing unit, and to promote in-service education programs among nursing personnel.

This classification method is also based on six factors, many of which are similar to the Office of Defense Mobilization method: physical or hygienic activities, observation of physical phenomena, medications and/ or treatments, instructional needs, diagnostic and therapeutic tests, and observation of patient's reaction toward illness. One interesting innovation employed in this method was the actual assignment of point values according to a four-point scale, which indicated the degree to which the patient possessed each of the six areas of nursing needs (see Table 12-5). This represents one of the few attempts in the development of patient classification methods to apply quantitative scaling techniques to the methodology.

A value of this quantification technique is that it provides a rather precise determination of the patient's category of nursing requirements. In the various studies in which this method was used—and it was tested in a variety of hospitals, chronic and convalescent as well as general hospitals—the scores were grouped into four patient care categories: intensive, moderate, minimal, and outpatient department type care. However, it would be possible with this methodology to have a greater number of categories, since 19 different scale values can be obtained.

University of Kentucky Method

During the latter part of the 1950s hospitals began to turn their attention toward a reorganization of hospital care that would provide a better matching of physical facilities and personnel resources to the requirements of patients. Plans for a regrouping of patients in terms of their nursing requirements began to be developed that were based on research findings. Central to the notion of grouping hospitalized patients in terms of their nursing requirements is the need for an instrument to measure these requirements. Some early work in the development of such an instrument was undertaken by Noback and his staff in their planning for the construction of the University of Kentucky Medical Center. It was hoped that this instrument could be used to determine the types of facilities needed, the amount and kind of nursing services needed for each type of facility, and the allocation of patients to the various types of facilities.

The methodology used in this study required that data be gathered on a number of factors representing patients' needs for nursing services.

The main portion of the forms was designed to permit recording of all services provided patients within the nursing unit. This included all items of

TABLE 12-4

Chart for Rating Patients Nursing Requirements: Overall, and for Specific Nursing Components

Class	Overall Needs	Observation	Emotional Support	Medications and/or Treatments	Assistance with Hygene	Tests	Teaching
1	*Intensive:* one or more components rated at class 1 level, or total of several components amounting to *nearly continuous nursing.*	Nearly continuous	Nearly continuous	Nearly continuous	—	—	—
2	*Moderately intensive:* one or more components rated at class 2 level, none higher, total *not* adding up to nearly continuous nursing.	Frequent	Frequent or protracted	Relatively complex and time-consuming	Complete or nearly complete	Relatively complex and time-consuming (for nursing personnel)	Very time-consuming. (Intensive.)
3	*Minimal:* one or more components rated at class 3 level; none higher.	Routine	Little	Moderately frequent and/or simple	Little other than assistance with A.M. and P.M. care	Occasional; limited	Some teaching and supervised practice
4	Could be met in an outpatient department: no component rated higher than class 4 level	None, or minimal, e.g. T.P.R.	None	(a) very infrequent (b) none	None	(a) Could be given in an outpatient department (b) None	(a) Intermittent widely spaced supervision (b) None

ODM-HRAC
Form approved Budget Bureau #98-5501

TABLE 12-5

Division of Nursing Resources Method of Classification

EVALUATION OF PATIENT'S NURSING NEEDS

Patient's Name: _____ Week of: _____

Diagnosis: _____ Unit: _____

Area of Need	Degree of Patient's Needs				Judgmental Evaluation Rating A = 18+ C = 10-13 B = 14-17 D = 6-9	Total Rating, All Areas				
						M	T	W	T	F
Physical or hygenic activities	Patient requires complete assistance Value = 4	Patient requires considerable assistance Value = 3	Patient requires some assistance and/or supervision Value = 2	Patient is responsible for his own care Value = 1	Daily Rating					
						M	T	W	T	F
Observation of physical phenomena	Patient requires constant observation due to serious nature of illness Value = 4	Patient requires frequent observation such as reaction to medications, changes in vital signs, etc. Value = 3	Patient requires periodic observation such as those accomplished on nursing rounds and general nursing care Value = 2	Patient requires little or no observation Value = 1	Daily Rating					
						M	T	W	T	F
Medications and/or treatments	Patient on continuous intravenous therapy—intubation therapy—receives numerous medications and/or dressings Value = 4	Patient on intravenous therapy—intubation therapy—receives frequent medications and/or dressings Value = 3	Patient receives some medications and/or dressings Value = 2	Patient may require an occasional medication and/or dressing Value = 1	Daily Rating					

Instructional needs	Patient requires intensive teaching and practice in activities essential for discharge or rehabilitation Value = 4	Patient requires teaching and supervision of activities in preparation for discharge or rehabilitation Value = 3	Patient requires and is able to receive limited teaching—verbal and/or observation of procedure Value = 2	Patient's condition inhibits his receptivity to teaching or patient does not have need for any specific teaching Value = 1	Daily Rating				
					M	T	W	T	F

Diagnostic and therapeutic tests	Patient receives time-consuming tests; considerable nursing assistance or observation is required Value = 4	Patient receives frequent tests; some nursing assistance or observation is required Value = 3	Patient receives occasional tests; minimal nursing assistance on observation is required Value = 2	Patient receives some tests or none; little or no nursing assistance or observation is required Value = 1	Daily Rating				
					M	T	W	T	F

Observation of patient's reaction toward illness	Patient requires constant observation for unpredictable behavior—delirium, hallucination, anxiety, excitement, depression, disoriented Value = 4	Patient requires frequent observation; appears anxious; irritable; apathetic Value = 3	Patient still seeks reassurance from nurse but appears to be adjusting to illness. Talks about his needs at home, willing to learn self-help Value = 2	Patient appears to have adjusted to illness. Performs activities with assurance Value = 1	Daily Rating				
					M	T	W	T	F

487

EDS—11/27/57

personal maintenance (such as washing, bed maintenance, and feeding), all diagnostic and therapeutic procedures (such as medications, oxygen, and naso-gastric tubes) and other attentions (such as intake and output recording, ob-servations, and instruction). In all, approximately one hundred and twenty items of information were called for on each patient.[9]

Based on an assessment of these detailed factors, the patients were grouped into four categories:

Critical care: These patients require a great many services. There was great urgency in providing these services, and very frequent observa-tions were commonly needed since life was often in jeopardy.

Intensive care: These patients require many services, but there is not the urgency as for critical care patients.

Standard care: These patients also require many services, but con-siderably fewer than those of the first two groups.

Minimal care: This group consists of patients who require some super-vision, are up at liberty, need few services, and often need only a few oral medications.

The classification of a group of nearly 200 patients according to this methodology resulted in the following distribution:

Patient Category	Per Cent of Patients
Critical care	9
Intensive care	11
Standard care	71
Minimal care	9

Comparison of these figures with data from the classification methods presented earlier shows a considerably lower proportion of patients in the two extreme groups with this methodology. This could be due to actual differences in the needs of the patients who were rated rather than meth-odological differences.

Progressive Patient Care Methodology

The methodology just discussed is different from any that preceded it in that the classification of the patients is based on an evaluation of a large number of factors. Also, the methodology is geared to making a deter-mination of the kind of nursing unit in which the patient could most efficiently be assigned. A similar and even more ambitious project, known as Progressive Patient Care, was undertaken at Manchester Memorial Hospital, Manchester, Connecticut, beginning in 1957 under the sponsor-ship of the U.S. Public Health Service's Division of Hospital and Medical

Facilities. (The authors served as principal investigator and biostatistician, respectively.) Progressive Patient Care has been defined as:

The organization of facilities, services, and staff around the medical and nursing needs of the patient. Its objective is that of tailoring services to the needs of the individual patient—whether in the hospital or the home. Patients are grouped according to their degree of illness and their need for care. The staff serving each group of patients is selected and trained, and the facilities are organized to provide the kind of services needed by that group.[10]

A hospital completely organized according to the principles of Progressive Patient Care has the following six elements.[11]

Intensive care: For critically and seriously ill patients who are unable to communicate their needs or who require extensive nursing care and observation.

Intermediate care: For patients requiring a moderate amount of nursing care.

Self-care: For ambulatory and physically self-sufficient patients requiring therapeutic or diagnostic services, or who may be convalescing.

Long-term care: For patients requiring skilled prolonged medical and nursing care.

Home care: For patients requiring skilled prolonged medical and nursing care.

Home care: For patients who can be adequately cared for in the home through the extension of certain hospital services.

Outpatient care: For ambulatory patients requiring diagnostic, curative, preventive, and rehabilitative services.

These six elements correspond to the categories in a patient classification method. In order to evaluate the placement of a patient in the first three categories, a checklist shown in Table 12-6 is used. Thus, this methodology illustrates the use of a classification system not only to assess a patient's requirements for nursing care, but also to determine his placement in that area of the hospital most appropriately suited to his needs. The contribution of this methodology to the development of patient classification systems is the delineation of a number of specific factors—16 are contained in Table 12-6—that are sensitive indicators of the nursing care needs of patients.

Johns Hopkins Method

Perhaps of all the patient classification methods thus far developed the one that has received the greatest amount of testing in terms of reliability and validity is the system developed at Johns Hopkins Hospital under the direction of Dr. Charles D. Flagle. Because of Flagle's participation in the Progressive Patient Care Project at Manchester Memorial Hospital, the Johns Hopkins' methodology is geared to the determination of patients

TABLE 12-6

Progressive Patient Care Method of Classification

Criteria for Evaluating Patients		Intensive Care	Intermediate Care	Self-care
T.P.R. and/or B.P.	More often than Q4h	A	C	C
	Q4h or less			
Hemorrhage	Constant-imminent	A	C	C
	Controlled	B	B	C
	None			
Stimulants	Needed			C
	Not needed			
Consciousness	Unconscious-unstable	A	C	C
	Unconscious-stable	B	B	C
	Conscious			
Isolation	Yes			C
	No			
Vomiting	Uncontrolled	B		C
	Occasional	B	B	
	None			
Motor activity	Overactive			C
	Withdrawn			C
	Normal			
Mood	Euphoric			C
	Depressed			C
	Normal			
Thought content	Disoriented			C
	Oriented			
Bath	By nurse	B		C
	Assisted	B	B	C
	Tub-shower			
Bathroom privileges	Not permitted	B		C
	Assisted		B	C
	Permitted			
Mobility	Bedfast	B	B	C
	Chair or walks with help		B	C
	Ambulatory without help	C		
Dietary	Fed	B		C
	Fed self		B	C
	Goes or could go to food	C		
Oxygen therapy	Needed	B	B	C
	Not needed			
Transfusion	Needed	B	B	C
	Not needed			
Suction	Needed	B		C
	Not needed			

Legend: A. Compelling indicator; B. Moderate Indicator; C. Contraindicator.
Source: U.S. Public Health Service, Division of Hospital and Medical Facilities, *Elements of Progressive Patient Care.* U.S. Public Health Service Publication No. 930-C-1. Washington, Government Printing Office, 1962, p. 10.

requirements for nursing services according to the three major "P.P.C." units: intensive care (or total care), intermediate (or partial care), and self-care. However, this method goes beyond patient assignment, and was the first instrument developed that gave a specific estimate of the nursing time requirements of patients who are rated by it.

The actual form used for the rating is shown in Figure 12-3, as well as the rules for categorization of patients. This is, of course, a factor evaluation system in which approximately a dozen factors are rated. Many of these factors are similar to those included on the previously discussed "P.P.C." checklist. When the checklist is filled out, the categorization of the patient is determined by applying the criteria shown in Figure 12-4.

Among the virtues of this system are its objectivity and simplicity. Since it deals primarily with readily observable physical characteristics, rater bias is kept to a minimum. In a reliability check of this instrument Levine[12] found a reliability coefficient of 0.92. As to simplicity, a head nurse can accurately fill out the form for all the patients on a 29-bed unit in five minutes.[13]

Another virtue is the ability to convert the patient's classification into a measure of nursing work load. In the study at Johns Hopkins it was found that, on the average, patients in the three categories required the following amounts of direct nursing care during the hours 6:00 A.M. to 12:00 midnight.[14]

Category of Care	No. of Hours
Self-care	0.50
Partial care	1.00
Total care	2.50

Multiplying the total number of patients classified in each category by these time requirements provides a measure of direct nursing time requirements. Thus, if a nursing unit has 5 self-care patients, 10 partial care patients, and 5 intensive care patients, total direct nursing care requirements would be 25 hours:

$$(5 \times .5) + (10 \times 1.0) + (5 \times 2.5)$$

Among the criticisms of this method is the strong emphasis on physical needs of patients. None of the factors deals with instructional needs or needs for observation or emotional support. However, it can be argued that for some patients the intensity of these needs is highly correlated with physical needs.

Another criticism is the short-range nature of staffing predictions based on this classification. Since the classification includes needs that can change rapidly within a short span of time, this method does not provide more

Check if YES

CLASSIFICATION OF PATIENTS
THE JOHNS HOPKINS HOSPITAL

CLINIC ______ WARD ______ DATE ______					AMBULATORY		UP IN CHAIR		BATHING				FEEDING				MISCELLANEOUS						EMOTIONALLY DISTURBED		SPEC. OF NEC.
									IN BATHRM.		AT BEDSIDE														
	Sex	Age	OR	RR	Self	With Ass't.	Self	With Ass't.	Self	Ass't. Nec.	Partial Self	Complete Ass't.	Self	Requires Food Cut	IV	Complete Ass't.	Incon-tinent	Suction	Q_2	Isolat.	Uncon-scious	Vision Inade-quate	Slight	Marked	

Fig. 12-3. Instrument for collecting data used in Johns Hopkins Hospital's method of patient classification. (*Courtesy* Robert J. Conner *et al.*: "Effective Use of Nursing Resources: A Research Report." *Hospitals,* J.A.H.A., **35:**30–39, May 1, 1961.)

Category I. Self-care

Any of the following combinations checked
(a) Ambulatory, or up in chair — Self (without assistance)
Feeding self, or requires food cut
Bathing in bathroom, or at bedside — Partial
Self (can bathe self except for back and perhaps extremities)
(b) Ambulatory — with assistance
Up in chair — Self
Bathing in bathroom, or at bedside — Partial
Self
(c) As in (a and b) with
Vision inadequate
Oxygen therapy
I.V. feeding
but no two of these factors simultaneously

Category II. Partial or intermediate care

Any of the following combinations checked
(a) Ambulatory — with assistance
Bathing in bathroom, or at bedside — Partial
Self
Feeding — Complete assistance (except I.V. feeding)

Vision inadequate ⎫
Oxygen therapy ⎬ optional (does not affect classification under these conditions)

(b) Up in chair — Self
Bathing at bedside — Complete Assistance
Feeding Self, or requires food cut or I.V. feeding
Oxygen therapy ⎫ optional
Vision inadequate ⎬
(c) As in (b) with the following changes
Up in chair — With Assistance
Bath at bedside
(d) Up in chair — With Assistance
Bath at bedside — Partial Self
Feeding — Complete Assistance
Vision inadequate ⎫ optional
Oxygen therapy ⎬
(e) Bath at bedside
Feeding — Self, or requires food cut, or I.V. feeding
Vision inadequate ⎫ optional
Oxygen therapy ⎬
(f) Being Specialed of Necessity (patient has continuous nursing assistance to the extent that meal relief must be provided for special duty nurse)

NOTE: Any patient who otherwise falls into Categories I or II, but who is under suction therapy or is in isolation, incontinent (including wound drainage necessitating change of bed linen), or markedly emotionally disturbed (needs almost constant observation, in single room, creates disturbance) will be dropped to the next category.

Category III. Intensive, or "total", care

All combinations not previously mentioned.

Fig. 12-4. Rules for categorization of patients in John Hopkins Hospital's method of patient classification. (*Courtesy Hospitals*, J.A.H.A., **35**:30–39, May 1, 1961.)

than a 24-hour forecast. However, this short-range prediction is characteristic of many of the other classification systems that rely primarily on physical phenomena.

Still another limitation of the method is the inability to predict needs according to the specific category of personnel that could meet them. The instrument obtains only a gross indication of the total amount of care required and does not indicate either the specific kinds of care needed or the specific categories of personnel who should provide the care.

Comprehensive Measurement of Patients' Needs

In 1959, Abdellah and Meyer* designed a research plan to develop a comprehensive system for determining patients' needs for nursing services

* Faye G. Abdellah and Burton Meyer. "Nursing Patterns Vary in Progressive Care." *The Modern Hospital*, **95**:85–91, August 1960.

that would assess not only physical needs but total requirements for nursing services. The needs of patients were perceived as comprising four categories of care: sustenal, remedial, restorative, and preventive. The research plan proposed to develop instruments to measure each of these four categories. By applying these measures to the patient an overall quantitative rating would be derived that would indicate how much specific nursing care is required by the patient.

The improvements that this method would make over previous approaches to the evaluation of patients' needs were several. First, it encompassed all aspects of nursing care requirements, nonphysical as well as

TABLE 12-7

St. Elizabeths Hospital Method of Classification of Psychiatric Patients Who Are Not Eligible for Immediate Discharge or Rehabilitation

   I. Chronically ill patients whose psychiatric difficulties are overshadowed by the severity of their physical disability. Such a patient is for the most part bedridden.

  II. This group of patients also suffer from chronic physical illnesses with psychological disabilities but not to such an extent that some success with simple rehabilitative efforts would be prevented.

 III. This group of patients may have physical disabilities but remain in the hospital primarily because of a chronic severe emotional disturbance. Such patients may be chronically or periodically disturbed or unpredictable and impulsive so that they become a danger to themselves or others.

 IV. This group of chronically dependent patients may be relatively free of symptoms but maintain a passive dependent adjustment to the hospital. With pressure to leave the hospital, they develop acute symptoms that defeat the rehabilitative effort.

  V. This group of long-resident patients do not show periodic exacerbations in their symptoms, and they make an excellent hospital adjustment. They would be able to live outside of the hospital providing there were available appropriate facilities in the community, such as nursing homes and foster homes, without which, prospects of discharge from the hospital would be unlikely.

 VI. This group of chronically ill patients may be relatively free of symptoms of a nature that would prevent their going into the community. They have been involved in a rehabilitative program for some period of time and with further improvement would be expected to be eligible for release in the forseeable future.

 VII. Acute admission—This refers to any patient on an admission service whose clinical picture is such that it appears that he could not be discharged directly from the admission service without an intervening transfer to another service.

VIII. M & S patients—There are the acutely ill patients being cared for in the medical and surgical service.

 IX. Prisoners—This group of patients have criminal charges.

  X. Children—Under 12 years of age.

 XI. Adolescents—12 to 18 years of age.

 XII. Mental defectives—This group of patients can profit from most of the above described treatment programs, but because they have intellectual deficiencies, special procedures over and above those previously described are indicated.

physical needs. Second, it attempted to derive a quantitative measure of needs, not just classification categories. Third, it provided a logical framework for assessing the needs of patients that departed from the conventional areas of physical care, teaching, observation, and so on.

No work has been done to date to implement this research plan. Undoubtedly, any attempts made to implement this plan would have encountered formidable methodological obstacles.

St. Elizabeths Hospital Method for Classifying Psychiatric Patients

All of the methods for categorizing patients according to their needs for nursing services thus far discussed have been geared to the acutely ill patient in the short-term general hospital. Some work has been done at St. Elizabeths Hospital in Washington, D.C., to classify patients in a psychiatric hospital. The complexity and diversity of the care needs of patients in a psychiatric hospital are seen by the fact that the classification instrument contains 12 distinct categories (Table 12-7). Many of the methods developed for patients in general hospitals have included only three or four categories. Further development of the St. Elizabeths method might result in a reduction in the number of categories as well as a shift from a strictly prototype system of classification to one that focuses on the individual needs of specific patients.

Oxford Regional Hospital Board Patient Classification Method

A patient classification system patterned after the Progressive Patient Care method was developed in England as part of a method of measuring nursing care, by Jeffery, James, and Logan.* Three care groups were defined as follows:

Care Group 1 (Self-care)

I. Patients aged 12–75 years, up at least four hours daily, and recorded as:
   (a) Ambulatory . . self
   (b) Bathroom . . . self
   (c) Toilet . . . . self
   (d) Feeding . . . . self

II. Patients aged 12–60 years, up at least four hours daily, and recorded as:
   (a) Chair . . . . self
   (b) Bathroom . . . self
   (c) Toilet . . . . self
   (d) Feeding . . . self

When patients are under 12 years of age or over 75 years and patients aged 60 years or more in chairs are considered in either care group 1 or 3.

* Gordon McLachlan (ed.), *Problems and Progress in Medical Care,* published for the Nuffield Provincial Hospitals Trust, London, Oxford University Press, 1964, pp. 77–92.

Care Group 2 (Intermediate Care)

All patients not classified as care group 1 or 3.

Care Group 3 (Intensive Care)

Patients recorded as:

I. Unconscious or
II. Specialled of necessity, or
III. Undergoing
Any three of the following six; any two if combined with marked confusion; or any two if patient is over 70 years of age.
(a) Tube feeding
(b) Intravenous
(c) Suction
(d) Oxygen
(e) Blood
(f) Drainage

This method is essentially an adaptation of the Johns Hopkins methodology. More recent methods, such as those developed by the Commission on Administrative Services in Hospitals, Medicus Corporation, and Community Systems Corporation, Ltd., and described by Giovannetti in the monograph cited in the update, are also variations of the Hopkins' method.

RESEARCH DESIGN FOR DEVELOPMENT OF SCALES TO MEASURE PATIENTS' NEEDS FOR NURSING

The research design for most of the classification scales that have been developed have followed approximately the same steps. These steps are similar to those employed in all types of methodological research and include:

1. State the purpose of the method to be developed. Is it to be used for total patient care planning, prediction of staffing needs, teaching purposes, evaluation of accomplishments, or as an instrument for use in further research?

2. Delineate the factors that have a significant influence on the requirements of patients for nursing services. These may be physiological, emotional, sociological, or administrative variables.

3. Incorporate the factors into an instrument that could be applied to patients to collect data concerning the degree to which they possess each of the factors.

4. Pretest the instrument on a group of patients with varying characteristics. In the pretest, check the reliability of the instrument by assessing the extent of agreement of independent ratings of the same patients. Check the feasibility of the instrument by seeing whether the ratings can be made within a reasonable period of time, that the method can be easily learned, and that it can be quickly and simply scored.

5. On the basis of the pretest, revise the instrument and develop its final format. Preferably, the final version should be printed and possess an attractive appearance.

The problem of developing a valid and reliable method to assess the needs of patients for nursing services has not been satisfactorily solved as yet. Considerably more work needs to be done in this area. The improvements that need to be made in existing methods include:

1. Scientific scaling of these methods: such techniques as the scalogram need to be applied to test the scales for unidimensionality. The methods need to be subjected to vigorous reliability checks and they should be validated in terms of external, meaningful criteria.

2. More effort needs to be applied to advance the scales beyond ordinal types. Attempts should be made to develop quantitative measures of the different factors included in the scale.

3. The scales need to have greater sensitivity than is possessed by those presently in use, many of which have only three or four limited categories of patient care requirements.

4. Scales need to have a larger range of applicability than those that have been developed. They should be able to predict patients' needs for nursing care not for just a 12- or 24-hour period, but for the total length of his stay in the hospital.

5. Scales need to be developed that are more comprehensive in their coverage of patients' needs than those currently being employed. Consideration needs to be given to the total range of care needs, not just the superficial ones. A model for such a comprehensive scale is the concept of "high level wellness" mentioned in an earlier chapter, with its focus on all components that compose an individual's health status and its concern with scientifically assessing departures from an ideal wellness level.[15]

Measurement of the Progress of Patients
Receiving Public Health Nursing Services

Roberts and Hudson[16] have developed a methodology for assessing the needs of patients under the care of public health nurses that is analogous to the previously discussed methods of evaluating the nursing care requirements of hospitalized patients. The major aim of this methodology is to gauge the extent to which public health nursing services provided to patients are accomplishing their purpose. Essentially, this is an evaluative tool to measure the effectiveness of nursing service. This is a somewhat different objective than the previously discussed assessment of patient care requirements in hospitals, which is primarily geared to forecasting staffing needs.

The basic instrument in the method for gauging the progress of patients receiving public health nursing services is a "patient schedule." This is a source document for making an initial assessment of the patient's needs for services, for recording the kinds of public health nursing services given over a period of time, and for evaluating the terminal status of the patient in regard to these needs at the end of this period.

The needs that are assessed by this methodology are categorized into five areas, which are further divided into subareas:[17]

1. Nursing care needs: In this section the nurse records those actual and potential health needs which are the primary responsibility of a nurse to help patients and families meet. These needs are subclassified or subgrouped into five areas: "physical care," "nutrition," "treatments," "emotional behavioral," and "other."
2. Immunization and tests: Here the nurse lists measures to achieve specific immunity from disease and also diagnostic examinations which may be necessary to determine a patient's health status.
3. Medical care needs: This part of the patient schedule is for recording health needs that are primarily the responsibility of a physician or dentist. Information is subclassified or subgrouped according to "diagnosed conditions or disabilities," "suspected illnesses or abnormalities," and "health supervision."
4. Social guidance and other health-related needs: Needs other than nursing or medical which affect the health or care of the patient are separated into four subclassifications: "social guidance," "economic assistance," "educational training," and "other health-related needs."
5. Self-care activity of chronically ill patients: For patients with long-term illness or disability, limitations in selected self-care activites are divided for reporting into four subclassifications: "locomotion," "bathing," "dressing," and "feeding."

Each patient's needs are assessed by the nurse responsible for the patient's care upon his entrance into service and again at the time the patient is discharged from nursing service. The initial assessment includes two evaluations, one reflecting the care needed by the patient and the other a prediction of the anticipated outcome for the patient in regard to his need. A scale for assessing both actual need and anticipated outcome is provided for each of the five areas of need. For example, the scale for nursing care needs is:

Care Status and Expected Outcome

1. Care not needed
2. Patient or family meeting need
   a. Through own resources
   b. Through outside resources
3. Patient or family need assistance
   a. Instruction needed
   b. Individual or family unable to give care
   c. Attitudes prevent family from assuming care
4. Patient in hospital or other institution
5. Patient deceased
6. Status unknown

In addition, the patient schedule provides for recording the types of nursing service provided during the period the patient is under care. Four major types of services are designated on the schedule:

Direct care
Instruction, counseling
Evaluation, supervision
Referral

The patient schedule, thus, is a very compact tool for assessing the needs of the patients, both initially and terminally, and for relating the services provided by the public health nurses to these needs.

The methodology includes another schedule called a "family schedule" listing all members of the patient's family, which serves as a control sheet for the patients being evaluated. Certain selected characteristics concerning the patient are entered on this schedule, such as program category (e.g., tuberculosis, maternity, mental health), age, source of referral of the patient to the health agency, the length of time from initial to terminal assessment, and the number of patient-nurse contacts.

The development of the schedules for this methodology followed the same pattern described for the patient classification instruments. The steps included selection and definition of areas of patient needs, development of a scaling of these needs, pretesting the schedules, and preparation of the final version of the methodology.[18] The pretest, which included a few hundred patients in several different public health agencies, provided a very thorough assessment of the method. In these studies a maximum period of 90 days was allowed for each patient from initial to terminal assessment.

This methodology has several commendable characteristics that represent significant improvements over many of the patient classification instruments previously discussed. First, it is totally patient-centered. It focuses attention on the specific needs of the patient rather than attempting to fit the patient into preconceived categories.

Second, it is very comprehensive. It includes not only the nursing needs of the patients, but medical and social needs as well.

Third, the instrument attempts to grade the intensity of each area of need in terms of an ordinal-type scale whose values are described operationally.

Finally, the instrument is concerned with changes in the patient's status over a period of time. Thus, it can be used to obtain an evaluation of the impact of the services provided to the patient as well as serving as a means of planning for his care.

Methodological Approach to Observe and Classify Child Behavior

Somewhat related to the patient progress methodology in its focus on the total needs of patients is Hook's study[19] concerned with child behavior. This research was directed at identifying the problems faced by children when they return from a psychiatric inpatient therapy service and also at gaining insight into the role of the nurse in the follow-up of these children.

Specific problems studied were those encountered by the child in his return to the home and community and the role of the nurse in helping the child and family.

A basic premise upon which this research is based is that "children shall be separated from their families for as short a time as possible" and that an essential part of the therapy is the continued maintenance of home and family relationships. This was a longitudinal study in which the research nurse made contact with the patient and his family through a home visit made prior to admission for treatment at a children's inpatient service. The nurse made observations of such variables as the child's behavior, the interactions between family members, characteristics of the home, neighborhood environment, physical health of the family. Home visits were scheduled just prior to the child's discharge and for periodic intervals over a two-year period.

A unique contribution of this study was the development of a method for classifying child behavior. The following five categories were developed:

1. Child—his behavior that could influence other peoples' interaction with him. Examples of his behavior included speech, gestures, poor toilet habits, noisy eating habits, isolated self, poor general behavior.
2. Family—their behavior concerning the child. Examples of behavior included discipline, isolation, antagonism, rejection of, or ashamed of, child.
3. Peers—interrelationships. Examples of behavior included isolation and getting along well with peers.
4. School. Attendance at school; exclusion from school; placement in wrong grade levels; attempts made by parents to place children in school.
5. Law. Involvement with law; admission to school by the court.

The role of the nurse was also explored, and her contributions were identified. For example, she learned as much as possible about the families, gave information, served as liaison between and among groups.

The study population included 53 subjects, of whom 48 were followed up by the research nurse. The subjects were all children from the psychiatric service. A total of 20 variables were studied, 15 of which were designated as "trend" variables that reflected changes that took place in the individual, his parents, the visiting nurse, or school personnel. A significant finding was that there was no single pattern of change that could be cited as being representative of change over a four- to six-month period of time. Eighty-five per cent of the problem areas remained unchanged.

The investigator made some major recommendations regarding the instrument which will be of value to other researchers wishing to perfect it. There was some concern that not all categories of the variable "child behavior" had been identified. Once this exploration has been completed, it is suggested that the categories be reduced to a "complete minimum" to produce an instrument that would cover all pertinent areas and at the same time be practical. In addition to the principal investigator, it is recommended that the visiting nurse, data analyst, and any others concerned with the interpretation and application of the findings be involved in the development of the list of categories.

A further finding showed that peer acceptance, amount of help needed, and the degree to which a behavior problem is present are not easily evaluated. Emphasis was placed upon the importance of describing the variable under study in such a way that it could be scaled along a continuum. It is proposed that a scale might be developed along which operational definitions of behavior are stationed at as near equal distances as possible on the continuum. The visiting nurse could then place a mark on this continuum according to her rating of the variable.

This study has helped to increase our understanding of the problems children have upon their return home after inpatient care at a psychiatric institute. Particularly valuable is a method for identifying and classifying these behavior problems.

METHODS OF STUDYING NURSING PERSONNEL

Many of the methods developed in the area of administration are concerned with personnel rather than patients. Several examples of these will be discussed: the nursing audit, methodology for studying the activities of nursing personnel, an evaluation of job satisfaction, measures of turnover, a tool to assess nursing administration, and a cost methodology.

Nursing Audit

The development of an important methodological tool is a nursing service audit,[20] which is "an official examination of nursing records for the purposes of evaluation, verification, and betterment." Deeken[21] developed a nursing service audit guide to serve as an aid in conducting the audit to appraise and improve the quality of patient care rendered.

In this study the immediate problem was to set up a guide for the nursing service unit that could show observable improvement in patient care. A thorough search of the literature in the field was made. Unlike the field of medicine, which reported a medical audit as early as 1918, little has been reported in the literature on a nursing audit. The basic principles in developing financial and medical audits were gleaned and used in the development of the nursing audit.

Theoretical Contribution   A basic concept in developing the nursing audit is that it must be recorded and made available on hospital forms. The theoretical principles upon which the nursing audit is based are that it must:[22]

1. Provide a systematic review of the nursing records of patients discharged from the hospital
2. Provide maintenance of a record of performance of each professional nurse on the staff
3. Provide a biographical index of the quality of nursing that each patient has received
4. Develop valuable and pertinent information for the physicians on the staff
5. Develop and improve the quality of nursing and nursing notes
6. Develop a means to reveal areas of strength and weakness in nursing service
7. Develop better cooperation between physicians and nurses as a result of an improved quality of nursing notes

Methodological Approach   The method, developed by Deeken to help appraise patient care rendered, is straightforward and involves the following seven steps:[23]

1. Appointment of a committee on a rotating basis
2. Establishment of a regular time of meetings
3. Qualitative auditing of nurses' clinical records
4. Grand rounds of the audit committee
5. Evaluation of the findings and preparation of the final report
6. Individual counseling of nurses who have been found deficient
7. Follow-up study of discharged patients to evaluate the effectiveness of the audit committee

The qualitative auditing of nurses' clinical records is achieved by the use of a specific list of coded factors which are recorded on a "Nursing Service Audit Observation Tally Sheet": (See Figure 12-5)
Examples of coded factors are:[24]

Were the physician's orders promptly and accurately carried out?
Were reasons given for delays in starting medications and/or treatments?
Was the nursing care plan adequate for each shift of personnel?
Were subjective or objective symptoms noted on admission?[25]

Nurse evaluation and counseling records and a follow-up patient service questionnaire were also developed.

Usefulness of Tool   The nursing service audit was designed to serve as an administrative tool for a nursing service director to help evaluate

Date of Audit _____ Service _____ Unit   Personnel observed:

Record reviewed by _____   Head nurse _____
                                                           Staff nurse _____
                                                           Student nurse _____
                                                           Practical nurse ___

Code No.	Record No.	Page	Tally Column	Name of Nurse

Fig. 12-5. Excerpt from "Nursing Service Audit Observation Tally Sheet." (*Courtesy* Sister Mary Helen Louise Deeken. "A Guide for the Nursing Service Audit." St. Louis, Catholic Hospital Association, 1960.)

quality of patient care by means of a nursing audit committee. A contribution of the study is that it includes the development of a simple procedure for carrying out the audit and standards for clinical recording. The nursing service audit is a means of broadening and strengthening the nursing service and improving hospital standards of care. The nursing service audit can be used as a criterion to determine if patients are receiving quality nursing care.

Bredenberg[26] also developed a nursing audit in the form of a "Hospital Nursing Service Checklist for Self-Appraisal." The checklist was built upon "tangible evidence" ordinarily found in a well-managed department of nursing service. Broad areas covered in the checklist include:

Philosophy and objectives
Organization
Policy manuals
Nursing procedures
Budgeting
Staffing
Appraisal of nursing service
Job specifications and descriptions
Personnel
In-service program
Hospital meetings

Methods of Studying Activities of Nursing Personnel

One of the most widely used administrative tools in nursing is the methodology for studying the activities of nursing personnel. The main purpose of such a study is to evaluate the extent to which nursing personnel are performing tasks that require their skill and the extent to which the tasks they perform could be done by others.

The impetus for such studies is the persistent problem of shortage of professional nursing skills. Determination of the extent to which tasks done by professional nurses could be performed by others provides a means of alleviating this shortage. The employment of auxiliary personnel, like ward clerks, to assume certain nonnursing tasks could serve to free the professional nurse for those duties requiring professional nursing skill.

The fundamental basis for all studies of activities of nursing personnel —also called function, utilization, or work sampling studies—is the time study approach developed by industrial engineers. The framework for the activity study methodology consists of two essential ingredients: (1) a scheme of classification of the activities of nursing personnel, and (2) a method for determining the amount of time personnel devote to each of the classes of activities during the period of study. The method does not attempt to evaluate quality of performance and is focused directly on what is being done, not why or how it is being done.

Activity studies in nursing differ from the typical industrial engineer's time study primarily in terms of the classification scheme for the activities. These have been very elaborate, as in a study entitled *Nursing Practice in California Hospitals,* which consisted of over 400 different categories of nursing activities,[27] or very concise, as in the work sampling methodology developed by the U.S. Public Health Service's Division of Nursing.[28]

Methodologies differ, too, in the types of personnel and the kinds of work situations they encompass. Some methods have been developed specifically for certain classes of personnel—head nurses, staff nurses, operating room nurses, nurses in the outpatient department, or public health nurses. Although many methods have been developed for nurses in short-term general hospitals, there are some techniques available for studying activities of nurses in psychiatric hospitals, nursing homes, industrial health programs, and schools of nursing.

Methods also differ in the ways in which the data are collected. Many require the use of the nonparticipant observer to record the activities observed. A few of the methods make use of the participant observer technique. A methodology developed by the Veterans Administration employs the diary device, in which the personnel studied record their activities.[29] Also some methods require a continuous observation of the activities performed in which the time required to complete each activity is recorded. Other methods employ work sampling, in which a sample is drawn of different time periods, and the activity performed at that time period is observed. The number of times each activity is performed is then converted into an estimate of the total amount of time spent on the various activities.

To illustrate the development of an activity study method, the Division of Nursing's work sampling study will be described briefly.

The method grew out of the work done by the Division in the early 1950's in studying, on a continuous observation basis, the activities of head nurses in general hospitals.[30] It was later expanded to include all personnel assigned to the nursing unit. The scheme of classification was broadly conceived to encompass all types of nursing personnel. By providing for collection of the data through work sampling, the method enabled a single observer to record the activities performed by each of the personnel on a nursing unit every 15 minutes.

The development of the scale of classification involved a considerable amount of pretesting. Careful checks were made on the reliability of the method as well as the validity and meaningfulness of the data collected through its use.

The classification scale for the method consists of describing each activity according to two nominally scaled variables: (1) the area of the activity, and (2) its level. The area of a nursing activity essentially describes its purpose. It consists of four main classes:

Patient-centered
Personnel-centered
Unit-centered
Other

The level of the activity defines the nature of the skill, training, and responsibility needed to perform the activity. Seven levels are differentiated:

Administration. Activities which involve responsibility for planning and providing effective patient care; for development of unit personnel; and for management and operation of the nursing unit

Nursing. Direct and indirect activities involved in giving nursing care to patients

Clerical. Activities concerned with counting, copying, ordering, and recording

Dietary. Activities involved in routine servings of fluids, food, and nourishment

Housekeeping. Activities concerned with the appearance of the unit environment, care of supplies and equipment

Messenger. Activities involved in transport services, escort services, and errands

Unclassified. Activities not classified under any other code level

The observer is provided with a carefully designed form on which to record the observations. The sampling scheme advocated is that of a systematic sample. Observations of all personnel assigned to the nursing unit are made every 15 minutes. Randomness of the sample is considered to be achieved by the random order of the activities performed by the personnel being observed.

The Division of Nursing's methodology has been widely used in hospitals throughout the nation. Although its primary use has been to gather data to make administrative changes in the assignment of duties, it has also been employed as a research tool. For example, in a study of the comparison of the floor manager plan of organization in a hospital nursing unit with the traditional head nurse form of organization, the activity study methodology provided a criterion measure of the extent to which each type of organization promoted the effective use of personnel.[31]

The objectives of the activity study tool are limited. It does not evaluate quality of care nor is it geared toward assessing the total administrative character of a nursing unit. With these limitations the activity study can be termed a success if the wide use to which it has been put is the criterion. However, need for further methodological refinement in this area does exist. One such refinement would relate the activities performed to the patients' requirements for services in order to balance staffing with the needs of patients.

Measurement of Job Satisfaction of Nursing Personnel

In 1956–1957, Wright[32] developed a 215-item questionnaire concerned with evaluating all aspects of working conditions that could affect the job satisfaction of nursing personnel in hospitals. Each item was designed in the form of statements to which the respondent could agree, disagree, neither agree nor disagree, or state that he does not know. The scale then is a Likert-Type. The items could be grouped into categories representing major areas of working conditions, such as pay and benefits, supervision received, physical facilities, equipment, assignments given, and so on, Some typical items include:

> The hospital does not operate smoothly and effectively.
> As long as I do good work, I can be sure of my job.
> I can usually get my vacation at the best time for me.
> Patient charts are often not adequate or clear.
> The doctors here seldom blame us for things beyond our control.
> Some of the equipment I use is not always in good condition.

The approach used to design this methodology was as follows: First, a conceptual framework was established encompassing the various components of the variable "job satisfaction." The framework was used ·to gather items concerning the different components. These were drawn from existing published sources and from interviews and questionnaires. The initial collection included over 1,000 items. Many of these were eliminated by inspection as being rewordings of other items.

The initial questionnaire contained several hundred items, which were then pretested among nursing personnel as to clarity and meaningfulness. An item analysis was performed on the pretest data in which each item was correlated with the total score to find out which items discriminated most sharply between those personnel who scored high on the total questionnaire and those scoring low. In other words, an item that discriminated well was one in which a respondent attaining a high score (high job satisfaction) on the total instrument consistently responded to it in a certain way (e.g., "the hospital is a part of me"—*agree*) while a low scorer (low job satisfaction) always responded to the item the opposite way—*disagree*.

Reliability of the items was tested by a comparison of the consistency of responses to items in which the content was identical but the wording was different. Unreliable items were considered to be those in which responses to similar content material contradicted each other—as, for example, a respondent agreeing with "As long as I do good work, I can be sure of my job," and disagreeing with "We are usually told where we stand."

In addition to the elimination of nondiscriminating and unreliable items, some items were screened out by a process of analyzing the correlations among responses to the items. This was accomplished by a short-cut method of factor analysis known as cluster analysis, in which correlation profiles were drawn for the items.[33] When several items were highly intercorrelated, and they dealt with essentially the same content, one of the items was selected from the cluster for inclusion in the form.

By these methods of screening the items and by further pretesting of the entire form for clarity of wording, a battery of 215 items was produced. The next step in the development of this methodology was to validate it. This was done by measuring the extent to which a score on this instrument correlated with the external criterion variable, "job turnover." The validation study was based on 411 subjects representing all levels of nursing. The study found only a small degree of correlation between turnover behavior and total scores for the 215 items.

A final step in the development of the instrument was to correlate responses to individual items with turnover behavior. On this basis of item validation a set of approximately 45 items was found to be most highly related to turnover. This shortened set of items not only would provide an instrument that would be of maximum validity but would also be simpler to administer.

A total score was computed for the 45 items and correlated with turnover behavior. This was done for four separate personnel groups: head nurses and supervisors, staff nurses, practical nurses, and aides and orderlies. The coefficient of correlations between the score on these items and turnover behavior ranged from 0.37 for staff nurses to 0.69 for practical nurses. This would suggest a fairly high degree of correlation, at least as high as in many tests used as preadmission screening devices in colleges and universities to assess an applicant's potential performance.

Although possessing fairly high predictive ability, this job satisfaction instrument has not been widely used, even though the purpose for its development was to provide a tool for nursing administration. Perhaps one of the reasons for its lack of popularity is that it may touch on sensitive areas that some administrators would rather avoid. Also, until more theoretically oriented research is done in the area of morale among nursing personnel, we cannot be sure how to interpret the data collected with such an instrument.

Measurement of Turnover Among Nursing Personnel

In the development of a criterion measure to validate the job satisfaction instrument just described, Levine and Wright[34] found that the traditional measurement of turnover behavior developed by the U.S. Bureau of Labor Statistics was not adequate for use in tests of statistical significance. The conventional measure of turnover is a ratio in which the total number of personnel who have terminated their employment during a period of time is divided by the average number of personnel employed during that same period. Since a test of the significance of the difference between two rates requires that the rates be true relative frequencies, this measure of turnover is not usable, particularly when computed for a fairly long time period, like a year. This is so because the denominator of the turnover rate is the average number of persons employed during the year—or the average number of filled positions. This figure is derived by adding the number of persons employed at the beginning of the year to the number employed at the end of the year and dividing by two. The average number of filled positions is not the total population exposed to the risk of turnover, since within the year some positions may be filled by several different people. Unlike a true relative frequency the turnover rate does not have a limit of 100 per cent, but may exceed that.

The rate developed to avoid this difficulty is called the *relative frequency of turnover*. In this rate the numerator is the number of personnel who terminated their employment during the time period studied—the same numerator as in the previous ratio. However, the denominator is the sum of the number of personnel who terminated their employment during this time period *and* the number who did not. Such a turnover rate is a true relative frequency and can be subjected to statistical tests of significance.

Another type of turnover rate developed at this time was the *instability rate.* This rate represents an attempt to add another dimension to the measurement of turnover among nursing personnel. A serious drawback of crude turnover rates is that they hide differences in length of service of employees. Two hospitals can have identical crude turnover rates, yet one hospital may be mainly staffed by employees with periods of short service and the other with personnel who for the most part have long periods of employment.

The instability rate was developed primarily to account for differences in the length of service of personnel. The rate is simply the percentage of persons employed at the beginning of the year who terminated their employment during the year. To illustrate how this rate supplements the turnover ratio,* consider a hospital that has no turnover within a 12-month period. It would have a turnover rate of zero and an instability rate also of zero. A hospital in which all positions turned over once would have a turnover rate of 100 per cent (assuming, of course, all the positions were refilled at the end of the year) and an instability rate also of 100 per cent. A hospital where all positions turned over twice would have a turnover rate of 200 per cent and an instability rate of 100 per cent. A turnover rate of 100 per cent and an instability rate of 50 per cent would mean, therefore, that half of the positions turned over twice.

The computation of such administrative measures as the turnover and instability rates requires that adequate records be kept on the employment of personnel. These records should show the number of personnel on the payroll of the agency and the number of accessions and terminations during the time period being evaluated.

Method for Examining the Total Character of Nursing Administration

Mullane, in her doctoral dissertation,[35] developed a methodology that could be used in assessing the overall quality of nursing service administration in a hospital. The purpose of her project was to identify criteria of excellence in the administration of hospital nursing service and to validate them in terms of the criterion of job satisfaction. Her hypothesis was that there would be a relationship between level of excellence of administration and the degree of job satisfaction in the hospital.

To develop the criteria, the first step was a thorough review of the literature. The inital set of criteria selected consisted of 19 criterion areas with 163 related indices. These were reviewed by a panel of judges and after a lengthy period of refinement reduced to eight main criteria:

Purpose
Organization
Staff

* The traditional turnover rate, not the relative frequency of turnover.

Conservation of energy and material
Budget
Appraisal of service
Planning
Reporting

Within each of the eight areas, indices were developed for evaluating the degree of excellence of the criterion area. For example, for the criterion "purpose" some of the indices were:

The director of nursing is conscious of goals more specifically defined than to "give good nursing care."
She involves the supervisors and/or head nurses in defining the goals of nursing service.
The specific objectives of nursing care are discussed periodically with the nursing staff.

The criteria and their indices were submitted to 54 experts who were asked to score them in terms of a three-point Likert-type ordinal scale. The scale assessed the importance of the indices to excellence of nursing service administration in a hospital:

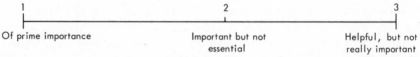

Fig. 12-6. Scale for assessing importance of indices of excellence of nursing service administration. (*Courtesy* Mary K. Mullane.)

On the basis of the scoring of the judges it was possible to obtain a rank ordering of the criteria and their indices. The rank ordering of the criteria are as follows:

1. Organization
2. Planning
3.5. Appraisal of service
3.5. Conservation of energy and material
5. Reporting
6. Staff
    6.1. Appraisal
    6.2. In-service education
    6.3. Assignment
    6.4. Conditions of service
    6.5. Participation
    6.6. Recruitment, etc.
7. Purpose
8. Budget

The validation of the instrument consisted of relating the criteria in 23 hospitals in Michigan to a measure of the job satisfaction of the personnel in the hospitals. Correlations between each of the criteria and the job satisfaction scores ranged from +0.42 for the criterion "purpose" to +0.70 for the criterion "staff."

As a method for appraising the total administrative character of a nursing service organization this methodology can be a useful tool. One of its virtues is that unlike some of the methodology now being employed in nursing service administration, it was developed especially for nursing.

Measurement of Costs of Providing Nursing Services

An important administrative criterion is that of the costs incurred in making an organization's product. In health agencies the product is patient care, and the costs of "making" the product are largely those related to the personnel services that compose patient care.

The costs incurred in producing an organization's product can serve as a useful criterion of effectiveness. Effectiveness can be said to have increased when the quantity (or quality) of output is increased while costs have remained the same. As a criterion measure costs are quantifiable, relatively easy to measure, readily understood, and pragmatically meaningful.

Several methods of cost analysis have been developed for nursing services. Ferguson[36] developed a method for determining the annual expenditures per work unit of small health agencies providing public health nursing services. Data are collected from existing records and from a time study of personnel activities extending over a period of a month. The work unit is defined as a home visit, office visit, clinic session, visit to a nursing home or day care center, visit to a school, or class or group teaching.

A manual has been published providing step-by-step instructions for the determination of the work unit expenditures.[37] The method includes five schedules which are used to record the necessary data and a work sheet for summarization of the data and computation of expenditures per direct service work unit.

Schedule	Purpose
1	Time study form to record number of minutes spent on each work unit area and in supporting services (meetings, other office work, personal and lunch), during the month of the study
2	Summary of time study data
3	Record of the number of direct service work units during the month of the time study and for the reporting year
4	Annual expenditures of the agency and calculation of charges to nursing service by object of expense (salary, travel, equipment, supplies, other)
5	Calculation of expenditure per direct service work unit

METHODOLOGICAL RESEARCH IN THE AREA
OF NURSING EDUCATION

Much of the methodology employed in the area of nursing education has been borrowed from other educational fields. This is particularly true of the methodology used to select nursing students. Many of the tests used to assess an applicant's aptitudes, personality, and interests are those that have been developed for fields other than nursing. Three examples of methodological research conducted specifically for nursing education will be briefly discussed. These cover such wide-ranging topics as measurement of attitudes of applicants to schools of nursing, assessing a student's perception of the needs of patients, and a method of evaluating the costs of nursing education.

A Method for Evaluating the Attitudes of Prospective Nursing Students

The loss of vital nurse-manpower through student withdrawal from schools of nursing is a persistent problem. The fact that one out of three students fails to graduate, many because of reasons not related to scholastic achievement, would suggest that psychological factors play an important part in attrition. Such was the thinking of Thurston[38] and his research team that led them to undertake a systematic and meaningful method of inquiry into the attitudes and emotional reactions of prospective nursing students.

As part of a six-year research program a battery of tests was administered to applicants of three schools of nursing and their performance analyzed. The Luther Hospital Sentence Completion Form (LHSC) was one of the instruments (attitudinal scale) devised by the investigators and used as one of the psychological tests. It is designed specifically for nursing students and applicants to schools of nursing.

The LHSC Form evaluates the attitudes and emotional reactions of students and prospective students in the following seven attitudinal areas:

1. The profession of nursing
2. Self
3. Home and family
4. Responsibility
5. Others
6. Academic areas
7. Love and marriage

The development of the LHSC instrument was based on over 400 incomplete sentence items assembled by the investigators from professional nurses, a clinical psychologist, and a review of the literature. The items were reduced to 150 which met the criteria of relevance, clarity, and potentiality for yielding "rich" responses. Further pretesting reduced the items to 90 sentences. The student expresses her attitudes and feelings in regard to nursing as a profession and other attitudinal areas by completing sentences of which the following fifteen are examples:

Nursing Sentence Completions

Directions: Below are a number of incomplete sentences. By completing these sentences you can express how you feel about many things. Try to do every one. Feel free to write whatever you wish.

1. When I go to nursing school, my family
2. In high school, I was happiest when
3. At home, I
4. Teachers
5. I feel sad if
6. When on a date, I
7. I like to help when
8. I'm different from other girls in that
9. My family
10. When someone tells me to do something
11. When with strangers, I
12. Supervised study periods
13. I pray
14. Ten years from now, I
15. Most people think that a nurse

Source: Nursing Sentence Completions, copyright 1964 by Thurston-Brunclik; excerpted from instrument by permission of the authors.

The proposed method is significant in that it is possible to make a psychological evaluation of the respondent without any other knowledge. The investigators stress that the instrument is most useful in opening up for exploration areas involving personality problems that would not be picked up through psychological testing or in an initial contact with the student. This technique would seem to be most useful in identifying problem areas before a student is accepted, or if admitted, to work out a program to correct the problem.

Methodology for Assessing Student Perception of Patients' Attitudes Toward Their Care

In 1960, Boyle published the results of a study in which a methodology was developed to determine the ability of nursing students to recognize the self-perceived needs of patients. Her report, *A Study of Student Nurses Perception of Patients' Attitudes,* contains a very complete description of the steps followed in the development of this methodology, including the problems encountered in the pursuit of the research objective and the rationale for decisions made at the various stages of development.[39]

Several hundred patients, students, and instructors and supervisory personnel in the hospitals in which the students were assigned participated in this methodological research. Three instruments were used to collect the data. These are summarized in Table 12-8. In the card sort, 34 items pertaining to three aspects of hospital care—physical and social environment, physical care, and information and assurance—were rated by patients and students according to two scales: whether the item was or was not true for the patient (yes-no scale), and the importance (very important, important, less important, not important) of the item to the patient. Thus for the yes-no sort, one of the items read: "I understand why I am getting my medicines." For the importance sort the same item read, "To understand why I am getting my medicines." In the analysis of the data the ratings of a patient were compared with those of the student taking care of him, and a score was determined that signified the extent of agreement between student and patient.

Students also responded to a questionnaire in which they were asked to rate the importance of a series of items corresponding to those on the importance card sort by imagining themselves as patients. These responses were matched with those on the importance sort to determine the extent to which the attitudes of a student deviated from those she ascribed to her patient. Students also were asked to respond to an open-ended question— "List the things that would be most important to you if you were a patient in the area of medical care, nursing care, or environment." These free responses were compared with the importance assigned to the items on the questionnaire as an additional assessment of the way in which the students perceived the importance of different aspects of patient care.

Finally, the instructors and the supervisory personnel assigned to the nursing units were asked to respond to the 34 items contained on the card sort in terms of their assessment of the importance of each item to "most" medical and surgical patients in their hospital. These responses were compared with those of the students to determine whether students were better or less able to predict the responses of particular patients than were the faculty and supervisory staff who responded for patients in general.

Among the findings of this study were the following: Freshman students perceived the importance of particular items of care to their patients as well as did senior students. Students estimated the importance of particular items of care to their patients more accurately than did the instructors and supervisors who responded in terms of "most patients." Most students tended to underestimate the importance to patients of physical care.

Methodologically, this study is interesting because of the attempt to develop ordinal scales to measure the closeness of agreement between the responses of different study subjects to the same phenomena. It also demonstrates the use in a single study of a variety of methods—interviews,

TABLE 12-8

Summary of Techniques Used in Study of Student Perception of Patient Needs

Instrument	Patients	Students	Instructors	Head Nurses and Supervisors	Scoring or Use
Card sort:					
1. "Yes-No" sort (would the patient answer "Yes" or "No" to each item)?	X	X			Agreement between student and patient responses provided a "Yes-No" or satisfaction score. (See p. 28.)*
2. "Importance" sort (How important is each item to the patient)?	X	X			Extent of agreement between student and patient response provided basis for "importance" score. (See p. 28.)
Questionnaires:					
1. "If I were a patient." (How important would each item be to you if you were a patient)?		X			Student response for self matched with her estimate of "importance" for her patient. Scored to indicate extent of agreement. Correlation determined between scores on "importance" sort and "If I were a patient." (See p. 29.)
2. "Most patients want" (How important would each item be to "most" medical and surgical patients)?			X	X	Determined average value assigned by each group of respondents. Ranked groups of respondents in relation to closeness to patients responses. (See p. 29.)
Free response: What things would be important to you if you were a patient?		X			Unstructured responses of students compared with "Importance" assigned to items in questionnaire—If I were a patient." (See p. 29.)

* Refers to pages in document cited below.
Source: Rena E. Boyle. *A Study of Student Nurse Perception of Patient Attitudes.* P.H.S. Publication No. 769, Washington, D.C., U.S. Government Printing Office, 1960, p. 31.

card sorts, questionnaires—to gather sufficient data with which to explore a research problem in depth.

Method for Determining Costs in a School of Nursing

In 1956, the National League for Nursing and the U.S. Public Health Service published a manual describing the methodology for determining the costs incurred in operating a collegiate school of nursing.[40] This, of course, is a more involved methodology than the previously described technique for determining expenditures for public health nursing in small agencies. Whereas only five schedules are employed in the latter method, approximately 50 different schedules are contained in the costs of education methodology.

Essentially this method consists of determining the costs for each *cost center,* which represents an activity, a function, or department of the school. Among the cost centers are staff benefits (salaries and wages), operation and maintenance of physical plant, general administration, library, student aid, and student services.

During the period 1958–1963 the National League for Nursing applied the cost methodology to a sample of baccalaureate, associate degree, and diploma schools of nursing in the United States to determine the costs of basic programs of professional nursing.[41] The data revealed considerable variability from school to school in the cost per student as well as variability among the three types of programs. On the basis of preliminary data the median gross costs in the three types of programs per student per year were:

Baccalaureate	$1,400
Associate	1,600
Diploma	2,500

METHODOLOGICAL RESEARCH IN THE AREA OF NURSING PRACTICE

There is a rich variety of methodological research in the area of nursing practice. Several such studies will be discussed. The first of these is an attempt to develop a model for the measurement of patient care. Another presents a theoretical framework for identifying the nursing problems of patients. Two studies deal with the development of methodological tools for evaluating nursing practice: one focusing directly on the patient, attempts to assess the effect of nursing care on the patient, and the other, focusing on the staff nurse herself, attempts to evaluate the quality of performance. In another study, the development of instruments to measure decubitus ulcers is discussed. The development of a method of assessing patient and personnel perception of unfulfilled nursing care needs, also known as a method of assessing satisfaction with patient care, will be discussed, as well as recently developed patient assessment tools. A method for systematically assessing the nursing care needs of patients will be presented. Finally, the development of a measure of the quality of nursing care will be described.

Development of a Measure of Patient Care

Howland and McDowell have adopted the concepts of homeostasis and cybernetics in the development of a hospital system model to measure patient care.[42,43,44] Basic to the understanding of the method of patient care measurement proposed by these investigators is that regulation is defined as the ability of a system to maintain an organism in specific survival states.

If a hospital system model is to function and provide ways of measuring patient care, it must provide a means of measuring decisions from community to bedside on the ability of the system to regulate patient condition. The intent here is to be able to predict patient states and thus preplan specific actions to equalize these states. The ultimate overall hospital system goal is that of a "high level wellness."[45]

Patient care is measured on the basis of the homeostatic regulatory capacity of the hospital. When homeostatic disequilibrium occurs, the hospital must provide the staff, equipment, and supplies to restore it. "Patient care, then, is a system performance measure, rather than a measure of any component."[46]

The investigators specify that the basic subsystem of the hospital that is responsible for maintaining patient states is the nurse-patient-physician triad. "Good" patient care would be a measure of the ability of the hospital system to respond promptly and accurately to changes in patient condition. Such a system would complement that of Progressive Patient Care, which groups patients by their common medical and nursing needs regardless of diagnosis.

The proposed method of measuring patient care provides a basis for further construction of formal hospital system models. The investigators have succeeded in moving closer to the frontier of patient care measurement. They recognize that much research still needs to be undertaken before the concepts of homeostasis and cybernetics can be stated in useful terms for hospital design and operation.

Methods of Identifying Covert Aspects of Nursing Problems

If professional nursing education is to prepare the nurse to identify and solve the nursing problems presented by patients, methods must be developed and utilized that are suitable to the development of skills in, and sensitivity for, solving all significant aspects of nursing problems.

Purpose of This Study   Abdellah[47] undertook a study that was concerned with an important aspect of the methodology of teaching in nursing —namely, the teaching of the art of the identification of *covert* nursing problems. The term "nursing problem" as used in this study is a condition faced by the patient or family that the nurse can assist him or them to meet through the performance of her professional functions. The study had as its purpose the exploration of three methods nurses might use to identify covert nursing problems, with a view to their immediate application in nursing education to improve methods of clinical teaching.

Rationale   Basic knowledge of the discipline of nursing and its distinct qualities appears to fall into five elements of nursing, an analysis of which shows clearly the need for a broader concept of professional nursing.

The first element is the continuous mastery of human relations, including the mastery of technical and managerial skills needed to take care of patients.

The second element is the ability to observe and report with clarity the signs and symptoms, and deviation from normal behavior, that a patient presents. This element would include the mastery of basic communication skills.

The third element is the ability to interpret the signs and symptoms that compose the deviation from health and that constitute nursing problems. The deviations from health usually are identified from one or more signs and symptoms the nurse has observed. They involve nursing problems. Thus, a nursing problem exists in a situation involving patient care, a possible solution to which is found through the services that are the functions of nursing.

The fourth element requires the analysis of nursing problems that will guide the nurse in carrying out nursing functions. It also requires that, as the nurse plans for total patient care, she also select the necessary course of action that will help the patient attain a goal that is realistic for him.

The fifth element is the organization of her efforts to assure the desired outcome. Effective patient care would thus result when the nurse is able to help the patient to return to health, or what can be considered approximate normal health for him.

In brief, the rationale for undertaking this study is based on the assumption that the *correct identification of nursing problems influences the nurse's judgment in selecting the next steps in solving the patient's nursing problems.*

Methodology   The three methods used in this study were picture story, free answer, and direct questioning. The study was carried out in two different test situations to collect the data (one research hospital and three home situations) and in a third test situation (one general hospital) to validate the data. Data were collected over a six-week period from a sample of patients and professional health workers.

Testing and validation of the three methods yielded the following results.

Picture Story Method The picture story method (modified TAT) produced the most physical (overt) nursing problems when the source was the nurse or the doctor. Although this method produced fewer emotional (covert) nursing problems than the free answer method when the source was the patient, nurse, or doctor, the type of emotional problem that was revealed was very often deep-seated and one which the subject was not apt to verbalize by other methods. Qualitative aspects of nursing problems were better identified by this method than by the others. Picture stories were not found to be very useful in getting at sociological problems presented by the patient. When picture stories were used in the home situation, the situation described by the interviewee produced about the same number of physical problems as did the free answer method.

In the hands of the untrained nurse, the picture story method has questionable value for identifying covert nursing problems. However, it is a promising research tool which should be tested further in a variety of situations. This method has great promise in the hands of the clinical nurse specialist, and may have a useful place in training professional nurses in skills in perception as a basis for practice and in preparation for teaching. It may also be used to validate nursing problems identified by other methods.

Free Answer Method The free answer method was found to be the most productive method for identifying all types of nursing problems, regardless of whether the situation was in the hospital or in the home. In the hospital situation this method produced the most nursing problems when the source was the patient or the doctor. This method also was useful in identifying the patient's emotional (covert) nursing problems when the source was the nurse or the doctor. A great many emotional nursing problems were verbalized by the patient when this method was used.

Direct Question Method Patients and professional health workers were able to verbalize fewer nursing problems when this method was used as compared to other methods. This method was helpful in identifying overt nursing problems but was found to have limited use in identifying covert nursing problems.

Regardless of method and source, 99 per cent of the physical nursing problems identified were *overt*. Over 98 per cent of the emotional and sociological nursing problems identified were *covert,* regardless of source.

The other sources of data studied—medical histories, daily log, and nursing notes—produced the fewest nursing problems. The few problems described were almost all overt. Covert problems were seldom described.

A significant finding revealed by this study was that patient interviewing was more likely to succeed if the interviewer was in uniform—in this case in the uniform of a nurse. Intensive interviewing of patients was most successful when carried out in conjunction with the giving of nursing care.

Perception of Problems   The perception of a patient's nursing problems varied according to whether it was done by the patient or by professional health workers. Patients in hospitals were able to perceive many more nursing problems than nurses, doctors, or social workers. Perception of all types of nursing problems increased when the free answer and picture story methods were used. In the hospital situation, nurses and doctors showed better agreement on nursing problems when the picture story and free answer methods were used. The direct questioning method in the hands of the hospital nurse showed high agreement with patient's perception of overt nursing problems, but both nurses and doctors completely missed many (80–84 per cent) of the covert, or emotional and sociological, nursing problems verbalized by patients.

In the home situation, the public health nurse, unlike her hospital counterpart, was able to perceive many more nursing problems than did the patient. However, she saw the overt and covert nursing problems in the same proportion as did the nurse in the hospital situation. Both public health and hospital nurses verbalized overt nursing problems readily but missed many covert nursing problems verbalized by patients. This seems to indicate that nurses and doctors do not perceive the same nursing problems as patients, and nursing problems that are vitally important to the patient are often missed by professional health workers.

The three methods described can be used successfully by nurses to identify *covert* nursing problems presented by patients. The free answer and direct questioning methods have immediate application in improving clinical teaching and in helping students to develop skill in identifying and correctly perceiving all types of nursing problems. The picture story method, as a research tool in the hands of a clinical nursing specialist, has great potential and when tested further may prove to be useful for identifying nursing problems not elicited by other methods.

Implications for the Curriculum   The position is taken that in order to gain the skills and master the knowledge necessary to the stated broad concept of professional nursing, the curriculum must provide the widest possible experience for the nursing student. Preparation based on the

problem-solving technique is essential. Skills in identifying o
covert nursing problems become imperative if the nurse is to
analyze, and select appropriate courses of action to solve these p
If methods to attain such skills were available, it is believed that e
could make better use of the problem-solving approach in teaching.

The findings of this study indicate that such an approach would provide
a setting in which (1) teaching is patient-centered rather than disease-
centered; (2) more emphasis is placed upon the student's responsibility
for her learning; (3) nursing practice is brought into its proper relationship with restorative and preventive measures; and (4) students will be
prepared to give better nursing care to patients.

Implications for Improved Clinical Practice   Introduction of the use of
methods for identifying covert nursing problems necessitates a coordinated
plan of approach by a number of schools if necessary steps are to be
taken for selecting professional nursing experiences based on nursing
problems. Such schools should have well-prepared faculties and university
resources at their disposal. Many encouraging steps have already been
taken in this direction.

The problem-solving approach is receiving wider recognition by schools
of nursing. Students must learn to solve a variety of nursing problems
before they can achieve professional competence.

Recommendations   Specific recommendations related to this study are
as follows:

1. Students should be trained in the use of free answer and direct
questioning methods while they give nursing care during their clinical
experience.

2. Students should be trained in skills in perceiving the true nursing
problems presented by patients. This might be accomplished through the
team and multidiscipline conferences where each participant has an
opportunity to communicate the nursing problems that he or she perceives.

Further Research Needed   The next steps to advance the research, as
seen by the investigator, are as follows:

1. Additional picture stories should be tested in a variety of situations,
both in the hospital and home. Further testing should be carried out of
ways in which to introduce picture stories to patients and professional
health workers.

2. Study should be made of the home situation to determine why, in
this study, the public health nurse was better able to identify nursing
problems and why she had a truer perception of these problems than did
nurses in hospital situations.

3. The methods proposed in this study for identifying covert nursing

problems need to be tested in additional situations—namely, mental hospitals, tuberculosis hospitals, nursing homes, and outpatient departments—to determine if the findings in this study also apply to those situations.

4. The picture stories and free answer questioning—the preferred methods for identifying nursing problems as found in this study—should be used to develop a list of recurring or persistent nursing problems that all nurses must know how to solve.

5. Once this list has been developed a classification system of nursing problems should be evolved that would classify nursing problems by type (physical, emotional, sociological, interpersonal, etc.), common elements of patient care, and level of nursing personnel best prepared to solve this nursing problem.*

6. As the research described above is completed, a fundamental core curriculum in nursing should be developed, in which the core is made up of persistent and basic nursing problems that all nurses must be able to solve.*

Measurement of Nursing Practice

A persistent and complex problem is how to measure nursing practice and its effect upon the consumer. Kaufmann[49] approached the problem by investigating the levels of autonomic activation as reflected by the electrodermal response, systolic blood pressure, and pulse rate in a selected group of patients following the administration of one comfort measure—the back rub.

The investigator adopted a technique from psychology—the electrical skin response—as it provided a measurement of the generalized response of the whole body. The systolic blood pressure and pulse rate were used as autonomic indices to provide a comparison with the electrical skin response.

The study population included 36 adult patients in a university medical center in a large metropolitan area. The patients were divided into four test groups. The independent variables were T1—back rub without conversation; T2—back rub with conversation; T3—conversation only; and Tx—no treatment. The latter served as a control group. The criterion measures were (a) the continuous electrodermal response recorded for the control and treatment test periods; (b) the systolic blood pressure recorded continuously through the control and test periods; and (c) the pulse count taken manually as a single recording at the beginning and end of both control and treatment test periods.

* These recommendations have been accomplished and are reported in reference 48.

A specific test schedule was worked out for treatment and control groups to undergo measurements of their autonomic activation on two successive evenings. The heart of the research was to find out if the physiological changes occurred to a greater extent as a result of treatment than without treatment.

The analysis of variance for each of the three measures showed no statistically significant difference as a result of treatment. However, an analysis of individual patient profiles showed an observable response in the degree of relaxation of patients that could not be picked up in the analysis of data.

An important conclusion drawn by the investigator is that when measures of physiological response are taken, a parallel study should be planned to permit measurements of the psychosocial and environmental dimensions of the relaxation and comfort producing aspects of patient care.

Measurement of Staff Nurse Performance

The three approved routes that a student can pursue to achieve the R.N.—namely, the diploma, associate degree, or baccalaureate routes—have raised many questions about the on-the-job performance behaviors of the graduates of these programs. It became evident to Spaney and Matheney[50] that only a comparative study of graduates of these three types of programs could form the basis for objective discussions of the merits of each program. This led to the development of an extensive study to evaluate graduates of the three programs on the job.

The immediate problem under study was to compare employers' expectations with staff nurse performance for graduates of basic baccalaureate degree, diploma, and associate degree programs.

Specific subproblems studied were:

1. What do "remote and "immediate" employers expect of staff nurse graduates of the three types of basic programs upon graduation?
2. How do the expectations of the "remote" and "immediate" employers compare with each other?
3. How do head nurses and supervisors who graduated from these three types of programs rate the performance of staff nurses who graduated from these same types of programs?
4. How do these ratings compare with the expectations of the raters?
5. How do these ratings compare with the staff nurse's self-rating?
6. What kind of norms can be established for staff nurse graduates of the three types of basic programs?

A detailed reference list is included in the study report on literature on nursing stereotypy. The list has been subdivided into helpful categories

Pseudonym _____
or
Identification No. _____

QUEENS COLLEGE

EMPLOYER EXPECTATIONS VS. STAFF NURSE PERFORMANCE PROJECT

Performance Expectations - Part I

Directions: Below you will find a list of behaviors classified under eleven categories. Some of the behaviors are included under more than one category. Behaviors in a given classification define effective performance in that classification. For each category indicate what proportion of graduates of basic baccalaureate, diploma, and associate degree programs in nursing you would expect to show effective behavior. Please use the following key and indicate your responses in the space at the right.

> 0 if you would expect it of less than 1/4 of the graduates
> 1 if you would expect it of about 1/4 of the graduates
> 2 if you would expect it of 1/2 of the graduates
> 3 if you would expect it of 3/4 of the graduates
> 4 if you would expect it of more than 3/4 of the graduates

Record answer here

	Bacc.	Dip.	A.D.

Category I: Observation of Health Status
  A. Recognition of deviation from normal
  B. Observation of key changes in patients that demand immediate action
  C. Observation of key changes in personnel that demand immediate action

Category II: Planning and Organization of Own Work
  A. Individual patient care
  B. Group patient care
  C. Emergency or stress situation

Category III: Direction of Work of Others
  A. Planning
  B. Assigning
  C. Teaching personnel
  D. Supervising
  E. Evaluating

Category IV: Use of Resource Materials
  A. Hospital records
  B. Medical records
  C. Reference materials
  D. Provision of equipment and supplies
  E. Care of equipment and supplies
    (except in direct patient care)

Category V: Teaching of Patients and Families
         (Including Explaining Procedures)
  A. Planned individual
  B. Planned group
  C. Spontaneous individual
  D. Spontaneous group

Fig. 12-7. Performance expectations—Part I. (*Courtesy* Emma Spaney and Ruth V. Matheney, *Employer Expectations vs. Staff Nurse Performance.* Section 2 of Manual. New York, Queens College of the City of New York. Sept. 1961.)

such as, "The Layman Looks at the Nurse," "The Hospital Administrator Looks at the Nurse," "Individual Nurses Look at the Nurse," "Literature on Stress Situation Tests."

It is from this vast literature search that the investigators have gleaned their concepts about the nursing stereotypy and broadened their knowledge about the available tests to measure behaviors in stress situations.

The study population included graduates from the Queens College Associate in Arts nursing program, hospital administrators and directors of nursing service (26); head nurses and supervisors (56); and staff nurses (155) from 27 hospitals in the New York City–Long Island area. The study also included graduates from other programs, including a baccalaureate degree program.

Two instruments were developed to measure employers' expectations and staff nurse performance. These instruments were based on a central core of 54 desirable nurse behaviors.

"Performance Expectations—Part I," consists of eleven behavior categories classifying the basic 54 items as follows:

    I. Observation of health status
    II. Planning and organization of own work
    III. Direction of work of others
    IV. Use of resource materials
    V. Teaching of patients and families
    VI. Use of personnel resources (exclusive or nursing personnel)
    VII. Skills of communication
    VIII. Gives emotional support to patient
    IX. Functions effectively in team relationships
    X. Problem-solving process
    XI. Nursing procedures—technical

Figure 12-7 contains an excerpt of the "Performance Expectations— Part I."

Staff Nurse Performance Rating, the second instrument, lists the 54 basic behavior items. Following is a facsimile from the rating scale.

Pseudonym_____
or
Identification No._____

QUEENS COLLEGE
EMPLOYER EXPECTATIONS VS. STAFF NURSING PERFORMANCE PROJECT
Staff Nursing Performance Rating

Directions: Write your pseudonym on each page in the space indicated above, and write the name of the staff nurse whom you are rating and the other information called for on the appropriate answer sheet. Now consider each behavior in relation to the staff nurse whom you are rating, and indicate what proportion of the time she has shown this behavior, based on your experiences with her. Then place the appropriate number on the answer sheet, on the line corresponding to the behavior, as follows:

> 4 if the staff nurse does it at all possible times
> 3 if the staff nurse does it about ¾ of all possible times
> 2 if the staff nurse does it about ½ of all possible times
> 1 if the staff nurse does it about ¼ of all possible times
> 0 if the staff nurse does not do it at all
> X if you have had no opportunity to observe

1. Notes changes in vital signs, etc., and promptly initiates appropriate action.
2. Notes any sudden or unusual expressions of anxiety or apprehension that represent a marked change in patient behavior, and promptly initiates appropriate action.
3. Is alert to changes in personnel, such as physical condition or emotional stress that call for intervention, and promptly initiates appropriate action.
4. Preplans care of patients in relation to their needs.
5. Assembles and arranges equipment and patient unit for easy functioning.
6. Practices economy of own motions and effort.
7. Plans time to meet patients needs.
8. Allows for and can adjust to emergencies.
9. Assigns patient care to personnel best suited to perform it.
10. Makes assignments clear to personnel.
11. Distributes work fairly among personnel under her direction.
12. Ascertains level of knowledge of other nursing personnel.
13. Follows through on performance of other nursing personnel and determines adequacy of performance and/or additional help or instruction needed.
14. Provides time and means for discussion and improvement of quality of personnel.
15. Consults patient's chart for his progress as a basis for planning care.
16. Consults references and current literature for information about new drugs, treatments, therapies, etc.
17. Notifies charge nurse or supervisor of needed supplies and equipment before stock supplies are exhausted.
18. Suggests new and/or added equipment for patient's comfort and safety.
19. Uses correct methods of care for all supplies and equipment.
20. Obtains pertinent information about the patient from family and/or friends.
21. Gives pertinent information about patient to family and friends.
22. Reports patient's problems and significant changes in condition to appropriate person.
23. Initiates or requests patient referrals to appropriate community agencies.
24. Uses accurate knowledge of hospital policies and routines to help other personnel.
25. Consults with all members of health team in coordinating the therapeutic plan for the patient.
26. Identifies the religious needs of the patient, and contacts appropriate clergy as indicated.
27. Identifies patient's teaching needs accurately.
28. Provides information on patient's level of comprehension.

29. Teaches patient procedures using equipment patient will have to use.
30. Teaches family how to participate in patient care when their assistance is desirable.
31. Tests patient's understanding of learning.
32. Introduces the patient to other patient groups when such contact is helpful.
33. Writes nursing notes that are clear, descriptive, and accurate.
34. Discusses and explains doctor's directions to the patient and his family.
35. Interprets hospital policies to patient and family.
36. Includes patient in all conversations about him which occur within his hearing.
37. Recognizes language and physical barriers to communication and is able to overcome them.
38. Takes appropriate action with patients who are anxious and apprehensive, such as providing for expression of emotions, listening, changing patient's location, giving explanations, notifying physician, etc.
39. Does not avoid or stay away from patient who is anxious or apprehensive.
40. Listens to co-workers and discusses differences in viewpoint with them calmly.
41. Recognizes worth of co-workers and gives praise when earned.
42. Investigates situation, and does not make snap judgments about co-workers.
43. Has a sense of humor and uses it appropriately.
44. Observes the patient and thoroughly surveys his physical and emotional status before giving care.
45. Carries out nursing care that is specifically planned for each patient.
46. Adjusts nursing care to meet patient's needs as conditions or patients' behavior change.
47. Performs procedures correctly using basic principles involved.
48. Uses good manual skills.
49. Uses good body mechanics.
50. Prepares unit and equipment before starting work.
51. Records and/or reports desirable and undesirable results of treatments or procedures.
52. Protects patient from exposure, strain or injury through positioning, draping, handling equipment, etc.
53. Cares promptly and accurately for specimens.
54. Exhibits appropriate professional behavior.

Fig. 12-8. Staff nurse performance rating. (*Courtesy* Emma Spaney and Ruth V. Matheney, *Employer Expectations vs. Staff Nurse Performance,* Sec. I, Summary. New York, Queens College of the City of New York, July 1962, Appendix I, pp. 9–11.)

"Performance Expectations—Part II: Nursing Situations" was developed by the investigators to measure the ability of the "two-year" nurse to handle emergencies. An excerpt of this instrument is contained in Figure 12-9.

"Performance Expectations—Part III" was developed to investigate how employers and staff nurses saw nurses and nursing. An excerpt of this instrument is shown in Figure 12-10.

Pseudonym _____
or
Identification No. _____

QUEENS COLLEGE

EMPLOYER EXPECTATIONS VS. STAFF NURSE PERFORMANCE PROJECT

Performance Expectations - Part II

Nursing Situations

Directions: Each one of the following situations describes a hospital emergency or problem. For each situation, decide which type of graduate would be most likely to exhibit appropriate behavior, and which type would be least likely to exhibit appropriate behavior. Mark your answer in the column at the right. Do not spend too much time on any situation - just indicate your first reaction. B.A. stands for "basic baccalaureate degree program graduate"; Dip. stands for "basic diploma program graduate"; and A.D. stands for "basic associate degree program graduate."

	Most Likely			Least Likely		
	B.A.	Dip.	A.D.	B.A.	Dip.	A.D.
1. A nurse reports for work on an active surgical unit with sixty patients, and only one other nurse is available to help her give patient care. Which graduate would you be most and least likely to choose as the other nurse?						
2. A patient is so acutely ill that he requires excellent nursing care. No private duty nurses can be obtained at the time, and someone must be selected from the staff. Which graduate would you be most and least likely to choose?						
3. The night nurse reports sick just before she is to go on duty. Someone must be selected to cover at least two wards for the night. Which graduate would you be most likely to choose? Least likely?						
4. A medical floor on the evening shift with a high census and limited staff receives two or three unexpected admissions. Which graduate would you expect to handle this situation without asking for help? Which graduate would be least likely to handle it well?						
5. An attempt is being made to introduce a team assignment on a ward where the team concept has not been used before. Which graduate would you be most likely to assign as a team leader? Least likely?						
6. A patient has a sudden severe visible hemorrhage. From which graduate would you expect the most effective performance? The least effective performance?						
7. An acutely ill patient says to the nurse, "I am going to die. Will you pray with me?" Which graduate could best handle this situation? Which is least likely to be effective?						

Fig. 12-9. Performance expectations—Part II. (*Courtesy* Emma Spaney and Ruth V. Matheney. *Employer Expectations vs. Staff Nurse Performance.* Part II, New York, Queens College of the City of New York.)

Performance Expectations – Part III

Directions: In each of the following situations, two
STAFF NURSES are commenting upon the person indicated. Complete what Staff Nurse A has started to say,
and then give Staff Nurse B's reply. Do not spend too
much time on any one item; just give your first reaction.

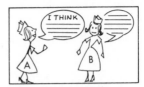

Please do not write here

Situation 1: Staff Nurses A and B are commenting about
their Director of Nursing Service, Miss S.

Staff Nurse A: "In my opinion, Miss S

Staff Nurse B: "

Situation 2: Staff Nurses A and B are commenting about
a supervisor, Miss T.

Staff Nurse A: "I think Miss T

Staff Nurse B: "

Situation 3: Staff Nurses A and B are commenting about
another staff nurse, Miss U.

Staff Nurse A: "Miss U

Staff Nurse B: "

Situation 4: Staff Nurses A and B are commenting about
a patient, Mrs. V.

Staff Nurse A: "I've noticed that Mrs. V

Staff Nurse B: "

Fig. 12-10. Performance expectations—Part III. (*Courtesy* Emma Spaney and Ruth
V. Matheney. *Employer Expectations vs. Staff Nurse Performance*. Part III, New
York, Queens College of the City of New York.)

Empirical validity of these instruments was determined by a series of
additional tests as the "Group Rorschach Study," and the "High vs.
Low Clinical Groups Study." Reliability of the instruments was determined by the use of the "Kuder-Richardson Formula 21 Reliabilities"
which the instrument calculated for the extremism and indecision scores
on "Opinions about Nurses and Nursing" for head nurses and staff
nurses. Figure 12-11 contains an excerpt from this instrument.

One significant finding of the study was that graduate nurses showed a

Pseudonym_____
or
Identification No._____

QUEENS COLLEGE
EMPLOYER EXPECTATIONS VS. STAFF NURSE
PERFORMANCE PROJECT

Opinions about Nurses and Nursing—Part I

Directions: Read each statement carefully. Decide whether you Strongly Agree, Agree, Are Undecided, Disagree, or Strongly Disagree. There are no "correct" answers; we are just interested in your opinions. Do not spend too much time on any one statement, but record your first opinion by making a check mark in the proper column on the right.

Strongly Agree	_SA		
Agree	_A	Disagree	_D
Undecided	_U	Strongly Disagree	_SD

	SA	A	U	D	SD
1. Nurses have satisfying lives.	1. —	—	—	—	—
2. Kindness and generosity are the most important qualities for a nurse to have.	2. —	—	—	—	—
3. The average nurse should not probe too deeply into her own and other people's feelings but take things as they are.	3. —	—	—	—	—
4. A nurse should be prepared to cut her moorings—quit home, family and friends—without suffering great regrets.	4. —	—	—	—	—
5. What nursing needs most, more than laws and political programs, is a few courageous, tireless, devoted leaders in whom people can put their faith.	5. —	—	—	—	—
6. Nurses should ignore other people's faults and make an effort to get along with everyone.	6. —	—	—	—	—
7. Nurses have considerable self-respect.	7. —	—	—	—	—
8. The happy nurse tends always to be poised, courteous, outgoing, and emotionally controlled.	8. —	—	—	—	—
9. Young nurses sometimes get rebellious ideas, but as they grow older they ought to get over them and settle down.	9. —	—	—	—	—
10. It is easy for nurses to take orders and do as they are told.	10. —	—	—	—	—
11. Most patients seem to like nurses.	11. —	—	—	—	—
12. The average nurse is not very well satisfied with herself.	12. —	—	—	—	—
13. Nurses are governed by normal prejudices and fears, but make an honest effort to overcome them.	13. —	—	—	—	—
14. Nurses feel that they are average persons in our society.	14. —	—	—	—	—

Figure 12-11. Opinions about nurses and nursing. (*Courtesy* Emma Spaney and Ruth V. Matheney, *Employer Expectations vs. Staff Nurse Performance,* Section 2, Manual. New York, Queens College of New York, Sept. 1961, Appendix AA-5a.)

general feeling of acceptance of various categories of personnel with whom they worked. The major identification of rejection was with staff nurses who were graduates of diploma programs. On the other hand, familiarity with graduates of associate degree programs in a work situation reduced the overt expression of rejection.

An important implication for nursing education is that a graduate of any of the three types of programs is a beginning practitioner who is competent to give nursing care within the area for which she has been prepared. It was also confirmed that preparation of nurses can be conducted by the junior or community college, that the educational principles of these colleges are sound, and that their graduates are safe practitioners of nursing.

The study provides a major breakthrough in making valid and reliable instruments available for the measurement of staff nurse performance. The investigators recommend replication in other settings to collect wider normative data.

Objective Measurement of Decubitus Ulcers

Verhonick[51] conducted one of the first studies in nursing to measure objectively the observations of decubitus ulcers. In order to accomplish this a criterion measure had to be developed. The necessary specifications for the criterion measure were (1) validity; (2) reliability; and (3) convenience or availability. Two data-collecting instruments were developed: "criterion measure for decubiti observations" and a "nursing diagnosis checklist."

Observations of patients with decubitus ulcers are made once a week and include the size or surface areas of induration, excoriation, necrosis, and scarring. Changes in the size of each of the areas indicate improvement or deterioration. The surface area measured is then plotted on a graph in square centimeters. (See Figure 12-12)

The changes in the color of the lesion are also observed as healing takes place. The investigator raises important questions about the significance of change in color to the rate or degree of healing. She points out that the existing color scales have limited use but can provide a record of frequency of occurrence.

Skin tone, skin condition, amount and type of drainage, subjective complaints of the patient concerning sensation, and infectious process were other types of observations recorded on the criterion measure.

The second measuring instrument, the nursing diagnosis checklist, was developed to help the ". . . observer look comprehensively at the patient in order to determine the best approach for this specific patient." (See Figure 12-13)

The investigator reports the need for the expansion of the criterion measure to include pH of the exudate of established decubiti. The relevancy of this research to the phenomenon of the settling of sludge in human patients is described later.

Assessing Patient and Personnel Satisfaction with Patient Care

How can one measure patient and personnel satisfaction with nursing care? Several approaches have been made to this problem. Many hospitals use a form letter to find out how patients feel about their care. This letter,

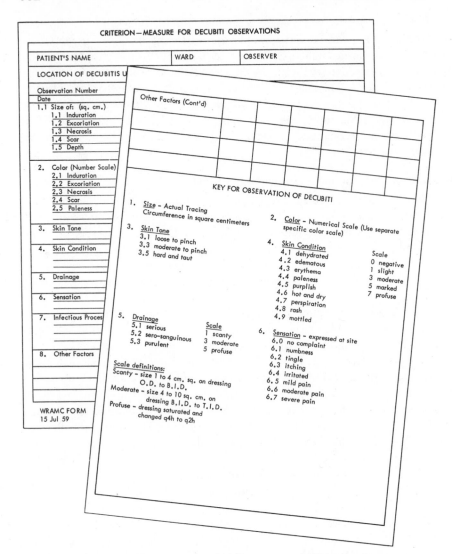

Fig. 12-12. Instrument to measure decubiti. (*Courtesy* Phyllis J. Verhonick. "Decubitus Ulcer Observations Measured Objectively," *Nurs. Res.*, **10**:211–14, Fall, 1961.)

usually signed by the hospital administrator, is given to the patient upon discharge. He is asked to indicate his feelings about the care he has received.

The American Hospital Association[52] has developed a questionnaire which is also given to patients upon discharge. This form asks such questions as, "Was there too much noise for you to get your rest?" "Were you

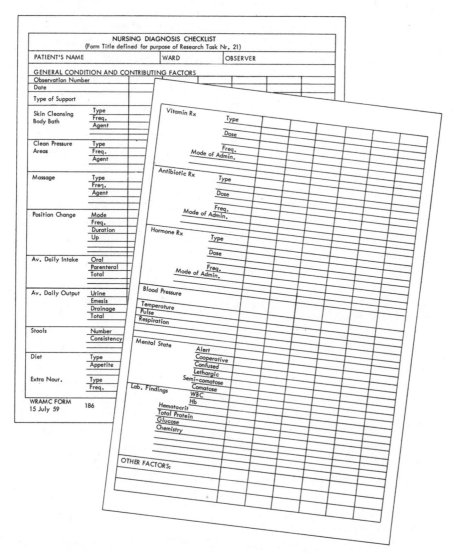

Fig. 12-13. Nursing diagnosis checklist. (*Courtesy* Phyllis J. Verhonick. "Decubitus Ulcer Observations Measured Objectively," *Nurs. Res.,* **10:**211–14, Fall, 1961.)

properly instructed in how to take care of yourself after you get home?" A companion form has also been developed specifically directed to questions about food.[53] It contains such questions as, "How about the coffee you get here?" The respondent then checks whether the coffee is "tops," "usually pretty good," "sometimes not so good," or "pretty bad all the time."

A hospital survey conducted by the British Ministry of Information[54] was more detailed than other questionnaires about satisfaction with care. A sample of patients discharged from the hospital was visited by an interviewer. Two questionnaires were given to each person: one was completed as the interviewer asked questions, and the second was left with the respondent and was returned by mail.

The individuals were asked to check such items as:

I was not told by my own doctor how long I might expect to be away from home. (Yes or No)
I was not told how long I might expect to be away from home. (Yes or No)

Although each of these instruments has value, the instruments used would need further validation before they could be used in a scientific study or as a methodological tool for evaluating adequacy of patient care.

It took the U.S. Public Health Service's Division of Nursing Resources (now the Division of Nursing) two years to develop a valid instrument to measure satisfaction with nursing care that it could use as a criterion measure in a study of the relationship between amount of nursing care provided and patient and personnel satisfaction with the care.[55] The initial impetus for the development of the instrument came in the fall of 1953, when the Cleveland Commission of Nursing invited the Division to try to find out why hospital personnel in the Cleveland area were continually feeling the pressure of "nursing shortage." These hospitals were giving relatively high hours of care at that time and were unable to explain why more nurses were needed. Some of these hospitals had undertaken management studies and, as a result, had experimented with a variety of staffing patterns. Nevertheless, hospital and nursing administrators and nurses themselves continued to express feelings of nursing shortage. In the spring of 1954, the Division sent a study team comprising a nurse, a psychologist, and a statistician to work with three hospitals that volunteered to participate in the development of the instrument.

Initial Development of Methodology   The team's objective was to try to develop an instrument that would measure patient and personnel satisfaction with nursing care by having each respondent record specific occurrences of nursing care that they observed. These occurrences were to be recorded in the respondent's own words on a form that was not much more than a blank sheet of paper. The patient forms were divided into two columns, one labeled "satisfactory," the other "unsatisfactory." Instructions were, "List events of care you have received that were either satisfactory or unsatisfactory."

Personnel forms contained only one column in which nursing care events were to be recorded. This was labeled, "Instances in which patient care might have been improved." Instructions were, "Include patient care that should have been provided and was not, as well as instances in which patient care might have been improved."

A sample of 100 patients and all nursing and medical personnel from each hospital were asked to participate in the study. Sixty of the sample patients in each hospital were given the forms to fill out four times a day for a period up to seven days. The remaining 40 patients in each hospital, in addition to completing the forms, were interviewed either individually or in groups by the study team. The interview had a dual purpose—to collect events that might not turn up on the written forms, and to check the reliability of events reported on the forms by having the patient describe in detail exactly what happened.

Completed forms were placed in sealed envelopes and collected from patients after dinner. The forms were checked in on a control list to assure completeness of returns. Personnel were asked to deposit their completed forms in a box located at each head nurse's station. Maintenance of the anonymity of the respondent was continually stressed.

When all forms were returned, analysis of the data proceeded by grouping reported events according to similarity of content. Groups of events were then tallied by the number of times each was reported by the respondents.

To validate patient and personnel reporting of events, personnel indicated on their forms the actual patient to whom the event referred. As the completed forms were checked, the study team frequently found that personnel and patients corroborated each other. For example, when a patient reported that his medication was late, a professional nurse would report the same event on her form by saying that she was unable to give the medication on time because of an admission or some other emergency. This cross-checking gave assurance that the events reported on the forms actually happened.

The open-ended forms, although successful in producing a generous number of comments about nursing care, could not serve as a final instrument. These forms were too time-consuming to fill out, too unwieldy to tabulate, and difficult to analyze. Development of a simple, completely directive, and unambiguous form became the objective of the study team.

The main use of the open-ended forms, therefore, was to collect statements of events in which patients' needs for nursing care were unfulfilled. The next step was to organize the open-ended material into two checklists —one for patients and the other for personnel—that would include a sample from the whole spectrum of nursing care events.

Field Tryout of the Checklists   The initial checklists consisted of 100 items. The study team returned to the same three hospitals in Cleveland to test them. All the patients and personnel who were able to participate

in the study were asked to fill out the checklists on a study day that was
selected. In addition, a sample of patients and personnel was selected to
rate each item on the checklists according to its importance to patient
satisfaction with care. A simple five-point scale was used ranging from
"not important" to "very important." This gave the study team two criteria
for selecting events—namely, the frequency with which the event was
reported, and its importance to patients and personnel.

Conclusions Relative to Development   The tryout of the initial checklists indicated that the final instruments could be reduced to 50 items each
to include events that were most frequently reported and/or rated highest
in importance. On the patient form, 47 of the events described omissions
in care and 3 described instances in which good care was provided. On
the personnel form all events portrayed omissions in care.

The time for recording was also reduced. It was found that one typical
day, usually one during the middle of the week, would yield a valid sample
of patient and personnel responses.

It was also concluded that the final instruments should be designed to
focus on nursing events. Events that related to the medical staff or other
departments were deleted. Examples of items and the frequency scale for
the patients' checklists are shown in Figure 12-14.

The final steps in the development of the instruments were to validate
them and to determine a numerical scale for the items. Three hospitals
were selected for this purpose.

To validate the checklists, interviews were held with a sample of patients and personnel to see if they understood all of the items on the
checklists. The investigator actually kept a record of the events reported
by patients and checked to see if what the patients reported actually happened. The same approach was used with personnel.

Event	This happened today	This happened some other day	This did not happen
1. Couldn't get anything from the nurse for pain			
2. My call for a nurse was answered promptly			
3. Food trays left in front of me too long			
4. Thermometer left in too long			

Fig. 12-14. Excerpt from instrument to assess patient satisfaction with care.

It was found that there was a very close relationship between what patients reported and what personnel reported. In nearly every instance what the patient reported was found to have actually happened. This also was true for personnel. Patients and personnel interviewed were also asked to interpret individual items. When events could not be explained, the difficulty was often due to misinterpretation of a word. All words causing difficulty were simplified, using language expressed by the patient. For example, "ventilation" was changed to "air." Each item was also checked against Payne's list of problem and multimeaning words.[56]

Scaling the Checklists Developing a numerical scale for the items proceeded as follows. The two checklists asked the respondents to record whether each of the 50 items included did or did not happen in the last seven days. One way of scoring the items would be simply to count the number reported as happening. The total number reported would be the score for the checklist. Thus, a total score of 50 would indicate that all items included on the checklist occurred during the past seven days; a score of zero would indicate that none of the events occurred. A short-coming of this method is that it assumes that all events have an equal numerical importance in determining a respondent's satisfaction with nursing care. Inspection of the content of the events indicated that some were more important than others. A numerical weight could be assigned to each event that would reflect its importance.

Although in the second phase of the Cleveland study each of the events was assigned a weight in terms of its importance in contributing to the satisfaction with patient care, there was concern that the method used to obtain the weights—a graphic rating scale—was too crude for use as a research instrument. A decision was made to derive a new scale. The "Q-sort" technique was used for this purpose.

For the Q-sort, sets of index cards containing the 47 unfavorable events from the patient checklist were given to each patient. He was asked to pick out the three cards containing the events that were most important to the quality of care he received and the three that were the least important. These six cards were placed to one side, and the patient was then given the remaining 41 cards. He was next instructed to pick out the 12 cards containing the events that were the most important to the quality of his care and the 12 that were least important. When this was done, 17 cards were left which were then placed in a "middle" group, giving a total of five categories of events: very most important—3 events; most important—12 events; middle group—17 events; least important—12 events; very least important—3 events.

The procedure for weighting the events included on the personnel form was identical with that used for the patient form. As there were 50 events on the personnel form, these were sorted into five piles containing 3, 12, 20, 12, and 3 events each. By averaging the sortings for all the respondents, a five-point scale was developed in which the three very most important events were given the weight of 5; those in the next group of events were given a weight of 4; the events in the next group, a weight of 3; the next group of events, a weight of 2; and the three least important events, a weight of 1. If an event was not reported as occurring by the respondent, the weight for the event would of course be 0. A total score on the checklist could thus vary between 0 to 150 for personnel and 0 to 141 for patients.

Three events that *patients* selected as being the very most important to the quality of care which they received were:

Couldn't get anything from the nurse for pain.
No answer to call for a nurse for a long time.
Had to wait a long time to use the bathroom.

Events assigned the very most important score by *personnel* were:

Postoperative or critical patient left unattended for a long time.
Patient did not receive needed medication.
Patient with communicable disease not properly isolated.

This methodology, published by the U.S. Government Printing Office in a manual entitled *Patient and Personnel Speak*,[57] represents an elaborate attempt to apply quantitative scaling techniques to the measurement of adequacy of patient care. Whether the scale is truly quantitative is subject to question. However, it does possess the properties of a refined ordinal scale. As such, it has proven to be a useful tool in numerous studies that have been conducted following its development.

PATIENT ASSESSMENT—ITS POTENTIAL AND USE

A historical perspective of the development of patient assessment tools derived from the need in hospitals at the level of the patient care unit to be able to distribute resources, manpower, and supplies to areas where they were needed.

In 1957, an early approach in patient assessment was undertaken by the U.S.P.H.S. using the concept of progressive patient care in which patients were classified into categories for appropriate placement to areas in the hospital where their needs could be met.[58]

As the interest in the development of patient classification systems occurred efforts were undertaken to extend the classification systems to long-term care facilities such as nursing homes and home care programs.

Patient Classification for Long-Term Care

The Bureau of Community Health Services and later the National Center for Health Services Research, U.S.P.H.S. supported a major effort of developing assessment and classification procedures for long-term care patients.

In 1968, a coalition was formed of researchers from Harvard, Case-Western Reserve, Johns Hopkins, and the Hospital Association of New York State.[59] A common language for long-term care and a set of objective descriptors of patients were developed. By 1971 the coalition had produced and field tested a classification system plus a manual and glossary for its use. The classification developed served multiple purposes; i.e., for use in individual patient care, resource allocation in single institutions, and the community as a whole, program evaluation, planning and policy determination, and research and teaching.

OARS—Multidimensional Function Assessment Questionnaire

This instrument was developed as part of the Older Americans Resources and Service (OARS) program of the Duke University Center for the Study of Aging and Human Development.[60] It was specifically designed to assess the functional status and need for service of the aging.

The OARS survey questionnaire takes 1¼ hours to complete by a trained interviewer and is designed to collect systematic information on the subject's functional state, knowledge of information regarding services, and perception of the individual's need for specific services. Each individual is assessed for mental health, physical health, social resources, economic resources, and capacity for the activities of daily living (ADL) representing major areas of functioning.

The data collected were consolidated by the interviewer into a single numerical score ranging from 1 to 6. The OARS instrument places more weight upon the areas of behavioral and social needs than do other patient assessment instruments. The instrument has proved to be useful in identifying individuals in a high-risk population who have a need or potential need for long-term care.

Patient Status Instrument

The Functional Outcome Measures developed by Katz was designed to measure disability in terms of an Index of Independence in Activities of Daily Living.[61] Items have been added to the instrument to take into account intangible characteristics of attributes of disability and severity of illness. The Patient Status Instrument is organized by the method to be used for data collection, i.e., information to be collected by interview and by patient assessment.

Some of the data can be collected by trained interviewers or clerical assistants, while others require professional judgment. The instrument is multidimensional, incorporates a patient profile, and describes functional status. Items of the instruments are categorized by functional status, social functioning, psychological functioning, impairment, medically defined conditions, and medical risk factor measurement. The Patient Status Instrument provides a method of obtaining a multidimensional profile that provides a basis for exercising clinical judgment.

Patient Appraisal and Care Evaluation (PACE) System

PACE is a systematic process for assessing health care. By using the PACE instrument, the appraiser (provider of care in a nursing home) observes and records data about patient characteristics and functional capacity, logically plans for the individual's goals, and determines whether or not those goals have been met. The system of PACE evolved in relation to the Department of Health, Education, and Welfare's survey/certification process of nursing homes.[62]

In recent years, there has been expressed dissatisfaction with the survey and certification process for long-term care facilities. Although there are established regulations regarding the proper conduct of such facilities for reimbursement purposes, most of these rely on the determination of whether or not a facility is *capable* of providing the needed service, not whether or not it, in fact, has delivered such service. The present form which the surveyor uses is, in effect, a checklist that does not identify whether the patient is receiving the service or making the progress that he should. The survey and certification process only evaluated paper compliance, not the quality of care rendered.

Phase I of the National Long Term Care Facility Improvement Plan recognized this limitation and had HEW teams carry out patient appraisal on a selected sample of patients in over 300 skilled nursing facilities. This part of Phase I documented that a patient appraisal mechanism could identify both met and unmet needs in physical, psychological, and social dimensions and whether or not services were being rendered to patients according to those needs. Phase I was limited to a one-time effort. In addition, patient assessment in itself does not afford an opportunity to improve the quality of care through care planning and evaluation.

In designing Phase II, an effort was made to determine the following answers:

1. Could nursing home personnel themselves carry out the patient appraisal, care planning, and evaluation effort?
2. Could the progress of an individual be measured?
3. Could the PACE instrument serve as an effective care planning and evaluation tool for nursing home personnel?

4. Could those who would be surveying the facility be able to determine the quality of care from the PACE program?

The feasibility study provided a "yes" to the first three questions. PACE was found to be systematic, continuous, objective, practical, and effective. It provides a base for measuring patient status, the care given, and the outcomes of care. PACE provided an opportunity to change the survey and certification process from one of paper compliance to one in which determination of compliance is on the basis of outcomes of care.

While PACE was being tested to determine whether or not it could be effectively used by nursing home personnel, a parallel activity has been started at the federal level. All regulations pertaining to Skilled Nursing Facilities and Intermediate Care Facilities are being reviewed with the goal of determining which of these are related to patient care and patient care outcomes. A second step in this review will include a review of survey and certification procedures that presently hamper the application of PACE in the field.

A third step will be to identify what changes in the survey and certification process would need to be made if the measurement of outcomes of care were used instead of the capability of the facility to provide such care.

The present goals of the PACE system are to:

1. Establish a system that can be maintained by nursing personnel within the facility and be kept current, objective, accurate, and complete, while effectively serving the nursing home personnel in the development of care planning based on patient or resident needs and established goals;
2. Provide an internal monitoring tool for the facility to modify its administrative practices and standards of care, and to improve the quality of care;
3. Provide a baseline information for external monitoring through survey and certification, quality assurance and quality improvement activities.

PACE provides a single, consistent, and current source of patient/ resident data including demographic descriptors; care need descriptors (including diagnoses, impairments, functional status, etc.); services provided; a continuous profile of a patient/resident that facilitates the establishment of measurable goals and sound care planning; a data source useful to facility administrators both within and outside the facility for resource allocation, determining the cost of care and program planning; accessible and measurable data on appropriateness of care as well as its outcomes both within the facility and to outside groups or individuals concerned with determination of quality of care; and a potential mechanism for instituting a system of appropriate patient/resident placement and continuity of care whether institutional or noninstitutional.

Initially, the PACE system is being limited to SNFs and ICFs, but will be expanded to hospitals and noninstitutional care settings. Expansion of PACE into hospitals could contribute to better placement of patients and thus reduce the 30 to 40 per cent of patients who are now inappropriately placed in nursing homes. To accomplish this will require support from health care providers and planners to provide the linkage between levels of care, both institutional and noninstitutional, and to assure that community support services are readily accessible.

Other approaches have been proposed to assess quality in long-term care.[63] For example, the Joint Commission on Accreditation of Hospitals (JCAH) instrument developers feel that regardless of the processes of care selected, health care practitioners can agree on and predict outcomes that patients should achieve with optimal care. The result is a problem-orientation method. The basic features of the system are a patient history and assessment, master problem list, patient care plan, and goal achievement analysis.

Still another approach is a process approach, a quality evaluation system (QES), developed by Rush-Presbyterian-St. Lukes Medical Center and Medicus Systems Corporation in Chicago. The QES instrument provides data on the functional competence of patients as determined by chart review and interviews with the patients and staff who know them well. Data are collected by two trained surveyors (two RNs or an RN and a social worker).

Common objectives of all patient assessment instruments are the use of common definitions in relation to mental and physical status and care problems and a common data base from which one can make an assessment of patient needs and identify outcome measures. The form the instrument takes becomes less significant provided these two common objectives are met.

Considerable progress has been made in the development of a Long-Term Care Minimum Data Set. This has been accomplished by a Long-Term Care Technical Consultant Panel of the U.S. National Committee on Vital and Health Statistics under the leadership of DHEW, PHS's National Center for Health Statistics. The panel was charged with the responsibility of the development and recommendation of a minimum data set to be incorporated into the data collection activities of the Cooperative Health Statistics System. The long-term care data set will be particularly useful to the needs of those at federal, state, and local levels who plan for, provide, and assess long-term care services and conduct research in this area.[64]

Fewer than thirty items make up the long-term care minimum data set and include uniform definitions related to demographic items, such as current labor force status, education and function, and illness items, such as vision impairment, hearing impairment, activities of daily living, social competence, behavioral problems, orientation/memory.

Determinations of what items to include in the minimum data set were based on the following criteria. Item must:

1. Be valid, reliable, relevant;
2. Make it possible to make a clear-cut decision and be definable, e.g., sex—female or male;
3. Differentiate between certain kinds of people with respect to services needed, e.g., can someone prepare meals? Someone who has pain vs. no pain?
4. Serve some useful purpose such as:
   - Items would generate data needed by case managers, care givers, individual clinical data for clinical decisionmakers.
   - Provide minimum data set for program and policymakers, e.g., character of the population to be served; services and treatments.
   - Provide research data to test hypothesis in that area but for only that area not a universal data.
5. *Not* include data for rare events, e.g., amputee, albino (it is suggested that the item must have a 5 per cent frequency before data are collected).
6. Permit as little branching as possible in response to the item. Multiple answers are permitted but not branching, e.g., Caucasian race would be one response not Caucasian, North, South, East, or West; and
7. Have specified a common definition for each item so that everyone handling the data knows what the language means and this is so stated in explicit glossaries, e.g., definition of nursing care.

SYSTEMATIC NURSING ASSESSMENT

The recent growth and sophistication of health care, proliferation of highly specialized health disciplines, and explosion of scientific knowledge have resulted in unprecedented changes and increased complexity in the provision of optimal patient care. In order to cope with the continual change and pressure, a hierarchy of functions has been created in nursing that has moved the nurse farther away from the most vital concern of the profession—the patient. Administration, rather than patient care, has become the focus of nurses' duties.

In many hospitals, information handling by the nurse has become the major problem that prevents her from caring for the patient. Nurses deal with large volumes of patient-centered information and base important judgments and decisions about patient care on this information. The methods nurses employ in collecting, recording, and communicating information, while patterned, are not systematic.

Ritualistic methods for gathering illness- or disease-related data have been developed in medicine over a long period of time. These methods make the collection of medical information more adaptable to standardization and computerization.

In order to reduce information handling, a new type of standardized and integrated record keeping was developed by Taylor and others at the State University of New York at Buffalo.[65] The project concentrated on seeking the contributions of practicing nurses in identifying the descriptive clinical information nurses need in order to give excellent patient care. The essential information was then organized into nursing assessment forms adaptable to machine processing.

Prior to development of the tools for patient assessment and information gathering, written and verbal communication patterns and the clinical content of nurses' notes and patients' records at several hospitals and health agencies were reviewed. The first phase of the study focused on standardizing the clinical data of surgical patients at the study hospital.

The following forms were developed for use with hospitalized adult surgical patients from admission to the time of discharge:

- Nursing assessment: basic patient information (social and health/ illness status upon admission);
- Nursing assessment: patient progress (physiological and psychological responses to illness and therapy);
- Nursing assessment: recovery from anesthesia (acute physiological and psychological responses to surgery and anesthesia);
- Nursing assessment: 8-hour intake and output (fluid balance and therapy, including responses of patient to therapy).

The project was extended to a second phase for developing and testing forms for use with hospitalized adult nonsurgical patients (no obstetrical forms) and with adult patients and their families cared for by community health agency nurses. The clinical information necessary for assessment of these patients was identified and incorporated into several forms that were appropriate to the collecting and recording of patient-family data by the community health nurse.

The forms were evaluated and revised to assure ease of use, validity of data, and adequacy and relevance of information for decision-making and planning patient care. Manuals of instruction for each form were developed. Inservice programs were conducted to prepare personnel to use the forms. Methods of communicating patient information from hospitals to community health agencies were developed.

A METHODOLOGY FOR MONITORING QUALITY
OF NURSING CARE

Phase I

The central objective for the first 12 months of the study, conducted by the staff of Medicus Corporation in Chicago was to develop a framework for monitoring quality of nursing care that would:

- Reflect the state-of-the-art in nursing research in the quality of care area;
- Incorporate all useful evaluative criteria in existing methodologies;
- Be internally statistically consistent and reliable;
- Be economically feasible to administer;
- Permit ready inclusion of relevant future research results.

The approach that was taken was to:

1. Thoroughly review all relevant literature, identify evaluative criteria for nursing quality, and synthesize these into a single master list;
2. Develop a unified conceptual framework of the nursing process in terms of overall objectives for the process and subobjectives within these into which the master list of evaluative criteria could be translated;
3. Develop a computer-based methodology for generating quality monitoring worksheets consisting of subsets of evaluative criteria systematically selected from the master list;
4. Monitor quality with the aid of these observation sheets on eight patient units in each of two participating study hospitals—Presbyterian–St. Luke's in Chicago and Baptist Medical Centers at Montclair in Birmingham, Alabama; and
5. Statistically analyze these observations and the quality scores computed from them to refine and revise both evaluative criteria and the structure within which they are applied.

All of these steps have been carried out successfully.[66] As a result, there now exists a methodology for evaluating quality of nursing care for medical, surgical, and pediatric patient units, including related intensive care units. This methodology is based on a master criteria list consisting of 230 criteria grouped under 28 subobjectives within six objectives for the process of nursing care.

Phase II

The objectives of Phase II of this project were to:

- Test in a range of hospitals the applicability of the quality-monitoring methodology developed in Phase I.

- Expand the methodology to newborn nurseries and recovery rooms.
- Analyze the influence of certain organizational factors and of educational background on nursing performance.
- Begin to relate nursing processes to measures of patient outcomes.

Experience with the quality-monitoring methodology developed and utilized in Phases I and II of the project led to certain refinements.[67] Criteria for quality evaluation were reworded for clarity, and the manner in which quality-monitoring worksheets containing representative criteria were generated was changed. The quality-monitoring methodology utilized in Phase I and expanded in Phase II is based on an objective and sub-objective structure into which the criteria for quality nursing care are classified. The structure allows the inclusion of criteria at a level of detail that reflects actual operational definitions of the nursing care process. Further, because the structure is in terms of objectives, it can be readily modified to include new criteria developed through future research or that reflects new procedures, equipment, and so forth. The criteria themselves are stated in objective, measurable terms, normally with dichotomous answers (often yes or no).

In April and May of 1974, data were collected in the nineteen hospitals on key variables thought to potentially affect the quality of care. These variables represented six general categories:

- Total hospital characteristics (e.g., size, complexity)
- Unit structural characteristics (e.g., nursing organization, staffing)
- Leadership style
- Unit staff perceptions and attitudes
- Supervisory staff perceptions and attitudes
- Nursing staff education

Analyses were performed using stepwise regression and other techniques. Correlations of these variable sets with one another indicated that total hospital characteristics were significantly correlated with all other sets. When analyzed by stepwise regression, no single set of variables provided a high R^2 value—an indication that many factors are involved in quality health care.

The project also involved an exploratory study of the relation of patient care outcomes to measured quality of the nursing process. Data were gathered in two Chicago hospitals on congestive heart failure and abdominal hysterectomy patients that met certain criteria such as lack of confounding complications. Patient selection was designed to maximize the likelihood that nursing effort, as opposed to general physical condition and other factors, had been the major contributor to observed differences in outcomes. Meeting these criteria for patient selection became a problem. In both pathologic categories together, only 28 acceptable patients were found over a period of several months.

Assessment instruments were designed specifically for the outcomes study and were used by three project nurses, either independently for each patient or by joint interpretation of questionable responses. Most of the findings for abdominal hysterectomy patients (18 observations) indicated that the process measures of nursing quality are positively related to patient health outcomes. For congestive heart failure patients (10 observations), however, the findings were less consistent, in that only the psychological status of the patients related positively, as expected, to quality measures of the specific part of the nursing process relevant to nonphysical patient needs.

Although the data do support the focus on outcome assessment, they also suggest that the relation between process and outcomes may be different for different types of patients and is almost certainly influenced by patient condition and nursing priorities. This would seem to indicate that for effective quality assessment, both performance (process) and effectiveness (outcomes) of nursing care should be monitored.

These findings have certain implications for nursing. They suggest

- That nursing management is important in unit organization, staff coordination, maintenance of a clinical orientation, and attitude determination—all of which are positively related to the quality of nursing care provided.
- That nursing management is important in controlling nursing processes on a regular basis and in gearing training and development activities to process management.
- That process monitoring has a role in quality assurance programs specifically because it addresses the entire scope of the nursing process and provides timely feedback on specific problem areas.
- That nursing education should have a broader focus in order to develop, at all levels of training, nurses competent in the complete scope of the nursing process and trained to take a more active role, in partnership with nursing management, in the development of nursing practice within the organizational setting of the patient care system.

The project results point the way to several fruitful areas for further research. The exploration of the relation between patient outcomes and nursing processes indicates that much further study of this relation is required. This project has identified numerous nursing unit organizational and attitudinal variables that are highly intercorrelated. A controlled study of these variables might better indicate which are the most important and which are causal. Attitudinal variables, for example, could either be causal or could be part of the effect of other conditions. A third possibility for further research would be the extension of the quality-monitoring methodology to the development of performance profiles for individual nurses in professional standards review.

Summary

This discussion has by no means exhausted the total range of method-ological research that has been developed in the field of nursing and patient care. Some examples of methods developed in the area of nursing administration, education, and practice have been described. These have pointed up the great variety of approaches that have been pursued in the methodological research that has been undertaken in nursing as well as the many different purposes to which this research has been put. The develop-ments in this area are particularly noteworthy when it is considered that most have occurred within the past ten years.

Methodological studies have been most widely undertaken in the area of nursing administration. For the future it is hoped that the area of nursing practice will receive increasing attention. One methodological subject in this area that is beginning to receive considerable attention is that of the application of automation and related labor-saving devices to nursing practice. This includes the use of electronic data-processing equipment in the storage and retrieval of information relating to the patient, the use of electronic devices for monitoring the patient, and the application of programmed instruction in the teaching of patients and personnel.

References

1. Eugene Levine, "Nursing Supply and Requirements—The Current Situ-ation and Future Prospects." In Michael L. Millman (ed.), *Nursing Personnel and the Changing Health Care System*. Cambridge, Mass., Ballinger Publishing Co., 1978.
2. National League of Nursing Education, *A Study of Pediatric Nursing*. New York, National League of Nursing Education, 1947.
3. Ethel Johns and Blanche Pfefferkorn, *An Activity Analysis of Nursing*. New York, Committee on the Grading of Nursing Schools, 1934.
4. National League of Nursing Education, *A Study of the Nursing Service in Fifty Selected Hospitals*. New York, The United Hospital Fund of New York, 1937 (reprinted from the *Hospital Survey for New York,* Volume II, Chapter V, pp. 355–429).

5. National League of Nursing Education, *A Study of Nursing Service in One Children's and Twenty-One General Hospitals*. New York, National League of Nursing Education, 1948.

6. "Criteria for the Assignment of the Nursing Aide." *Am. J. Nursing,* **49:** 311–314, May 1949.

7. Marion Wright, *Improvement of Patient Care*. New York, G. P. Putnam's Sons, 1954.

8. Esther Claussen, "Categorization of Patients According to Nursing Care Needs." *Military Med.,* **116:**209–214, March 1955.

9. Richardson K. Noback, "An Approach to Health Problems in Kentucky." *J. Kentucky State Med. A.,* **56:**33–37, January 1958.

10. Jack C. Haldeman and Faye G. Abdellah, "Concepts of Progressive Patient Care," Parts I and II. *Hospitals, J.A.H.A.,* **33:**38–42, 142, 144, May 16, 1959; **33:**41–46, June 1, 1959.

11. U.S. Public Health Service, Division of Hospital and Medical Facilities, *Elements of Progressive Patient Care*. U.S. Public Health Service Publication No. 930–C–1. Washington, Government Printing Office, September 1962, p. 2.

12. Eugene Levine, "A Comparative Analysis of the Administration of Nursing Services in a Federal and Non-Federal General Hospital." Unpublished Doctoral Dissertation. Washington, D.C., American University, 1960, p. 31.

13. Robert J. Connor *et al.,* "Effective Use of Nursing Resources: A Research Report." *Hospitals, J.A.H.A.,* **35:**30–39, May 1, 1961.

14. John P. Young, *A Method for Allocation of Nursing Personnel to Meet Inpatient Care Needs*. Baltimore, Operations Research Division, Johns Hopkins Hospital, October 1962, p. 8.

15. Halbert L. Dunn, *High Level Wellness*. Arlington, Va., R. W. Beatty Co., 1961.

16. Doris E. Roberts and Helen H. Hudson, *How to Study Patient Progress*. U.S. Public Health Service Publication No. 1169. Washington, D.C., Government Printing Office, 1964.

17. *Ibid.,* pp. 11–12.

18. Doris E. Roberts, "How Effective Is Public Health Nursing." *Am. J. Pub. Health,* **52:**1077–1083, July 1962.

19. Majorie J. Hook, "Report on Nurses' Follow-up of Children from Psychiatric Service." University of Nebraska, Nebraska Psychiatric Institute, 1961 (U.S.P.H.S. Grant GN–4796).

20. Maria C. Phaneuf, "A Nursing Audit Method." *Nursing Outlook,* **12:**42–45, May 1964.

21. Sister Mary Helen Louise Deeken, *A Guide for the Nursing Service Audit*. St. Louis, Catholic Hospital Association, 1960.

22. Ester C. Pfab, "An Analysis of the Nursing Audit as a Tool for the Improvement of Nursing." Unpublished master's thesis, Dept. of Nursing Education, DePaul University, Chicago, Illinois, pp. 4–5.

23. Deeken, *op. cit.,* p. 18.

24. *Ibid.,* p. 19.

25. *Ibid.,* p. 21.

26. Viola Bredenberg, *Nursing Service Research*. Philadelphia, J. B. Lippincott, 1951, p. 170.

27. California State Nurses' Association, *Nursing Practice in California Hospitals*. San Francisco, California State Nurses' Association, 1953.

28. Division of Nursing, U.S. Public Health Service, *How to Study Nursing Activities in a Patient Unit*, rev. ed. U.S. Public Health Service Publication No. 370. Washington, D.C., Government Printing Office, 1964.

29. Veterans Administration, Department of Medicine and Surgery, *Program Guide, Nursing Service*, G-7, M-2, Part V. Washington, D.C., Veterans Administration, 1961.

30. Apollonia F. Olson and Helen G. Tibbitts, *Study of Head Nurse Activities in a General Hospital*. U.S. Public Health Service Monograph No. 3. Washington, D.C., Government Printing Office, 1951.

31. Ruth Gillan and Eugene Levine, "The Floor Manager Position—Does It Help the Nursing Unit?" *Nursing Res.*, **3**:4–10, June 1954.

32. Stuart Wright, "Turnover and Job Satisfaction." *Hospitals, J.A.H.A.*, **31**: 47–52, October 1957.

33. John G. Peatman, *Descriptive and Sampling Statistics*. New York, Harper and Row, 1947, pp. 491–502.

34. Eugene Levine and Stuart Wright, "New Ways to Measure Personnel Turnover in Hospitals." *Hospitals, J.A.H.A.*, **31**:38–42, August 1, 1957.

35. Mary K. Mullane, "Identification of Excellence in the Administration of Hospital Nursing Service." Doctoral Dissertation. Chicago, University of Chicago, 1957.

36. Marion Ferguson, *How to Determine Nursing Expenditures in Small Health Agencies*. U.S. Public Health Service Publication No. 902. Washington, D.C., Government Printing Office, 1962.

37. *Ibid.*

38. John R. Thurston *et al.*, "A Method for Evaluating the Attitudes of Prospective Nursing Students." *J. Nursing Education*, **2**, No. 2, May–June, 1963 (U.S.P.H.S. Grant NU–00018).

39. Rena E. Boyle, *A Study of Student Nurse Perception of Patient Attitudes*. U.S. Public Health Service Publication No. 769. Washington, D.C., Government Printing Office, 1960.

40. Leslie W. Knott, Ellwynne M. Vreeland and Marjorie Gooch, *Cost Analysis for Collegiate Programs in Nursing, Part I, Analysis of Expenditures*. New York, National League for Nursing, 1956.

41. Harold R. Rowe and Hessel H. Flitter, *Study on Cost of Nursing Education, Part I, Cost of Basic Diploma Programs*. New York, National League for Nursing, 1964 (U.S.P.H.S. Grant NU–00009).

42. Daniel Howland and Wanda E. McDowell, "The Measurement of Patient Care: A Conceptual Framework." *Nursing Res.*, **13**:4–7, winter 1964.

43. Daniel Howland, "Approaches to the Systems Problem." *Nursing Res.*, **12**: 172–174, summer 1963.

44. Daniel Howland, "A Hospital System Model." *Nursing Res.*, **12**:232–236, fall 1963.

45. Dunn, *op. cit.*

46. Howland and McDowell, *op. cit.,* p. 5.

47. Faye G. Abdellah, "Methods of Identifying Covert Aspects of Nursing Problems." *Nursing Res.,* **6:**4–23, June 1957.

48. Faye G. Abdellah, Irene L. Beland, Almeda Martin, and Ruth V. Matheney, *Patient-Centered Approaches to Nursing.* New York, Macmillan Publishing Co., Inc., 1973.

49. Margaret A. Kaufmann, "Autonomic Responses as Related to Nursing Comfort Measures." *Nursing Res.,* **13:**45–55, winter 1964 (U.S.P.H.S. Grant GN–7981).

50. Emma Spaney, Ruth Matheney, *et al., Employer Expectations vs. Staff Nurse Performance.* New York, Queens College of the City of New York, July 1, 1962 (A three-part report, U.S.P.H.S. Grant GN–4872).

51. Phyllis J. Verhonick, "Decubitus Ulcer Observations Measured Objectively." *Nursing Res.,* **10:**211–214, fall 1961.

52. American Hospital Association, "We Wish We Could X-ray Your Opinion About Your Hospital Experience in. . . ." Chicago, American Hospital Association, 1954 (A.H.A. Questionnaire Form).

53. American Hospital Association, "How About Your Food?" Chicago, American Hospital Association, 1954 (A.H.A. Questionnaire Form).

54. British Ministry of Information, *Hospital Study—Social Survey Section.* London, British Ministry of Information, 1954 (unpublished).

55. Faye G. Abdellah and Eugene Levine, "Developing a Measure of Patient and Personnel Satisfaction with Nursing Care." *Nursing Res.,* **5:**100–108, February 1957.

56. S. L. Payne, *The Art of Asking Questions.* Princeton, N.J., Princeton University Press, 1951.

57. Faye G. Abdellah and Eugene Levine, *Patients and Personnel Speak,* rev. ed. U.S. Public Health Service Publication No. 527. Washington, D.C., Government Printing Office, 1964.

58. Department of Health, Education, and Welfare, *The Progressive Patient Care Hospital, Estimating Bed Needs.* Rockville, Md., U.S.P.H.S., DHEW, Pub. No. 930–C–2, 1963.

59. Edith W. Jones, B. J. McNitt, and E. M. McKnight, *Patient Classification for Long-Term Care: Users Manual,* Rockville, Md., DHEW, Pub. No. (HRA) 74–3107, 1973.

60. Eric Pfeiffer, "Generic Services for the Long-Term Care Patient." In J. Murnaghan (ed.), *Long Term Care Data,* Report on a Conference, *Med. Care,* **14** (No. 5) (Suppl.), May 1976.

61. Sidney Katz *et al.,* "Patient Status Instrument Project: for Functional outcome Measures." Rockville, Md., DHEW, Grant #1501059–01, July 1, 1973 to June 30, 1974 (unpublished).

62. Faye G. Abdellah *et al.,* "The Long-Term Care Facility Improvement Campaign: The PACE Project." *ARN Journal,* **1** (No. 7): 3–4, November–December 1976.

63. Janet Plant, "Various Approaches Proposed to Assess Quality in Long-Term Care." *Hospitals, JAHA,* **51:**93–98, September 1, 1977.

64. Jane H. Murnaghan, "Long-Term Care Data." *Report of the Conference on Long-Term Health Care Data.* New York, J. B. Lippincott Co., 1976.

65. Deane B. Taylor and Onalee H. Johnson, *Systematic Nursing Assessment: A Step Toward Automation.* DHEW Publication No. (HRA) 74–17, Washington, D.C., Government Printing Office, 1974.

66. Richard C. Jelinek, R. K. Dieter Haussmann, Sue T. Hegyvary, and John F. Newman, Jr., *A Methodology for Monitoring Quality of Nursing Care.* DHEW Publication No. (HRA) 76–25. Washington, D.C., Government Printing Office, 1974.

67. R. K. Dieter Haussmann, Sue T. Hegyvary, and John F. Newman, Jr., *Monitoring Quality of Nursing Care. Part II. Assessment and Study of Correlates.* DHEW Publication No. (HRA) 76–7, Washington, D.C., Government Printing Office, 1976.

Problems and Suggestions for Further Study

1. How is the process of developing methodology for research different from developing methodology for practice? How is it similar? What are the advantages and disadvantages of using a methodological tool that has been developed for a research study as a tool for practice?

2. Briefly, how would you go about developing a method for accomplishing the following purposes?
   a. A rating of quality of performance of a nursing aide
   b. A measure of a patient's self-help ability
   c. A method of assessing the efficiency of a nursing home
   d. A tool for teaching family members how to care for patients who are sick at home
   e. A method for screening candidates to a school of nursing who are likely to drop out for reasons other than academic performance
   f. A measure of productivity of the nursing staff
   g. A method for evaluating a patient's level of anxiety
   h. A health education program on the subject of weight control

3. Some of the advantages of a valid and reliable instrument to assess patients' requirements for nursing services have been presented in this chapter. Can you think of any possible disadvantages or limitations to the use of such a tool? What are the ways in which a patient's nursing requirements are determined without the use of such a tool? Could not forecasting of nursing requirements be done by an electronic computer?

4. Why is it important to pretest a methodology on subjects who are representative of the population to which the methodology will be applied? What are the guidelines for determining the number of subjects to be included in such a pretest? Should a pretest be conducted for each revision of a methodology before it is put into final form?

5. Write a brief critique on the following methodological studies that have been reported in the literature.
   a. William A. Gorham, "Methods for Measuring Staff Nursing Performance." *Nursing Res.*, **12:**4–11, winter 1963.
   b. Cynthia Kinsella, "Educational Television for a Hospital System." *Am. J. Nursing*, **64:**72–76, January 1964.

    c. Anne K. Kibrick, "Drop-outs in Schools of Nursing: The Effect of Self and Role Perception." *Nursing Res.,* **12:**140–149, summer 1963.

    d. J. Richard Simon and Marion E. Olson, "Assessing Job Attitudes of Nursing Service Personnel." *Nursing Outlook,* **8:**424–427, August 1960.

    e. Silvia Bakst, "What We Did About Patient Complaints." *Mod. Hosp.,* **98:**110–114, 146, April 1962.

    f. Mary T. Grivest, "A Personnel Inventory of Supervisors, Head Nurses, and Staff Nurses in Selected Hospitals." *Nursing Res.,* **7:**77–87, June 1958.

    g. Morris F. Collen *et al.,* "Automated Multiphasic Screening and Diagnosis." *Am. J. Pub. Health,* **54:**741–750, May 1964.

    h. Carol A. Lindeman, "Measuring Quality of Nursing Care. Part One." *J. of Nurs. Admin.* **6:**7–9, June 1976.

    i. Jean Wyman and Kathy Fernau, "Developing a Criterion-Referenced Tool." *Nurs. Outlook,* **25:**584–586, September 1977.

6. What are the disadvantages, if any, in using methodology, either in research, teaching, administration, or practice, that has been developed in another field? Are there any advantages in using such methodology? If you needed such a methodological tool, how would you go about finding out if a suitable one already existed?

7. Read the article by E. H. Noroian, "Efficiency and Effectiveness" (*Nursing Outlook,* **12:**46–48, May 1964). How does the author distinguish between these two concepts? Discuss some criterion measures that could be developed for these variables.

8. Does methodological research largely fall under the heading of applied research? Can you conceive of any methodological studies that might be considered as basic research?

9. In the article, "Methods for Assessing Nursing Care Quality," by Mark Blumberg and Jacqueline A Drew (*Hospitals, J.A.H.A.,* **37:**72–80, Nov. 1, 1963) the authors discuss several methods for assessing nursing quality. Critically evaluate these methods. Which of these can be developed and tested through a research approach?

10. In her article, "Myth and Method in Nursing Practice" (*Am. J. Nursing,* **64:**68–72, February 1964), Dorothy M. Smith states, "one of the reasons that many nurses enjoy giving medications or carrying out medical orders may be because these are systematized, there is a prescribed procedure to follow, and there is therefore not much need to worry about whether the right or wrong thing was done. We have not yet carried out enough knowledge in other areas of nursing care to develop similarly effective systems" (p. 71). What might some of these other systems be? How can methodological research help to develop these systems?

11. In what ways is methodological research different from other types of research? In what ways is it similar? Does methodology always have to be developed through the process of research in order to be valid? How is the validity of a methodological tool or procedure assessed?

12. Read the article by Donald L. Patrick, "Constructing Social Metrics for Health Status Indexes." *International Journal of Health Services,* **6:**443–453, 1976. Explain how health status indicators can be useful in nursing research.

Update Note

A very valuable methodological study which brings together 140 instruments that have been used in nursing research is Mary Jane Ward, Carol A. Lindeman, and Doris Bloch (eds.), *Instruments for Measuring Nursing Practice and Other Health Care Variables*. Washington, D.C., Government Printing Office, 1979.

An update of patient classification methods can be found in Phyllis Giovannetti, *Patient Classification Systems in Nursing: A Description and Analysis*. DHEW Publication No. (HRA) 78–22, Washington, D.C., Government Printing Office, 1978.

A manual combining study of nursing activities and patient classification is entitled *Methods for Studying Nurse Staffing in a Patient Unit*. DHEW Publication No. (HRA) 78–3, Washington, D.C., Government Printing Office, 1978.

A wealth of information on methodologies applicable to nursing research as well as nursing practice and education is found in the following three publications:

Myrtle K. Aydelotte, *Nurse Staffing Methodology. A Review and Critique of Selected Literature*. DHEW Publication No. (NIH) 73–433, Washington, D.C., Government Printing Office, 1973.

Effie S. Hanchett, *The Problem Oriented System: A Literature Review*. DHEW Publication No. (HRA) 78–6, Washington, D.C., Government Printing Office, 1978.

Richard C. Jelinek and Lyman C. Dennis, *A Review and Evaluation of Nursing Productivity*. DHEW Publication No. (HRA) 77–15, Washington, D.C., Government Printing Office, 1976.

Chapter Thirteen

DESCRIPTIVE STUDIES

THE AIM of descriptive research is to uncover new facts about the situation under study. In nursing and patient care, descriptive studies represent the most common type of research. Such studies have covered a very wide range of subject matter. Some, perhaps the largest number, have focused on nurses themselves and have described who nurses are, how they got into nursing, what they do, and, in great detail, their physical, social, psychological, and economic characteristics. Other descriptive studies have focused on the characteristics of patients, while some have described the facilities in which nursing care is given, the supplies and equipment used in the provision of nursing care, and the administrative and organizational patterns for the provision of care.

A number of descriptive studies have been concerned with nursing students, and a few with persons trained as nurses who are no longer active in nursing. In recent years descriptive studies have been increasingly directed toward the content and methodology of nursing administration, education, and practice, a shift of focus from the nurse herself.

Descriptive studies range widely, too, in their methodology. The vast majority of such studies have been nonexperimental in their design. The very few examples of experimental descriptive studies have attempted to study nursing care under highly controlled conditions. As to methodology for collecting data, many have employed the questionnaire approach, while some have gathered their descriptive facts by the interview method or through an observer. Some of the studies have employed probability sampling, while others have used nonrandom sampling methods or have not employed sampling at all.

Descriptive studies have varied in their scope. Some, particularly those undertaken by a governmental agency or by a professional organization, have been national in scope, while others have been more local, restricting themselves to a particular geographic area—a region, a state, or a city— or even to a single institution, such as a hospital, school of nursing, or public health agency.

555

The remainder of this chapter will present an analysis of selected descriptive studies in nursing which have been grouped according to experimental and nonexperimental designs. These studies are drawn from the areas of nursing practice, education, and administration.

NURSING PRACTICE STUDIES IN NONEXPERIMENTAL FIELD SETTINGS

Study of Quality of Nursing Care

Reiter and Kakosh (1950–1954)[1] pioneered in conducting a field study to establish valid and reliable criteria to appraise the quality of nursing care.

The study extended over a four-year period and utilized several methodological approaches. Like most field studies where the emphasis is placed upon exploration and description there was less concern with establishing controls. The study combines descriptive and methodological aspects and could be classified under both headings.

An initial step was to explore nursing situations broadly and then to select those situations that might be fruitful in providing measures that could be used to appraise nursing practice.

An operational definition of the function of nursing was developed. The critical incident technique was used to collect descriptions of "best nursing care." A poll of observations of nursing care was made to identify and illustrate those aspects of nursing practice that were considered to be valid. These components were then placed into categories of "increasing value to patients."

During the second year of the study the research team concentrated its efforts on the development of an "observation guide" limited to the specification of qualities of safety and effectiveness of three types of nursing care. The three types were categorized under (1) providing personal hygiene, (2) administering treatment measures, and (3) nurse-patient relationships.

The third year led to further refinement of the instrument and the differentiation of those nursing operations which are distinctly professional in nature. The observation guide also underwent rigorous field testing. By the fourth year the researchers were able to translate critical questions into statements of criteria based on the nature of the nursing care and the nurse operations observable within each of three types. Nurse operations were also clustered around four major nursing operations: ministrations, observation, communication, and teaching, all within the function of nursing management of patient care.

The instrument resulting from this field study—the observation guide— is a useful tool that can be used by nurses to sense differences in the quality of nursing practice. The researchers point out that the instrument does focus attention upon the quality of *direct* nursing care through the use of critical questions stated in terms of nurse operations and/or patient responses.

Study of Home Visits of Public Health Nurses

Emphasis in this study was placed upon the verbal behavior of public health nurses and patients in face-to-face contacts.[2,3] This is an exploratory investigation with two general aims, one descriptive and the other explanatory. The investigators sought to determine the range and amount of the content and dynamics of home visits and to identify control mechanisms. Also important to the study was the identification of possible factors that might help to clarify or increase understanding of reasons for differences in nurse and patient behavior in face-to-face contact. No hypotheses were formulated because of the exploratory nature of the study.

The investigators classified verbal behavior according to what is discussed (subject matter), how much it is discussed, who discusses it, who dominates, the mechanisms of communication, the expressions of affect, criticism and praise between participants, forms of reassurance, instances of laughter, and evidences of humor.[4]

No attempt was made to study the effects of verbal communication on subsequent patient behavior or on the degree of improvement in health resulting from the verbal efforts of the nurse.

An important contribution of this study is that an approach to measurement of home visits is presented, centered around "topics" that are discussed during the visits:

Classification System of Topics[5]

I. *The Physical Status of the Patient*
   A. Bodily states, processes and symptoms (e.g., respiratory states, pain)
   B. Treatment and control measures (e.g., diet, weight control)
   C. Implementation measures (e.g., implementation of prescribed therapy, contacts with physicians, procurement of medications)

II. *The Physical Status of Other Household Members*
    (similar categories as for the patient)

III. *Other Topics About Household Members and Household Environment*
   A. Occupation and income
   B. Housing
   C. Household roles
   D. Household equipment and household objects
   E. Interpersonal relations between members
   F. Personality and behavior characteristics of individual household members not classified above

IV. *All Other Topics*

A model or series of models of home visit behavior might be developed wherein topics for further investigation might be specified in advance. Measures of frequencies of topics can offer promising indices for the measurement of quality nursing care.

The researchers point to the need for further study of existing data and refinements and extension of studies of verbal behavior. Their research has provided new insight into understanding why nurses and patients behave as they do. Generalized theories, hypotheses, and concepts about human behavior need to be adapted to the recurrent situations in nursing, testing these in the empirical situation and studying them to see how they predict or fail to predict relevant forms of behavior.[6]

Problems of Field Studies[7]   Much can be learned about field studies from the one just described.

1. Empirical-observational studies requiring the active participation of human subjects have unique methodological problems related to finding, selecting, and obtaining cooperation of subjects to be studied.

2. Field studies may be longitudinal and require two or more sets of observations on the same subjects at two or more points of time. There is invariably a loss of subjects for the second and subsequent sets of observations.

3. When the subjects of a study are patients, written permission from the physician and family is needed for their participation in the study.

4. Timing of interviews presents a problem, particularly in the Johnson study when the spouse of the patient had to be interviewed before the patient was discharged from the hospital.

5. Multiple interviews require rigid criteria for the selection of patients and families to control possible extraneous variables.

6. The selection of the sampling technique has to be related to the aims of the study. Some field studies use probability sampling, but if a scientific sample is not deemed essential, a nonprobability sample can be used. In the Johnson study certain restrictions on the population from whom the participants were drawn were specified, such as selecting patients from large hospitals only.

7. Case finding may be the only course open to the study of some kinds of problems. All units found may have to be studied, with appropriate allowances for time and effort required to locate the units of study. Case finding can be costly in terms of the time and effort of the research staff.

8. Field studies of human populations, particularly longitudinal studies, require attention to procedures to reduce the loss of subjects. For example, the provision of a free physical examination to obtain morbidity data could enhance participation in the study. Other factors contributing to losses are migration, mortality, and nonresponse.

9. A systematic plan for case finding by the research team is a crucial requirement. The reduction in the number of cases may make tests of borderline hypotheses obscure or uncertain.

10. No general rules can be specified for making assumptions about the extent of bias introduced by the nonobserved segment of the population.

Nursing and Psychological Needs of the Elderly Ambulatory Patient

A monumental study in nursing that might well be referred to as a landmark descriptive study in nursing research is the study undertaken by Schwartz and her research team.[8] The report provides documentary evidence of the many realistic problems encountered when studying human populations, a variety of methodological approaches used in the collection of data, and multiple hypotheses that might be tested in subsequent studies.

The research was conducted by an interdisciplinary team made up of a professional nurse, a physician, and a social worker.

The initial research concerned itself with the study of a random sample of chronically ill patients over the age of 60 years drawn from a general medical clinic. Nursing histories were taken on all patients in the sample, but only half of the histories were made available to the nurses working in the clinic. The histories for the remaining half of the patients were filed. These patients were to continue to be cared for in the clinic in the traditional way. A follow-up with the nurses working in the clinic permitted the investigators to assess the needs of the entire patient group— both study and control. Thus, the research team hoped that the nurses' knowledge of patients' nursing needs and the action they had planned or taken could then be viewed against the background of the facts and attitudes obtained when these were looked for and when a discerning nurse skilled in observation took the time to take and record a history.[9]

Half the patients were seen first by the public health nurse on the research team and the other half by the social worker. The investigators originally hoped that their study might be set up as an experimental study with control and experimental groups. However, it was soon realized that this was not feasible because of the difficulty in controlling the biases by the nurses caring for patients in both groups. That is, there was no practical way of preventing the nurses in the experimental group from influencing the nurses in the control group.

The study design was modified to provide a factual documentary description of the clinic population from which the sample was drawn randomly. Here then for the first time was descriptive, documentary evidence of patients' activities of daily living that cannot be obtained from present medical records in a general hospital's unselected clinic population.

Interviews were held with patients in the clinic as they came for regular visits and with those who could no longer come to the clinic. Interviews provided two kinds of data: information from the respondents' answers with no interpretation placed on them, and the nurse or social worker's judgments based on the hospital record, the knowledge of the respondent gained at the interview, and professional insights and experience.[10]

High turnover of nursing personnel required changes in the original research design as many of the study patients were unknown to some members of the staff. It became necessary for the study group to postpone all staff nurse follow-up until the close of interviewing. The research was later extended over a four-year period.

Much can be learned from this study about the nursing needs of patients. "Never take anything for granted, no matter how simple," when it has to do with patients are words that will long be remembered by all those concerned with the improvement of patient care.

Nurses must know the nature and range of patient needs that exist. Likewise, the need for obtaining information systematically about what a patient is doing or plans to do, and what he understands or thinks he understands, becomes clearer to the individual nurse who is giving care. Surely these words of Doris Schwartz and her research team will guide many nurse researchers as they pursue research questions important for the improvement of nursing practice.

Descriptive studies of this nature that are well conceived and documented are greatly needed and will help to achieve major breakthroughs in nursing practice.

Utilization of All Classifications of Nurses Caring for the Sick at Home

The Visiting Nurse Service of New York undertook a project directed by Holliday[11,12] to study the best possible use of all categories of nursing personnel who are caring for the sick at home.

The investigators recognized the need for an exploratory study before a comprehensive study was undertaken. Methodologically this reasoning was sound in that an exploratory study increased the investigators' familiarity with the phenomena to be studied. They were able to establish priorities for further research, to determine what kind of a comprehensive study should be carried out, and to identify those problems that were crucial to the investigator and the staff.

The respondents included all levels of nursing personnel, nurse physical therapists, and nonnurse physical therapists. The study found that patients 60 years of age or over provided the greatest satisfaction to personnel. The most satisfying nursing care was found in the realm of "general care and health supervision."

The exploratory study was valuable in that it was found that the field staff nurse could identify important variables in relation to nurse utilization. This led to a clearer definition of the research problem—namely, to describe in an analytical way the present utilization of staff nurses at the Visiting Nurse Service of New York. It was also perceived important to include patients and human resources (i.e., members of families) in the comprehensive study.

The methods of procedure involved the development and use of an instrument that would give descriptive information on the present utilization of nursing personnel. Questionnaires and interview schedules were developed. An interview guide was also constructed to assess patient and family reaction to the agency's nursing care. Interview schedules were developed to interview selected patients and selected human resources, regarding home nursing care.

The exploratory period permitted the investigator to move more closely toward securing factual description of patient/family care and staff nurses' opinion concerning their own skills.

In a later study the nurse investigator studied staff utilization in three sub-populations of the Visiting Nurse Service of New York. She explored the following question: Are visiting nurses being utilized on the basis of what they are trained and educated for—nursing? A significant finding was that, contrary to the general belief, visiting nurses assume a major professional role where they are untrained and uneducated—namely physical therapy.

Rehabilitative exercises were found to consume the major portion of the nurses' time and they could not give adequate nursing care. It did not matter to the patients if the nurses giving the care were professional or practical nurses.

Intensive Nursing Care of the Patient with Acute Myocardial Infarction

Meltzer and others[13] at Presbyterian Hospital in Philadelphia undertook a study that may well prove to be one of the most significant studies for nursing practice in this century. The research was designed to ascertain if the fatality rate from acute myocardial infarction can be significantly reduced by constant bedside care by specialized nurses aided by a continuous evaluation of the patient's status as reported by electronic monitoring devices. Planned, uninterrupted observations were made by the research team to identify factors significant in sudden death that might trigger an arrhythmia. Professional nurses were taught to apply countershock therapy within two to three seconds after the detection of the arrhythmia (such as a pacemaker). In the first year of the research, several lives were saved, clearly attributed to nursing intervention.

Instruments were also developed to study the patient's emotional reaction to illness, his reaction to constant nursing care and the use of electronic monitors, and his reaction on transfer from the coronary care unit at the end of hospitalization. Tape recorders were used to record the patient's orientation to the coronary unit and to permit a continuous documentation of the patient's reactions throughout his hospitalization.

Nursing Care of the Hospitalized Cardiac Patient

Nite and Willis[14] have attempted to identify criteria that can be used to test the effectiveness of a special type of nursing care that can be given to a selected group of patients. This was essentially a descriptive study of 69 adult hospitalized cardiac patients in one 200-bed hospital. It also included an explanatory phase that was conducted experimentally.

The investigators used Henderson's definition of nursing (1958), which served as a basis for the development of an operational philosophy of nursing. The nursing process that was used involves four steps: (1) identifying nursing problems; (2) specifying nursing goals or objectives from the nursing problems; (3) designing and administering nursing care directed to attain the nursing goals; and (4) evaluating the nursing care.[15]

Participant observation was the essential method used to collect data. From these data, criteria were derived for the experimental phase of the study. The dependent variable of concern to the investigators was the therapeutic effect of a special type of nursing care on a group of adult patients with myocardial infarction. The experimental group was compared with a similarly diagnosed control group. The special type of nursing care did not require an increase in the number of nursing personnel on the unit and could be taught to existing personnel.

Important findings of the study showed that the experimental patients had significantly less change in occupation, general productivity, and income than did patients in the control group. Statistical significance was evident in differences between the two groups in relation to cardiac signs and symptoms and compliance with sleep and rest prescriptions.[16] Other criteria tested were increase in sleep and reduction in defecation difficulties.

The investigators recognize that the criteria are verbal and have limitations. Likewise, it is difficult to relate such things as patients' reports of activities, positive comments about treatment, and complaints to the actual behavior demonstrated. "Until dependable relationships are established between patients' verbalizations and their nonverbal behaviors, the use of verbal criteria in patient care studies will be of limited value."[17]

The publication provides a very useful annotated bibliography for all those interested in research on patient care.

Ritualistic Behaviors in Nursing

Nurses' notes were selected for analysis as a way of studying ritualistic behavior. Walker and Selmanoff[18] define ritualistic behavior operationally as repetitive acts which are judged by nursing services in the university hospital to be dysfunctional—e.g., unnecessary, useless, undesirable, or harmful in achieving adequate patient care. Not all ritualistic behaviors are harmful. Some can serve useful purposes.

Nurses' notes were selected, as they represent the recorded, professional judgment of the nurse and are an important aspect of the special contribution of the professional nurse in the determination of the patients' medical and nursing diagnosis and therapy.

Data were obtained through interviews with professional nurses, practical nurses, and interns. Observations were also made by members of the research team of the time spent in writing and the incidence of referral to the nurses' notes made on medical and surgical wards. The accuracy of the nurses' notes was studied by observing patient care actually given on several wards of the university hospital.

Nurses' notes were found to be relatively unimportant by the majority of the medical and nursing personnel interviewed. Doctors and supervisory nurses made minimal use of nurses' notes. Nurses spent little time in writing nurses' notes and an analysis of the content of these notes showed a high incidence of omission of essential information. The chart is still recognized as the primary means of communication of those aspects of a patient's condition and progress not recorded elsewhere.

Crying as a Physiological State in the Newborn Infant

Johnson[19] undertook an exploratory investigation to examine the changes in the neonate in the heart and respiratory rates which precede, accompany, and follow crying episodes.

The heart beats and respiratory cycles of 28 normal newborn infants were recorded continuously over a one- to two-hour observation period under conditions of active and inactive sleep, wakefulness, and during crying. The investigator found a high degree of regulation of the heart rate during crying toward definite fixed values, under the definitions of stabilization and specificity used. The evidence for regulation of the respiratory rate was not as clear.

Stabilization was defined to be a point at which conditions are relatively well defined and unchanging for a period of time, and when the smallest meaningful time unit is employed. The cardiac rate was found to accelerate immediately with the onset of crying and continue its acceleration to the point of stabilization, around which it oscillates until the cry closes, then returns to a lower rate. The stabilization level was found to be an individual, specific value independent of the sleeping or awake values, the absence of body movement, or the duration of the episode.

A significant research question raised by this study is the relationship between body movement, with and without crying, the frequency of respirations, and respiratory air volumes.

This type of research is an example of the basic descriptive research that must be done in nursing before nursing theories can be identified and a nursing science defined.

Faculty Development Grants—A Way to Stimulate Research

Very often nurses are hesitant to undertake studies no matter how small. The hesitancy is due to lack of research training, insufficient time, and/or lack of supporting personnel and resources. As part of a long-range effort to encourage research training as well as small pilot studies, the Division of Nursing in 1959 initiated a Faculty Research Development Grant (FaReDeG). Nineteen universities have now been awarded such grants, and tangible results are beginning to emerge. Examples of such studies affecting nursing practice resulting from this type of grant at Ohio State University, School of Nursing, are summarized below.[20]

The participants in the project at Ohio State were interested in finding how nurses make nursing diagnoses, the steps they follow, and the manner in which nursing diagnoses can be validated.

An initial step was to undertake an exploratory study to obtain data about the intentions and expectations of doctors in writing P.R.N. medication orders. The instrument developed was an interview guide structured to gain a broad sampling of doctors' opinions of nurse judgment and action in carrying out the orders. Representatives of each group were purposively chosen by the investigators rather than by a random method.

The results of the exploratory study showed that doctors did read nurses' notes; they expected to be called if there was a question about effectiveness of P.R.N. pain medications; they expected nurses to exercise considerable judgment in using P.R.N. orders; and they were essentially unaware of the value of nursing measures in the relief of pain.

A second study[21] focused on the problem of P.R.N. orders from another aspect—namely, what are nurses likely to encounter with reference to P.R.N. medication orders in one hospital setting.

A third study[22] dealt with the observable nurse action in the administration of the analgesics, Darvon and Darvon Compound. The hypothesis tested was that there is a pattern of observable action taken by the medication nurse in response to a stated or interpreted need for an analgesic. This consisted of checking the Kardex and/or doctor's order book, reviewing the patient's record for information, and preparing and administering the medication, provided the existing requirements are met.

Observers with previous experience in the use of process recording observed graduate professional nurses assigned to the administration of medications. All the activities of the medication nurse in a specified time period were observed. An instrument for recording the observations was developed to provide for a consistent way of recording the data.

The hypothesis was not supported by the findings. "There were no observable patterns of nurse action associated with the administration of Darvon and Darvon Compound prescribed as P.R.N. medication." A significant problem identified was that the analysis of the nurses' conversation revealed little evidence that can support the thesis that the professional nurse utilizes communication skills in her effort to assist the patient with a problem of pain.

A fourth study[23] concerned itself with decision making in relation to the administration of P.R.N. medications to children. Data for the study were obtained from a survey of charts of currently hospitalized children in one children's hospital. It was found that the young child and the critically ill child do have fewer numbers of P.R.N. medications ordered as well as fewer types of drugs.

The four studies described provide a useful way of assessing existing data and permitting the study team to formulate possible research questions that might later be explored in more depth. These were reported at the American Nurses' Association 1964 Convention clinical sessions in monograph 3, *Evaluation of Nursing Intervention*.

Relating Concepts of Social Sciences and Psychiatry to Teaching

Gifford (1960)[24] reported a significant experiment that related social science and psychiatric concepts to nursing at the University of North Carolina, School of Nursing. The study provides descriptive data on the changes observed in the faculty, curriculum, and students as a result of the experimental teaching program.

The theoretical basis for the study is ". . . that the social, psychological and biological aspects of human functioning are inextricably interwoven and that good nursing care must attend simultaneously to all these levels."[25]

Seminars for students and faculty provided an opportunity to bridge the gap between the academic and clinical practice experiences of the students. As students advanced educationally, their expectations of patients were less stereotyped and more realistic. Students learned to understand patient behavior and were helped to perform nursing activities.

Once students had completed the junior year experimental program they developed a questioning attitude toward existing practices and were highly motivated to pursue their questions by conducting simple studies.

The investigators concluded that nursing care should be a unity; ". . . learning proceeds through several stages before such a unity is achieved, staged in which the physical and emotional aspects of care are thought of and dealt with separately."[26] Likewise, if students learn to change their attitudes toward patients, they may find it difficult to gain acceptance in the social system of the hospital. The clinical setting must provide a model of the kind of nursing that is being taught.

Studies of Attitudes Toward Practice and Patient Care

Meyer (1960)[27] reported data gathered in the Los Angeles area describing nursing as being in transition between two poles: tenderness (patient-centered care) and technique (technique and colleague-centered).

Four classifications of present-day nurses were described:

Type I.   The ministering angel
Type II. The patient-oriented
Type III. The colleague-oriented
Type IV. The technical-administrative-oriented

The initial descriptive study aimed at exploration of social influence as it exists in the nursing situation. It later became a study of attitudes of nurses and of student nurses, together with information about prevalent social perceptions among nurses.

Significant agreement was found among nurses on the four types of present-day nurses, particularly in relation to nurses' attitudes about giving supervision to others. Beginning students placed high value on Type I. However, as the nurse's educational level progressed upward, a gradual shift of attitude from Type I toward Type IV occurred. The terminal effect showed that the graduates of the baccalaureate program remained in Type II category (patient-oriented); diploma graduates moved toward Types III and IV; and the graduates of the associate degree program showed the least shift and were spread among the four types.

Some significant questions still need to be explored—namely: What would longitudinal studies show of shifting values? Can the four types described be validated in practice? What effect(s) does each type have on patient care?

Longitudinal studies exploring this research problem further would help to provide a theoretical foundation for the knowledge gained in this area.

The intent of theory in research is to be able to go beyond common sense. The ideal is to make a prediction contrary to common sense and have it prove out. Such theory and such predictions require sitting with the same problem for a long period of time until you know more than meets the casual eye.[28]

The Inaccessible Patient

Coleman and Dumas (1961)[29] observed that about half of the patients who visited a psychiatric clinic turn away after one encounter. This led the investigators to conduct an exploratory study of the problem of the inaccessible patient—one who attends clinic once but does not return.

The project was set up to see if a specific nursing activity or group of activities could supplement existing skills that were highly relevant to the needs of patients who come to a clinic. The skilled nursing activities were intended to help patients deal with their illness, therapy, treatment personnel, or environmental situations.

The "special" nursing process made it possible for the nurse to explore with the patient ". . . the meanings of his troubled communications, recognizing that the nurse's own response is an aspect of the system of the patient's communications."[30] Dumas worked with 74 clinic patients. Home visits were made if the patient failed to keep his clinic appointment. The exploratory project proved successful in that the nurse was able to make a contribution in dealing with the delinquent patient by adopting a socially established role in which the nursing process, "defined as a particular method of nurse-patient interaction, helped to bring out and relieve certain distresses in the patient's clinic experience."[31]

Predictors of Success in Nursing

A very useful descriptive study was undertaken by Taylor and Nahm[32] to find out the current procedures used in schools of nursing to select students, including prediction studies. The investigators were concerned about evaluating the present status of knowledge about predictors of grades in formal academic courses in nursing school; predictors of grades and other measures of performance in clinical practice; predictors of on-the-job success; amount of agreement among present testing programs in nursing; overlap of variance of tests in currently used batteries; other new predictors used successfully in other fields; and criterion studies that have been or could be made of specific areas in the field.

Information was obtained by questionnaire from all known schools of nursing in the United States and Puerto Rico. Approximately 67 per cent of the questionnaires were returned. All states participated and a 50 per cent or better return was received from each state.

The investigators found that high school grades and tests of learning ability can predict, with a high degree of accuracy, academic success in nursing school. The predictors found to be most stable were obtained from weighted battery scores derived from multiple correlation studies: ". . . the most consistent prediction appears to occur where each predictor is weighted according to its specific contribution in predicting the criterion."[33]

No studies were identified that could predict on-the-job success in different types of nursing activities. The researchers stress the need for studies in this area. Schools of nursing showed little agreement in the use of testing programs but did place considerable weight upon test scores in their selection programs.

Biographical information was found to be a useful predictor, and in one school situation many hypotheses for further study were identified.*

* Dr. Calvin Taylor has subsequently developed a *Biographical Inventory* and scoring key for the National Aeronautics and Space Agency (NASA) that has proved highly successful in identifying creative scientific talent. It is hoped that the instrument can be adapted to identify creative nurse-scientists.

Another void uncovered by the investigators was the lack of studies to establish criteria for specific clinical areas at the baccalaureate level or areas of specialization at the graduate level.

The researchers leave little doubt that the studies accomplished to date have been of little help to the problem of differential prediction within nursing. Urgently needed is the development of instruments to measure on-the-job nursing performance.

DESCRIPTIVE STUDIES—A.N.A. CLINICAL SESSIONS 1962

In 1962, the American Nurses' Association pioneered in organizing clinical sessions at the convention in Detroit, Michigan. A milestone for nursing research, 21 clinical sessions were held in which nurse researchers were given an opportunity to present their clinical papers.

A special advisory committee was set up to select the papers several months prior to their presentations. Criteria used by the Advisory Committee were:

A clinical paper is one that derives from the direct nursing practices of a professional nurse which:

describes, interprets or explains nurse-patient occurrences, and modes of intervention in a single case in any setting; or

presents generalizations from empirical study of several cases of the same clinical nursing problem in one or in different settings (e.g., hospital, home); or

presents findings resulting from research, experimental or action types, investigating a particular clinical nursing problem; or

shows the application of new or very recent knowledge from a basic or applied science to a particular clinical nursing problem; or

describes and in a new way clarifies one aspect of the total work role of the nurse (e.g., teaching techniques showing the relation of this aspect to described instances of patient behavior with respect to one clinical problem.)[34]

Following are examples of descriptive studies presented at the clinical sessions in Detroit. These papers were published as a series of 21 monographs and are available separately or as a total series from the American Nurses' Association. The number in the reference cited refers to the number of the monograph in which the study was reported.

Ray, Ruth M. "Independent and Dependent Judgments of the Nurse in the Care of Selected Surgical Patients." No. 21.

The investigator undertook an investigation of the nursing care of peptic ulcer patients who required surgical treatment, for the general purpose of determining the existence of a unique body of knowledge in nursing. This particular disease condition was chosen because of its prevalence and increasing incidence in present-day society and its possible serious consequences for the patient.

Two areas were considered: (1) nursing care requiring independent judgments and activity by the professional nurse; (2) nursing care requiring dependent judgments and activities, in which the nurse shares responsibility for medical problems through delegated authority.

An independent judgment, as used by the investigator, is an autonomous estimate or conclusion in matters affecting action and discretion in nursing care, and a dependent judgment is an estimate or conclusion subordinate to medical direction in matters affecting such action and discretion. If there is a unique body of knowledge in nursing it would seem to be the knowledge essential for independent judgments and activities by the professional nurse.

The data were obtained by the investigator's participation in their nursing care, observation of the care given by other nursing personnel, study of the patients' clinical records, and cumulative recording of the information.

The cumulative data were analyzed to identify the nursing problems involved in care, the areas of nursing practice requiring independent judgments and activities of the nurse, and the areas in which she shared responsibility through delegated authority. Particular attention was given to the physician's orders in the patient's clinical records as an aid to identifying those areas in which dependent judgments were required of the nurse.

It is significant that numerous independent judgments were essential in providing nursing care for these patients. Both the independent and dependent judgments implied that the professional nurse must have the requisite knowledge, skills, and attitudes to make wise decisions and to act judiciously.

The data implied that the dependent judgments identified required technical skills, administrative ability, and objective observations. The independent judgments demanded ability in identifying nursing problems, planning nursing care, making subjective observations, providing psychological support, and teaching the patient and his family. These observations would concern the covert aspects of the patient's condition and behavior. Skill in making and interpreting such observations could be expected to vary greatly among nurses. The two types of judgments are interwoven in nursing practice, and the dividing line is seldom sharply delineated.

McDowell, Wanda S. "Nurse-Patient-Physician Behavior: Nursing Care and the Regulation of Patient Condition." No. 21.

Problem: To explore and describe direct patient care in a selected hospital setting utilizing a conceptualization of nurse-patient-physician behavior.

Methodology: The study was conducted by observing nurse-patient-physician behavior and recording a sequence of time-varying events focused on the regulation of patient condition. The hospital setting for the study was the recovery room of University Hospital, The Ohio State University, Columbus. Continuous observations were made of 20 patients—11 men and 9 women from 18 to 70 years old—and their care during the postanesthesia recovery period. The observation periods ranged from 100 minutes to 4 hours. The criterion for selection was that the patient had had a major surgical procedure under general anesthesia.

The collected data were organized and then examined for regularities and repetitiveness so that the triad model (discussed in an earlier chapter of this book) could be described in terms of (1) system input information; (2) system output information—patient condition as a multidimensional vector made up of selected variables which change in value over time; (3) the occurrence and consequence of monitor, control, comparator, and regulatory activities; and (4) the utilization of regulatory strategies to regulate patient condition.

The behavior of nurse, patient, and physician was described by the triad model. Nurse and physician behaviors were identifiable in terms of monitor, regulator, and control functions. The patient's behavior was identified in terms of states that changed in value over time. Patient states were combined to form a three-dimensional vector of essential variables. The essential variables selected as vector components were blood pressure, airway patency, and pain.

Findings: The following inferences were made from the data: (1) the essential variables that composed the patient vector in the recovery room setting and that initiated nurse-physician action were systolic blood pressure, airway patency, and pain; (2) the patient's age, sex, and operative procedure did not influence the initiation of the nurse-physician action or the utilization of regulatory strategies as a consequence of patient disequilibrium; (3) measurements of the patient's temperature, pulse, and respiratory rates did not elicit nurse-physician action.

Conclusions: It was concluded from the study that conceptualization of the triad was a useful model.

This research re-emphasizes the concept that patient care is dependent upon information about patient condition. This concept holds implications for establishing a rigorous basis for developing patient educational programs. Medical and nursing programs, too, should consider the incorporation of information-processing procedures in their curriculums as information requirements are specified for particular patient care settings.

Smith, Mary Margo. "Nursing Knowledge and Activity in Relation to the Period of Anticipation of Pain in the Adult." No. 20.

The purpose of this study was to devise a scientific conceptual framework for the nurse to use in determining the adult's immediate nursing care needs in the anticipation of pain. Related nursing knowledge and activity were derived from the conceptual framework. The study focused only on the immediate situation of anticipation of pain and on the one-to-one relationship between the patient and nurse.

The method of the study was to examine the literature in the physical, behavioral, and nursing sciences in search of theories and principles of use to the professional nurse in the pain-anticipation period. It was felt that such an approach might be valuable for problem solving in nursing.

The first part of the framework dealt with concepts and related nursing knowledge of similarities and differences in adult patients anticipating pain. The second part dealt with concepts on which nursing activities are based.

It was found that the patient's anxiety and tension during the period of pain anticipation may be relieved through some combination of the following nursing activities: remaining with the patient, providing for physical contact, providing for learning, encouraging verbalization, utilizing the patient's physical activity, administering an analgesic, and arranging for the performance of the painful procedure as soon as possible.

Alley, Janet Ann. "Nurse Actions During Hemorrhage in the Child." No. 1.

Problem: To determine the cause of a four-year-old boy's reaction to hospitalization and surgery for the reconstruction of his external right ear.

Methodology: A case study which included the child's history and the child's reactions to all treatment and hospitalization from the time he was three years nine months old to five years of age.

Findings: The child's reaction was more pronounced than that of many children whose history appears to be equally stressing. Although at the time the child hemorrhaged his stresses were both physical and psychological, the cause of his reaction remains undetermined.

Newsom, Betty H. and Oden, Gloria, "Nursing Intervention in Panic." No. 1.
Problem: To describe the difference between panic and anxiety.
Methodology: Ths paper has abstracted pertinent nursing principles from clinical examples of patients at the different states of panic: the prepanic state (rise of anxiety), the panic state (culminating anxiety), and the postpanic state (lowering of the anxiety). The patient's behavior is the nurse's clue to the patient's anxiety plateau. The principles of nursing intervention, formulated for each plateau, are applicable regardless of the patient's diagnosis.

Hickey, Mary Catherine. "Nursing Care for Patients in Hypothermia." No. 3.
Problem: To identify the physiological basis of hypothermia which might modify the nursing care of patients who received this treatment.
Methodology: Data were collected from November 11 to December 22, 1961, on three neurosurgical patients who were hospitalized in the intensive care unit of the Robert Long Hospital, Indiana University Medical Center, Indianapolis. Room temperature in the unit throughout the study was maintained at 80° F. The method of collecting the data was not stated in this paper.
Limitations of the study include (1) the number of patients studied; (2) the patients studied all had neurosurgical diagnoses; (3) the external method of inducing hypothermia was used for all three; and (4) a limited amount of time was available to administer and/or observe nursing care.
Conclusion: A high quality of nursing care for these patients requires (1) knowledge of the physician's therapeutic plan and its application to the patients; (2) development of a nursing care plan within the framework of the physician's therapeutic plan, including those tasks that fall within the realm of nursing and are nursing responsibilities; (3) knowledge of hypothermia as a method of treatment, the methodology of its use, its effect on the patient, and responsibilities of the nurse in relation to it; (4) understanding of the physiological principles and pathological changes that lead to the symptoms upon which the nursing care plan is based; and (5) knowledge of the individual patient's needs which may require adaptations and modifications of nursing approaches.

Largey, Lillie B. "Knowledge, Understanding and Skill Necessary to Meet the Nursing Needs of the Adult Patient Who Has Undergone Open-Heart Surgery." No. 30.
Problem: To gauge the knowledge, understanding, and skill needed by nurses to give effective nursing care during the first eight hours postoperatively to the patient who has undergone open-heart surgery.
Methodology: The five male and five female patients in the study, ranging in age from 14 to 50 years, were selected without regard to the method permitting visualization of the open heart. Hypothermia alone or combined with the pump oxygenator was the method utilized in the large general hospital in Maryland where the study was conducted from April through August 1959. The surgical procedure and the patient's reactions were observed and recorded in a running account, which provided a picture of his operating room experience from the viewpoint of the nurse. The investigator helped transfer the patient from the operating room to the recovery room and cared for him during the next eight

hours. All physical care was recorded on the Composite Nursing Record Form P.H.S. 2225. Some nurse-patient interaction was recorded, also, on a form, but it was not possible to record all because of the amount of physical care required. Each of the patient's postoperative experiences was analyzed for the following factors: the needs he was able to express and the time expressed postoperatively; phases of the operative experience that had significance for his postoperative nursing care and the time following surgery that they were utilized; and nursing action essential to help meet the patient's needs and the time that the action was carried out.

Smiley, Dorothy M. "Nursing the Patient Who Is Experiencing Chronic Pain." No. 9.

Problem: To identify the observable manifestations of pain and comfort, to analyze the patients' reactions to acute and chronic pain, and to determine how this knowledge could be utilized in planning and administering nursing care.

Methodology: Two patients with advanced breast carcinoma were observed intermittently from 8:00 A.M. to 2:00 P.M. on Saturday, Sunday, and Monday by a ward nurse assigned to patient care. Both patients were 44 years of age, mothers, and their husbands were living and well. At the time of the study both patients were on palliative therapy, including symptomatic relief of pain, anxiety, and depression. The observer identified the observable direct and indirect manifestations of pain and comfort, recording on a prepared data sheet those symptoms classfied as comfort, moderate pain, or severe pain, at half-hour intervals or more often if indicated, and noting factors in the medical and nursing care that seemed to influence the patients' responses. Also noted were environmental factors and relevant miscellaneous data such as statements of the patients' feelings toward their illnesses and statements of others regarding the patients' behavior.

Findings: The findings indicated the ways in which the patients handled chronic pain and how they perceived pain loss; data analysis also revealed a relationship among anxiety, pain, and activity in the patients. The analysis of physiological and behavioral symptoms of acute pain and chronic pain, particularly identification of the activity-pain-anxiety cycle, has implications for nursing care. Some nursing activities appeared to aggravate the patients' cyclic reactions.

Abreu, Xenia A., Anderson, Barbara L., Bean, Margaret A., Krahn, Frances A., Yoshida, Mabel T., "An Experience in Nursing Care of Selected Patients on Electronic Monitors." No. 5.

Problem: To determine the effect of the use of monitoring devices on the patient and nurse, and the physical and/or mechanical factors that influence the reliability and use of the monitor.

Methodology: The observations were based on a study of two types of electronic monitors in use on a trial basis in an intensive care unit for approximately four weeks. The nurses participating in the study included the writers, who were members of the nursing staff of the intensive care unit. A simple form was used to record the data—nursing activity, reactions, and comments. Monitor use was restricted to patients on vital signs of 30 minutes or less. If alert and conscious, the patient was given preparation and a simple explanation of the equipment's function. Attending physicians and residents were consulted on use of the monitors. The study was limited to adult patients, as pediatric-size sensors were not available.

Conclusion: From their use of two physiological monitoring devices, the authors describe the problems they encountered and observations on their use, but do not generalize from them, since the study was confined to only two specific machines. They offer their experience as one small step in the new era of automation in nursing.

Brown, Myrtle Irene. "Implications of Cultural Change for Maternal and Child Health Nursing." No. 18.

Problem: To study the relationships between variability in the extent of use of professional maternity and infant health services, and changes in the social situation and sociocultural behavior of Puerto Rican–born women who had moved to New York City. This investigation was undertaken to gain further understanding of the process underlying variable behavior in one cultural complex and to find out how this variable behavior was related to change in sociocultural behavior in many areas of living.

Methodology: The study consisted of a series of intensive case studies of 30 Puerto Rican–born women living in New York City who had just completed a pregnancy of at least 28 weeks' duration. Only those who had lived in Puerto Rico and New York City were asked to participate. Further selection criteria were used, so that the group of 30 was made up of two subgroups of 15 each: subgroup A, whose members had medical supervision regularly from the first trimester of the most recent pregnancy, and subgroup B, whose members had no professional health services until the last trimester of pregnancy or, in some cases, not until labor was established. This utilization of professional maternity care for the current pregnancy was controlled to provide two groups of 15 women each whose behavior in this respect varied sharply.

The women, who were selected for interview during the postpartum period in two Manhattan hospitals, were visited repeatedly at home by the investigator, where data were collected using these methods: extensive guided interviews, unstructured interviews, planned observation, free observation, participant observation, and a Spanish test of reading literacy. The structured interviews, guided by schedules prepared in both English and Spanish by the investigator, dealt with the history of each woman's childhood in Puerto Rico, the educational experiences and aspirations of the subject and her various relatives, the circumstances of migration, her life experiences in New York City, her present beliefs and practices regarding her role behavior in the family and in other social groups, her reproductive and health history, and her use of professional health care throughout her life. Checks for consistency were built into the structured interviews. Data collected by other means served to test the reliability of verbal responses.

These data were analyzed by case summaries and by comparison of data on variables among the subjects. While seeking commonalities and differences in the total sample of 30 subjects and in the subsamples A and B, as well as in other subgroups that emerged in the analysis, an effort was made to preserve the integrity and uniqueness of the individual cases.

Historical material given by the women, corroborated by the extensive literature on Puerto Rican culture and history, were compared with data collected concerning the present situations and behaviors of the women. This permitted comparisons of two generations—each subject with her mother.

Findings: The study yielded a wealth of social and cultural facts about these Puerto Rican–born women who had moved to New York City; generalizations about the continuing process of enculturation in the midst of sociocultural change; and hypotheses for research and field demonstrations.

This report is limited to a brief summary of the reproductive histories of the study subjects, the patterns of use of professional maternity care, and some generalized findings of relationships between sociocultural experiences and the behavior of the study subjects and their patterns of maternity care usage. The report concludes with some of the implications that these findings would seem to have for nurses and health agencies.

Schmalzried, Georgia L. "Effects of Continuity in the Nursing Care of Emotionally Disturbed Children." No. 17.

Problem: To investigate what is supportive and what is nonsupportive to the emotionally disturbed child during early morning care.

Methodology: Two boys on a ward of a multidisciplined, residential treatment center for emotionally disturbed children were randomly selected for detailed observation of their behavior. At the time of the study 16 boys and 9 girls between the ages of 6 and 16 occupied the ward. The days for observation of each child were also randomly selected. The data were collected for four mornings, by direct observation of his behavior between 7:30 A.M. and 9:00 A.M.

Findings: The principal findings of the study are as follows:

1. The responses of the boys indicated that the early morning time was a period of adjustment.
2. The structured program of routines did not provide adequate support; both children needed the support of interaction with adults.
3. Consistency (assigning the same child-care worker to the child) and uninterrupted interactions were supportive in starting the day.
4. Lack of individual attention was nonsupportive and resulted in particular behavioral responses from each child.
5. The number and variety of interactions influenced the child's behavior when he did not have the support of an adult.

The supportive factor in nursing care of the child during the early morning routines was consistent interaction with a significant adult. The nonsupportive factors were the lack of consistency in interaction; interrupted interaction; nature of assignments of child-care workers due to the physical structure of the ward; absence of the workers in particular situations, especially when the children had free time; and the number and variety of unsupervised interactions among the children.

Rose, Patricia Ann. "Identification and Application of Psychiatric Principles in the Nursing Care of Maternity Patients." No. 14.

Problem: To identify psychiatric principles inherent in the nursing care of a selected group of maternity patients.

Methodology: The research method used was the descriptive survey, and the participant observation method was used to collect data. Process recordings were made by the nurse investigator of interactions between herself and the patient during the observation period. Six maternity patients in the third trimester of pregnancy, selected at random on admission to the hospital in labor, composed the population for the study. These patients were given total nursing care from the time of admission through labor and delivery, eight hours per day, for two to three days postpartum. The investigator acted in the capacity of a staff nurse so that the patient would not be aware of being observed. Process recordings were analyzed by the investigator to determine psychiatric principles inherent in the nursing action. A panel of ten nurses was asked to consider the completed analysis of interactions, to determine how the analysis might be strengthened and whether the principles inferred were operating in the interactions and were correctly stated.

Conclusions:

1. The method described was useful in identifying psychiatric principles in the nursing care of a selected group of maternity patients.
2. The method described helped the investigator to become increasingly aware of her own behavior in interactions with patients.
3. Many of the same principles were applicable in the nursing care of all six patients studied. Additional principles were related to problems specific for individual patients.

McWalters, Beverly H. "The Relationship of Attitudes to Nursing Practice." No. 11.

Problem: To determine whether nurses' attitudes affected the nurse-patient relationships in a prenatal clinic setting and, if so, in what way.

Methodology: The study involved 12 nurses and nursing students who visited a prenatal clinic weekly, primarily to acquire more skill in interviewing techniques, to learn to use anticipatory guidance, and to gain more experience in teaching and influencing patients through instruction. The instruction centered on general health measures, and special care during pregnancy, childbirth, and the postpartum period. The nurses were questioned about their own feelings and attitudes toward pregnancy, breastfeeding, natural childbirth, the clinical experience itself, and the patient's using the clinic's facilities.

Findings: The interviews showed that the nurse's attitude had a great effect on the nurse-patient relationship; and that her views of patients and the attitudes she communicated in her work could alter the efficiency of nursing service. There seemed to be a correlation between the nurse's prejudiced attitude and the degree to which she viewed her nursing service as successful. This small study seemed to support the theory that attitudes are communicated interpersonally.

Allen, James Constance. "A Psychodynamic Approach of the Nurse in Combating Denial of the Disease—Tuberculosis." No. 12.

Denial, a problem in the treatment of tuberculosis, was explored. The investigator defines denial as a mental mechanism operating without conscious awareness and employed to resolve emotional conflict and allay anxiety by denying one of the more important elements. The investigator found that a person's premorbid personality determines the form of denial he uses rather than a specific lesion located in a particular area along the nervous system. Other determining factors are interpersonal relationshps, general environmental climate, the individual defect or disability, and the individual's past experience and mode of handling stress situations. To briefly review the predominant form of adaptation and the characteristics of patients displaying explicit and implicit denial, there seemed to be a decided need in both groups for security and prestige, and both groups had formed attitudes in regard to illness based on social and cultural factors. When obtaining information on the personality histories of patients, it was found that not only the patient denies, but so do the family, nurses and doctors.

A case study, with which the investigator was familiar, was presented as an example of the manifestations of denial developing after hospitalization and to show how interpersonal relationships and attitudes enter into the picture involving denial. To combat denial, the nurse must first accept denial as a problem and then learn all she can about it so that she can detect it in her patient, co-workers, and herself.

Johnson, Dorothy E. "The Meaning of Maternal Deprivation and Separation Anxiety for Nursing Practice." No. 2.

Problem: To determine the meaning for nursing practice of maternal deprivation and separation anxiety caused by the child's separation from his parents through hospitalization.

Methodology: The investigator explored briefly the present knowledge of the problem and cited specific cases of children from which she suggested specific nursing practices.

Findings: The specific nursing practices suggested in the examples are the following:

1. Continuity in contact of a limited number of nursing personnel with the child
2. Genuine interest and involvement by these personnel in the child's current experiences
3. Frequent body contacts
4. Provision for variation in sensory stimulation of the child
5. Establishment of the nurse as a bridge between mother and child

These practices require systematic study if greater certainty about their value and effectiveness is to replace impressions.

Meurer, Sister Mary Christopher. "Working with the Mother to Improve Nursing Care of the Child with Leukemia." No. 2.

Problem: To identify and clarify the nurse's role in the care of leukemic children.

Methodology: The study was limited to nurses who had had experience in caring for leukemic children, and mothers who had lost a child to leukemia. It was conducted at Cardinal Glennon Memorial Hospital for children in St. Louis, Missouri, a general pediatric hospital in which leukemic patients are not segregated. A structured interview was prepared and used in a pilot study involving three professional nurses. A revised form of the interview was used in the study with 29 full-time professional nurses then employed at the hospital in order to investigate their reactions to leukemia and explore their attitudes toward parent-child, parent-nurse, and child-nurse relationships. A questionnaire was sent with letter to mothers whose leukemic children had died at this hospital from 1956 through 1960 in order to evaluate the nurse's supportive role as perceived by them. Questionnaires were completed by 47 mothers. The data from interviews and questionnaires were analyzed for common responses and were interpreted in the light of material from the literature.

Findings: The role of the nurse in the care of children with leukemia is largely a supportive one predominantly concerned with the psychological aspects of nursing care. Both the nurses and the mothers stressed the importance of the nurse's meeting each child's personal needs in a loving motherly manner. Both also thought that there is a definite place for parental participation in the total picture of the nursing care of children with leukemia.

EXPERIMENTAL STUDIES

Descriptive experimental studies that describe the behavior of certain phenomena may not have immediate application to patient care but are indicative of the kinds of highly controlled fundamental observations that must be made before possible solutions to problems can be deducted. An example of a descriptive experimental study is the pioneering work of Knisely and Harding in the settling of sludge in animals and in human beings.[35,36] Knisely[37,38] was the first to report the settling of blood-cell masses during life, a phenomenon that was thought to occur only in death. Much of Knisely's early work was done with animals. Matteis[39] was later to make the first observation of the settling of blood masses in living human beings.

Knisely and his research team observed a group of phenomena that are a part of pathological circulatory physiology and not a part of the physiology of health. "In healthy animals and men, the red cells are not agglutinated; they are separate from each other, freely suspended and, in vessels wider than capillaries, tend to be carried rapidly in an axial stream of cells concentrically surrounded by a peripheral layer of plasma."[40] After ten years of study with animals Knisely observed that the settling phenomena did not occur in completely healthy animals or human beings.

The analysis of the settling phenomena required many detailed steps before any possible significance could be attached to the observations. It was first necessary to isolate and to attempt to evaluate the significance of individual biological and physical factors in "the summations of this particular constellation of pathologic circulatory phenomena." Examples of biological and physical factors considered were low circulating blood volume, low red cell count, depth of anesthesia, rates of blood flow, and the length of time settling is permitted to continue.

Observations were next made in vessels of healthy normal human beings and in human patients. The sludging phenomena (settling of masses of agglutinated blood cells to the gravitationally lower sides of vessels) were observed by the investigators with microscopes aimed in the horizontal direction. This was in contrast to the usual way of aiming microscopes vertically downward. The bulbar conjunctiva and the sclera were observed from the side, regardless of the position of the patient, in 14 healthy normal people who had unagglutinated blood, and in 57 patients with sludged blood suffering from a variety of diseases. Each case study was described in detail and schematic drawings made of the observations.

During the observations of the subjects the sludging phenomena were observed to occur in living human beings, but no attempt was made to determine the possible consequences of the sludging. However, another important observation was made—namely, that as a consequence of the sludging of the blood cells, separation of blood plasma from blood cells occurs. It was next necessary to return to the laboratory to study this aspect of the phenomena in detail in frogs.

After several years and multiple case studies in animals and human beings the investigators were now ready to summarize the essential concepts drawn from their observations. Examples of these concepts are as follows:

1. No settling has thus far been observed in healthy persons having unagglutinated blood cells.
2. A mass wide enough to fill a vessel cannot settle in that vessel; masses must be narrower than a vessel in order to settle in it.
3. A slight contraction of a vessel which contains sludge can completely stop the flow in that vessel. The slight increase in vasomotor tone, which thus stops the flow of sludged blood, would but slightly throttle down the flow of healthy normal unagglutinated blood. It seems necessary to conclude that sludge thus directly upsets the precision of vasomotor control of blood flow to each and every functioning histological unit of the body.
4. Settling of sludge occurs in some sick people ante mortem. Settling can no longer be considered merely a post mortem phenomenon.
5. In sick persons having heavily agglutinated blood, small differences in rate of blood flow have a sharp effect upon the settling of blood-cell masses. In healthy persons with unagglutinated blood cells, small differences in rates of flow have no observable effects on the suspension of blood cells.[41]

Having completed detailed observations of the sludging phenomena and extracting essential concepts from their observations, the investigators were now ready to pose several deductions (hypotheses). These stem from the basic question: What are the direct consequences of the settling processes?

1. Does the settling contribute to the formation of venous thrombi?
2. Does settling contribute to the formation of cadaver coagula?
3. Does the settling of blood-cell masses help reduce the red cell count of the circulating blood in some patients?
4. Does the settling of large numbers of blood-cell masses contribute to some types of circulatory shock?[42]

The investigators have indicated many possible studies that might be undertaken. The direct application of their findings to nursing practice is as yet not known, but already Verhonick,[43] at the Department of Nursing,

Walter Reed Army Institute of Research, explored some of the sludging concepts in relation to decubitus ulcers and wound healing, described in Chapter 12.

The work of Knisely and Harding provides an excellent example of how research in theory development is undertaken. The steps in theory development described in an earlier chapter were followed—namely, operational definition of the research problem; observation of the phenomena; specification of concepts; and statement of deductions or hypotheses for further study.

As descriptive experimental studies are undertaken in research in nursing, major breakthroughs in the development in nursing theories can be envisioned.

SURVEY OF CLINICAL RESOURCES FOR NURSING EDUCATION

Formulation of the Problem

Providing adequate clinical experience for professional nursing students is a perpetual problem faced by nurse educators. Hospital administrators as well as directors of nursing service are also concerned with this problem. Previous studies[44] have shown that nurses are more apt to seek employment in hospitals and health agencies that are close to home, particularly where they have had experience.

Another pressing need apparent to the investigators was that of exploring other means of providing public health nursing experience that might be supplemental to the usual type of public health affiliation in a health agency.

The fact that approximately two-thirds of general hospitals in this country have 100 beds or less and have clinical facilities that might be used for student experience led the investigators of this research project to explore the following problem:[45] To determine what variety of nursing problems patients in hospitals of different sizes provide for student nurses. The study combined aspects of descriptive, explanatory, and methodological research.

Two additional major problems were inherent in the overall problem: (a) how to provide nursing students with a sufficient variety of experience, and (b) how to distribute nursing services so that they will be available to all who need them.

Early in the research the investigators had to specify what they meant by nursing problems. Restrictions had to be set about who was to identify these problems and determine the necessary course of action. This, then, involved making a diagnosis—specifically, a nursing diagnosis. The decision was made that the identification of a nursing problem was the prerogative of the professional nurse. It became apparent that nursing problems presented by patients also encompass members of a family or even an entire family. For example, the coronary patient who is a bread-winner of a family faces his illness with not only his own problems but also the problems resulting from the effect of his illness upon his family. If the nurse is to help the patient she needs to visualize the patient as a total family unit.

The following definition of a nursing problem resulted:

A nursing problem is defined as a condition faced by the patient or his family, which the nurse can assist him to meet through the performance of her professional functions.[46]

The investigators sought to go beyond the identification of nursing problems, for they recognized that a list of nursing problems would have little meaning unless one looked at each problem in relation to the other. It became apparent that a typology of nursing problems grouped by a variety of conditions presented by patients had to be developed. Such a typology would have to meet specific criteria if the classification was to be of any use in planning meaningful experiences for students.

Since the investigators were interested in the practical application of their research, they were also faced with the problem of developing a method that nurse educators could use to identify nursing problems and classify them by meaningful criteria that could be used in selecting clinical resources for student experience.

Formulation of a Framework of Theory

Size of hospital continues to be used as an important criterion in select-ing clinical resources for the professional student nurse. Underlying this criterion is the assumption that the larger the hospital, the more adequate the clinical resources for student experience that can be provided with the most economy of faculty time. Superficially, this criterion would seem to be valid, but the investigators questioned it by hypothesizing that if it were possible to develop a typology of nursing problems that grouped patients by common criteria of need, the quantity of clinical resources would no longer be the determining factor. Furthermore, if nursing problems pre-sented by patients were found to be related regardless of their specific diagnosis, then would it not be possible to find groups of patients with common nursing problems in small hospitals similar to those in large hospitals? As the overall problem was one that has existed from the be-ginning of the establishment of the first school of nursing, the investigators found that some exploration of the problem had been made. Some states, such as Colorado, Michigan, and Minnesota, have had considerable ex-perience in using the rural community hospital as a way of attracting more nurses to work in small hospitals.

Several previous attempts had been made to appraise clinical resources in hospitals, but the findings of the studies were found to be of limited value. Most of the hospitals included were large urban institutions, the diagnostic groupings were too broad, and the data were not available by size of hospital. The status of existing knowledge about the appropriateness of using clinical resources in small hospitals and the development of a typology of nursing problems grouped by common needs remained vague and ill defined.

Hypotheses That Might Be Tested

Search of the literature to find what was known and the identification of concepts and theories held by nurse educators regarding the use of clinical resources for student experience enabled the investigators to formulate several hypotheses that might be subjected to testing: (a) the clinical resources available in hospitals of different sizes continue to be one of the major sources of student experience; (b) when diagnoses involve similar nursing problems, experience in caring for patients with each disease entity is not necessary; (c) information about the number of patients discharged, by diagnosis(es) for which they were treated, provides basic data from which nursing problems can be identified; and (d) identification of common elements of nursing care will result in more effective utilization of clinical resources.

A crucial problem was the source to be used for the identification of the nursing problem. It was recognized that patients very often have multiple diagnoses that could present sources of nursing problems. Moreover, what diagnoses would be considered—admission, provisional, or discharge? When patients are admitted they usually are given an admitting or provisional diagnosis. Some are admitted with only a symptom or manifestation recorded. The final diagnosis is reported on the chart often after the patient is discharged and after laboratory reports or autopsy reports are made. Obviously, then, the final diagnosis would tend to be the most accurate. The final diagnosis, in turn, presented a whole new series of problems to be considered. How long would it take to obtain a sufficient quantity of final diagnoses to make it possible to draw inferences from the data? How long a delay is there between the discharge of the patient and the recording of the final diagnosis? This is recorded by the attending physician, and one is all too familiar with the pile of uncompleted charts in the medical records office. Another problem to be faced was the method of recording the diagnosis. Was the commonly accepted Standard Nomenclature and more recent International Statistical Classification used by a sufficient number of hospitals to obtain uniform data?

Hypothesis (d), which sought to test the efficacy of the identification of common elements of nursing care against the criterion measure of more effective utilization of clinical resources, was dependent upon several factors. Particularly important was the method used to identify and classify the nursing problems. This had to be developed and tested for reliability and validity. The method would then have to be tested against the criterion measure of effectiveness.

Definition of Variables

Each step in the research design brought the investigators closer and closer to the narrowing of the problem to a point where it was researchable. Definition of variables brought the problem into specific focus.

The variables considered were (a) the accessibility and availability of the number of discharge diagnoses, by size and location of hospital; and (b) the degree to which the reported diagnoses could be translated into categories that portray the nursing problems involved in the care of patients.

Selection and Development of Measuring Instruments

An important step that had to be considered was the development of an instrument that would provide a reliable way of providing needed data to determine the variety of nursing problems available for student nursing experience in various-size hospitals. The decision was made that patients with diagnoses that nurses need to care for in general hospitals of varying size were to be used as a source of nursing problems. One might speculate as to whether diagnostic data were appropriate sources of nursing problems. Certainly one would not argue that a diagnosis provides all the needed basic information about the patient essential to providing nursing care.

Diagnostic data were used for two purposes: to determine nursing problems that nurses need to know how to solve, and as a basis for a guide to be used by nurse educators in selecting clinical resources for student experience. The investigators were emphatic to point out that no attempt was made to analyze the student's total experience. Recognizing and stating the limitations quite early in a study help to define the scope of the study and further delimit the research problem.

Now an important problem had to be faced—namely, what form should the measuring instrument take? After several trials and pretesting, a four-page form was prepared for collection of the data. Columns were provided for the date of admission, discharge, diagnosis, and record of operations performed. The latter was an important addition, as patients undergoing surgery were separated from those with similar diagnoses but not undergoing surgery. Thus, it was recognized that problems related to surgery might be the determining factors in classifying patients in one group instead of another.

Six small boxes in the diagnosis column were provided for coding purposes, but the hospitals were not asked to code the information. This provided an important control over the data, as not all hospitals have registered medical librarians who use the Standard Nomenclature of Diseases and the International Statistical Classification. Since a registered medical record librarian might not always be available, caution was taken to include specific instructions for filling out the form and recording the final diagnosis.

When an instrument is developed the mechanics of filling out the form need to be given careful thought. In this case, the investigators pretested the instrument and found that an average of 20 minutes was required to make the entries for one day. Any longer period in recording needed data would have reduced the number of hospitals participating in the study.

Selection, Control, and Allocation of Study Subjects

The study was limited to a total of 1,000 discharged patients from a representative sample of 30 general hospitals in Virginia. This was thought to provide a sufficient number of patients. Approximately 200 patients were apportioned among five size groups ranging from a daily census of 50 to 400 patients and over. The state was divided into three geographic regions, and an equal number of hospitals (nine) was randomly selected from each region. Analysis of previous discharge data from the general hospitals in Virginia showed that it was possible to obtain 200 discharge diagnoses in each size group if data were collected over a period of four days. Such knowledge prior to the data collection can be invaluable. The design permitted the inclusion of the maximum number of hospitals and at the same time kept the consecutive days of participation of each hospital to a minimum.

The data-collection period was controlled by a series of field visits made by one of the investigators to 19 of the 30 hospitals. This helped to validate the data being collected by assuring uniformity in data collection, facilitating understanding by the person filling out the schedule, and correcting the reporting of the data in terms of a true primary diagnosis.

Methods of Analyzing Data

The 1,915 diagnoses reported by the 30 hospitals for the 1,000 patients were first coded according to the International Statistical Classification. Coding was done by two experienced coders from the National Office of Vital Statistics. The diagnoses were then classified into 58 groups according to similarity of nursing problems they presented. The classification into groups took the greatest amount of time and required a detailed study and analysis of thousands of diagnostic conditions. Only the primary diagnosis reported for each patient was used, as it was found that, for the most part, the additional diagnoses offered no new nursing problems.

The method of classifying the diagnoses into the nursing problem groups was as follows.

A preliminary test of diagnostic conditions from which nursing problems could be selected was prepared from morbidity data. Diagnoses were grouped topically and coded according to the Standard Nomenclature of Diseases and the International Statistical Classification. Childhood communicable diseases were omitted.

Diagnostic conditions involving surgery were included in the preliminary list. These conditions presented a variety of new nursing problems that need to be considered in planning the patient's total care; hence, operations that were likely to be associated with any diagnostic condition were included as separate diagnoses. The preliminary list was then abridged to eliminate (a) those operations which presented no *new* nursing problems other than those already identified by the diagnostic conditions, and (b) those conditions which presented nursing problems common to all surgical patients. From the abridged list, a final list of diagnostic conditions was prepared by eliminating all diagnoses that would not provide any new nursing problems.

Four criteria were used in setting up the diagnostic groups. Diagnoses were grouped together when (a) the major physical needs of the patient were similar; (b) emotional problems, such as anxiety, depression states, and adjustment situations, were similar; (c) rehabilitative measures involved in the therapeutic plan presented similar nursing problems; and (d) the diagnostic condition presented nursing problems similar to those of one of the diagnostic categories, but the disease syndrome was so important for the student to recognize that it had to be singled out and placed in a separate diagnostic group.

After the diagnoses had been arranged in groups that presented similar nursing problems, the groups were evaluated by three experienced nurse educators. This helped to avoid the introduction of any biases on the part of the investigators in classifying the problems.

The 1,915 diagnoses were classified into 58 nursing groups. Tabulations were prepared to compare the proportion of discharges in each of these groups in small versus large hospitals. Differences among hospitals were quite pronounced in the proportion of multiple diagnoses reported and in the average length of stay. The larger hospitals reported a high proportion of multiple diagnoses. Two of the three hospitals with an average daily patient census of 200 or more were teaching institutions for both medical and nursing students, which may account for the greater proportion of multiple diagnoses reported.

The average length of hospital stay of discharged patients increased directly with the size of the hospital. The length of stay in the largest hospital was twice that in the hospitals in the smallest size group. In the smallest hospitals, nearly half of the patients were discharged in less than four days as compared to only one-quarter of the patients discharged within this time in the largest hospital.

To simplify the comparison of discharge rates among the different size hospitals, 12 of the 58 diagnostic groups having the highest frequency of patient discharges were analyzed. According to these groupings clinical resources for nursing education in small hospitals were very similar to those available in large hospitals, even though the differences were significant at the 5 per cent level in a chi-square test of statistical significance.

In all sizes of hospitals, the per cent of patients discharged who had diagnoses in the 12 diagnostic groups was higher than the per cent of *patient days* falling into these groups. This meant that such commonly occurring short-stay diagnoses as deliveries and tonsillectomies and adenoidectomies tended to become less important when evaluated in terms of the actual number of days of patient care they require.

A comparison was also made of the discharge rates by diagnostic groups in small (under 100 census) urban versus rural hospitals. This showed very close agreement between the two groups. One difference noted was a smaller proportion of tonsillectomies and adenoidectomies in the rural hospitals.

MANPOWER SURVEYS IN NURSING

The term "manpower survey" refers to the measurement and analysis of the personnel resources of an occupational field. Such surveys are essentially descriptive. They are directed toward the quantitative description of the numbers of personnel in the occupational field, the demands for these personnel, and their utilization, educational level, and mobility. Manpower surveys are also concerned with the manner and extent to which new personnel enter the occupational field as well as the attrition from the field through retirement, death, and transfers to other occupational fields. Finally, such surveys may be concerned with the economics of the occupation, including salaries and wages, nonmonetary incentives, and assessment of the productivity of personnel, including losses of productivity through sickness and absenteeism.

In many occupational fields there is a great interest in the collection of manpower data. This is particularly true in a field like nursing where severe and chronic personnel shortages have existed for many years. Some manpower surveys are directed toward the description of personnel shortages as well as an assessment of the reasons for the shortage.

Manpower surveys serve several purposes. Their value is essentially administrative in that the data they yield can be useful for program planning and evaluation. For example, descriptive data on nurse staffing patterns in hospitals can assist directors of nursing service in planning the staffing for their own institutions. Data on attrition rates in schools of nursing can be useful to directors of nursing education in evaluating the effectiveness of their own student selection procedures.

Descriptive manpower surveys can also be useful in generating problems, theories, and hypotheses for further research. Studies concerned with the description of the role, functions, self-images of professional nurses, conducted in the early 1950's with stimulation from the American Nurses' Association, have served to generate explanatory studies to test hypotheses suggested by the descriptive data. Also, some of the early surveys of nursing needs and resources, conducted by the U.S. Public Health Service, produced data indicating that a shortage of nursing services was not necessarily indicative of a numerical shortage of nursing personnel. To further explore this finding, a number of research projects were undertaken dealing with various factors that could influence a shortage of services, such as utilization of personnel, stability of staff, adminstrative efficiency, and attitudes of personnel toward patient care.

Manpower surveys also have had important methodological implications on research in nursing and patient care. Many of these surveys have employed random sampling techniques, some of a fairly complicated design, which have served as guides for their use in other research. The questionnaire and the interview method of data collection have undergone considerable development in descriptive manpower surveys. Indeed, much can be learned from these surveys for application in explanatory research.

The Spectrum of Manpower

Figure 13-1 contains a schematic representation of the scope of manpower surveys in nursing. The horizontal scale can be considered as representing the dimension of time, beginning at the point at which a young girl begins to think seriously about the kind of career she will pursue—perhaps during her early teens—and ending at the point at which the nurse practitioner permanently leaves the field of nursing because of age, health, or other reasons. At various places along this scale, the subject matter for different kinds of manpower surveys is suggested. At the pre-student stage, for example, descriptive studies can be made of the factors influencing the selection or rejection of nursing as a career. At the student stage, studies can be made of the characteristics of students in training, the facilities in which training is provided, and the faculty providing the training. At the practitioner stage, where most manpower surveys have been conducted, a great variety of useful studies are possible: the characteristics of the practitioners, their functions and utilization, their mobility and attrition, just to name a few.

The overriding consideration in the analysis of manpower data is, of course, the question of needs for personnel. This would include not only *how many* personnel are needed, but also the *kinds* of skills, training, personality, and other characteristics they should possess. The ultimate determinant of needs is, of course, the patient. Until good measures become available of patients' needs for nursing services and the extent to which

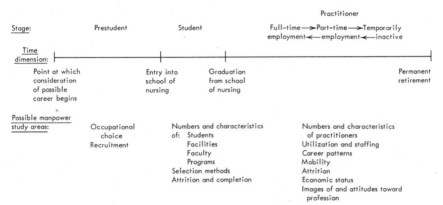

Objective of Manpower: To meet the needs for patient care

Fig. 13-1. The spectrum of manpower.

the existing supply fails to meet these needs, such assessments will have to be based on indirect and rather crude criteria: vacant positions in institutions employing nurses, "standards" expressed as ratios of personnel to the population they serve, and attitudes of the satisfaction of patients and personnel toward the care provided.

Complexity of Manpower Studies in Nursing

Two factors contribute to the complexity of the manpower situation in nursing. One is the very large number of personnel in this occupational field, and the other is the complicated distribution of these personnel among the many agencies that employ them. If we were to add together the total number of individuals falling within the purview of the spectrum of manpower contained in Figure 13-1, we would have a sizable group indeed. For the latest year (1978) in which data are available we have the following estimated counts of nursing personnel and students for the United States as a whole:

Total, All Personnel and Students		*3,617,000*
Professional nurses, actively employed in nursing		1,011,000
Professional nurses, not actively employed in nursing		587,000
Maintaining current registration	387,000	
Not maintaining current registration	200,000	
Practical nurses, actively employed in nursing		498,000
Nursing aides, attendants, orderlies		1,112,000
Professional nursing students		250,000
Practical nursing students		59,000
Volunteers providing some nursing services		100,000

Source: U.S. Public Health Service, Division of Nursing.

Nursing personnel are employed by a large variety of agencies. Although no exact figures are available, the following is a rough count of the number of different agencies employing nursing personnel in 1978:

Total, All Agencies	120,800
Hospitals	9,000
Clinics and other outpatient facilities	1,500
Nursing homes	22,000
Public health agencies (including visiting nurses' associations)	11,200
Elementary and secondary schools	30,000
Schools of nursing	2,600
Industrial plants and offices	8,500
Physicians' and dentists' offices	36,000

Source: U.S. Public Health Service, Division of Nursing.

Nursing personnel are thus distributed among nearly 121,000 different employing agencies. This large number creates difficulties in trying to assess accurately the manpower situation nationally. Some of these difficulties will become apparent in the following discussion of two major descriptive surveys of our nation's nurse-manpower situation. The first of these is the attempt to obtain a periodic count of the total number of nurses in the United States. The second is actually a series of surveys whose purpose was to gather detailed data on the characteristics of professional nurses employed both full and part time, and those who are no longer active in nursing but who maintain current registration.

Survey of the Total Nurse Supply

Unlike some other professions, there does not exist for nursing a single source of data that provides an up-to-date, continuing, and reliable count of persons in the profession. For example, data on physicians are available from the American Medical Directory, published periodically by the American Medical Association. Similarly, the American Dental Association regularly prepares the American Dental Directory which provides a count of dentists.

Data on nurse supply are obtained from three main sources:

1. Decennial Census of the United States Bureau of the Census
2. Annual estimates prepared by National League for Nursing, American Nurses' Association, American Hospital Association and Public Health Service (Interagency Conference on Nursing Statistics)
3. Inventories of registered and practical nurses

Decennial Census   Every ten years the federal government's Census Bureau gathers data on the characteristics of our population, including occupational field. Census data pertaining to nursing for the years 1910 to 1970 are contained in *Health Manpower Sourcebook; Nursing Personnel* [DHEW Publication No. (HRA) 75–43, 1974] and also in the various editions of the Amercan Nurses' Association's *Facts About Nursing.*

Because of reporting errors, considerable adjustments have had to be made to improve the accuracy of census data. The 1970 census count of nurses was 841,000, which is considerably higher than the Interagency estimate of 722,000 for that year. There is reason to believe that much of the higher census count is due to errors in sampling and reporting since the occupational data in 1970 were obtained by a sampling of persons who were self-enumerated. In addition to inaccuracies, other limitations of census data as a source of nurse supply data are:

1. Does not categorize supply by field of employment.
2. Is not available frequently enough to provide current data or to be useful in trend analysis.

Interagency Estimate Since 1952, representatives of the National League for Nursing, American Nurses' Association, and Public Health Service have been meeting regularly to prepare estimates of the number of registered nurses employed in the United States by field of practice. This group, which is part of the Interagency Conference on Nursing Statistics, released nurse supply estimates for the even-numbered years 1954 to 1964 and annually thereafter. These are published in the American Nurses' Association's *Facts About Nursing,* and in the Division of Nursing *Source Books.*

The Interagency estimate is prepared from data for specific fields of nursing that are obtained from various sources. For some nursing fields, supply counts are obtained from employers of nurses through ongoing surveys conducted by professional or governmental organizations:

Field	*Source of Data*
Hospitals	Annual survey of hospitals, American Hospital Association (nursing data discontinued in 1960 but gathered in special surveys conducted from 1962 to 1972. Latest survey conducted in 1979.)
	Survey of osteopathic hospitals, American Osteopathic Hospital Association
Public health (including school nursing and occupational health)	Biennial survey of public health agencies, Public Health Service (latest survey conducted in 1979 after a gap of five years).
Nursing education	Biennial survey of schools of nursing, National League for Nursing (since 1960).

For other fields of nursing—private duty, office nursing, nursing homes —periodic surveys are not undertaken. A variety of methods are used to estimate the number of nurses in these fields.

The advantage of the Interagency Conference on Nursing Statistics' estimate is that it provides the only current estimate of nurse supply. Since an estimate has been made since 1952, it provides a useful time series for analyzing trends.

Inventories of Registered and Practical Nurses   Initiated by the American Nurses' Association in 1949, in which the state licensing system was used as a vehicle for collecting national, state, and county nurse supply data, the inventories have served as a major national data base for descriptions of the supply of nurses. The inventories have been conducted at irregular intervals. For registered nurses data from inventories are available for the years 1949, 1951, 1956–58, 1962, 1966, 1972, and 1977. For practical nurses data are available from national inventories for 1967 and 1974.

Some states have supplemented national inventories by doing their own nurse supply surveys using the licensing system. Although state inventories have certain limitations, such as the exclusion of some nurses working and/or living in the state who may be licensed in another state, they do provide a useful estimate of a state's nurse supply.

Surveys of the Characteristics of the Professional Nurse Supply

During the past twenty years the U.S. Public Health Service's Division of Nursing has supported a number of manpower surveys aimed at describing in detail and characteristics of the professional nurse. Some of these studies include:

1. *Survey of the Educational Preparation and Educational Goals of Professional Nurses.* To determine the educational preparation of all professional nurses in the United States who were actively employed as nurses and to assess their needs for further educational preparation.
2. *Survey of the Part-Time Nurse in the General Hospital.* To determine the actual number of hours per week worked by nurses employed for less than a full-time work week in general hospitals and the reasons for working on a part-time basis.
3. *Survey of the Nurse Who Is Not Working in Nursing but Maintains Current Registration.* To determine the reasons for inactivity in nursing and to estimate the extent to which these nurses can be expected to return to active practice in the future.

4. *Survey of Registered Nurses Employed in Physician Offices.* To obtain data on office nurses, the settings in which they work, the activities they perform, and the nurses' opinions about this type of nursing and their future role.
5. *Evaluation of Employment Opportunities of Newly Licensed Nurses.* To secure information about the job-seeking experience of newly licensed registered and practical nurses.
6. *RNs One and Five Years After Graduation.* To obtain data from nursing school graduates on nursing careers one and five years after graduation.
7. *Longitudinal Study of Nurse Practitioners.* To obtain data from students and graduates of nurse practitioner education programs on prior background and training, previous work experience and income, degree of satisfaction in previous roles, stimuli to enter nurse practitioner programs, and employment after graduation.

Methodology of Surveys Manpower surveys have employed similar methodology in that the data were gathered by the use of questionnaires mailed to the study subjects. Items included on the questionnaires, of course, differed, but many were identical, such as questions relating to the personal characteristics of the nurses: age, sex, marital status and family status, experience, and education.

The sampling designs for the studies varied. For example, the educational preparation study employed a stratified random sample. Lists of the names and addresses of registered nurses were obtained from the state boards of nurse examiners. The lists were stratified by the nurses' state of residence and other characteristics, and a random sample was drawn from each strata.

For the part-time nurse survey, a two-stage cluster sample was drawn. First, all short-term general hospitals in the United States were stratified by the number of part-time nurses employed, and a sample of hospitals was selected at random from the different strata. Each of the sample hospitals was asked to provide a listing of nurses they employed part time. A simple random sample of the nurses was selected from the list. The physician office study was also two-stage, with physicians being the first stage.

All studies employed similar mechanisms for obtaining a high response rate for the mailed questionnaires. Letters accompanying the questionnaires stressed the importance of the survey and the need to obtain as high a response as possible. Several follow-up letters were sent to respondents who failed to return their questionnaires. As a result, the following rates of return of the questionnaires were achieved in each of the surveys:

Educational preparation survey	75 per cent
Part-time survey	91 per cent
Inactive nurse survey	78 per cent
Office nurse survey	55 per cent
Newly licensed nurses	81 per cent
RNs one and five years after graduation	84 per cent
Nurse practitioners	85 per cent

Findings   One of the important descriptive facts that emerges from analysis of the data from manpower studies is the interesting career pattern pursued by many professional nurses. This pattern consists of full-time employment for a year or two after graduation from a school of nursing, marriage during this period, retirement from active practice at the end of the period for purposes of child-rearing, return to employment in nursing on a part-time basis when children reach school age, return to full-time status when children are grown. The detailed descriptive findings from each of these studies have been published extensively in the literature.[47-55]

Implications for Further Research

Numerous studies are suggested by manpower surveys. One possible fruitful area is the degree of commitment to nursing as a career by a group as transient as some of the part-time and inactive nurses appear to be. Questions relating to the utilization of such personnel need to be explored, including the problem of maintaining a high level of quality of patient care when staffing consists of highly mobile and short-term personnel. Another area of possible study is a descriptive study of those nurses who are no longer active in nursing and who do not maintain current registration. To what extent are these nurses permanently out of the manpower pool in nursing? To what extent have they left nursing to work in other fields?

Earlier in the manpower spectrum a study needs to be done concerning how young people decide to enter nursing as an occupational field. At what age levels are firm decisions made? What are the influences on the decision? More study needs to be made of how to recruit students most effectively to schools of nursing, as well as the best method of selecting the students. Once the student has been selected, data are needed on the reasons for attrition from schools.

After the student graduates from a school of nursing, research on the career patterns of nurses needs to be undertaken similar to the study being conducted by the National League for Nursing.[56] Finally, descriptive data are needed on the mobility of nurses, including rates of turnover from various types of institutions and for various categories of nursing personnel, the extent to which nursing personnel progress from one level of position to another in the organization hierarchy, the rate of movement in and out of the active labor force in nursing, and the rate at which nurses permanently retire from the profession.

Summary

Descriptive research represents the most frequent type of research that has been undertaken in the field of nursing. Descriptive studies are important because not only can they yield data that can be useful in program planning, but they can generate hypotheses for explanatory studies. For this latter purpose, descriptive studies are essentially exploratory studies. They have also been helpful in providing a means of developing and testing such research methodology as questionnaires, interviews, sampling designs, and data-processing procedures.

Most descriptive studies in nursing have been nonexperimental in design. In recent years a few experimental studies of a descriptive nature have been undertaken.

The focus of descriptive studies has been shifting significantly. Studies undertaken in the early 1950s were primarily concerned with describing the characteristics of the nurse. Today more and more descriptive studies are concerned with nursing, particularly the practice of nursing and its impact on the patient. Such studies should contribute much to the generation of fruitful hypotheses for explanatory research.

References

1. Frances Reiter and Marguerite E. Kakosh, *Quality of Nursing Care, A Report of a Field-Study to Establish Criteria,* 1950–1954. (U.S.P.H.S. Grant RG–2734.) Institute of Research and Studies in Nursing Education, Teachers College, Columbia University.

2. Rhoda Abrams, "Patterns in Public Health Nursing Home Visits." *Am. J. Nursing,* **63:**102–104, March 1963.

3. Walter L. Johnson and Clara A. Hardin, *Content and Dynamics of Home Visits of Public Health Nurses,* Part I. New York, The American Nurses' Foundation, Inc. (U.S.P.H.S. Grant GN–4512), 1962.

4. *Ibid.,* p. 11.

5. Johnson and Hardin, *op. cit.,* p. 51.

6. Johnson and Hardin, *op. cit.,* p. 106.

7. Walter L. Johnson, "Longitudinal Study of Family Adjustment to Myocardial Infarction." *Nursing Res.,* **12:**242–247, fall 1963.

8. Doris Schwartz, Barbara Henley, and Leonard Zeitz, *The Elderly Ambulatory Patient: Nursing and Psychological Needs.* New York, Macmillan Publishing Co., Inc., 1964.

9. *Ibid.*, p. 5.

10. *Ibid.*, p. 7.

11. Jane Holliday, "Public Health Nursing for the Sick at Home" (U.S.P.H.S. Grant NU 00045), June 1964.

12. Jane Holliday, "The Exploratory Study Method." *Nursing Res.*, **13:**37–44, winter 1964.

13. Lawrence C. Meltzer, F. G. Abdellah, and J. R. Kitchell, *Concepts and Practices of Intensive Care for Nurse Specialists.* Philadelphia, The Charléss Press, 1969.

14. Gladys Nite and Frank Willis, *The Coronary Patient: Hospital Care and Rehabilitation.* New York, Macmillan Publishing Co., Inc., 1964.

15. *Ibid.*, p. 280.

16. *Ibid.*, p. 279.

17. *Ibid.*

18. Virginia H. Walker and E. D. Selmanoff, "A Study of the Nature and Uses of Nurses' Notes." *Nursing Res.*, **13:**113–121, spring 1964. See also: *Ritualism in Nursing and Its Effect on Patient Care.* Indianapolis, Indiana University Medical Center, November 1964 (U.S.P.H.S. Grant NU–00040).

19. Dorothy E. Johnson and Margo M. Smith, "Crying as a Physiological State in the Newborn Infant." (U.S.P.H.S. Grant NU 00055–01.) University of California at Los Angeles, School of Nursing, June 1, 1962–August 31, 1963.

20. Helen Dorsch *et al.*, "Doctors' Expectations of Nurse Action and Judgment in the use of PRN Pain Medication Orders." Ohio State University, School of Nursing (U.S.P.H.S. Grant NU 00043). Convention Clinical Sessions, *Evaluation of Nursing Intervention,* Monograph 3. New York, A.N.A., 1964, p. 26.

21. Wilda G. Chambers and Geraldine G. Price, "A Survey of PRN Medication Orders Prescribed for Medical-Surgical Patients." Ohio State University, School of Nursing (U.S.P.H.S. Grant NU 00043). Convention Clinical Sessions, *Evaluation of Nursing Intervention,* Monograph 3. New York, ANA, 1964, p. 17.

22. Ann J. Buckeridge *et al.*, "A Study of Overt Nurse Action When Darvon or Darvon Compound Are Prescribed for PRN Administration." Ohio State University, School of Nursing (U.S.P.H.S. Grant NU 00043). Convention Clinical Sessions. *Evaluation of Nursing Intervention,* Monograph 3, New York, ANA, 1964, p. 44.

23. Gwendoline Bellam, "The Effect of Age and Severity of Illness on the Number and Type of PRN Medications Ordered for the Pediatric Patient and Their Consequent Impact on the Number and Types of Decisions to Be Made by the Pediatric Nurse." Ohio State University, School of Nursing (U.S.P.H.S. Grant NU 00043). Convention Clinical Sessions. *Evaluation of Nursing Intervention,* Monograph 3, New York, ANA, 1964, p. 4.

24. Alice J. Gifford (ed.), *Unity of Nursing Care.* Chapel Hill, N.C. University of North Carolina, School of Nursing, 1960.

25. *Ibid.*, p. 173.

26. *Ibid.*, p. 178.

27. Genevieve Rogge Meyer, *Tenderness and Technique: Nursing Values in Transition*. Los Angeles, Institute of Industrial Relations, University of California, 1960.

28. Norman A. Polansky, "Interpersonal Influence and the Nursing Function" (unpublished paper). Highland Hospital, Ashville, N.C.

29. Jules V. Coleman and Rhetaugh Dumas, "Contributions of a Nurse in an Adult Psychiatric Clinic: An Exploratory Project." *Mental Hygiene,* **46:** 448–453, July 1962.

30. *Ibid.,* p. 450.

31. *Ibid.,* p. 452.

32. Calvin W. Taylor and Helen Nahm *et al., Selection and Recruitment of Nurses and Nursing Students*. Salt Lake City, University of Utah Press, 1963 (U.S.P.H.S. Grant GN–6330).

33. *Ibid.,* p. 55.

34. American Nurses' Association, A series of 21 monographs on Clinical Sessions (1962 A.N.A. Convention), 10 Columbus Circle, New York, N.Y., 10017, Monograph 1, p. 1.

35. Fann Harding and Melvin H. Knisely, "Settling of Sludge in Human Patients." *Angiology,* **9:**317–341, December 1958.

36. Melvin H. Knisely, Louis Warner, and Fann Harding, "Ante-Mortem Settling." *Angiology,* **2:**535–588, December 1960.

37. Melvin H. Knisely, E. H. Bloch, T. S. Eliot, and L. Warner, "Sludged Blood." *Science,* **106:**431, 1947.

38. Melvin H. Knisely, *The Settling of Sludge During Life*. New York, S. Karger, 1961.

39. F. de Matteis, "Elementi Biologici di Diagnosi della Reumatica Nell'Infauzie." *Recenti Progr. Med.,* **18:**457, 1955.

40. Harding and Knisely, *op. cit.,* p. 317.

41. *Ibid.,* pp. 328–329.

42. *Ibid.,* p. 330.

43. Phyllis J. Verhonick, "Decubitus Ulcer Observations Measured Objectively." *Nursing Res.,* **10:**4:211–214, fall, 1961.

44. Eugene Levine, Maurice E. Odoroff, Margaret G. Arnstein, and John W. Cronin, "Sources of Nurse Supply for New Hospitals." *Pub. Health Rep.,* **70:**356–361, April 1955.

45. Faye G. Abdellah and Eugene Levine, *Appraising the Clinical Resources in Small Hospitals*. Public Health Monograph No. 24, U.S.P.H.S. Publication No. 389, Washington, D.C., Government Printing Office, 1954.

46. *Ibid.,* p. 3.

47. Arthur Testoff, Eugene Levine, and Stanley Siegel, "Analysis of Part-time Nursing in General Hospitals." *Hospitals, J.A.H.A.,* **37:**54, 56, 58, 60, September 1, 1963.

48. Arthur Testoff, Eugene Levine, and Stanley Siegel, "Part-time R.N.'s: A Growing Force in Nursing." *R.N.,* **26:**88–91, September 1963.

49. Arthur Testoff, Eugene Levine, and Stanley Siegel, "The Part-time Nurse." *Am. J. Nursing,* **64:**88–89, January 1964.

50. Dorothy E. Reese, Stanley E. Siegel, and Arthur Testoff, "The Inactive Nurse." *Am. J. Nursing,* **64:**124–127, November 1964.

51. U.S. Public Health Service, Division of Nursing, *Nurses for Leadership.* U.S. Public Health Service Publication No. 1098, Washington, Government Printing Office, 1963.

52. Division of Nursing, *Survey of Registered Nurses Employed in Physicians Offices.* DHEW Publication No. (HRA) 75–50. Washington, D.C., Government Printing Office, 1975.

53. Patricia M. Nash, *Evaluation of Employment Opportunities for Newly Licensed Nurses.* DHEW Publication No. (HRA) 75–12. Washington, D.C., Government Printing Office, 1975.

54. Lucille Knopf, *RN's One and Five Years After Graduation.* New York, National League for Nursing, 1975.

55. Harry A. Sultz, Maria Zielezny, and Louis Kenyon, *Longitudinal Study of Nurse Practitioners.* DHEW Publication No. (HRA) 76–43. Washington, D.C., Government Printing Office, 1976.

56. In addition to the publication cited in reference 54 also see the following two publications by the same author *From Student to RN.* DHEW Publication No. (NIH) 72–130. Washington, D.C., Government Printing Office, 1972, and *Graduations and Withdrawals from RN Programs.* DHEW Publication No. (HRA) 76–17. Washington, D.C., Government Printing Office, 1975.

Problems and Suggestions for Further Study

1. Can a study be purely descriptive? Does not every study have at least some explanatory aspect? Would a purely descriptive study be a somewhat sterile exercise?

2. Discuss some of the methodological problems that might be encountered in undertaking the following descriptive studies:

   a. The number of patients in the United States who need home nursing care.

   b. At what age do young girls become interested in pursuing nursing as a career?

   c. How many hospitals in the United States use the team plan of nursing service organization?

   d. The vacancy rate among positions in schools of nursing.

   e. The socioeconomic status of nurses in the United States.

   f. How many industrial plants in the United States employ nursing personnel?

3. What are some of the reasons why descriptive studies undertaken in the early 1950s were concerned with the characteristics of nurses rather than nursing? Can you cite any descriptive studies completed prior to the 1950s that were concerned with the practice of nursing?

4. Discuss the following remarks by Herbert Hyman in his *Survey Design and Analysis* (New York, The Free Press of Glencoe, 1955): ". . . the central theoretical problem for the analyst of a descriptive survey is the *effective conceptualization* of the phenomenon to be studied. Otherwise any description actually obtained may be incomplete or may distort the nature of the

phenomenon. It is the complexity of the phenomena the survey analyst is usually called upon to describe that makes for this difficulty in conceptualization" (p. 92).

5. What would be the role of a test of significance in a descriptive study? When would confidence intervals be computed for the statistics gathered for a descriptive study? Explain the difference between a confidence interval and a test of significance.

6. Critically discuss the descriptive data contained in the following reported studies. What kinds of interpretations would you make from the data that have been presented?

   a. James T. Nix, "Study of the Relationship of Environmental Factors to the Type and Frequency of Cancer Causing Death in Nuns, 1963." *Hospital Progress,* **45:**71–74, July 1964.

   b. Arthur M. Master and Richard P. Lasser, "Blood Pressure After 65." *Geriatrics,* **19:**41–46, January 1964.

   c. Dorothy E. Reese, D. Ann Sparmacher, and Arthur Testoff, "How Many Caps Went on Again." *Nursing Outlook,* **10:**517–519, August 1962.

   d. Barbara L. Tate, "Attrition Rates in Schools of Nursing." *Nursing Res.,* **10:**91–96, spring 1961.

   e. Harold L. Wilensky, "Mass Society and Mass Culture, Interdependence or Independence?" *Am. Sociol. Rev.,* **29:**173–197, April 1964.

   f. William H. Stewart and Virginia V. Vahey, "Nursing Services to the Sick at Home in Selected Communities." *Am. J. Pub. Health,* **54:**407–416, March 1964.

   g. Shizuka Chino, "Nursing in Japan." *Internat. Nursing Rev.,* **11:**19–26, January/February 1964.

   h. Joan Peterson, Mary Jackle, and Carolyn Ceronsky, "Nursing Students' Experience in Critical Care." *J. Nursing Education,* **16:**3–9, September 1977.

   i. Rebecca Bergman, Nelu Shovett, Lea Zevanger, Rena Sharon, and Mashl Brocha, "Work-life of the Graduates of Schools for Practical Nurses in Israel." *Int. J. Nursing Studies,* **14:**163–198, 1977.

7. Why do you think that descriptive studies are the most common type of study in nursing research? Are descriptive studies less difficult to perform than other types of research? Are descriptive studies less important than explanatory studies?

8. Discuss five uses to which data from descriptive studies can be put. For some suggestions on these uses read Chapter 12, "The Survey," in Tyrus Hilway's *Introduction to Research* (Boston, Houghton Mifflin, 1956, pp. 175–198).

9. Read the study by Frank A. Sloan, *The Geographic Distribution of Nurses and Public Policy* [DHEW Publication No. (HRA) 75–53. Washington, D.C., Government Printing Office, 1975]. Is this essentially a descriptive study? Are any aspects of this study explanatory?

Update Note

Many of the abstracts and bibliographies mentioned in Chapter 5, in the section on "Review of the Literature," cite descriptive studies in nursing. The

Research Conferences, sponsored by the American Nurses' Association and the Western Interstate Commission on Higher Education in Nursing, also referenced in Chapter 5 contain many examples of descriptive studies.

Updates on manpower surveys are contained in the following references:

Eugene Levine and Henry D. Kahn, "Health Manpower Models," in Larry J. Shuman, R. D. Speas, Jr., and J. P. Young (eds.), *Operations Research in Health Care*. Baltimore, Johns Hopkins University Press, 1975.

Jessie M. Scott and Eugene Levine, "Nursing Manpower Analysis: Its Past, Present and Future," in Dale L. Hiestand and M. Ostow (eds.), *Health Manpower Information for Policy Guidance*. Cambridge, Mass., Ballinger Publishing Co., 1976.

American Nurses' Association, *Facts About Nursing, 76–77*. Kansas City, Mo., The Association, 1977.

National League for Nursing, *Nursing Data Book*. New York, The League, 1978.

Pauline Gingras (ed.), *Analysis and Planning for Improved Distribution of Nursing Personnel and Services: National Conferences*. DHEW Publication No. (HRA) 77–3, Washington, D.C., Government Printing Office, 1976.

Chapter Fourteen

EXPLANATORY STUDIES

As has been discussed in Chapter 12, explanatory research has as its aim, evaluation, prediction, or the determination of causal relationships. Evaluative research is probably the most practical type of explanatory research. It is concerned with the assessment of alternative courses of action, programs, products, or procedures.

Since nursing is a very practical occupation, the abundance of evaluative studies is not surprising. These studies have been primarily concerned with investigating the comparative merits of alternative programs or procedures. They have been pursued in the areas of nursing administration, education, and practice, with increasing emphasis on the practice area.

A recent major concern of evaluative studies in nursing has been an assessment of the effects on patients of the provision of nursing care. In this relationship the independent variable "nursing care" has taken different forms:

Amounts of nursing care available to patients
Organization of nursing care (team plan, functional assignment, case method, primary nursing)
Types of nursing procedures
Composition of the nursing team
Psychosocial orientation of members of the nursing team
Facilities in which nursing care is provided

Most evaluative studies in nursing have been performed on-the-job, so to speak, in natural settings. Few have been conducted in highly controlled experimental settings. One that has been, Hasselmeyer's study of premature infants, was able to achieve a high level of control because the natural environment was itself a highly controlled one.

Other experimental studies in patient care have been able to exert only partial controls over the total research process. Since such controls as randomization, the placebo, and the double-blind are often impractical to apply in many important areas of study in nursing, the difficulty of attaining the same purity of explanation as in research in the physical sciences must be recognized. To overcome this limitation in research design, methods of getting the most mileage from the study data through sophisticated analysis and interpretation must be pursued.

Because of the difficulties in controlling all aspects of the study design in many important research areas in nursing, it is doubtful whether significant causal relationships will be established in the near future. This should not preclude the discovery of such relationships as a goal for explanatory research in nursing. Such a goal can have a salutary effect on the improvement of research design and the acquisition of valid and reliable research data.

The following pages contain examples of explanatory research in nursing. These have all been undertaken in the past twenty years. They are mostly in the area of nursing practice. They are all evaluative in purpose, and most are partially experimental in design.

There is no question that all of these studies easily meet at least one criterion given in Chapter 5 for determining whether research should be undertaken or not. This is the criterion of *importance*. Many of these studies are concerned with the undeniably important topic "the improvement of patient care."

THE RELATIONSHIP BETWEEN NURSE STAFFING AND PATIENT WELFARE

Relationship Between Nursing Care Provided and Satisfaction with Care

Formulation of the Problem   During the past decade, the number of professional nurses and nonprofessional nursing personnel employed in general nonfederal hospitals has increased faster than the patient population. Nevertheless, shortages of nursing personnel, particularly professional nurses, continue to exist. These shortages are perhaps even more severe today than ever. Abdellah and Levine sought to find an explanation for this paradox through a rather elaborate study.[1]

This knotty problem is typical of the complex problems frequently encountered in nursing. The descriptive facts that the investigators had to face included:

1. Patient services had quadrupled since the end of World War II.
2. The increased complexity of service placed greater responsibilities on the professional nurse.
3. Hospitals with high hours of nursing care reported personnel shortages with the same urgency as did hospitals with low hours of nursing services.
4. Hospitals conducting work simplification and management studies reported large numbers of nurse vacancies.

What then was the problem? The investigators might have approached it by studying the organizational and administrative patterns of short-term general hospitals, but they already had evidence to show that management studies were not the solution. They might have carried out an extensive study of personnel practices, but hospitals with outstanding personnel policies were faced with the same shortages as those with weak policies.

Some investigators might have been content to accept facts 1 and 2 previously stated and assume that these were the causes of the increased shortages. These factors, although true, were not accepted by the investigators as being the fundamental causes of the shortages.

As the investigators narrowed the problem, it seemed to center on feelings of inadequacy of nursing services rather than on the numerical shortage of nursing personnel. Feelings of inadequacy were defined as factors in the hospital work situation that impaired the full-time effectiveness of nursing personnel and decreased the amount of nursing services that would otherwise be available. No previous research had been done that would scientifically test the relationship of the number of nursing personnel employed in hospitals and the feelings of inadequacy of nursing services.

Formulation of a Framework of Theory   Although the phenomenon of a nursing shortage had been reduced to one of testing its relationship to inadequacy of feelings, many unresolved questions had to be faced. A most urgent question to be explored was to determine how feelings of inadequacies arise.

In exploring this question decisions first had to be made about how to determine the different sources of feelings. Feelings of inadequacy can arise from many sources in hospitals—from patients, families, physicians, nurses, administrators—or they might stem from a variety of sources not related to numerical adequacy of nurse staffing, such as poor patterns of work utilization that reduce the effectiveness of the nurse.

Previous studies had shown that patients and personnel may not verbalize their feelings about care directly.[2,3] Very often these feelings are expressed indirectly and are covert. In these studies, shortages of nursing personnel were found to be symptomatic of deep-seated problems.

Hypothesis Tested   The purpose of the research was to see whether differences in numerical staffing of nursing personnel in hospitals affect feelings of inadequacy of staffing. The specific hypothesis to be tested was stated as a null hypothesis—namely, "There is no relationship between total nursing hours available and number of unfulfilled needs reported by patients."

Definition of Variables   The investigators were concerned with testing the hypothesis in a way that the data could be quantified. Therefore, a mathematical model was designed to express the relationship between number of nursing personnel and amount of feeling of inadequacy of care.

One might ask why a mathematical model was necessary. It has been pointed out that quantification of the findings was essential if one were to get objective data and, most important, if inferences were to be drawn from the findings. Many opinionnaire studies had already been completed providing subjective data from which it was not possible to make any generalizations to other hospitals.

The main independent variable in this study was the number of hours of care available per patient per day in a hospital. The inadequacy of services was to be the dependent variable. Expressed mathematically $(y = k x)$ this would state that when the number of hours of nursing services changed, feelings of inadequacy of nursing services changed proportionately. Determining the value of k was a crucial part of the study, since the aim was to determine the closeness and form of the relationship between the dependent and independent variables.

To determine the value of k was not a simple one for the investigators, as they were interested not only in the effects on feelings of inadequacy of nursing services of the total number of hours of nursing care provided, but, most important, in the effects of the number of hours of a particular kind of care—professional nursing hours. The independent variable was therefore expanded to include professional nursing hours as well as total hours of care. Also, the size and ownership of hospital were treated as additional independent variables. Thus, the model was in the form of a *multiple regression equation.*

Many other variables might also have been included, such as the size and shape of patient units, hospital policies and procedures, and so on. The decision to exclude these variables was made because to include them would have increased the complexity of measurement and statistical analysis beyond the resources available for the study.

Why did the investigators choose a multiple regression equation to express the relationship between the variables studied? This type of equation permitted the investigators to determine the relative importance of each of the independent variables.

The independent variables considered were, therefore, the average daily patient census of the hospital, ownership of the hospital, average daily hours of total nursing care available in the hospital, and the average daily hours of professional nursing care in the hospital. The dependent variable was satisfaction with the adequacy of nursing service as expressed quantitatively. The development of this criterion measure is fully discussed in Chapter 12.

Briefly, satisfaction with nursing services was measured by two check-lists, one for patients and the other for personnel. Each contained 50 items describing omissions in nursing care that could occur in a general hospital. Each item had a quantitative weight, so that a total score was obtained for a respondent by summing up the weights for all the checked items.

Selection, Control, and Allocation of Study Subjects   An important decision that had to be made was to determine the basic unit of sampling in this research. This was determined to be the hospital. Faced with a target population of over 7,000 hospitals in the United States, decisions had to be made to narrow the sample to those hospitals meeting the study specifications. What were these decisions?

1. Size of hospitals would be restricted to those between 100 and 500 daily average patients. This made the target population more homogeneous and eliminated hospitals that presented variables that could not be easily controlled.

2. The sample would be limited to nonfederal hospitals, as federal hospitals have patient populations very different from those of the non-federal short-term hospital.

3. The sample would be restricted further to general hospitals, as the items included on the check lists evolved from patients and personnel in these types of hospitals. The methodology is applicable to other types of hospitals, but the events would have to be modified to include omissions in nursing care that could occur in mental or tuberculosis hospitals.

4. The geographic scope of the hospitals to be studied would restrict the area to seven states that were homogeneous with respect to standards of hospital care. These states were in the midwestern and eastern areas of the United States. States in the southern region were not included, as certain value concepts held by patients and personnel regarding care seemed to be quite different from other regions. For example, in the South it is part of the culture for as many persons as possible to visit the sick patient. It is not unusual to find as many as a dozen visitors in a patient's room at one time. Thus, the problem of handling visitors would be perceived differently in the North as compared with the South.

The target population was narrowed down to 450 general hospitals in the seven-state area meeting the above criteria. The investigators took advantage of data made available by the American Hospital Association to group the 450 hospitals into hours of nursing care available per patient, according to those providing high, medium, or low nursing hours. These hospitals were further subdivided into size and ownership groups, forming 27 basic strata. A total of 60 hospitals was randomly selected from the 27 strata.

How could the investigators be assured of the participation of the hospitals selected in the sample? The fact that the American Hospital Association co-sponsored the study helped to secure a higher response because of the known reputation of this association to participate in studies that would benefit all hospitals. All but 10 of the 60 hospitals originally selected agreed to participate. These hospitals were replaced through substitutes chosen by random selection.

The large number of study subjects included in the study necessitated that the investigators direct their attention to certain controls on the data to be collected. Attention to these controls helped to assure the validity of the data. One such control to assure uniformity in the administration of the study was the appointment in each hospital of a full-time member of the nursing staff as study director. Another important control was the decision to assign three members of the study team to personally visit each hospital. Each team member assumed the responsibility for approximately 20 hospitals and oriented the study director to all phases of the study. To help in this orientation, a manual was prepared describing each step in the study.[4]

Why were field visits by team members an important control? The validity of the data depended upon these visits. Each team member making the visit had to be sure that the study director was given the correct information concerning the study. Likewise, the field researchers could be alerted to any hospital personnel with an axe to grind who might want to use the data for their own purpose. The visit also helped to avert any attempts to withhold information. Advance preparation afforded by the field visit could allay any fears the study director might have.

Another important control was the assignment of a study day by the researchers. This avoided conducting the study on a weekend or a high surgical or admission day, which could introduce extraneous variables.

When completed by the study subjects, each checklist was placed in an envelope and sealed by the respondent. These were collected and mailed directly to the Public Health Service for processing. Mailing the checklist to an outside agency helped assure the respondent that the information was confidential.

Additional validity checks regarding hours of care available were provided in the form of daily and weekly time sheets submitted by each study director.

The instructional manual, the study director in each hospital, the field visits, and the provision of a carefully worked out mechanism to distribute, collect, and mail the checklists, all helped to assure that the study would be conducted with a minimum of complications.

Methods of Analyzing Data   The punched-card machine method was used to compute the data for the regression analysis. The number of checklists obtained from patients and personnel were extensive. Some 20,000 were processed, making machine tabulation a necessity.

How were the data analyzed? Two types of data analyses were selected. One analysis was concerned with the testing of the significance through the analysis of variance of the relationship between hours of nursing care and feelings of the inadequacy of the nursing service.

The second analysis focused on the relative occurrences of the individual events on the checklists as reported by different respondents in the sample hospitals. These data were available for each of the 60 hospitals and an analysis was made separately for each hospital. The individual reports to hospitals were not essential for the research but were valuable in helping hospitals plan action programs to reduce the number of omissions in nursing care.

Separate tests of the relationship between hours of nursing care and feelings of inadequacies were made for each type of respondent. Obstetrical patients were separated from other patients, as they were found to have different needs for nursing care.

Interpretation of Findings   The conclusion is drawn by the investigators that no matter how much nursing care a hospital has available, there will still be some groups within the hospitals that will express the feeling that the hospital is omitting certain aspects of nursing care.

Findings of the research substantiated the original null hypothesis posed by the investigators—namely, there was found to be no relationship between *total* nursing hours and the number of unfulfilled needs reported by patients. However, a significant finding was that patients in hospitals providing higher *professional* nursing hours reported fewer unfulfilled needs than patients in hospitals with lower professional nursing hours. The obstetrical patient, on the other hand, reported the same volume of unfulfilled needs regardless of the number, or kind, of nursing hours provided.

What significance do these findings have for patients? One can only pose additional questions that need to be tested. For example, patients' needs are better fulfilled when they receive professional nursing care. Orientation of personnel to patients' needs, better utilization of nursing skills, and higher standards of nursing care might be explored as variables resulting in fewer unfulfilled needs reported by patients.

Doctors, orderlies, and aides reported the same proportion of unfulfilled needs regardless of the nursing hours provided. Is this because they observe fewer patients' needs, or is the instrument not sensitive enough to pick up their observations?

A startling finding was that with the exception of aides and orderlies all other nursing personnel, including student nurses, reported fewer unfulfilled needs of patients when *total* nursing hours were higher, but there was no relationship between the unfulfilled needs reported by these personnel and the amount of *professional* nursing care available.

These findings seem to support other hunches—namely, that the addition of hands and feet may be a temporary or superficial relief of the nursing shortage. The data suggest that adding hands and feet will not reduce the number of unfulfilled needs reported by the patients themselves. For patients, unlike for personnel, the number of professional nursing hours available does seem to make a difference as to whether they perceive their needs as having been met or not. Here then is the significant finding of the study.

Study of Variations in Staffing Patterns

New[5] (1956–1957) undertook an experiment with staffing patterns focused on two independent variables: the ratio of staff nurses to auxiliary personnel and the ratio of all nursing personnel to patients. The study was designed to answer two questions:

1. When the total nursing hours per patient are varied, how does the proportion of nursing time spent with the patient vary, and what happens to the attitudes of both patients and nurses concerning the new situation?
2. When the composition of a nursing team is varied, how does the proportion of nursing time spent with the patient vary, and what happens to the attitudes of both patients and nurses concerning the new situation?

Answers to these questions were sought by staffing two units in each of two hospitals for nine consecutive weeks, with nine different combinations of nursing personnel. The proportion of staff nurses was varied from 25 to 75 per cent of the total number of personnel, and the average hours of nursing care provided per patient ranged from 2.1 to 5.1. Each variable had three possible alternatives, resulting in nine possible combinations. The research thus employed a factorial design. Each combination of staffing was tried out for one week and evaluated. The procedure used for observing nurse activities was adopted from time-sampling methods developed by the Public Health Service's Division of Nursing. Attitudes of patients and personnel were evaluated from questionnaires and interviews. The study was a logical sequel to the nurse utilization studies that had been done previously.

Questions have been raised about the validity and practicability of subdividing the independent variables into so many different subgroups and then making an assessment of change in one week's time. In spite of the weaknesses in the research design, valuable clues are provided about nurse staffing patterns that need to be tested further. For example, in experimental "situation 8," which was a high total hours nursing staff combination, many of the nurses felt uneasy and tired because of insufficient work to do. In other words high levels of nurse staffing could have negative consequences, or, as the investigators conclude, too many nurses may be worse than too few.

Patient Welfare as a Criterion Measure

Multiple experiments were conducted at the State University of Iowa* Hospitals by Aydelotte[6] and her research team to test the validity of the hypothesis that increases in the amount or the quality of nursing care will produce improvements in patient welfare. The hypothesis was tested in two ways: (1) increasing the size of a ward nursing staff; and (2) introducing an in-service education program designed to increase the amount and quality of nursing care given by a ward staff. Five experiments were conducted in which variations in ward staffing patterns were made.

The patient welfare measures were categorized into three groups: clinical measures (e.g., number of hospital days, fever days, postoperative days, doses of narcotics); scaled measures (e.g., patient's mental attitude, physical independence, mobility, skin condition, opinion of nursing care); patient activity sampling measures (e.g., percentage of time spent in bed, in a chair, up, and in communication and occupied leisure). Work sampling techniques were used to collect data for the latter variables.

A significant finding was that neither incrementing the staff nor introducing an in-service education program resulted in any detectable improvement in patient welfare.

The investigators believe that the instruments were sufficiently sensitive to measure changes in patient welfare. The reasons provided to support this conclusion are that the measures detected differences among individual patients and among groups of patients classified by age and general condition. The measures also detected improvement in groups of patients during their hospital stay.

Effects of Minimal Conditions on Nursing Activity

An important replication of some aspects of the Iowa study was conducted by Bryant,[7] testing the effects of minimal nursing care.

Three null hypotheses were subjected to testing:

1. There will be no significant differences in the number of omissions and completions in nursing tasks among the various staffing patterns employed.
2. There will be no significant differences in the number of omissions

* Now the University of Iowa.

and completions in nursing tasks among the various levels of nursing hours per patient.

3. The degree of care required by the patients on the experimental wards will have no significant effect on the omission of required nursing tasks.[8]

According to the data, hypotheses 1 and 2 were rejected and hypothesis 3 was accepted.

THE EFFECT OF PROGRESSIVE PATIENT CARE
ON PATIENT WELFARE

Progressive Patient Care is defined as the organization of facilities, services, and staff around the medical and nursing needs of patients.[9,10] Six elements make up Progressive Patient Care: intensive care, intermediate care, self-care, long-term care, home care and out-patient care.

A 200-bed community hospital that was in transition toward becoming a Progressive Patient Care hospital was selected for study of the effects of P.P.C. on patient welfare. This was the only hospital within a radius of ten miles. The hospital administrator and board of trustees, faced with a nursing shortage and a long waiting list of patients, decided to experiment by reorganizing the hospital facilities.

All critically ill patients were grouped on an intensive care unit, regardless of diagnosis, sex, or economic status of the patient. A selected number of patients were placed in a self-care unit. The self-care patients were all physically able to care for themselves but required hospital services such as x-ray or laboratory or needed additional help in learning to live with their limitations. Those patients with chronic diseases and those with fractures requiring hospitalization for more than 30 days were grouped in another unit for long-term care. All other patients not fitting into these three categories were placed on three intermediate care units.

A research team was established to conduct the study which consisted of members from numerous disciplines, such as: nurses, physicians, hospital administrators, industrial engineers, statisticians, behavioral scientists, architects, dieticians, medical records librarians, and cost accountants.

The task of the research team was to study this hospital situation to determine what factors, if any, affecting medical practices, nursing practices, dietary practices, costs, and patterns of patient recovery, might be attributed to Progressive Patient Care.

Progressive Patient Care (P.P.C.) is a phenomenon made up of many variables resulting in multiple effects, thus increasing the complexity of conceptualization. When dealing with such a broad phenomenon like P.P.C., it is often necessary first to carry out a descriptive survey to determine which differences may be attributed to it. These differences can be further scrutinized by means of a comparative study to identify significant factors (criterion measures) that are related to the phenomenon. Once these criterion measures are identified they can be subjected to more intensive analysis, refinement, and verification through experimental research. This is often the sequence in research approaches.

Identifying Major Components

During the initial phase of the study, each discipline represented on the research team had to prepare a description of the situation one year prior to and for one year after the P.P.C. program was initiated. This is sometimes referred to as retrospective experimentation and is useful where changes have already occurred that prevent prospective experimentation.

The architect used original hospital blueprints to sketch the physical renovations that had been made. The hospital administrator, the physician, and the dietitian reviewed previous practices and spelled out those practices in their areas that had to be introduced as a result of P.P.C. The cost analyst prepared a new basis for estimating costs, one based on patient services rather than by type of services or facility.

In nursing, nurses and a biostatistician obtained time sheets and computed hours of nursing care per patient on each unit prior to and after the P.P.C. program was initiated. The biostatistician also computed turnover rates for each category of nursing personnel before and after P.P.C. was initiated. Nurse utilization studies were carried out on units affected to determine the kinds of nursing practices that were being provided. Studies of patient and personnel satisfaction were made to determine the present attitude toward P.P.C.

Interviews were held with patients, physicians, and nurses to determine their perception and feelings about P.P.C. Characteristics of professional nurses were studied to determine why nurses were selected for specific units.

After several months of intensive study of this one situation, the major components composing the phenomenon of P.P.C. were isolated. If these components could be spelled out in a series of items, from which hypotheses could be elicited and attributed to P.P.C., and later tested for validity and reliability, they might serve as dependent variables to measure the effects of P.P.C.

The five major components (criterion measures) resulting from the introduction of P.P.C. that were isolated and the hypotheses that might evolve concerning them follow:

Major
component: 1. Faster patient recovery.
Hypotheses: 1.1 Belief that time factors related to the rapidity with which medical procedures can be carried out have a direct bearing on patient recovery.
                 1.2 Belief that time factors related to the rapidity with which nursing procedures can be carried out have a direct bearing on patient recovery.

1.3 Belief that complications related to patient care are reduced. (For example, incident reports, I. V. infiltration.)

1.4 Belief that consultative visits are reduced because of a higher level of patient care and reduction in complications.

1.5 Belief that the patient's length of stay can be reduced.

1.6 Belief that the patient is able to return home and to work at a faster rate.

Major
component: 2. Positive acceptance of Progressive Patient Care program by patient, family, community, and hospital personnel *after* the introduction of this program.

Hypotheses: 2.1 Belief that doctor, patient, and family relationships have improved.

2.2 Belief that medical, interstaff, departmental and trustee relationships have improved.

2.3 Belief that nurse-doctor relationships have improved.

2.4 Belief that nurse-patient and family relationships have improved.

2.5 Belief that patient satisfaction has improved.

2.6 Belief that the nurse's satisfaction with her work situation has improved.

2.7 Belief that patients on intensive care units assign greater importance to medical and nursing care than to their physical surroundings.

Major
component: 3. Reduction in cost to patient, family, and hospital.

Hypotheses: 3.1 Belief that it is more economical to patient, family, and hospital to have Progressive Patient Care programs than the usual type of service found in general hospitals.

3.2 Belief that self-care units can be furnished with home furnishings at a greater reduction in cost than present hospital furnishings.

3.3 Belief that personnel services can be provided on the self-care unit at a reduction in cost.

3.4 Belief that equipment can be concentrated in specific areas at a reduced cost to hospital operation. (For example, oxygen only in intensive care units instead of piping throughout hospital.)

Major
component: 4. Effective utilization of Progressive Patient Care units by type of patient, physician, and nurse.

Hypotheses: 4.1 Belief that medical, surgical, and emotionally disturbed patients can be cared for on P.P.C. units.

4.2 Belief that the self-care unit should be utilized by convalescent patients and not limited to patients receiving diagnostic workups.

4.3 Belief that minimal and optimal nurse staffing patterns can be determined for each type of progressive patient care unit based on medical and nursing needs of patients.

4.4 Belief that nurses on intensive care and self-care units have more time to spend with patients.

4.5 Belief that progressive patient care permits an effective classification of patients based on patients' needs.

4.6 Belief that intensive care units should be staffed with one professional nurse and one nursing aide to six patients.

Major
component: 5. Efficient operating plant.

Hypotheses: 5.1 Belief that future designs of hospitals must include intensive care areas and self-care areas.

5.2 Belief that self-care areas should be separate from the main hospital plant with a connecting archway.

5.3 Belief that intensive care areas should be so located as to permit easy movement of patients from one area to another.

5.4 Belief that intensive care areas should be set up so that each area is self-sufficient in terms of equipment, medications, supplies, and linen.

5.5 Belief that all equipment in intensive care areas should be recessed into the wall.

5.6 Belief that the furniture in intensive care areas should be limited to the patient's bed.

Testing a Major Component

Specific hypotheses under three major components were selected for intensive study by the research team during the second phase of the study. One component related to cost, the second to efficiency of the operating plant, and the third to the effective utilization of P.P.C. units by type of patient, physician, and nurse. How the study of the hypotheses under the third major component were approached will be discussed briefly.

A specific hypothesis related to the utilization component was selected for investigation. This was the hypothesis that minimal and optimal nurse staffing patterns can be determined for each type of P.P.C. unit based on medical and nursing needs. To test this belief two studies were set up. The first was an empirical study to determine nurse staffing patterns and reasons for variability in general hospitals having one or more types of P.P.C. units throughout the country. This phase of the study provided information about practice in general hospitals with and without P.P.C. units concerning nurse staffing patterns.[11]

Such information can be helpful in evaluating the relevancy and adequacy of a criterion measure. For example, analysis of these data showed that fixed staffing patterns that are absolute cannot be set up for each unit. If there is a great deal of open-heart surgery or neurosurgery performed in a hospital, a staffing pattern designed for a general medical and surgical floor would be unrealistic. One would probably need a ratio of one nurse to one patient with such a work load.

The second study, exploratory in nature, was carried out in a large metropolitan hospital and was directed at identifying: (a) a conceptual framework from which concepts of nurse staffing patterns might be derived (described previously as an example of a nursing model); (b) criterion measures to measure the effect of nursing services on patient progress; and (c) levels of nursing skills required to carry out the services.

The key hypotheses being tested were:

1. Nursing services should be determined by the patient's needs.
2. Patient's needs change during 24 hours, and hence a daily evaluation of these needs should be made by the professional nurse and physician directly responsible for the patient's care. (This may be done by a team leader and resident or intern.)
3. There are four needs for care that can be identified. These are the

patient's needs for sustenal care, remedial care, restorative care, and preventive care.

4. Evaluation is a type of service that is continuous.
5. There are three levels of skills required in meeting the needs of patients. These are coordinating, technical, and custodial.

A sample of medical and surgical patients was studied from the time of admission until discharge. Some phases of nursing care were given by the hospital staff. Aspects of nursing care that were not given to patients under study were provided by one other nurse and the investigator from the research team.

The most crucial aspect of this study was the identification of valid and reliable dependent variables, which when translated into scores could be used as criterion measures to determine the effect of nursing services upon patient welfare.

The latter study differed from the descriptive study in that an attempt was made to develop nurse staffing patterns based on what nursing services should be provided to meet patient needs rather than upon nursing services that were actually being provided. The descriptive study showed that facilities for patients had changed but nursing practices had not. One hypothesis evolving from the descriptive study that needs further testing is that there are nursing practices being omitted that are essential to the patient's progress.

Once the functions, levels of skills, and criterion measures have been identified, experimentation with various levels of nursing personnel needs to be carried out to determine those groups that can perform adequately the nursing services based on patients' needs. This will next lead to testing the utilization of various categories of nursing personnel (professional and nonprofessional) to determine the effectiveness of nursing practices in meeting the needs of patients. Effectiveness would be measured by criterion measures identified while actually caring for a sample of patients.

MEASURING THE EFFECTIVENESS OF CLINICAL NURSING PRACTICE

Study of Closed-Circuit Television

Griffin, Kinsinger, and Pitman (1962)[12] undertook an experiment with closed-circuit television to see if individualized clinical instruction might be possible through the use of this medium. The experiment proved highly successful. The closed-circuit television was also used in a large classroom to show a nursing demonstration conducted at the bedside of a patient.

The study was extended to develop criteria for measuring the quality of nursing care, to develop evaluation instruments based on these criteria, and to test them for validity and reliability. A closed-circuit television system equipped with a video tape recorder made it possible for the investigators to obtain objective data on which such measures would be based. The usefulness of such a system for improving nursing practice was also tested in the next phase of the study.

Expert nurse practitioners observe an actual nursing practice by closed-circuit television and use criteria developed by other investigators to rate the quality of the practice observed. The reliability and validity of the criteria were established by reviewing the video tapes, and the evaluation instruments were adapted as indicated.

Freshman student nurses in an associate degree program were assigned to experimental and control groups on a random basis to serve as subjects for this part of the study. The experimental variable consisted of immediate playback of a video tape of the student's own performance in carrying out actual patient care responsibilities, with an analysis of her performance by the instructor. At the conclusion of the experimental period, a final examination on clinical practice was video taped and evaluated by the instrument(s) previously developed. The experiment was replicated once, and the rating of the performance in the examination was done by members of the nursing faculty who taught only sophomore students and who had no prior contact with the experimental subjects.

Patients' Reaction to Stress

Another example of an explanatory study in the area of nursing practice is that of Meyers[13] who explored ". . . the effects of three different conditions of communication on the impact and resulting cognitive structuring of an unfamiliar and moderately stressful situation."

The procedure, designed to produce a mild stressful situation for the patient, consisted of the investigator carrying a covered tray containing test tubes. One of three conditions of communication was given as the investigator swabbed the patient's forearm with tap water and covered it with gauze. The skin area was observed by the investigator but could not be seen by the patient. After one minute the gauze was removed.

The three types of communication were (1) structured communications, (2) no communication, and (3) irrelevant communication. Seventy-two hospitalized patients participated in the study and were assigned to these three groups.

Each subject participated in a postexperimental interview to find out the patient's response as to what he thought did happen. The results were analyzed to provide five scores: an accuracy score, a blood-needle score, and overestimation, underestimation, and talkativeness scores.

The investigators found that there was less tension created when the patient was given specific information upon which he could prepare for the impending stress.

If a measure of the stress a patient feels upon hospitalization is related to the deprivation he experiences, then it follows that the "communication" approach will negate or at least minimize some of the stress inherent in hospitalization.[14]

Study of Postoperative Vomiting

A small, well-designed experimental study in nursing practice was carried out by Dumas and Leonard[15] at Yale University.

The conceptual basis for the study was that the emotional reactions of surgical patients to their illness and treatment have important consequences for their postoperative course. The relief of emotional stress of the patient is considered to be part of the professional nurse's role. The hypothesis tested was that the use of an "experimental" nursing approach in the care of surgical patients would reduce the incidence of postoperative vomiting. The experimental treatment was a process of nursing directed toward helping the patient attain a suitable psychological state for surgery. The following were specified:[16]

1. The nurse explores with the patient her observations of his behavior to determine whether he is experiencing distress.
2. The nurse explores further to find out what is causing the distress and to determine what is needed to relieve the distress.
3. The nurse uses the information in the first two steps to select an appropriate course of action to relieve the distress.
4. The nurse checks with the patient to see if the action relieved the distress.

The experimental patients, in addition to routine physical preparation, were seen by the investigator one hour before surgery. The control patients received only the routine preoperative physical preparation from hospital nursing personnel.

A pilot study followed by two actual experiments was conducted. The findings were substantiated in the experiments. The investigator found that by using the experimental nursing process, she was able to relieve the distress of 70 per cent of the experimental patients. Twenty per cent of the distress of control patients was relieved by nurses who gave care to this group. None of the patients vomited who either experienced no distress or whose distress was relieved.

The experimental research design used in this study provides one approach to testing hypotheses dealing with the improvement of nursing practice. It is only when many studies of this type are conducted that nursing theories can be developed.

An Experimental Study in Breast Feeding

Disbrow[17] conducted a study to explore the significance of selected sociocultural factors of the breast-feeding practices of primiparas in one university medical center.

The investigator hypothesized that demographic determinants played a crucial part in successful breast feeding. For example, the primiparas who have some college education will be more successful in breast feeding than those with less education; mothers with a high socioeconomic status will be more successful in breast feeding than those with a lower socioeconomic status; and 20–29-year-old mothers will be more successful than those in other age groups.

A sample of 200 primiparas meeting specified criteria were selected for study. Data were collected through interviews during the first three days after delivery, and a second interview was held with 122 mothers of the original sample in their homes between four to eight weeks after delivery. A third contact was made with 175 mothers by telephone or interview at the termination of breast feeding.

No significance was found in the relationship between the mother's education and her success in breast feeding. Mothers under 20 years of age were found to be less successful in breast feeding than the 20–29-year-old mother. The influence of family and friends on the success or lack of success of breast feeding was much greater after the mother was discharged.

A significant finding of this study was that nurses and doctors did not prepare the mothers for the problems that they will likely encounter in the early weeks of breast feeding at home. This was found to be the most crucial feeding period affecting the success or lack of success of breast feeding.

An Experimental Approach to Testing Patient Response

Thornton and Leonard[18] designed an experiment to test the effectiveness of three ways of presenting a hospital request to a patient.

Included in the experiment was a 25 per cent sample of patients discharged from postpartum units on the days selected for the experiment who composed one of the experimental groups, and another 25 per cent who were assigned to a different experimental treatment. The remaining patients formed the control group. Each day, the investigators alternately assigned the patients to one of the three groups as their names appeared on the discharge list. A total of 120 patients participated in the experiment.

The instrument used was a questionnaire on the baby's condition given to postpartum patients who were instructed to mail it back two weeks after discharge from the hospital. The study tested the extent of patients' cooperativeness in mailing back the questionnaires.

Three different approaches were used to ask the patient to return the questionnaire. Those patients in the control group were simply handed the questionnaire on discharge (38 per cent returned it).

A second approach was unfocused, in which the experimental nurse used a "friendly" approach to the patient with no specific reference to the hospital (52 per cent returned the questionnaire).

The third approach focused on the hospital request, explored the patient's reactions, and explained its purposes (67 per cent of the patients in this group returned the questionnaire).

The investigators point out that their experiment can provide a simple but useful method to test the effects of various nursing approaches.

RELATIONSHIP BETWEEN NURSING CARE AND THE BEHAVIOR OF PREMATURE INFANTS

Another in the series of studies concerned with the relationship between nursing care and patient welfare was reported by Hasselmeyer[19] in 1961. This study was directed toward the care of the premature infant. Its immediate purpose was to test whether a specific nursing procedure— namely, the provision of continuous support to the infant through the placement of a diaper roll at his back or side—could influence his well-being.

Importance of the Study

The importance of the problem of prematurity can be easily demonstrated. As indicated by the investigator:

Prematurity is the leading cause of death among infants in the neonatal period. In the city of New York during 1959, the mortality rate of infants weighing less than 2,500 grams at birth was 15.5 per 100 live births in contrast to a rate of 0.6 per 100 for infants weighing more than 2,500 grams.[20]

The nurse has an important role to play in the care of premature infants. In addition to being responsible for assisting the infant in feeding, breathing, and maintaining a stable body temperature, she can take the initiative in providing needed emotional support, although this is restricted by the practice of minimal handling of premature infants.

Rationale for the Study

The idea for this study originated in observations made by the investigator in the care of premature infants. It was noted that in collecting stool specimens from the infants, the placement of a rolled diaper at the back of the infant tended to quiet him. Infants continually supported by the diaper roll appeared to gain weight at a faster rate than unsupported infants.

Various reasons were conjectured for this relationship. One was physiological—if a baby was quieter, his energy output would be less and therefore his rate of weight gain would increase. More fundamental was a psychological relationship. The support provided by a diaper roll would provide the infant with needed security. He would, therefore, be less restless, he would sleep more, conserve energy, and gain weight faster. These effects would be beneficial, since at higher weight levels the infant's chances of survival could well be enhanced.

Hypotheses for the Study

The independent variable was the dichotomized nursing procedure: provision of support to the infant through a diaper roll, withholding the diaper roll support. As the criterion measure for evaluating the effects of the support, the most desirable measure would be the survival rate of the infants. However, the investigator decided that this would not be a sensitive or practical criterion, since many deaths occur during the first days of the infant's life—too soon for the effect of the diaper roll to make itself felt. Moreover, deaths among premature infants are frequently caused by certain conditions that would override and tend to obscure the effects of the diaper roll support.

As dependent variables, a group of six criterion measures were developed. A relationship between each of these and the independent variable was formulated in a series of six hypotheses to be tested in the study:

Time required to regain birth weight
Rate of weight gain
Sleep behavior
Crying behavior
Bodily movements
Eating ability

The investigator hypothesized that infants supported by a diaper roll would exhibit more favorable behavior on each of these variables than unsupported infants. That is, they would regain weight faster, sleep better, and cry less than unsupported infants. Except for the hypothesis concerning bodily movements, all were stated in the form of the expected relationship, not as null hypotheses. The tests of significance would, however, employ the null hypothesis.

Measurement of Variables

The variable, weight, is of course measurable by a scientific instrument, a quantitative weight scale. For the other variables, measures had to be developed by the investigator. As seen in Table 14-1, the scales that were finally developed were all essentially ordinal scales. The infant was rated on each of the scales through a detailed checklist completed by an observer at stated intervals (see Table 14-1).

The development of the measuring instruments for these four variables occupied a great deal of the time and effort spent on the research. Because of the crucial need to make valid, reliable, and sensitive measurements of these variables, this effort was considered to be well justified. If existing measures had been available, they undoubtedly would have been used.

Even with the great effort expended in developing criterion measures for this study, the best that could be achieved were ordinal type qualitative scales. However, some of these scales had a quantitative counterpart. For example, sleep behavior was measured not only in terms of quality of sleep according to the scale shown in Table 14-1, but also in terms of the amount of time spent sleeping. Also, feeding behavior could be quantitatively measured by caloric intake.

The reliability of all the scales used in the study was carefully assessed.

TABLE 14-1

Scales Used to Measure the Dependent Variables—Sleep Behavior, Crying Behavior, Bodily Movements, and Eating Ability— in the Premature Infant Study

Sleep Behavior

If infant is in incubator or bassinet not attended by any person, the following classification is to be used:

Sleep—Eyelids are closed and remain closed with no evidence of opening of eyelids. Infant usually lies quietly in crib but there may be a slight movement of an extremity or head.

Eyelids slit—Eyelids are not fully closed, but there is no movement of eyelids.

Undecided—Infant appears to be fluctuating between sleep and wakefulness. His eyes open and close involuntarily. His expression is dull. Bodily movement may be present. Crying or whimpering is not present.

Awake—Eyes are definitely open, and facial expression denotes wakefulness. Vocal sounds may be absent. However, if infant is whimpering or crying, although eyes are closed, he is considered awake.

If infant is being cared for by nurse or doctor, the following classification is to be used:

Eyes closed

Eyes opened or evidence of an opening or closing of lids

Vocal Behavior

No sounds

Grunts, moans

Crying, whimpering—weak, whining sound

Crying—tense, forceful, not necessarily loud

Bodily Movement

No movement.

Movement of one or more extremities but trunk not involved in the movement. (Do not record movements of hands or feet which do not include arms or legs.)

Relaxed movement of body, shift in position, or stretching, which is slow, easygoing, but involves head, trunk and/or more than one extremity.

Vigorous extension and flexion of all extremities, trunk and head involved; movements tense, rigid.

TABLE 14-1 (continued)

Feeding Behavior
Pattern

A —Interest in eating in both the first and second half of the feeding. Stimulation and encouragement not required.
B —Similar to *A* in first half of feeding, although the quality of suck and grasp on nipple not necessarily as powerful as in the *A* pattern.
C —"Middle-of-the-road" eating ability.
D —Marked changes in behavior would occur between first and second halves of feeding. While the first half of the feeding might resemble pattern *A* or *B*, the second half would represent poor eating behavior. Effort and encouragement would be needed to feed the infant in the second half.
E —Effort and encouragement would be needed to feed the infant from beginning to end of the feeding. The feeding was seen as beginning unsuccessfully and ending in the same manner because of extreme lethargy, marked evidence of fatigue, and inability of the infant to suck.

Variable	*Frequency of Measurement of Infants*
Weight	Once a day before 10:00 A.M. feeding
Eating ability	Recorded after each feeding
Sleep behavior	
Vocal behavior	Every 10 minutes, 24 hours a day
Bodily movement	

Source: Eileen G. Hasselmeyer, *Behavior Patterns of Premature Infants,* U.S. Public Health Service Publication No. 840. Washington, D.C., Government Printing Office, 1961.

The observers received a lengthy period of training. After the training period, the observers and instructors made simultaneous observations of the same infants. Correlations between these independent observations were very high.

Experimental Design

The research design was essentially a matched-pair type of experimental design. A total of 59 infants at the Bellevue Hospital Center's Premature Nursery, New York City, were randomly allocated to one of two groups Thirty infants were assigned to the experimental group, in which backs were continually supported by a diaper roll. Twenty-nine infants were assigned to the control group, from which diaper roll support was withheld. All other conditions—amount of handling, type of clothing, feeding —were kept constant for the two groups.

Infants were admitted to the study within 96 hours after birth. Criteria for admission included weight between 1,000 and 1,999 grams and absence of illnesses or abnormalities.

Matching was accomplished in terms of three variables: weight, which had four levels, and sex and race, each of which had two categories. This made a total of 16 matching cells ($4 \times 2 \times 2$).

Weight Group	
I	1,000–1,249 grams
II	1,250–1,499 grams
III	1,500–1,749 grams
IV	1,750–1,999 grams

Sex—male, female
Race—white, nonwhite

A random start assigned the first infant to either the experimental or control group in one of the 16 cells according to its characteristics. The next infant was assigned to the opposite study group in the appropriate cell. As reported by the investigator, the assignment procedure was such that:

Placement of a single born infant in the experimental or control group in each of the 16 cells was opposite to the group in which the preceding infant had been placed. For example, if the last infant for white females with a birth weight between 1,750 grams and 1,999 grams had been an experimental subject, then the next white female of this birth weight group would be a control subject. If twins were admitted to the study, one was placed as an experimental subject, the other as a control.

A similar procedure was used when starting cells previously unoccupied. The first infant in any cell was placed in the group opposite to that occupied by the first infant in the last cell to be started. In other words, if the first infant to be admitted to the cell for nonwhite males, weighing between 1,250 grams and 1,499 grams, had been placed in the experimental group, then the next infant who showed characteristics for a cell as yet completely unoccupied would be a control subject.[21]

The matching procedure insured that the subjects in the alternative groups were equalized as closely as possible on the three main organismic variables.

Administration of the Study

Each of the 59 study infants was observed for a period extending from less than 96 hours after birth until the age of 42 days or upon reaching the discharge weight of 2,500 grams, whichever came first. The earliest discharge date was at the twenty-first day of life. This primarily included infants in the higher birth weight groups.

The number of infants admitted to study varied between 13 and 16 a month. To obtain the required number of study subjects in each group took a period of 32 weeks of observation, 24 hours a day.

Various techniques were used to keep the study as tightly controlled as possible. This included, in addition to the randomization and matching procedures, a thorough training period for the observers, careful control over the administration of the diaper roll support to keep it uniform from infant to infant, carefully designed instruments to gather data on the dependent variables, and control over the total study environment to eliminate possible effects of extraneous variables.

Such a high degree of control is possible in a study setting like a premature nursery, which is naturally a highly controlled one. Few patient care areas present such capabilities for control. In addition to nurseries, other highly controlled natural settings in a hospital include the operating room and the recovery room. Settings like these simplify the problems of executing experimentally designed studies.

Findings

The significance of the relationship between the diaper roll support and the dependent variables was tested by a series of *t*-tests. These tests assessed the significance of differences between the experimental and control groups in the values of the criterion measures for each of the six dependent variables. Tests used were two-tailed. *None* of the tests indicated that the diaper roll support produced effects among the experimental infants that differed significantly from the controls.

Conclusions

Although the findings of the study were not in the expected direction, the research had several important outcomes. First, much descriptive data was produced by the study that could be of value in the care of premature infants. For example, weight curves were derived that could be helpful to nursing personnel in evaluating the progress of prematurely born infants.[22]

Second, the study had methodological significance. It produced instruments for measuring important behaviorial variables of infants such as eating, sleeping, and crying. Perhaps even more important, the study demonstrated that a tightly controlled experimental design can be used to evaluate effects of nursing care on patient welfare.

Finally, it provided a framework for pursuing further research in the area. One study, undertaken by the director of the project, was concerned with the relationship between handling of premature infants and such variables as incidence of morbidity, weight gain, vocalization, and bodily movements.[23]

A question can be raised about any possible shortcomings in the study design that could have influenced the findings. With all the careful controls employed in this study it may seem surprising that no significant differences were found between the experimental and control groups. One possible shortcoming of the study is the sensitivity of the criterion measures. Perhaps with more refined measures—say, the employment of numerical scales rather than the cruder ordinal scales that were used—

significant differences might have been detected. However, one could question whether such differences would have had any practical importance.

The investigator herself raised questions about possible limitations of her research in her report. One of these is the "Hawthorne effect"—the reaction of the study subjects to the *process* of change rather than to the substantive change itself. Since the introduction of the diaper roll produced no significant effects detectable by the researcher, this is not an issue. If significance was found, the possibility of psychological bias could be raised, since the study design did not employ a placebo or the double-blind technique.

Also there is a question about the tests of significance employed—the *t*-tests of significance of the difference between mean scores for the alternative groups. It may well be that an analysis of variance would have been a more powerful test to use in that it might have been more sensitive to any differences between the alternative groups studied.

In retrospect, many changes could be suggested in the study design to simplify the data collection and to yield more sensitive data. For example, the observations could have been made through a television camera. This would have reduced the number of observers required considerably, lowering the cost of the study as well as reducing effects of observer bias.

These suggestions for improvement demonstrate that there is no perfect research design. Only by analyzing what previous researchers have done and by profiting from their experiences can we hope to improve our methodology and enhance the validity and sensitivity of the data we gather through research.

STUDY OF THE EFFECTS OF SKILLED NURSING CARE

Measurement of the effects of nursing care is extremely difficult to do at the present time, as few precise measuring instruments are available. Brown[24] and her research team at Washington University, St. Louis, and Simon[25] at the University of Iowa have provided a major breakthrough in the development of methods to measure the sociological aspects of care and to test the effects of nursing care on this measure.

Brown proposed to investigate the hypothesis that by the effective implementation of the skills of nursing personnel, the personalization of chronically ill aged patients could be significantly enhanced. It was anticipated that a patient would become more active and would do more things for himself as personalization takes place. The patient was expected to take over things the nurse formerly did for him, and the nurse in turn would become less active in his care.

The research problem was to investigate the effects upon a variety of behavioral indices of personalization that might be produced by providing the aged patient with skilled nursing care. Comparisons were made between patients receiving skilled nursing care (experimental group) and those receiving care standard to the institutions in which the patients were lodged (control group).

The method developed was used to test the following hypotheses:

1. In those situations wherein the experimental nurse is present with the experimental patient, and regular nursing personnel are present with the control patient, the frequency of active participation will be greater for the experimental patients than for the control patients.
2. In the experimental group when the nurse and the patient are involved as a dyad (pair), the patient will be active a greater proportion of the time than will the nurse, but when nursing personnel and patients in the control group are involved as a dyad, the reverse will be true.
3. The frequency of both verbal and nonverbal communication will be greater in the experimental group than in the control group.
4. Time spent by patients in moving or walking will be greater in the experimental group.
5. The frequency with which the patient employs suggestions and directions with positive effect will be greater for the experimental patients.
6. The frequency with which the patient is involved in nonverbal, nondistorted components of biosocial functions will be greater in the experimental group.

Skilled nursing care was viewed as a process of verbal and nonverbal interaction directed toward the attachment of a patient to his social system. The skilled nurse was defined as one with a minimum of one year of specialized clinical preparation at the master's level and who has received training in handling of the aged patient. She possesses skills to attach the patient to the social system by perceiving variations in a patient's complete situation and giving appropriate individual care.

Other operational definitions important to the research were: *Personalization*—attachment of an individual to his social system (that which

Research Method

Independent Variable	Dependent Variable
Skilled nursing care	Personalization of older patient as measured by: 1. greater initiative–active interactional participation 2. greater verbalization 3. greater nonverbal functions and communications 4. greater control of the environment as indicated by the employment of suggestions 5. greater reality orientation as measured by employment of nonverbal, nondistorted biosocial functions

represents society in an individual). *Depersonalization*—depriving a person of those factors that attach him to his social system.

A split-plot type of experimental design, a type of factorial design, was used in which a series of small experiments were arranged. Each experiment provided for two small paired groups of subjects: one of these paired groups receiving skilled nursing care, the other not. There were three replications, each containing six matched pairs of patients who were randomly assigned to the alternative groups. The experimental patients on one unit received treatment Monday, Wednesday, and Friday; the other unit Tuesday, Thursday, and Saturday. Five nurses participated in collecting data so that each contributed equally to the experimental and control groups. Each of three replications was performed in a different institution and environment. Each institution was rated for tolerance for personalization:

Replication	I	1,450 bed public hospital in a large city
	II	100 bed private nursing home. Charges: $225 and up/mo.
	III	107 bed private nursing home. Charges: $132–$150/mo.
Replication	II	Highest tolerance for personalization (enriched environment)
	I	Second highest tolerance (type of environment between two extremes)
	III	Lowest tolerance (deprived environment)

Five nurses were employed: Three available each day to provide skilled nursing care to the experimental patients while observing them, and two nurses available to observe the patients in the control group. The five nurses were rotated so that at times they served as observers of the control patients or gave skilled nursing care to the experimental patients.

Skilled nursing care was given one and one-half hours, three times per week over a six-week period; the control group was observed over six weeks, three times per week at 20-minute sessions (20 minutes was justified in terms of greater behavioral homogeneity).

Data Collection

Participant observation was the primary method used for data collection. During each replication the nurses assigned to give skilled nursing care dictated their own participant observations in narrative form immediately upon leaving the patient. Nurses observing control patients did so in narrative form at time of occurrence. Concurrent observations were made by a second nurse observer on some of the nurse-patient interactions in both groups.

Classification of Observations

The observations were classified according to several dimensions. One of these was readiness to interact. This variable increases with personalization. The components of this variable are:

1. Persons involved
2. Role with respect to others
3. Stereotypy
4. Verbalization
5. Mobility
6. Frequency and duration

Findings of the Study

The main findings of the study were as follows:

1. Introduction of skilled nursing care in institutional settings caring for aged patients *does* contribute to the personalization of the patients.

2. Institutional settings vary markedly with respect to the degree to which they foster personalization independent of the amount of skilled nursing care provided.

Conclusions to Be Drawn

A significant conclusion of this research was that the effect of skilled nursing care was greatest in a deprived environment and least in an enriched environment. A significant contribution of this study is the method it provides for measuring the personalization process of older patients.

As to the limitations of the study, one might raise the question of the "Hawthorne effect" in that the patient was aware of the differential treatment. As has been discussed in Chapter 6, it is extremely difficult to control this type of bias in studies like these.

CONTINUED CARE BY NURSES AND DOCTORS: AN EXPERIMENT

Ford, Katz and Adams[26] conducted a controlled, longitudinal, study of the effect of regular visits by a public health nurse on the status and function of chronically ill patients. This is one of the first types of controlled studies of this kind.

Subjects included patients discharged from a university chronic disease rehabilitation hospital who were assigned randomly to one treatment and two control groups of 75 patients each. Treatment (experimental) groups were visited regularly by a visiting nurse over a three-year period; control patients had planned follow-up care other than the usual discharge report to the referring physician.

Observations of physical, psychological, and social functions were made every three months of the experimental and one of the control groups by a team of observers who were separate from the care personnel. Criteria to assess these functions were objective data and indices that have been shown to be sensitive to change in previously conducted longitudinal studies at this hospital. A second control group was observed only initially and terminally as a control for possible effects of regular visits by the observers.

HOSPITAL CULTURE, THE NURSE, AND PATIENT CARE

Wooden (1964)[27] extended his work to include the study of the nursing function in relation to the hospital and to the patient. The investigator interprets his research as social research which ". . . is concerned with exploring the way human beings behave when they work in a group, at a given location, in pursuance of some defined goal."

The research focused on assessment of the impact of care management patterns on the hospitalized patient. The investigator hypothesized that present approaches do not necessarily produce the most desired or most functional results from the standpoint of the patient's well-being, nor do they achieve an "interactive or supportive environment." The study had three specific aims—namely, (1) to devise a pattern of making hospital operation more flexible; (2) to determine what effect such flexible operation has on the physical, the social, and the psychological well-being of the patient; and (3) to determine what effect this kind of flexibility has on hospital personnel, particularly nursing personnel.

Hypotheses tested were:

1. A general reduction of patient anxiety will result from increased information flow and increased understanding.
2. If the patient's anxiety is reduced, his recovery rate will be speeded up and his level of recovery may be raised.
3. A hospital setting that is interactive will lead to giving more comprehensive care.

Several independent variables were introduced on the experimental unit. Examples of these are: the use of long-range, in-service instruction of personnel in behavioral science principles as they relate to patient care; introduction of a team approach to nursing; modification of current patterns of routinized nursing procedures; formal and informal instruction to convalescing patients and to members of the family; development of a permissive daily life routine approximating the patient's customary patterns of life routine.[28]

Patients admitted by the six attending physicians participating in the study assigned patients to the experimental and control areas. No changes were introduced in the latter area.

Possible significant outcomes point to a definition of the elements and relationships in a program of care that is *patient-centered* rather than hospital-centered; identification of "certain personality qualities" of people that seem to contribute to the care process; access to information that nurses who currently find themselves struggling to give care lack; and the availability of instruments to measure the impact of care management patterns on hospitalized patients.[29]

EXPLANATORY STUDIES REPORTED AT THE A.N.A. CLINICAL SESSIONS 1962

Following are examples of *explanatory* studies reported at the American Nurses' Association Clinical Sessions in 1962. The numbers refer to monographs in the series.

Bochnak, Mary A., Rhymes, Julina P., and *Leonard, Robert C.* "The Comparison of Two Types of Nursing Activity on the Relief of Pain." No. 6.

Problem: To test the relative effectiveness of an automatic and deliberative nursing process in relieving those patients whose complaints were interpreted by the staff as meaning "pain," and for whom medication for pain was ordered to be given at the nurse's discretion. The essential difference between these two processes lies in the nurse's approach to a patient's complaints. The nurse using the deliberative nursing process makes a deliberate effort to determine the patient's needs before supplying the help needed.

Methodology: The study was conducted in an urban 660-bed general hospital in a university medical center. Data were collected on 19 patients. In two randomly selected matched groups, 10 patients were assigned to control treatment (automatic nursing) and 9 to the experimental treatment (deliberative nursing). The control patients were given care by the staff nurse who happened to be on duty. All experimental patients were cared for by the principal researcher, who was specially educated in the art of deliberative nursing. A qualified person observed and recorded exactly what took place in the nurse-patient interactions of both groups.

Findings: All the control patients were given pain-relieving medication by staff nurses in response to complaints of pain. None experienced marked relief. Eight of the nine experimental patients had marked relief; the remaining one attained some relief. Only four of these nine patients required pain medication.

Mertz, Hilda. "Nurse Actions That Reduce Stress in Patients." No. 1.

Problem: To test the relative effectiveness of an automatic and deliberative nursing process in relieving patients' distress as seen in blood pressure readings and pulse rates. The essential difference between these two processes is that deliberative nursing includes an exploration of the patient's behavior to determine how he is experiencing his illness and treatment.

Methodology: The criterion for selection for the study was that all patients be emergency cases. Patients were assigned alternately to the control group (automatic nursing) or to the experimental group (deliberative nursing). There were 11 patients in each group. Data were collected in the emergency unit of a large urban hospital by the investigator. Blood pressure readings and pulse rates were used as objective measurements of the result of nursing care and were taken at the beginning and end of the 45-minute observation period for each patient. The investigator also recorded detailed descriptions of patients' behavior and nurses' activity in both groups. A qualified person independently recorded the same data for a sample of patients; her records confirmed the accuracy of the investigator's data.

Findings: The comparison of the two processes in this study provides evidence that nursing activity incorporating exploration of patients' needs can lead to improved patient care.

Tryon, Phyllis A. "The Effect of Patient Participation in Decision Making on the Outcome of a Nursing Procedure." No. 19.

Problem: To test the following hypothesis: If the patient participates in decision making, the outcome of the procedure will be more effective under the assumption that participation gives the patient a basis for giving consent for the procedure to be carried out.

Methodology: The study sample consisted of 25 labor patients in the experimental group and 25 labor patients in the control group. A soapsuds enema had been ordered for all 50 patients. In the experimental group the investigator gave the enema. The idea of having the enema presented to the patient and its meaning were explored. Nursing action was based on the patient's response. The results of the enema were assessed by graduate and student nurses on the staff. Neither group received special nursing treatment. The nurse-patient interactions in both groups were immediately reconstructed by the investigator from memory. The results of the enema were judged to be effective, ineffective, or to have had an adverse effect. Two major characteristics were evaluated—physical effectiveness, and acceptance of the enema by the patient.

Findings: The data showed that the outcome was effective in the experimental group 24 per cent more often than in the control group. These differences are significant at the .025 level using Fisher's exact probability test. The following differences were found in the study groups:

Experimental Group

1. Focus was on the meaning of the procedure to the patient.
2. Nurse used exploration to find the meaning to the patient of what she was experiencing.
3. Nursing action was based on a combined decision of patient and nurse.
4. Patient's consent to the nursing procedure was obtained.

Control Group

1. Focus was on the procedure itself or on distracting the patient's attention from the enema.
2. Nurse sometimes explored but often did not use the information gained.
3. Nursing action was an order and the patient had to accept it.
4. Nurse does not necessarily obtain the patient's consent to the procedure.

Bowen, Rhoda G. "The Effects of Organized Instruction Given by Registered Professional Nurses for Patients with the Diagnosis of Diabetes Mellitus." No. 10.

Problem: To determine whether improvement in well-being could be demonstrated in a group of diabetic patients under routine medical care who participated in a planned program of organized instruction taught by registered professional nurses.

Methodology: Data were collected through use of two techniques: (1) tests of patients' knowledge, skills, and attitudes given during individual interviews, and (2) systematic analysis of the patients' medical records, with attention to selected clinical indices. The following criteria were used in the selection of patients for the study:

1. Known to have diabetes for at least the past two years
2. Self-injections of insulin daily
3. Self-use of the Clinitest for the presence of sugar in urine
4. Prescribed calculated diabetic diet
5. In the 25–70 year age range
6. Educability

Sixty-nine patients were assigned at random to the two groups, 34 to the control group and 35 to the experimental group, with some adjustment made according to the extent of their ability to participate. Attrition for various reasons left 51 patients—23 in the experimental group and 28 in the control group—who were comparable in age, formal education levels, and duration of disease.

The four categories in the test were the patient's familiarity with (1) diabetes mellitus, (2) insulin, (3) diet and food exchange, and (4) personal hygiene.

Tests of skill were concerned with (1) self-administration of insulin, and (2) use of the Clinitest.

The categories of attitudes represented an attempt to evaluate the patient's attitude toward the disease, employment, recreation, acceptance of the prescribed therapeutic regime, and social acceptance of diabetes.

Total scores and subscores (knowledge, skills, and attitude) were computed for each patient and appropriate comparisons made between control and experimental groups. Improvement in the scores was considered indicative of improvement in patient well-being.

In collaboration with the physician who served as medical consultant, the following clinical indices were selected as indicators of each patient's condition:

1. Blood sugar valuation recorded in mg. per cent
2. Urinalysis for sugar and acetone recorded as 0, trace, 1+, 2+, 3+, 4+
3. Weight recorded in pounds
4. Incidence of commonly associated complications—infection, neuropathy, periods of uncontrolled diabetes; physicians' comments relative to patient's dietary indiscretion and/or evidence of control or lack of control of the illness.

It was assumed that reduced glycemia and less fluctuation in the four blood sugar measurements, decreased glycosuria, and acetonuria, weight reduction, and fewer complications would all indicate improvement in patient well-being.

The planned teaching program consisted of five 45-minute instruction and/or demonstration sessions, each followed by a 30-minute question and answer period. Classes were scheduled each week for five weeks. The concept that the patient, in addition to having essential knowledge, must be motivated to follow a way of life compatible with diabetes mellitus was basic to the development of the educational program.

Findings: The findings revealed that patients in the experimental group showed a significantly greater gain in knowledge about their disease and skill in carrying out treatment than did control patients. They exhibited more knowledge of insulin and of necessary personal hygiene measures and more skill in self-administration of insulin. Differences in attitude changes in the two groups as measured by a simple scale were not demonstrated.

CREATIVE THINKING AND ITS RELATION TO NURSING

An explanatory study—a first for nursing in the area of creativity and its relation to nursing performance—was undertaken by Hart[30,31] at Indiana University. The investigator was interested in determining what effect, if any, creative thinking ability of nurses had upon the effectiveness with which the nurse performed within the nursing setting. Another intriguing question pursued in this study was to find out if faculty in a basic collegiate school of nursing could recognize "the differences in the creative ability of nursing students."

A sample of 53 senior students of a basic baccalaureate school of nursing was chosen to participate in the study. Two tests from a battery of tests of the Minnesota Tests of Creative Thinking developed by Paul Torrence at the University of Minnesota were administered to the subjects to measure their creative thinking abilities. One area covered in the tests was that of verbal ability, which involved creative thinking processes of ideational fluency, spontaneous flexibility, originality, elaboration, and adequacy. Faculty members also rated the nursing students on a six-point scale of creativity.

For the purposes of analysis, the investigator divided the nursing students into two groups—those rated as the more effective members of the sample in the performance of nursing functions; and those who had been rated as the less effective in the performance of nursing functions. Mean scores for each group were calculated for total verbal ability, total nonverbal ability, and individual tasks. The t-test (described in Chapter 9) was applied to test the significance of the difference between the various mean values.

Part of the analysis included a comparison of the two groups in terms of the differences between the mean scores for the specific creative thinking factors. Only the creative thinking factor of elaboration discriminated between Group I and Group II at the .05 level of significance.[32] Differences between the means of the groups tested on the verbal creative thinking factors of ideational fluency, spontaneous flexibility, originality, and adequacy were not significant at the .05 level.

The investigator concluded from her study that there was no "consistent" evidence that the verbal creative thinking ability influences the effectiveness with which the nurse performs within the nursing setting. The nonverbal creative thinking ability of nurses was found to be significantly high. The creative thinking factors of spontaneous flexibility, originality and elaboration were found to be significantly associated with nursing performance.

Nursing faculty were not able to discriminate between the more creative and less creative students of nursing. The investigator concludes that faculty members do not consider creativity as being important in judging nursing performance.

The investigator urges replication of her study in other situations and recommends that a longitudinal study be undertaken to determine the degree to which a school of nursing fosters or inhibits the creative thinking abilities of students.

The study just discussed, although exploratory in nature, presents several significant hypotheses that need to be tested. If the hypotheses are substantiated, present patterns of nurse recruitment, nursing education, and nursing service (including measurement of performance) would require major changes.

Summary

To some, explanatory research is considered to be the most important form of research. Such research can help nursing establish a scientific body of knowledge. As Hempel[33] has said:

> The explanatory and predictive principles of a scientific discipline are stated in its hypothetical generalizations and its theories; they characterize general patterns or regularities to which the individual phenomena conform and by virtue of which their occurrence can be systematically anticipated.

To date, much of the explanatory research in nursing has been evaluative in purpose. It has had a strong practical orientation and has been concerned with ways of improving patient care. This practical inclination is understandable when the urgency with which many problems in nursing demand solution is considered. Such problems as the nursing shortage, the most desirable pattern of nursing education, and the effect of nursing care on patient welfare cannot patiently await for their solution the thorough, highly controlled, and cautious approach that often characterizes basic research. However, until such research is stimulated and undertaken in nursing it will be difficult to establish a systematic and comprehensive body of scientific knowledge.

A major problem in establishing a scientific body of knowledge in nursing is the dynamics of the nursing situation. How can generalizations from research have any long-term relevance when patient care is continuously undergoing change? What is practice today may be outmoded tomorrow. In such a fluid situation it is difficult to conceive of a stable set of principles, laws, or theories. Nevertheless, beneath this surface instability there are some scientific truths to be found that can serve to enhance the quality of nursing care and promote patient welfare. It is a function of explanatory research to find them.

References

1. Faye G. Abdellah and Eugene Levine, *Effect of Nurse Staffing on Satisfactions with Nursing Care.* Hospital Monograph Series No. 4. Chicago, American Hospital Association, 1958.
2. Faye G. Abdellah, "Methods of Identifying Covert Aspects of Nursing Problems." *Nursing Res., 6:*4–23, June 1957.
3. Ernest Dichter, "A Psychological Study of the Hospital-Patient Relationship: What the Patient Really Wants from the Hospital." *Mod. Hosp., 83:*51–54, 136, September 1954.
4. Faye G. Abdellah and Eugene Levine, *Patients and Personnel Speak.* U.S. Public Health Service Publication No. 527. Washington, D.C., Government Printing Office, 1957.
5. Peter Kong-Ming New, Gladys Nite, and Josephine M. Callahan, *Nursing Service and Patient Care: A Staffing Experiment.* Kansas City, Mo., Community Studies, Inc., Publication No. 119, November 1959.
6. Myrtle K. Aydelotte, "The Use of Patient Welfare as a Criterion Measure." *Nursing Res., 11:*10–14, winter 1962.
7. W. D. Bryant, S. J. Miller, and S. B. McConnel, *The Occupational Pattern of Nursing Personnel at a Community General Hospital.* Kansas City, Mo.) Community Studies Inc., 1963. See also: S. J. Miller and W. D. Bryant. *A Division of Nursing Labor. Experiments in Staffing a Municipal Hospital.* Kansas City, Mo., Community Studies Inc., 1965.
8. *Ibid.,* Summary.
9. Faye G. Abdellah, "Criterion Measures   for Research in Nursing." in Veronick, Phyllis J. (ed.), *Nursing Research II.* Boston, Little Brown Co., 1977, pp. 3–31.
10. U.S. Dept. Health, Education, and Welfare, Division of Hospital and Medical Facilities, *Elements of Progressive Patient Care.* U.S.P.H.S. Publication No. 930-C-1, Washington, D.C., 1962.
11. Faye G. Abdellah: "Criterion Measures in Nursing." *Op. cit.*
12. Gerald J. Griffin, Robert E. Kinsinger and Avis Pitman, "New Dimensions for Improvement of Clinical Nursing: Development of Criteria to Measure the Effectiveness of Clinical Nursing Practice." Bronx Community College, New York (U.S.P.H.S. Grant NU 00116).
13. Mary E. Meyers, "The Effect of Types of Communication on Patients Reaction to Stress." *Nursing Res., 13:*126–131, spring 1964.
14. *Ibid.,* p. 131.
15. Rhetaugh G. Dumas and Robert C. Leonard, "The Effect of Nursing on the Incidence of Postoperative Vomiting." *Nursing Res., 12:*12–15, winter 1963.
16. *Ibid.,* p. 12.
17. Mildred A. Disbrow, "Factors Involved in Successful Breast Feeding." University of California at Los Angeles (U.S.P.H.S. Grant GN 7901).
18. Thelma N. Thornton and Robert C. Leonard, "Experimental Comparison of Effectiveness and Efficiency of Three Nursing Approaches." *Nursing Res., 13:*122–125, spring 1964.
19. Eileen G. Hasselmeyer, *Behavior Patterns of Premature Infants.* U.S. Public

Health Service Publication No. 840. Washington, D.C., Government Printing Office, 1961.

20. *Ibid.,* p. 1.

21. *Ibid.,* p. 25.

22. Eileen G. Hasselmeyer *et al.,* "A Weight Chart for Premature Infants." *Nursing Res.,* **12:**222–231, fall 1963.

23. Eileen G. Hasselmeyer, *Handling and Premature Infant Behavior.* Doctoral dissertation. New York, New York University, 1963.

24. Martha Brown, *Effects of Skilled Nursing Care upon Personalization of Older Patients.* Washington University, School of Nursing, 1962.

25. J. Richard Simon, "Effects of Age on the Behavior of Hospitalized Patients." *J. Gerontol.,* **19:**364–369, July 1964.

26. Amasa B. Ford, Sidney Katz, and Mary Adams, "Continued Care by Nurses and Doctors: An Experiment." Western Reserve University, Benjamin Rose Hospital (U.S.P.H.S. Grant NU 00067).

27. Howard E. Wooden, "Hospital Culture, The Nurse and Patient Care." St. Mary's Hospital, Evansville, Indiana, Progress Report, February 1964 (U.S.P.H.S. Grant NU 00035).

28. *Ibid.,* p. 69.

29. *Ibid.,* p. 76.

30. Ann M. Hart, "A Study of Creative Thinking and its Relation to Nursing." Doctoral dissertation. Bloomington, Indiana University, 1962.

31. Calvin W. Taylor, Paul Torrence, Morris Stein, and other psychologists have made many contributions to the field of creativity. For several years the University of Utah has sponsored conferences on creativity under the leadership of Calvin W. Taylor. See *Creativity, Progress and Potential,* by Calvin W. Taylor (ed.). New York, McGraw-Hill Book Co., 1964.

32. Hart, *op. cit.,* p. 73.

33. Carl G. Hempel, "Fundamentals of Concept Formation in Empirical Science." *International Encyclopedia of the Unified Science,* Volume II, No. 7. Chicago, University of Chicago, 1952, p. 1.

Problems and Suggestions for Further Study

1. Discuss five problem areas in nursing whose solution might be approached through explanatory research. Briefly sketch the design for such studies.

2. Compare the findings of the following four studies that were directed toward testing the relationship between nursing care and patient welfare. To what extent do the findings corroborate each other? To what extent do they contradict each other? Can you give some reasons for any contradictions?

   a. Myrtle K. Aydelotte and Marie E. Tener, *An Investigation of the Relation Between Nursing Activity and Patient Welfare.* Iowa City, State University of Iowa, 1960.

   b. Faye G. Abdellah and Eugene Levine, *Effect of Nurse Staffing on Satisfactions with Nursing Care.* Hospital Monograph Series No. 4. Chicago, American Hospital Association, 1958.

   c. Beverly J. Safford and Rozella M. Schlotfeldt, "Nursing Service Staffing and Quality of Nursing Care." *Nursing Res., 9:*149–154, summer 1960.

   d. Peter Kong-Ming New and others, *Nursing Service and Patient Care: A Staffing Experiment.* Kansas City Mo., Community Studies, Inc., Publication No. 119, November 1959.

3. Read the article by Ellwynne M. Vreeland, "Nursing Research Programs of the Public Health Service" (*Nursing Res., 13:*148–158, spring 1964). What are some of the programs and trends in nursing research that are cited by the author that would tend to stimulate the undertaking of explanatory research?

4. Why do you think that so few fully controlled, explanatory experimental studies have been undertaken in nursing? Considering the difficulties often encountered in undertaking experimental research, do you think it is worth the effort to apply experimental designs to problems in nursing?

5. Critically review the following explanatory studies that have been reported in the literature. What are the main conclusions to be drawn from these studies? Can the findings be generalized beyond the study settings? Why do you think these studies have been classified as explanatory research?

   a. Leonard I. Pearlin and Morris Rosenberg, "Nurse-Patient Social Distance and the Structural Context of a Mental Hospital." *Am. Sociol. Rev., 27:*56–65, February 1962.

   b. Frank J. Whiting, "Patients' Needs, Nurses' Needs and the Healing Process." *Am. J. Nursing,* **59:**661–665, May 1959.

   c. Beverly N. Dunston, "Pica Practice: Its Relationship to Hemoglobin Level and Perinatal Casualties." *Nursing Sc.,* **1:**32–39, 64–69, April–May 1963.

   d. Howard J. Lockward, George A. F. Lundberg, Jr., and Maurice E. Odoroff, "Effect of Intensive Care on Mortality Rate of Patients with Myocardial Infarcts." *Pub. Health Rep.,* **78:**655–661, August 1963.

   e. Eugene E. Levitt, Bernard Lubin, and Marvin Zuckerman, "The Student Nurse, the College Woman, and the Graduate Nurse: A Comparative Study." *Nursing Res.,* **11:**80–82, spring 1962.

   f. Judith E. Gray, Barbara L. S. Murray, Judith F. Ray, and Janet R. Sawyer, "Do Graduates of Technical and Professional Nursing Differ in Practice?" *Nursing Res.,* **26:**368–373, September–October 1977.

6. What is the function of a test of significance in explanatory research? How does a test of significance help to explain the findings of a study? How does the test assist in establishing a causal relationship?

7. To be widely useful does an explanatory study have to be an elaborate and costly study, with many study subjects and taking a long time to complete? Can a small study yield useful explanatory findings? What are some aspects of research design that can enhance the value of an explanatory study?

8. Comment on the following remarks by Lucile P. Leone in "Research in Nursing and Nursing Education" (in Loretta E. Heidgerken (ed.), *The Improvement of Nursing Through Research.* Washington, Catholic University of America Press, 1959, pp. 17–28): "Sometimes, we nurses want to fall back on research for the solution of problems which common sense could solve. Surely, we sometimes need research to tell us how to change action, but changes can be made in accordance with sound judgment. It is when we want to explain why the action is good, or find another change

which may be better, or measure results of change, that research is more fully justified" (p. 23). How do these criteria for determining when research needs to be undertaken compare with those given in this book in Chapter 5?

9. Read the article, "The Nature of the Hypothesis," by James K. Feibleman (*Nursing Forum,* 1:46–60, winter 1961–1962). Discuss the author's criteria for a good hypothesis. How does a good hypothesis assist in the undertaking of explanatory research?

10. The controversy over the relationship between smoking and lung cancer is based largely on explanatory studies, either experimental or nonexperimental. Read the article by Theodor D. Sterling, "A Critical Reassessment of the Evidence Bearing on Smoking as the Cause of Lung Cancer" (*American Journal of Public Health,* **65**:939–953, Sept. 1975) and comment on the author's statement that ". . . perhaps we should start by asking how population survey and statistical studies can contribute to our understanding of the possible complex courses of lung cancer, or, in fact, any cancer?" (p. 950).

Update Note

Explanatory studies can be found in most of the nursing journals, particularly *Nursing Research.* Use of the indexing and abstracting services listed in Chapter 5 is a good way to locate such studies. Also rich in explanatory studies are the research conference compilations such as those supported by the Western Interstate Commission on Higher Education. For example, Volume 9, entitled *Nursing Research in the Bicentennial Year* [M. V. Batey (ed.), Boulder Colo, WICHE, April 1977] contains brief reports of at least six very interesting explanatory studies, e.g., Mary Regina Gill Nolan, "Effects of Nursing Intervention in the Operating Room as Recalled on the Third Postoperative Day," (pp. 41–50) and William P. Osborn and Martha A. Thompson, "Variables Associated with Student Mastery of Learning Modules" (pp. 167–179).

Other rich sources of explanatory studies that can be used as case examples are in nonnursing journals such as *American Journal of Public Health, Medical Care,* and *Inquiry.* Journals in the fields of psychology and sociology are also excellent sources of case studies.

4

FUTURE OF NURSING RESEARCH

The chapters in this, the final part of the book, will examine the current status of nursing research, the future directions of research in nursing, and the role of the federal government in stimulating and supporting nursing research. Although some of this material has been touched on in previous chapters, most of the discussion in this chapter will cover new ground. For example, previous chapters have from time to time given suggestions for further studies that might be undertaken in nursing, these chapters will synthesize and expand these suggestions.

Previous chapters have dealt largely with the purpose, rationale, and method of research. The discussion has been somewhat general, and references to actual studies have been used to illustrate certain methodological or conceptual aspects of the research process. Part IV is quite specific in the material it presents, and its main purpose is to point the way to the initiation of productive research efforts in the area of nursing.

Chapter Fifteen

ROLES OF THE FEDERAL GOVERNMENT IN FURTHERING NURSING RESEARCH

THE EVOLUTION of nursing research must be viewed in context with the evolution of medical research. The contribution of the federal government to medical research in the early 1900's was negligible. In fact the federal government's participation traces back to only 1887 when a laboratory of hygiene was established at the Staten Island Marine Hospital (now the United States Public Health Service Hospital).[1,2,3] Emphasis was placed upon the study of bacteriological diseases brought back by merchant seamen, such as cholera, tuberculosis, diphtheria, typhoid fever. In 1891 the laboratory was moved to Washington, D.C., where it was known as the Hygienic Laboratory. In 1930 it was renamed the National Institute of Health—a name which was finally changed in 1948 to the present National Institutes of Health.

THE FEDERAL GOVERNMENT

The role of the federal government in furthering the support of medical research became significant in 1938 through the establishment of grants-in-aid to universities and other research institutions under the newly established research grants program.

The Public Health Service Act of 1944 provided the Surgeon General with broad authority for the conduct and support of all kinds of medical research. The act provided that:

. . . the Surgeon General shall encourage, cooperate with and render assistance to appropriate public authorities, scientific institutions and scientists in the conduct and coordination of research, investigations, experiments, demonstrations and studies relating to the cause, diagnosis, treatment, control and prevention of the physical and mental diseases and impairments of man.[4]

Special mention must be made of the Division of Research Grants (D.R.G.) of the Public Health Service, which is responsible for the overall grants management of extramural grants and awards programs for all segments of

Chronological List of Dates in the Development of United States Public Health Service Programs Affecting Medical and Health-Related Research[5]

1887   First research laboratory supported by federal government established at the Marine Hospital, Staten Island, New York.

1891   Hygienic Laboratory moved from Staten Island to Washington, D.C.

1902   First Advisory Board for Hygienic Laboratory formed. This was later renamed the National Advisory Health Council.

1912   Public Health and Marine Hospital Service renamed Public Health Service.

1930   Hygienic Laboratory renamed National Institute of Health.

1937   National Cancer Institute authorized by Congress.

1938   National Institute of Health establishes headquarters at Bethesda, Maryland. First research fellowships authorized.

1944   Public Health Service Act, giving Surgeon General broad research authority.

1945   First research grants awarded.

1946   First training grants awarded. Mental Health Act passed by Congress.

1947   Division of Research Grants established.

1948   National Institute of Health renamed National Institutes of Health. National Heart Institute and National Institute for Dental Research authorized by Congress. Other existing laboratories were reorganized to form Microbiological Institute, and Experimental Biology and Medicine Institute.

1949   Mental hygiene program expanded and organized as the National Institute of Mental Health.

1950   Two new institutes established: National Institute of Neurological Diseases and Blindness and National Institute of Arthritis and Metabolic Diseases (which included the former Experimental Biology and Medicine Institute).

1953   Federal Security Agency becomes Department of Health, Education, and Welfare. The Public Health Service represents the Health component of the new department. Clinical Center opened as first federal clinical research laboratory.

1955   Nursing Research Grants and Fellowship Program of the Division of Nursing established.
        National Microbiological Institute renamed National Institute of Allergy and Infectious Diseases.

1957   Health Research Facilities Act passed by Congress, authorizing matching grants for research construction in nonfederal institutions.

1958   Division of General Medical Sciences established, responsible for providing the scientific review processes for all noncategorical grants, including nursing.

1960   Public Health Service Act (1944) amended to provide for general support of research and research training programs in universities, hospitals, and other nonprofit institutions.
        International Health Research Act passed by Congress permitting the expansion of N.I.H. international programs.

1961   The Bureau of States Services–Community Health, Office of Research Grants was established and given primary responsibility at the bureau level, for leadership, coordination, and assistance in extramural research grants and research training grants. The office is responsible for: (1) the creation of national participation by competent scientists, state and local public health agencies, practitioners, and educators in research and training for research in community health; (2) the establishment of policies, organization, procedures, budget, reporting and control techniques, and effective project review and grants administration within Divisions, Bureau, and in relation to P.H.S. and departmental systems; (3) the analysis of scope and content of research and research training, progress toward defined goals, and utilization of findings in Bureau, State, and local health programs; (4) assistance to regional offices in program promotion and grants management for research and research training; (5) the representation of B.S.S.–Community Health program in operating relationships with N.I.H., other service and departmental components. The office also has continuing responsibilities for staff services to the National Advisory Community Health Committee in connection with its review of research and research training grants applications.

1962 Public Health Service Act amended to provide the establishment of two new institutes (Public Law 87-838, 87th Congress, H.R. 11099).

Establishment of the Institute of Child Health and Human Development for the conduct and support of research and training relating to maternal health, child health, and human development, including research and training in the special health problems and requirements of mothers and children and in the basic sciences relating to the processes of human growth and development, including prenatal development. Establishment of the Institute of General Medical Sciences for the conduct and support of research and research training in the general or basic medical sciences and natural or behavioral sciences that have significance for two or more other institutes, or are outside the general area of responsibility of any other institute, established under or by this act.

1962 Division of Research Facilities and Resources established to assume responsibility for activities authorized under the Health Research Facilities Act.

1963 Transfer of Division of Nursing, Extramural Research Program from the Institute of General Medical Sciences to the Bureau of States Services–Community Health.

1967 Division of Nursing became part of the Bureau of Health Manpower.

1968 Division of Nursing, Bureau of Health Manpower transferred to The National Institutes of Health.

1969 Bureau of Health Manpower renamed Bureau of Health Professions Education and Manpower Training.

1973 Division of Nursing moved to the Bureau of Health Resources Development, Health Resources Administration, which also included the National Center for Health Statistics and Bureau of Health Services Research and Evaluation (now the National Center for Health Services Research).

1975 Bureau of Health Resources Development reorganized into the Bureau of Health Manpower and Bureau of Health Planning and Resource Development, Health Resources Administration (HRA).

1978 Health Resources Administration reorganized into three Bureaus: (1) Planning, (2) Health Facilities Financing, Compliance, and Conversion; (3) Health Manpower with Division of Nursing in the Bureau of Health Manpower. A Division of Manpower Analysis was established in this Bureau to conduct manpower research.

---

the Public Health Service. Its staff numbers over 500 scientific, administrative, and clerical personnel. An important responsibility of D.R.G. is the management of 51 study sections, one of which was the Nursing Research Study Section, covering the basic sciences, major disease areas, environmental health, and community health. Each study section appoints one of the group as chairman, and the D.R.G. provides a scientist-administrator as executive secretary.[6] This mechanism provides the initial scientific review of research project grants.* The second review is provided by several health councils which review applica-

* Study Sections also have the responsibility of surveying the status of research in their fields to determine which research activities should be initiated or expanded. Neglected areas of research are uncovered and research efforts furthered through the stimulation of conferences, workshops, or publications. See James H. Cassedy, "Stimulation of Health Research," *Science,* 145:897–902, August 28, 1964.

tions for their significance to the nation. The National Advisory Health Council was the main council responsible for review of nursing applications. In April 1963, the National Advisory Community Health Committee was established, which will review, advise, and make final recommendations concerning applications for community health research, including nursing.

Although the Division of Nursing has had authorization since 1955 to award research project grants, research fellowships, and in 1961, nurse-scientist graduate training grants, the first appropriation specifically passed for research grants, fellowships, and graduate training grants for the Division of Nursing under Public Law 301 was July 1963. The purposes of these programs are to support needed research and research training in nursing; to stimulate and promote interest in studies to improve nursing practice; and to identify scientific talent and resources to achieve these purposes.

Research Training

Good research is dependent upon those doing the research. This requires that the investigators have a thorough knowledge of the pertinent substantive information and skill in the appropriate techniques of research investigation.

In an effort to increase and improve research training in the basic biomedical and health-related sciences, the Research Training Branch of the Institute of General Medical Sciences, N.I.H., provides funds to public and private nonprofit research institutions, such as schools of basic medical sciences, medical schools, and universities. The training programs are designed to help meet the requirements for trained scientific manpower in areas represented by the fields basic to medicine and health, such as the anatomical sciences, the behavioral sciences, biochemistry, biophysics, developmental biology, endocrinology, genetics, physiology. The research fellowships are for both predoctoral and postdoctoral study.[7]

The research training program in nursing, administered by the Public Health Service's Division of Nursing, is designed to strengthen research institutions and increase their potential for training nurse-scientists; to assist in the continuing research training of competent professional nurses through the graduate schools of universities; to expand the opportunities for intensive training of predoctoral and postdoctoral nurse candidates in research institutions; and to promote greater utilization of nurses with research training in the science fields to improve the teaching and training functions of universities and research institutions.

Nursing Research Grants and Fellowships

The Nursing Research Grants and Fellowship Programs of the Public Health Service were established in 1955. The authorization for these programs stemmed from the Public Health Service Act of 1944. This gave the Surgeon General research authority to encourage, cooperate with, and render assistance to appropriate public authorities, scientific institutions, and scientists in the conduct and coordination of research and investigations relating to the cause, diagnosis, treatment, control, and prevention of the physical and mental impairments of man.

Research grants and training grants for medical and allied health research have been made since 1945 and 1946. Appropriations for nursing research and fellowships were not available until July 1955, making the nursing research program a reality. From 1955 to 1976, approximately $39 million have been awarded for nursing research project grants; $7.7 million for nursing research fellowships; and $8 million for nurse-scientist graduate training grants.

Until July 1963, responsibility for the Nursing Research Grants Program was shared jointly by the Division of Nursing and the Institute of General Medical Sciences of the National Institutes of Health. The Division of Nursing has now been transferred to the Bureau of Health Manpower, Health Resources Administration.

Objectives 1. The purpose of research project grants is to encourage and support research and investigations in medical and allied health research related to nursing with emphasis upon research important to the improvement of patient care.

2. Research project grants also support studies of the development and utilization of nursing services, facilities, and resources.

3. Research project grants in nursing are intended to expand research activities throughout the country and to encourage nurse and nonnurse investigators to undertake research in the health fields important to nursing.

Methods of Attaining Objectives Through extensive programming efforts, the professional nursing staff of the Nursing Research Branch of the Division of Nursing, P.H.S., provides consultation to potential investigators throughout the United States and in selected international areas prior to the submission of research grant applications. New research areas are identified and stimulated to encourage research needed immediately and in the next five to ten years.

Research project grants in nursing are also supported by other institutes such as heart, cancer, and mental health.

It is anticipated that the volume of significant studies of patient care and nursing practice with different kinds of patients, in various settings, will increase considerably as a result of the full-time nurse research fellowship program and the nurse scientist graduate training program described later. These programs are making available more scientifically trained and motivated nurses, to undertake research in nursing.

As a direct attempt to bring nursing research into sharper focus, the Division of Nursing of the Public Health Service in July 1963 assumed the total responsibility for the research grants program. Several hundred nursing research projects have been awarded through this program. Projects are national and international in scope. All projects have relevancy to nursing and seek to foster significant improvements in patient care. Many deal with the improvement of nursing practice, nursing education and research development.

Special Predoctoral and Postdoctoral Fellowship Programs in Nursing

Problem The supply of competent nurse investigators trained in the biological, physical, and social sciences of importance to nursing and in the methodologies of research in education and administration must be increased. Their training makes possible an expansion of scientific research activities in the health fields throughout the country and encourages research in hitherto neglected areas, such as nursing care of patients that systematically complements the physician's care; the administration and economics of nursing care within complex organizational settings; and systematic evaluation of the various nursing curricula. Systematic investigation in these fields is not generally as accessible to other scientists. Other professional groups expect that 1 per cent of the active members of the profession be prepared to do research. There are now over 1 million active professional nurses, which would mean that 10,000 should have this preparation. As of 1979, approximately 1,500 nurses throughout the country have had extensive research preparation.

Objective Special predoctoral fellowships in nursing research are intended to provide support for research training in the sciences related to nursing leading to the development of independent research.

The nurse research fellowship program of the Public Health Service is a companion program to the nursing research grants program. This is designed to prepare professional nurses with a minimum of a baccalaureate degree to do independent research, to collaborate in interdisciplinary research, and to guide others in research in nursing. They are for nurses interested in research training in any of the health sciences at the predoctoral and postdoctoral levels.

Similar to the nursing research grants program, this fellowship program was also a shared responsibility of the Division of Nursing and the Institute of General Medical Sciences until July 1963 when the Division of Nursing assumed full responsibility. A Nurse-Scientist Graduate Training Committee was established in 1963 to provide scientific review of applications.

Special Developmental Research Training Grants*

Problem The limited participation of some universities, schools of nursing, and health agencies in the research project grant program is due to a paucity of project applications rather than to a high disapproval rate.

Many nurses, highly motivated to do research, are in full-time teaching and service positions with little or no time permitted for research activities, nor is released time made available for research training.

Objective The purpose of this program is to stimulate research capabilities among faculty in schools with advanced nursing programs as well as in selected basic nursing programs that have high potential for, but are not now actively engaged in, research.

Method of Attaining Objective Faculty Research Development Grants (FaReDeG's) are made to eligible universities and professional schools of nursing as a direct means of stimulating research capabilities in those institutions which have training responsibilities in scientific fields related to health but are not actively engaged in health research. This is achieved by releasing full-time faculty in the school of nursing part time to secure research training or depth of competency in a science area. Funds from the grant also make it possible for faculty from other departments to meet the nursing faculty in seminars where small pilot studies can be initiated.

Eligibility for these grants is determined, in part, by the research resources available to the school of nursing—i.e., medical, health-related or basic science disciplines within the university setting are heavily committed to or actively engaged in research. The commitment of nursing faculty to research is also an important criterion.

Nurse Scientist Graduate Training Grants

Problem More nurses must receive preparation in the basic sciences related to nursing (biological, physical, and social) to increase the supply of competent nurse scientists while at the same time maintaining their identity in nursing. Research in nursing practice has been limited primarily because of the extreme shortage of professional nurses who have been prepared at the doctoral level in the basic sciences. Nurse scientists are needed to delineate new nursing knowledge and to participate productively in interdisciplinary research. A nursing science will develop. It is the nurse scientist who will determine what the scientific basis for nursing should be.

Nurses have recognized that effective nursing is based upon theories, laws, and principles developed or discovered within the basic sciences. This places upon nursing the responsibility of having selected members of

* Also referred to as Faculty Research Development Grants.

the profession obtain preparation in the basic sciences so that they can identify and organize knowledge basic to nursing practice and have the necessary scientific preparation to pursue crucial nursing questions through systematic inquiry. Every learned profession has its body of scholars that includes a nucleus of scientists. The nursing profession has reached a degree of maturity that necessitates that attention be given to the development of this group. The nurse scientist graduate training program is conceived as a long-range investment in the future of nursing leadership and consequently in the health care of the nation. It should help to insure that in the future the nation will have high-quality and scientifically oriented leadership in nursing. The nurse scientist as a scholar and leader in the nursing profession must develop a means for more effectively improving health care throughout the world.

Nurse scientists will compose the university nurse faculty of the future. They may find present employment as junior or senior investigators on medical and health-related research projects; as nurse faculty members in universities; as research collaborators on interdisciplinary health research teams; and, on the staff of research hospitals, particularly those with experimental research laboratories. Some may wish to pursue postdoctoral study in universities, institutions, laboratories, and similar agencies.

Objective Nurse scientist graduate training grants are intended to increase the number of nurses available for research and academic careers who are competent in the basic sciences and who can contribute to the solution of health problems of the community, state, nation, and world through the application of knowledge in its most recent state of discovery.

UNIVERSITY RESEARCH VERSUS FEDERAL RESEARCH

The inevitable question must be faced as to the role of universities and the federal government in research. Universities continue to provide a major site for research and the major source for the preparation of scientists. It is in the university setting that man's freedom to seek knowledge and challenge our cultural and political systems can be safeguarded. This freedom must be safeguarded at wholesale cost. It is for this reason that universities must continue to maintain top priority as the most suitable milieu for research to thrive.

The federal government, on the other hand, cannot ignore its responsibility for research. Maintaining the national defense and safeguarding human welfare necessitates that the federal government become involved in scientific research whether this research is conducted in federal laboratories or financed in other laboratories with federal funds.[8]

It would seem that universities and the federal government need to continue their cooperative endeavors. The university system is dependent upon the federal government for support, in spite of the generous contributions of foundations and private philanthrophies; the federal government is dependent upon the university for its human resources.

Approximately 90 per cent of all federal funds for research and development (training) and 99 per cent of federal funds for research activities are provided under the statutory research charters of five agencies. These are the Department of Agriculture, the Public Health Service, the National Science Foundation, the Department of Energy, and the Department of Defense.[9]

It must be recognized, too, that most of the federally financed research is administered by operating organizations whose primary function is not research.

The federal government's objective in supporting research in universities is to make certain that an activity vital to the national defense and/or welfare of people is carried out. This is achieved through contract research in which research services are purchased to achieve specific aims determined by the government as essential, or through supported research which is a grant to a nonprofit university, institution, or agency in which the research is carried out by nonfederal personnel.

Each federal agency is an autonomous unit. Controls are exercised through Congress and the appropriations process as well as in hearings and reports of House and Senate Committees. In addition each agency has its own review mechanism. For example, the Public Health Service's Division of Research Grants has more than 50 study sections made up of scientists qualified to review projects in a specific area. One of the reviewing groups is the Nursing Research Study group, made up of nurse scientists, social scientists, physicians, hospital administrators, and biostatisticians who meet three times a year to review research applications in nursing on the basis of their scientific merit. In addition, applications then receive a second review by an appropriate council—for nursing it is the National Advisory Council on Nurse Training, which reviews all applications for their significance to the country and determines which priority level of payment will be possible in view of available funds.

The role of the university is the preservation, the transmission, and the creation of knowledge in a climate that provides a high degree of freedom for the investigator. The university is committed to teaching, research, and service.

The role of the federal government in research is the extension of knowledge that will benefit the nation and mankind. Through the provision of federal funds the freedom of individual scientists can be extended through support for research time to carry out their research without control by the federal government.

Major breakthroughs have been made in synthetizing new drugs and enzymes and in reproducing diseases for study in animals. For example, for many years scientists have surmised that at least one or more forms of cancer may be caused by a virus. Scientists have been successful in producing a viral agent associated with mouse leukemia that acquires such a high potency in serial passage in tissue culture that it can produce multiple primary tumors in mice and sarcomas in hamsters and rats.[10] Many new vital discoveries will continue to be made that will benefit mankind. The whole field of cybernetics and systems research as it applies to hospital practice is just being explored. Research endeavors in instrumentation and automation are beginning to have their impact in operating, recovery, and intensive care units.

The years ahead may be expected to see advances in tissue and organ transplants, continued search for the causes of cancer, heart diseases, and other major killers. The behavioral sciences, so important to medical and nursing research, can be expected to contribute even more to our understanding of man. Studies of aging, human ecology, and genetics are largely untouched by nursing research and open up new horizons to be explored.

Bridging the gap between research and the application of research is a challenge that must be faced.[11] Foundations and nonofficial health agencies can make a major contribution to medical research by closing this gap.

References

1. Dale R. Lindsay and Ernest M. Allen, "Medical Research: Past Support, Future Support, Future Directions." *Science,* **134**:2017–2024, December 22, 1961.
2. Charles V. Kidd, "The Effect of Research Emphasis on Research Itself," in *Research and Medical Education,* Julius H. Comroe, Jr. (ed.) *J. Med. Ed.,* **73**:95–100, December 1962, Part II.
3. Jerome B. Wiesner, "Federal Research and Development: Policies and Prospects." *Am. Psychologist,* **19**:90–101, February 1964.
4. U.S. Public Health Service, *Grant and Award Programs of the Public Health Service,* Vol. I, *Policy and Information Statement of Research Grants.* U.S. Public Health Service Publication No. 415, Washington, D.C., Government Printing Office, 1959.
5. *Basic Data Relating to the National Institutes of Health 1962.* Office of Program Planning, Bethesda, Md., N.I.H., January 1962, pp. 26–28.
6. Marion Oakleaf, "DRG's Supporting Role in the Drama of Health Research." *DRG Digest,* **5**:2–6, January 15, 1963.
7. U.S. Department of Health, Education, and Welfare, *Public Health Service Grants and Awards, Fiscal Year 1963 Funds.* U.S. Public Health Service Publication No. 1079, Part II, 1963.
8. Charles V. Kidd, *American Universities and Federal Research.* Cambridge, Mass., Belknap Press of Harvard University Press, 1959.

9. *Ibid.,* p. 3.

10. Dale R. Lindsay and Ernest M. Allen, *op. cit.*

11. Calvin W. Taylor, et al., "Bridging the Gap Between Basic Research and Educational Practice." *Nat. Ed. A. J.,* **51:**23–25, January 1962.

Suggestions for Further Reading

1. Howard E. Freeman, *The Strategy of Social Policy Research.* Reprint Series #7. Reprinted from The Social Welfare Forum, 1963. Boston, Brandeis University, 1963.

2. National Academy of Sciences, *Federal Support of Basic Research in Institutions of Higher Learning.* Washington, D.C., National Academy of Sciences, National Research Council, 1964.

3. James A. Shannon, "Sciences and Federal Programs: The Continuing Dialogue." *Science,* **144:**976–982, May 22, 1964.

4. U.S. Department of Health, Education, and Welfare, Public Health Service, *Resources for Medical Research.* Report No. 4, U.S.P.H.S. Publication No. 1068, Washington, D.C., Government Printing Office, August 1963.

5. Daniel J. Greenberg, "Congress Looks at Science." *Am. Psychologist,* **19:** 102–104, February 1964.

6. U.S. Department of Health, Education, and Welfare, Public Health Service, *The Public Health Service Today.* Washington, D.C. U.S. Government Printing Office, DHEW Publication No. (OS) 76–50048, September 1976.

Chapter Sixteen

CURRENT STATUS OF RESEARCH IN NURSING: THE DRAMA OF NURSING RESEARCH

IMPROVEMENT OF PATIENT CARE THROUGH NURSING PRACTICE AND NURSING EDUCATION

KNOWLEDGE is needed about the specific effects of nursing practice upon patient care. This can be obtained only through extensive research. The reasons for the success or failure of nursing practices must be determined. In order to do this, more research is needed of the physiological and psychological mechanisms that are influenced by nursing practice. The identification and development of measures to evaluate nursing practice are crucial if these practices are to be changed or improved. Finding valid and reliable criteria of nursing practice requires a series of long-range studies.

The behavior patterns of patients affecting nursing care is another important aspect of the problem of improving nursing practice.

In the last quarter century, in spite of major investments of the federal government (Table 16-1) and foundations in preparing nurse researchers and supporting research endeavors in nursing, few nursing schools have made remarkable progress toward achieving institutional commitment to science and inquiry.[1] Schlotfeldt states that, "the key predictor of nursing's eventual fulfillment of its potential as a socially significant, scientific, humanistic learned profession is commitment to research."[2]

Since 1964, several major efforts have been undertaken to prepare a "state of the art" analysis in nursing research making considerably easier for the researcher endeavoring to find out what has been undertaken in the field and the identification of specific gaps.

On the following pages references to "state of the art" summaries will be made rather than citing specific examples of studies. The gaps in nursing research produced by these summaries and analyses will also be identified.

TABLE 16-1

Total Annual Expenditures 1956-1976 for Research and Research Training in Nursing in the U.S. Department of Health, Education, and Welfare, Public Health Service, Health Resources Administration, Bureau of Health Manpower, Division of Nursing, Nursing Research Branch[1]

Type of Grant	Expenditures	Number of Awards[2]
Research grants	$39,330,323 (For 309 grants)	961
Fellowships	$ 7,693,939	1,963
Training grants	$ 8,020,115	96
Total	$55,044,377	3,020

[1] From the Nursing Research Branch, Division of Nursing, Health Resources Administration, June 30, 1976 (unpublished memo).
[2] Not including supplementals.

1964   Simmons and Henderson prepared the publication, *Nursing Research: A Survey and Assessment*, initiated by the National Committee for the Improvement of Nursing Service. This provided the first extensive guide to nursing studies.[3] A major part of the effort was devoted to a review and assessment of research in selected areas of occupational orientation and nursing care. Major emphasis was placed upon surveys of nursing needs and resources conducted by the Public Health Service; image, role, and function studies; and studies of social and cultural factors that influence the future of nursing. An overview is also included of investigations in all clinical specialties.

1972   Henderson completed her monumental work *Nursing Studies Index*, published in four volumes covering 1900–1959. This work provides an annotated guide to reported studies, research methods, and historical and biographical materials in periodicals, books, and pamphlets published in English.[4]

1970   Abdellah provided an overview of nursing research 1955–1968 of completed and ongoing studies in nursing research supported by the U.S. Public Health Service.[5] Approximately 175 nursing research projects were analyzed: to identify the major gaps in health services to which nursing research can make a contribution through continued and intensified investigation; to specify the knowledge now available from completed research projects that might contribute to the resolution of these problems; to identify the gaps in knowledge that need to be filled; and to suggest research techniques applicable to these problems.

The research projects were classified using the following typology:

Classification Of United States Public Health Service Supported Research

I. Clinical Research of Problems Related to Nursing Practice
    Cardiac Nursing
    Intensive Care Nursing
    Nursing in Chronic Illness
    Community Health Nursing
    Geriatric Nursing
    Mental Health and Psychiatric Nursing

Companion publications to the overview of nursing research appeared in 1969[6] and 1973[7] which provided descriptions of investigations and identified any publications resulting from the research.

1977   *Nursing Research* celebrated its silver anniversary by devoting all issues with feature articles to cover nursing research in the United States and abroad. The reader will find all six issues particularly valuable in getting a broad overview of nursing research undertaken by federal sources, foundations and professional, regional, and scientific societies. Following are a few of the major efforts reported in *Nursing Research* during the anniversary year:

- Gortner and Nahm provide an overview of nursing research in the United States covering historical perspectives, the development of nursing research in education, the contribution of nursing research to practice and research resources.[8]
- Abdellah describes the contribution of the U.S. Public Health Service to nursing research.[9] Three periods of nursing research are described: (1) The developmental period (1955–1968) when nursing research was conducted primarily by behavioral and social scientists and systems engineers. There was also a major emphasis on the preparation of nurse researchers and launching of the American Nurses' Association research conferences. (2) The clinical nursing period (1969–1972) when emphasis in research in the organization, distribution, and nursing services continued as well as research in areas of recruitment, selection, and education of

nurses. As more nurse researchers were prepared there was a decided shift to studies related to clinical nursing research. (3) "The outcomes" of nursing care period (1973-1976) which reviews efforts to measure quality of nursing care and the implications of Professional Standards Review Organizations (PSROs) for the identification of outcome measures in nursing.

- Cross describes the contribution of the Veterans Administration to nursing research.[10] The Veterans Administration Nursing Service (VANS) early recognized the importance of clinical nursing research and was one of the first federal services to establish nursing research positions within nursing service. The concept of establishing research as a vital part of nursing service is one to be emulated. This has resulted in a strong commitment to nursing research within the many VA hospitals. A variety of nursing research activities involve nursing service personnel such as research conferences and seminars and clinical research projects.

- Nursing research in the Army, Navy, and Air Force as told by the historian Kalisch describes the development of nursing research as these efforts paralleled the great wars.[11] Expenditures for research also paralleled the growth of modern industry and the development of new technologies mushroomed. The application of operational research techniques found a receptive home in the armed forces. The Air Force Aerospace Medical Division through its research efforts expanded the bank of information which could be applied in designing systems and the development of criteria for selection and care of military men to maintain an efficient and viable force. The Naval Medical Research Institute provided a locus for consultation, reference, and basic research in the biomedical sciences. Nurses in the Navy Nurse Corps conducted research aspects of the organization and administration of nursing service, orientation, and in-service programs. Nursing practice also served as a basis for nursing investigations.
Nurses in the Army Nurse Corps had a unique opportunity to conduct research through the Walter Reed Army Institute of Research which established a Division of Nursing in 1957. The Institute was charged with evolving a research-education program for the Army Nurse Corps. The Institute was to conduct several important clinical nursing research projects and research conferences to stimulate research.

- The regional compact groups such as the Southern Regional Education Board (SREB), the Western Council on Higher Education for Nursing (WCHEN) made significant impacts upon nursing research. SREB focused upon graduate education and research and conducted several regional research projects which stimulated individuals to conduct research and tested a process for developing ongoing faculty research.[12] The Committee on Research established its goal to have more ongoing research directed toward improving nursing practice and nursing education with the purpose of improving patient care. An extensive survey of research activities in participating SREB states provided useful baseline information upon which to project future research needs and resources.
WCHEN early on pioneered in conducting several significant regional research conferences.[13] Such milestones in research as "Defining Clinical Content— Graduate Nursing Programs," "Investigation of Nursing Content—Baccalaureate Nursing Programs," and the project, the "Investigation of Effectiveness of a Leadership Program in Nursing," served to stimulate a number of research projects. The nursing research conferences through communication of ongoing research and critiques of research conveyed a level of research sophistication that other regions in the country were to follow. Particularly noteworthy has been WCHEN's efforts to support the development and evaluation of models for facilitating the use of research findings, continued generation of experimental research to improve the quality of care, and the establishment of a regional information and development unit.

- The American Nurses' Association (ANA) has always included research activities as part of its program.[14] Particularly noteworthy were the nine research conferences conducted between 1965 and 1973 and the establishment of the ANA Commission on Nursing Research and Council of Nurse Researchers. The ANA's

Blueprint for Research in Nursing outlined six categories of research to be used as a long-range guide for the Association. The categories included nursing and its practice, nursing in the social milieu, communication and decision making in nursing, organization and operation of nursing services, education for nursing, and ANA as a professional organization.

In 1970 the Commission on Nursing Research was formed as a structural unit within ANA and had as one of its main functions the formulation of professional policy in such areas as research conduct and support and human subjects' rights. By 1971, the Commission established the first Council of Nurse Researchers to advance research activities, provide for the exchange of ideas, and recognize excellence in research.

The Commission published several significant documents helpful to nurse researchers, e.g., *Human Rights Guidelines for Nurses in Clinical and Other Research* (1974), *Research in Nursing: Toward a Science of Health Care* (1976), *Preparation of Nurses for Participation in Research* (*1976*), *and Priorities for Nursing Research* (1976).

The American Nurses' Foundation (ANF) established by ANA in 1955 to increase the public knowledge and understanding of professional and practical nursing and of the sciences and arts upon which the health of the American people depends.[15] The ANF both engaged in and supported studies, surveys, and research, and provided scholarships and fellowships.

- The research programs of the National League for Nursing (NLN) collect useful data for the benefit of nursing and examines issues to aid in the formulation of policy.[16] In 1959, a research and studies department was created to centralize the administration of projects and to provide needed expertise in the conduct of research and studies. Examples of significant studies include "The Nurse Career Pattern Study," "The Open Curriculum Study," "The Student Selection Process Study," "The State Board Test Pool Examination Validation Study."

- The silver anniversary issue for *Nursing Research*, May–June 1977, includes excellent resumés of research in the practice areas of medical-surgical nursing, community health nursing, maternal-child nursing, and psychiatric nursing.

SEARCH FOR THEORY IN NURSING

A major deterrent to research in nursing is the lack of a theoretical basis of nursing practice, namely, a nursing science.[17] A nursing science is a body of scientific knowledge from the physical, biological, and social sciences that is uniquely nursing.

As nurses become prepared as clinical investigators there are more concerted efforts to bring theory and practice closer together. "At this point in time, however, the conceptual framework of models, and particularly their application into practice, has not yet evolved into an articulate, well-defined, and integrated discipline of study."[18]

Riehl and Roy have developed a very useful publication pulling together a variety of conceptual models for nursing practice.[19] Also included in the publication is a discussion of the nature and history of models; conceptual models in nursing research, education, and service; and the implementing of models into practice.

Jacox provides an overview of theory construction in nursing with pros and cons for theory development in nursing.[20]

Theory building in nursing requires sticking to a particular area of inquiry long enough to produce related findings or contrasting explanations of phenomena and then to formulate links among them.[21]

A long-range study to develop the scientific basis of nursing in all clinical fields was undertaken by the Western Interstate Commission on Higher Education.[22] The research effort brought together clinical specialists in public health nursing, psychiatric nursing, and medical and surgical nursing to meet each summer to conduct research on the basic science content and the clinical content of master's degree programs in the western region. The research was directed toward seeking a synthesis of the basic sciences, medicine, and current nursing knowledge to provide a sound theoretical foundation for research in nursing practice and nursing education. A parallel study at the baccalaureate level was also undertaken.

A specific example of a study that explores the theoretical basis of nursing practice is that conducted by Hasselmeyer.[23] In this research the investigator explored the kinesthetic theory as it relates to the nursing care of premature infants.

The infant kinesthetic need theory was further substantiated by Kramer (1975) in that there was a significant difference in the rate of social development of premature infants as a result of extra tactile stimulation.[24]

Another example is the development of concepts and theories in relation to leadership.[25] Leadership is viewed as a separate entity, although it may be in combination with administration, management, and supervision.

RESEARCH ON NURSING PROBLEMS IN OTHER LANDS

Nursing research on the international front emphasizes research of the status of women and changing social forces.[26] The selection of research strategies and priorities is clearly determined by the status of women.

The practice of nursing has undergone radical changes, particularly since World War II, yet the public image of the nurse is the same as it was at Florence Nightingale's death' in 1910. The role of professional nursing has changed so rapidly that many nurses themselves and physicians find the present role of the nurse unclear and disturbing.

Selected Examples of Studies Completed or in Progress

In order to understand the underlying forces that can affect the public image of the nurse, there has been some development of research concerned with problems of nursing in other nations. The needs of nursing students from technically underdeveloped countries are studied in reference to their skills in communication and social adjustment to the United States.[27]

This study has significance in that approximately one-half of international nursing students pursuing graduate study in the United States come from technically undeveloped areas and from different cultures. These nurses often return to their own countries to fill important leadership positions in the health field. It is therefore important that a university know which methods are most helpful in providing assistance to these nurses.

The occupational status of nursing in Turkey was studied during a period of pronounced social change. This project was intended as part of a series of studies of the growth and potentialities of nursing as an occupation in a variety of countries. The research program provided adaptation of methodologies from other fields in analysis of nursing problems. This research was specifically aimed at defining the public and professional "image" of the nurse in Turkey and how the nurse views herself, her work, and opinion of her work.[28]

In 1968, the World Health Organization (WHO) consultant group suggested priorities in nursing practice research such as studies of manpower, organization, utilization, the quality of health care, costs, information and research systems, and community response studies.

Another significant step in international research was taken by the International Council of Nurses (ICN) in 1976 when it issued a nursing research statement and guidelines for nursing research.

Continued active liaison between ICN and WHO is essential if meaningful research strategies for developed and developing countries are to be initiated and implemented. Particular attention needs to be given to the education and preparation of nurses for nursing research assuring that educational settings in foreign lands encourage scientific freedom and inquiry. Research conferences and forums communicating research findings need to be given high priority. The *International Nursing Index* is a significant beginning that needs to be supported.

GAPS IN NURSING RESEARCH

Measurement techniques and methodologies of quality care for all practice fields in nursing continue to move slowly. This is one of the major contributing factors to the dearth of clinical nursing research projects.[29] Measurement scales need to be developed that discriminate among different levels of patient response. For example, drug absorption patterns in the elderly are quite different because of the slower metabolic and physiological processes. Criterion measures of patient care and precise instruments to measure the effects of nursing practice upon patient care represent major gaps in nursing research.

Several direct recommendations have been made for nurse researchers to undertake research in gerontology. During the next five to ten years, it is estimated that the individuals 65 and over will double, yet there is very little research going on by nurses in gerontology.[30]

For various reasons nurse researchers tend to avoid replication of completed research to validate the reliability of methods employed, nor do they build upon existing studies. There are literally hundreds of completed studies in nursing in need of replication with different populations before generalizations to other groups can be made. Assumptions need to be challenged as they often are untested covert hypotheses upon which studies are built. ". . . thoughtful examination of one's logic can begin to unfold a conceptual model with high probability of payoff for the researcher and practitioner."[31]

The rapid rise of hospital costs demand that most patients in the future be cared for through ambulatory services and extra-hospital-based facilities, yet little is known about effective organizational patterns of these facilities.

Nursing needs to focus on health strategies to activate, develop, or enhance a care recipient's achievement of a sense of well-being.[32] Thus, nursing needs to explore research within the boundaries of nursing practice and beyond to embrace health care. Large numbers of investigators are confronted by problems of students, faculty, staff, and organizational management and manipulation and tend to do their research in those areas rather than selecting real world problems in practice settings for their research. Access to human and animal subjects is not always readily available but persistent efforts can have a payoff if it is recognized that nurse researchers have their right too to have access to subjects. The right to be researched also means accountability for the nurse researcher who must be concerned about human rights and welfare. Likewise, the right not to be researched is a principle to be respected.[33] Informed consent of participating subjects, thus, must be considered and obtained.

There are major gaps in methods of research that are applicable to the study of organizational patterns of patient care systems. There is need for greater accuracy and control of questionnaires, interview schedules, and observational methods. The increased costs of health care necessitates the study of the organization and delivery of health services. The researcher is faced with the insurmountable problem of studying the effect of medical and nursing care as measured by common health indices of morbidity and mortality which have yet to be proven to be reliable and valid.

There is a positive trend for interdisciplinary research. Field studies of human populations, particularly longitudinal studies are ideal for interdisciplinary teams of researchers.

The emerging new practice roles of primary care practitioners, family nurse practitioners, hospice nurse, and so forth, need to be studied in light of the effect of these changing roles on patient care, medical care, and patient acceptance of these roles.

Another gap is the lack of predictors of success in clinical performance. New variables to measure success need to be explored.

Some progress has been made in developing a theoretical base for nursing practice to further the development of a nursing science, but vigorous efforts in this area need to continue.

There is a growing proliferation of doctoral programs in nursing. The number of nurses, however, with doctorates will not make an impact in the research field unless these nurses are prepared rigorously in formulating significant researchable questions and in appropriate methodology.[34]

Postdoctoral preparation needs to become more commonplace if the gaps in research are to be reduced. The Institute of Medicine, National Academy of Sciences, recommends that as qualified nurses seeking research training become available that up to 15 per cent of the total number of research training awards be made at the postdoctoral level.*

Regional programs of nursing excellence need to be fostered and provide a milieu for nurse researchers to undertake and replicate research.

NURSING RESEARCH PRIORITIES

The process ordering of priorities provides an essential sequential ordering of nursing research topics, problems, or events to be studied. This process is particularly important with the overall reduction of resources and qualified nurse researchers. The final selection of priorities should provide the maximum nursing research effort to achieve the goal of improved quality of care.

Nurse researchers should seek out opportunities to gain input into the decision process of selecting priorities. It is proposed that the determination of nursing research priorities be made at three levels: personal priorities at the individual level based upon the nurse researcher's interests, education, capabilities, and personal goals; priorities at organizational or institutional levels by mutual consent of individual researchers; and priorities determined at the level of the nursing profession based on the overall goals of the profession.[35] Nurse researchers have an obligation to select priorities that serve choices made by individuals, organizations, and the nursing profession.

Lindeman used the Delphi technique to identify 15 high priority areas for clinical nursing research.[36]

Priorities at best can only serve as guidelines. The ordering of priorities will change periodically when such factors affect them as major trends in health care, legislative commitments, public needs and demands for services change, new scientific knowledge becomes available.

* National Academy of Sciences, *Personnel Needs and Training for Biomedical Research*, Vol. I. 1977, p. 161.

The following framework suggests some research priorities in nursing. Individuals, organizations, and the nursing profession may choose to re-order the priorities.

Research Priorities in Nursing[37,38]

- Studies in long-term care of the elderly, mentally retarded, and developmentally disabled with particular attention to the design of quality assessment tools that will take into account functional status and the limited patient outcome goals and complex treatment processes characteristic of much long-term care.
- Studies of clinical problems related to nursing practice, especially descriptive studies of physiological and behavioral responses of patients with various diagnoses in varied settings, both institutional and noninstitutional.
- Studies to develop instruments to measure patient care directly.
- Studies to identify the criterion measures needed to study the effect of nursing care.
- Studies to develop models and theories of nursing practice.
- Studies of effects of technological advances on the functions of nursing service personnel.
- Studies of the organization of patient care systems; health services delivery systems that maintain quality of care and are cost effective.
- Studies to develop tools to measure effectiveness of health services.
- Studies in preventive health care to determine how best to change individuals' behavior and attitudes.
- Studies in nutrition to determine how healthful food consumption practices can be fostered.
- Studies of genetics of human diseases to prevent and better understand the degree to which genetic factors underlie susceptibility to such diseases as psychoses, diabetes, high blood pressure, coronary heart disease, and lung cancer.
- Studies to improve the outlook of high-risk parents and high-risk infants.
- Studies of life-threatening situations, anxiety, pain, and stress.
- Studies of manpower for nursing education, practice, and research.
- Studies of contraceptive and social science research to explore ways to prevent unplanned pregnancies and to develop a systems approach to strengthen comprehensive health, education, and social services.
- Studies in mental health to determine ways of preventing psychosocial disabilities.
- Studies using epidemiologic techniques to understand the mechanisms and sites of action as a result of toxic substances.
- Historical research in nursing using the vast number of primary resources maintained in individual schools of nursing, universities, the Library of Congress, the National League for Nursing, historical documents at the National Library of Medicine in Bethesda, Maryland, and the U.S. Archives.
- Studies of ways to standardize medical and nursing records for computerization.
- Studies of patient care using monitoring systems and computer-aided diagnosis.
- Studies of communication of nursing information in relation to organization patterns of nursing service in the hospital, home, and community.
- Studies of methods of incorporating new scientific and technological advances into the nursing curriculum.
- Studies to develop criteria of job performance and measures for evaluation.
- Studies to define success in nursing and to develop tools to measure this.

DEVELOPMENT OF REFERENCE MATERIAL FOR RESEARCH IN NURSING

In addition to the important problems of training scientific personnel for research in nursing, there is also the crucial problem of developing basic reference materials that can report completed studies in a way that they can be readily available.

Selected Examples of Tools Available

Volunteers from several schools of nursing throughout the country convened periodically to abstract reports of studies in nursing. This resulted in two volumes of *Nursing Research,* one that reported studies in public health nursing, and a second volume devoted to studies in other areas of nursing. This abstracting service proved to be so effective that it is being continued until 1978.[39,40,41]

Another monumental effort to make studies known to investigators was the work directed by Henderson[42] at Yale University. The investigators have prepared a comprehensive annotated index of the analytical and historical aspects of nursing literature published in English, covering 1900–1959.

Taylor prepared a bibliography on nursing research covering 1950–1974 categorized by 22 broad classifications.[43]

References

1. Rozella M. Schlotfeldt, "Nursing Research: Reflection of Values." *Nursing Res.,* **26:**4–9, January–February 1977.
2. *Ibid.,* p. 8.
3. Leo W. Simmons and Virginia Henderson, *Nursing Research: A Survey and Assessment,* New York, Appleton-Century Crofts, 1964.
4. Virginia Henderson, *Nursing Studies Index.* Philadelphia, J. B. Lippincott Co., Vol. I, 1900–1929, published 1972; Vol. II, 1930–1949, published 1970; Vol. III, 1950–1956, published 1966; Vol. IV, 1957–1959, published 1963.
5. Faye G. Abdellah, "Overview of Nursing Research 1955–1968." *Nursing Res.,* Parts I, II, III, **19:**6–17, January–February 1970; **19:**151–162, March–April 1970; **19:**239–252, May–June 1970.
6. DHEW, USPHS, *Research in Nursing, 1955–1968.* Bethesda, Md., Public Health Service, Publication No. 1356, 1970.
7. DHEW, USPHS, *Research in Nursing, 1969–1972.* Bethesda, Md., DHEW Publication No. (NIH) 73–489, 1973.
8. Susan R. Gortner and Helen Nahm, "An Overview of Nursing Research in the United States." *Nursing Res.,* **26:**10–33, January–February 1977.
9. Faye G. Abdellah, "U.S. Public Health Service's Contribution to Nursing Research—Past, Present, Future." *Nursing Res.,* **26:**244–249, July–August 1977.
10. E. Deana Cross, "Nursing Research in the Veterans Administration." *Nursing Res.,* **26:**250–252, July–August 1977.

11. Philip A. Kalisch, "Weavers of Scientific Patient Care: Development of Nursing Research in the U.S. Armed Forces." *Nursing Res.*, **26:**253–271, July–August 1977.

12. Audrey F. Spector, "Regional Action and Nursing Research in the South." *Nursing Res.*, **26:**272–276, July–August 1977.

13. Jo Eleanor Elliot, "Research Programs and Projects of WCHEN." *Nursing Res.*, **26:**277–280, July–August 1977.

14. Elizabeth M. See, "The ANA and Research in Nursing." *Nursing Res.*, **26:**165–171, May–June 1977.

15. Ann Hyde, "The American Nurses' Foundation's Contributions to Research in Nursing." *Nursing Res.*, **26:**225–227, May–June 1977.

16. Walter L. Johnson, "Research Programs of the National League for Nursing." *Nursing Res.*, **26:**172–176, May–June 1977.

17. Martha E. Rogers, "Some Comments on the Theoretical Basis of Nursing Practice." *Nursing Sc.*, **1:**11–13, 60–61, April 1963.

18. Joan P. Riehl and Sister Callista Roy, *Conceptual Models for Nursing Practice.* New York, Appleton-Century Crofts, 1974, p. ix.

19. *Ibid.*, 1–299.

20. Ada Jacox, "Theory Construction in Nursing: An Overview." *Nursing Res.*, **23:**4–13, January–February 1974.

21. Florence S. Downs, "Nature of Relationship Between Theory and Practice," in *Translation of Theory Into Nursing Practice and Education,* Shake Ketefian (ed.). New York University Continuing Education in Nursing, Division of Nursing, School of Education, Health, Nursing, and Arts Professions, 1975, p. 7.

22. Helen C. Belcher, "Identification of Commonalities in Four Reports Defining Clinical Content of Graduate Nursing Programs." Boulder, Colorado, Western Interstate Commission for Higher Education, June 12, 1962 (U.S.P.H.S. Grant NU-00019).

23. Eileen G. Hasselmeyer, "Handling and Premature Infant Behavior." Doctoral Dissertation. New York, New York University, 1963.

24. Marlene Kramer, et al., "Extra Tactile Stimulation of the Premature Infant," *Nursing Res.*, **24:**324–334, September–October 1975.

25. Helen Yura, *et al.*, *Nursing Leadership: Theory and Process.* New York, Appleton-Century Crofts, 1976, p. 76.

26. Helen Preston Glass, "Research, an International Perspective." *Nursing Res.*, **26:**230–236, May–June 1977.

27. Marie Farrell and Esther L. Brown, "Improvement of Education of International Nursing Students." Boston University (U.S.P.H.S. Grant GN-5047).

28. Leo W. Simmons, "Role Images and Opportunities for Nurses in Turkey." Teachers College, Columbia University (U.S.P.H.S. Grant NU-00033).

29. Faye G. Abdellah, "Overview of Nursing Research, 1955–1968." *Nursing Res.*, **19:**15, January–February 1970.

30. Rheba deTornyay, "Nursing Research—The Road Ahead." *Nursing Res.*, **26:**404, November–December 1977.

31. Marjorie V. Batey, "Bridging the Gap: Problems and Progress," in *Communicating Nursing Research. Is the Gap Being Bridged?* Vol. 4. Boulder,

Colorado, Western Interstate Commission for Higher Education, July 1971, p. 162.

32. Rosemary Ellis, "Fallibilities, Fragments, and Frames." *Nursing Res.*, **26:** 177–182, May–June 1977.

33. Patricia M. MacElveen, "Critical Issues in Access to Data," in *Communicating Nursing Research. Critical Issues in Access to Data*, Vol. 7. Boulder, Colorado, Western Interstate Commission for Higher Education, January 1975, p. 3.

34. deTornyay, *op. cit.*, p. 406.

35. Dorothy L. McLeod, "Nursing Research Priorities: Choice or Chance," in *Communicating Nursing Research, Nursing Research Priorities: Choice or Chance*, Vol. 8, Boulder, Colorado, Western Interstate Commission for Higher Education, March 1977.

36. Carol A. Lindeman, "Delphi Survey of Priorities in Clinical Nursing Research." *Nursing Res.*, **24:**439, November–December 1975.

37. Abdellah, *op. cit.*, p. 14.

38. American Nurses' Association, *Priorities for Research in Nursing.* Kansas City, Mo., ANA, Publication Code No. D-51 3M, May 1976.

39. R. Louise McManus, "Abstracting of Reports of Studies in Nursing." New York, Teachers College, Columbia University, (U.S.P.H.S. Grant GN-4970).

40. Hortense Hilbert, "Abstracts of Studies in Public Health Nursing." *Nursing Res.*, **8:**43–144A, spring 1959.

41. Hortense Hilbert, "Abstracts of Studies in Nursing." *Nursing Res.*, **9:**51–117, spring 1960.

42. Virginia Henderson, *Nursing Studies Index, op. cit.*

43. Susan D. Taylor, "Bibliography on Nursing Research, 1950–1974." *Nursing Res.*, **24:**207–225, May–June 1975.

Suggestions for Further Reading

1. James Dickoff and Patricia James, "A Theory of Theories: A Position Paper." *Nursing Res.*, **17:**197–203, May–June 1968.

2. Rosemary Ellis, "Characteristics of Significant Theories." *Nursing Res.*, **17:**217–222, May–June 1968.

3. B. G. Glaser and Anselm Strauss, *The Discovery of Grounded Theory.* Chicago, Aldine Publishing Co., 1967.

4. Robert K. Merton, *Social Theory and Social Structure.* New York, Free Press, 1968.

Chapter Seventeen

FUTURE DIRECTIONS OF RESEARCH IN NURSING

A DECADE of intensive work has made some discernible inroads in nursing research, but we are still on the periphery of uncovering the vast amount of knowledge that must become known before any major breakthroughs can be made in nursing practice. Studies in nursing education, occupational orientation, and career dynamics have been given major focus during this period.[1] Less attention has been given to studies that might be classified as patient care research or clinical research.

If one were to look beyond the periphery of existing biomedical knowledge as it affects nursing practice, what are some of the areas that might be rewarding to explore? What are some of the research questions that need to be studied in more depth? On the following pages the authors discuss some of these research opportunities. There is no attempt at complete coverage of these opportunities, but rather our intent is to raise questions to stimulate thought.

NEW HORIZONS IN NURSING RESEARCH

Evaluation and Improvement of Nursing Practice

During the next decade, major breakthroughs that will result in the improvement of nursing practice will come from research in the biological sciences and social sciences. Studies need to be undertaken that are concerned with gross physical and psychological signs that are directly relevant to nursing practice. Included here are descriptive and analytical studies of characteristics of gross behavior in relation to the nature and stages of illness; assessment of the value of visual and other sensory observations and prodromal signs (cues to impending disaster for the patient); and studies of the relative reliability and risks entailed in automated instrumental monitoring as compared to monitoring by a nurse.

Those concerned with research in nursing agree that the major focus of the research effort should be on inquiries concerned with patient care.[2]

The evaluation of patient care should be based upon nurse actions. Observations of nursing practice need to be based upon scientific inquiry and conceptual frameworks that draw heavily upon physiological, biological, and psychological principles.

In the area of patient care, criteria need to be identified and developed that measure the effects of nurse actions upon physical and emotional care, teaching of patients, observation and communication of observations to nurses and others, teaching and supervision of nursing personnel, and participation with health team members in planning community health programs.[3]

Measurement of patient care at present is a difficult problem that must be solved. Instrumentation that can read and measure a greater variety of things, more accurately and automatically should provide some answers to the problem. If research in nursing is to advance scientifically, measurements must be precise and not based solely on subjective observations. An example of a major breakthrough in medical research is the electron microscope, which has advanced the whole field of cell biology.[4] Electronic computers are just beginning to show their value in medical research and open up many avenues for the correlation of complex physiological data. Instrumentation yet to be developed that will permit continuous measurement of body processes concurrently can help us to understand such phenomena as stress and pain.

Nursing practices will surely undergo many changes as research moves ahead to find ways of successfully achieving tissue and organ transplants and the regeneration of tissues.

The study of man and his environment and the interactions between human populations, and interactions of these with other populations of animal and plant life on this and other planets, provides avenues for research for many years.

The amassing of data that one day will mean the eradication of cancer and some circulatory diseases will permit further concentration on the fundamental reproductive, aging, and mental processes.

Possible Research to Further the Evaluation and Improvement of Nursing Practice

1. Identification of criterion measures of nursing practices that are both physiological and psychological
2. Establishment of the scientific bases for nursing practices
3. Description of behavior patterns of patients with different types of diagnoses in different settings
4. Assessment of the nurse's observational power to predict prodromal signs
5. Adaptation of instrumental monitoring devices in furthering the analyses of patient care data important to predicting nurse actions
6. Adaptation and development of instruments to measure the effects of nurse actions upon patient welfare.

ORGANIZATION AND DELIVERY OF NURSING SERVICES

Many crucial problems in this area still plague nursing practice. Some progress has been made by studies of problems of nurse utilization and facilities. Yet to be explored are problems basic to nursing resources and logistics fundamental to patient care problems, problems of communication of nursing information about the patient's progress, and problems of the organizational patterns of nursing services in the hospital, home, and community.

In the area of demand for service and utilization of facilities Flagle[5] emphasizes the need to study the incidence of illness and accidents and the intensity and duration of need for hospitalization or occupancy of clinical facilities. Included here are studies of the phenomena of expressed need for service and the duration of service.

Still to be explored are problems dealing with the creation and distribution of resources to meet demands.[6] How can patients be moved from one area to another? How can supplies such as drugs and blood reach the right area when they are needed?

Instrumentation, including the use of computers, promises many changes in the area of organization and delivery of nursing services—for example, computer-aided diagnosis and electronic monitoring of patient's physiological changes. As progress is made in the storage, retrieval, and analyses of complex medical data, new avenues to the communication of vital information important to patient care should become available.

"Adequacy" of nursing care has yet to be defined. How much and what level of nursing care should specific types of patients receive?

Possible Research to Further the Organization and Delivery of Nursing Services

1. What elements of patient care (in this case, organization and delivery of nursing services) have an effect upon patient care?
2. What are optimal and minimal levels of nursing care services for different types of patients in different settings?
3. How can the methods of operations research be used in the decision making problems related to establishing the upper limits of capacity of facilities?
4. What are the common nursing needs of patients for care, regardless of diagnosis?
5. How can completed research be replicated and applied to other test situations?
6. What communication channels are necessary for planning patient care? How can effective communication essential to patient well-being and personnel satisfaction be achieved?
7. How can experimental changes employing or utilizing social facilities in the physical planning and arrangements in the hospital be measured?

Nursing as an Occupation

Promising areas for exploration are studies of the ecology of the nurse; longitudinal studies of career patterns that seem to be the most promising for success in nursing; studies of competing occupations when men and women have equal opportunities; studies of why nursing as a career is not selected by more men; and studies of the public image of nursing and ways in which it might be changed.

Little is known about the impact of research upon students and curriculum. Research in nursing schools should deal with broad questions of health that are patient-centered and not disease-oriented. One needs to look for the results of this experience upon students rather than the kind(s) of experience to which they should be exposed. Exposure to research in the undergraduate curriculum can help the student to develop an approach to dealing with the unknown or with the unfamiliar.

Research is needed to find out why students possessing the high qualities that we profess to be important for success in nursing find nursing schools less challenging and satisfying than do students of lesser talent. Why do nursing schools continue to ignore independent study programs that have proved highly successful in many liberal arts colleges, and some high schools? Are we deliberately ignoring the highly qualified students? Why do so many of these students withdraw from nursing schools for non-academic reasons? One possible solution to this problem is to offer a minor or a second major for selective students in a science area. A combined experimental R.N.-doctoral program at the undergraduate level should also be explored.

A crucial area for research is to find ways in which nursing students can be motivated to exercise their critical faculties and their problem-solving skills. It is easy to say that the good nurse practitioner should solve nursing problems presented by the patient in a scientific way, but what does this mean and how can it be taught? Research is needed to show how the scientific method can be applied to the kinds of difficult problems with which the nurse must deal.

Nurse educators agree that the student must acquire a certain minimum of information and skills. If the nursing school is to play an important part in the education of nurses for services to the individual and the community, it should provide the student with a core of basic knowledge and skills in the biological as well as in the behavioral and social sciences. What this basic core is has yet to be defined in a way that it relates to the effective nurse practitioner.

Unexplored areas needing research include the modernization of pedagogic methods such as the use of television and teaching machines, approaches to clinical teaching, and the role of the nursing school and postgraduate, and/or continuing education.

The application of television, teaching machines, and other automated devices as laboratory tools in the classroom and clinical situation offers fruitful exploration. Present teaching methods are outmoded. Research is needed to see how these tools can be interrelated with the teacher, and nurse practitioner, in using these technical skills, and in the teaching-learning process. The demonstrated value of audiovisual techniques in motivating the exceptional as well as the retarded student needs to be explored in nursing both in the classroom as well as in the clinical situation.[7]

Research in the educational processes of nursing provides a fertile field for investigation. In the area of graduate education, one can find several tenets contrary to opinion that need explanation.[8] Why, for example, do we compare educational qualifications of faculty employed in various types of nursing programs with one another instead of with faculty members in non-nursing programs at a similar level of preparation? Why in graduate education do we tolerate those without research training guiding those seeking this training? Why is a common yardstick used to measure those who receive professional and technical education? Why is the R.N. student exempt from certain course requirements in the baccalaureate program and the basic student not?

Much research has already been completed on problems related to the role of the professional nurse. The same problems still exist and are more acute. Has the approach to role conflict been peripheral? What steps must be taken to resolve the problems in this area?

Possible Research to Further Clarify Nursing as an Occupation

1. In order for television, teaching machines and other automated devices to serve nursing education and nursing practice with maximum effectiveness in teaching-learning, how can interaction between teacher and student be achieved?
2. Is there a concept of nursing that can be clearly defined? What are the essential learnings that must be communicated to students?
3. What are the role conflicts faced by nurses? What are their consequences in institutional practices?
4. What conflicts exist between role expectations and role performance?
5. What are the conflicting role expectations held by nurse educators and nurse practitioners? In what ways can they be resolved?
6. As the nurse becomes a contributing member of the health and/or research team the role conflicts she must face are maximized. How can the nurse deal with these conflicts? What research needs to be undertaken?

Development of Theories in Nursing and a Nursing Science

Why should we be so concerned about the development of theories in nursing? Theories in nursing form the basis of nursing practice and contribute to the formulation of a nursing science. "Nursing science is a body of scientific knowledge characterized by descriptive, explanatory, and predictive principles about the life process in man."[9] Typologies of nursing problems and nursing treatments are the principles of practice and constitute the unique body of knowledge that is a nursing science.[10]

Professionalization of nursing requires that nurses identify those nursing problems that depend for their solution upon the nurse's use of her capacities to conceptualize events and make judgments about them. Nurses need to become skilled in recognizing nursing problems, in analyzing them in terms of relevant principles, and in working out courses of action by applying principles of nursing practice.

Rogers[11] describes the professional practice of nursing as the process by which this body of scientific knowledge (nursing science) is used for the purpose of assisting human beings to achieve maximum health. The process is evaluative and diagnostic as well as interventive.

There are essentially five elements of nursing practice that are dependent upon a nursing science.[12] First is the continuous mastery of human relations, including the mastery of technical and managerial skills needed to take care of patients. Second is the ability to observe and report with clarity the signs and symptoms and deviation from normal behavior that a patient presents. Third is the ability to interpret the signs and symptoms that comprise the deviation from health and constitute nursing problems. Fourth is the analysis of nursing problems that will guide the nurse in carrying out nursing functions, and the selection of the necessary course of action that will help the patient attain a goal that is realistic for him. Fifth is the organization of her efforts to assure the desired outcome. Nursing practice may be considered to be effective when the nurse is able to help the patient to return to health or what can approximate health for him.

Konlande[13] describes a patient with hyperthyroidism as an example of the importance of utilizing the principles of the biological sciences in the treatment of this patient. The nurse must know how the body responds to excess thyroxin in order to provide nursing care that is effective. For example, large quantities of thyroxin may increase the metabolic rate as much as two to two and a half times. The patient loses a lot of weight in spite of a hearty appetite, feels uncomfortably warm because of the increased heat production, and is more excitable because of the increased activity of the nervous system. With this knowledge in mind, the nurse is better able to develop and carry out an effective nursing care plan.

Basic concepts in physics can readily be applied to nursing care[14]—for example, gravity exerts an effect on the circulation of the blood in the human body. In shock this concept comes into play when the patient is placed in a Trendelenburg position. Patients with edema of the extremities can be relieved considerably by elevating the extremities. Where there is reduced or impaired circulation in the extremities, this can be improved by changing the position of the patient. Patients following surgery are placed in a position to maintain a patent airway. In each instance the concept of gravity is fundamental in planning the nursing care for the patient. Scientific principles related to fluid and electrolyte balance are basic to maintaining a state of homeostasis.

Possible Research to Further the Development of Theories in Nursing and a Nursing Science

1. Development of a typology of scientific principles to coincide with the typology of nursing problems already developed[14a] to comprise a body of scientific knowledge
2. Development of theories in nursing that have a specific effect upon nursing practice
3. Evolvement of a nursing science based upon a scientific body of knowledge

International Health Research

An important untouched horizon for research in nursing is in the international field. Much can be learned about practice and nursing education in other countries where the level of development is not as complex as in this country. Many of the knotty problems plaguing nursing, such as patterns of nursing education, ratio of nurses to patients, and role image of the nurse, have so many intervening variables that one has to study these problems in a setting where there are fewer variables affecting the situation.

Glaser[15,16] has shown how the nonmedical culture and social structure of a country affect its medical services. Likewise, patterns of hospital and nursing administration in other countries as compared to ours can provide many valuable insights.

The preceding pages have described some of the new horizons for nursing research that directly or indirectly affect patient care. Freeman[17] in a report of a symposium of patient care research has described patient care as varied phenomena that are interrelated and refer to a wide range of objects, events, and people that have to do with health and illness behavior.

Patient care [is] regarded as a process which involves recognizing actual and potential health problems, delineating possible courses of action, deciding what should be done, providing personal health services built around an individual, and assessing the impact of these activities upon the public health. It represents a synthesis of three components: (1) the way in which people cope with their actual and potential health problems—what happens to them when they become patients, receive care, and relinquish their patient status; (2) the patterns of practice followed by the health professions singly and together; and (3) the ways in which the values, perceptions, and skills of patients and health personnel affect one another.[18]

The seven broad classes of patient care problems that were identified in which nursing research plays a key role provide a summary of needed research in patient care:[19]*

* See also: American Nurses Association, "Expanding Concern with Research," *Am. J. Nursing*, **62**:45, August 1962.

Possible Research to Further the Development of International Health Research

1. Why do American hospitals have more nursing employees per patient than do foreign hospitals? Can the effects of nursing care upon patients show any differences in the varied patterns in different countries?
2. American hospitals have many more categories and levels of nursing personnel than do foreign countries. What effect does this have on patient care? Have American hospitals succumbed to Parkinson's law? Are so many categories needed? Does the delegation of tasks in American hospitals contribute to role conflicts nonexistent in foreign hospitals?
3. The cost of nursing services far exceeds other personnel services' costs in both American and foreign hospitals. Do these costs truly reflect nursing services to patients? Is this a catchall category for related hospital services such as housekeeping, dietary, messenger services?
4. Nurses perform many more activities for patients in American hospitals as compared to foreign hospitals. This contributes to higher operating costs, but most important, do the increased activities for patients result in improved patient care?
5. What is the role of the director of nurses in American hospitals as compared to other countries? Is the lay nurse administrator an emerging concept of nursing service?
6. Nursing education in some foreign countries, particularly England, is changing slowly from an apprentice-type training to an educational program. How are these changes brought about? Will more than one pattern of nursing education emerge? How can American nursing schools consolidate existing patterns? What can be learned from developing patterns in other countries?
7. The hierarchical structure of hospitals in America and foreign countries differs markedly. What is the role of the nurse in these various hospitals? What are the role relationships of the nurse to her peers, to her supervisors, to physicians?
8. Recruitment, career development, and job satisfaction are complex problems facing American nursing, which if studied in foreign countries might provide a better understanding of contributing factors that bring about desirable and undesirable effects. The role of women in American and foreign cultures warrants study and could form the basis of many fruitful studies in human ecology.
9. Catholic hospitals compose approximately two-thirds of general hospitals in American countries. Professional nurses are unhappy that nursing nuns are sometimes placed into top supervisory positions in preference to equally qualified nurses who are not nuns. It would be helpful to study this problem in countries with a high percentage of church hospitals to determine the contributing factors to this dissatisfaction and to find appropriate ways to resolve this problem.
10. Nurses in America have greater opportunity for decision-making, as the nurse is the only member on the health team who is continuously with the patient. Nurse action in dealing with the patient's problems is crucial and is one of the decisive differing factors between American and foreign nursing. Therefore, when one speaks of professional nursing, is the conceptual basis for nursing practice closer to that of a nursing science as practiced in America as compared to foreign countries?

I. *Sociocultural Contexts of Patient Care*

1. Concepts of wellness and their relation to cultural patterns.
2. Cultural and social factors in perception of changes in physiological, personal, or social functioning as symptoms of illness. This includes differences between lay people and members of the health professions in the way they define illness.
3. The types of sick roles and well roles which the culture makes available.

4. The kinds of arrangements for care which are defined by the culture and provided by the society, such as scientific and lay medicine, the variety of practitioners and agencies giving care and the conditions governing access to them and their use.
5. The assumptions and value systems of the health professions and the lay public as they impinge on matters of health, other than their concepts of health and illness per se.

II. *Dynamics of Patient Care Systems*

1. The process by which people come to be defined by themselves and others as sick, to select from among alternative sick roles, and to secure endorsement of the role selected.
2. The influence of symptoms and other factors on the process whereby sick people become patients and select a source of care.
3. The kinds of health problems patients bring to family physicians, to internists, to gynecologists, to pediatricians, to public health nurses, to pharmacists, to chiropractors, and so on, and how these practitioners perceive the problems and what they do about them. (This would be the beginning of a descriptive classification of illness and disordered behavior based on patients' symptoms, patients' folklore, assumptions, values, and language, as a supplement to the nosology developed by contemporary Western health professions.)
4. How people move through the patient care system and how they are separated, by themselves and others, from the sick role.
5. Longitudinal, or natural history, studies of medical and patient care could determine what happens to cohorts of patients with particular problems or living in particular social environments in terms of seeking or not seeking help, and the results of this behavior, expressed in terms of "health," or "social productivity," or "dollars." Such studies eventually could contribute to the development of criteria for measuring the quality and efficacy of the work of the health professions for both communities and individuals.
6. Cross-cultural, cross-national, and historical comparisons of the routes people take to obtain health services, and the factors which influence this.

III. *Communication*

1. The language of patient care: symptoms as the language of illness, professional students' jargon, and so on.
2. The influence of health education and other channels of formal and informal communication from health personnel to patients upon patients' behavior—their use of patient care facilities, compliance with medical advice, and so forth.
3. Interprofessional communication, both formal and informal—the effects on professional practice of the form and content of personal, institutional, and mass communication among members of different professions.
4. Intraprofessional communication, both formal and informal—the effects on professional practice of the forms and content of personal, institutional, and mass communication among members of the same profession.

IV. *The Diagnostic Process*

1. Fashions in diagnoses—individual, professional, and cultural—and the diffusion of knowledge problem. (A patient cannot have a disease, let alone die of it, unless his physician or someone else can name it.)
2. The relation between the purpose or the purposes for which a diagnosis is made and the way diagnosis proceeds, the procedures undertaken, and so on. (A diagnosis for purposes of prevention is quite a different process from a diagnosis for therapeutic purposes. This again is a different process from a diagnosis for restorative purposes or rehabilitation. In addition, there is the traditional investigative "medical" diagnosis of the type conducted in many university hospitals where the object frequently is to satisfy the clinical investigators's curiosity and to improve the long-range health of society, not necessarily that of the particular patient undergoing investigational diagnosis. A program of therapy, of course, generally is initiated on the basis of the investigative diagnosis. All four are different processes and they involve different personnel.)
3. What conditions influence the usefulness of different types of diagnosis? Prediction of future performance, identification of genetic, dynamic, predisposing, precipitating, perpetuating, and/or ameliorating factors, and so on?
4. Evaluation of the patient's total problem: the multiprofessional aspects of diagnosis; the social diagnosis; the evaluation of the patient's health problems in the context of his life situation.
5. The involvement of the patient in the diagnostic process. The influence of his expectations of different sources of care upon their participation in the process.
6. The determination of the level of personal and social competence which is maximal for the patient and the selection of a course of action which will help him to achieve and maintain this level of competence.

V. *Quality of Patient Care*

1. Perspectives of the different health professions regarding the quality of patient care.
2. How can the quality of care be measured? "Best practice" is one approach to measurement, but it is important to know what some, or all, professional people think should be done, and to know which of the alternatives is thought to be best practice, and who says so. Other approaches include prerequisites of care, elements of performance, and end results.
3. How can scientific advances in understanding disease processes be translated into practice? What is the influence of communication and values in motivating lay individuals, professional people, and the community to adopt innovations?
4. How can patient factors, professional factors, and the interactions between them be identified and manipulated to produce better outcomes for patients and greater satisfaction for members of the health professions?
5. How do a patient's expectations of a source of care and the professional's approach to him influence the outcome of care?

VI. *Influence of Various Characteristics of Patient Care Organizations upon Professional Practice*

    1. The effect on professonal practice of the policy of the organization regarding the type of job specification used—whether job assignments provide for differentiation of functions or overlap of functions.

    2. The effect on professional practice of formal and informal specialization among personnel.

    3. The effects on professional practice of the form and content of personal, institutional, and mass communication among personnel in the organization.

VII. *Influence of Organizational Characteristics upon the Movement of Patients into and Through the Organization*

    1. How do the assumptions of health personnel regarding health, disease, and patient care affect the movement of patients into and through organizations providing care?

    2. The consequences for patient movement of variations in the role of members of the patient care team.

    3. The effects on patient movement of the form and content of personal, institutional, and mass communication among personnel of the organization.

    4. The effects on patient movement of the complexity of the way in which the work of patient care is organized—of the diversity and specialization of occupational roles.

    5. For what categories of personnel is the patient the desired, reluctant, or abhorred focus of work, and what are the consequences of this combination of circumstances for the patient?

    6. How does the coordination of activities of the patient care agency with those of other groups in the community affect patient movement?

    7. How is the utilization of the care provided by one agency influenced by the functions which other community agencies perform?

    Two other classes of patient care problems were identified, but not further developed. They are the *economic aspects of patient care* and the *design of facilities for patient care.*

Future Directions

Over the past 25 years there has been a significant increase in federal support for biomedical and behavioral research. By 1975, 36 per cent ($1.5 billion) of all health-related research and development in the nation was performed at academic research institutions. In addition, men and women well-prepared in research became available largely as the result of PHS-supported training programs. Where, then, can nurse researchers make their greatest impact in biomedical and behavioral research?

Long-Term Care Nurse researchers can make tremendous inroads in the area of long-term care. Although researchers do not ordinarily choose to do their research in this area, long-term care—which includes the needs of the elderly, developmentally disabled, and mentally retarded—represents limitless opportunities for nurses through their research efforts to have a direct effect upon improving practice (American Academy of Nursing, 1976).[20] The elderly alone represent 23 million individuals in the United States. By 1980, it is estimated that there will be 25 million Americans over 65. Particularly needed are special research efforts to design quality assessment tools that will take into account the limited patient outcome goals and complex treatment processes characteristic of much long-term care. Research in this area also needs to be addressed to health financing, systems for delivery of services, and methods that provide access to services.

Long-term care is the provision of that range of services—physical, psychological, spiritual, social and environmental, including economic— needed to help people attain, maintain, or regain their optimum level of functioning. It includes health maintenance throughout the life span as well as care during acute and protracted illness and disability. Long-term care affects patients, residents, families, and communities.

In long-term care, patients often experience overwhelming effects of disease, residual pathology, and irreversible disability.

Until individuals everywhere are convinced that helping people maintain optimum health takes precedence over other types of care, the country will continue to be faced with expensive illness and disability that could be prevented. Until we accept that premise, long-term care at best will be a catch-up effort rather than a direct attack on the problems. What are some of these problems that need to be researched?

Health Care Assessment Health care assessment efforts should be designed to address the unique needs of the chronically ill. We know that many individuals, particularly the aged, have several chronic conditions. Thus, health care assessment must not be limited to only diagnostic— specific criteria—but must use functional status as a measure. The long-term nature of the patient's condition and frequent fluctuations in physical and mental states require that treatment and care plans vary. Patients/ residents may require differing levels of care within a short period of time, ranging from acute hospital care, skilled nursing services, intermediate care services, home health services to periodic office visits. Health care assessment needs to include all sources of care and should consider the impact of care on the patients'/residents' expected and actual ability to function in daily life.

One direct way of improving patient care is to obtain and refine a mechanism by which an individual patient's care outcome can be measured systematically at regularly scheduled intervals. This would provide a method for determining the allocation of resources in a facility and whether the services provided are those actually needed by the patient.

A Patient Appraisal, Care Planning, and Evaluation (PACE) system discussed previously is one such approach.

The patient appraisal system will have important implications in the provision of care in long-term care facilities, in hospitals, home health agencies, and ambulatory care settings. It will be necessary to provide the linkage between levels of care both institutional and noninstitutional to assure that services are readily accessible.

Increased efforts need to be made to link nursing homes with home-care programs, day care centers, congregate living facilities into an integrated program that assesses the quality of care provided by the total health system. In this way an integrated review of the total range of services can occur. Anything less than this will be based on evaluation of care from the fragmented view of individual facilities or programs and would perpetuate the inefficient and costly services that currently exist.

Health care assessment is based on health outcome despite the limitations of current measures. Patient satisfaction is recognized as one indicator of outcome.

Health care assessment uses a multidisciplinary approach in which several disciplines, such as physicians, nurses, pharmacists, therapists, nutritionists, and social workers, join with their patients/residents in establishing realistic time-limited outcome objectives and examining reasons for success or failure to meet them.

Welfare Reform Individuals needing long-term care represent all age groups and the major portion of that care will not be institutional. Noninstitutional care as well as institutional care needs to be made a part of any benefit package of health care financing. State and federal reimbursement policies for long-term care need to be reformed.

The increase of medical costs in the United States has risen from 3.5 per cent of the gross national product (GNP) in 1929 to 9 per cent in 1978. The national hospital bill, which now accounts for 40 per cent of total health expenditures, has been rising even more quickly than the total health care bill. The biggest rate of increase, however, has been in nursing home care. As various payment systems are analyzed, greater emphasis will be placed upon approaches to cost control of governmentally reimbursed health care programs.

Controlling the System Coordinated management and improvement of institutional and noninstitutional long-term care services are essential if the needs of the elderly and developmentally disabled are to be met.

Control of the system needs to be shared by providers, consumers, state and federal agencies. No one group should control the system. Particularly needed is increased consumer involvement in the planning, management, and evaluation of health care programs.

The future delivery of long-term care services needs to fit within a range of services to be provided by hospitals, nursing homes, home health care programs, community mental health centers, day care centers, health maintenance organizations—all linked together by interlocking systems. This would require that long-term care services be managed efficiently and that patients/residents be appropriately placed within the system.

Federal and state barriers would have to be removed to permit integrated management of long-term care services. Attention also needs to be given to:

- Alternatives to institutional care such as home care, day care centers, community mental health centers;
- Increased effectiveness of Medical Review (MR), Independent Professional Review (IPR), and Utilization Review (UR) to assess patient/resident needs to assure proper placement;
- Inclusion of long-term care facilities (institutional and noninstitutional) in the activities of PSRO;
- Activating nationwide the Patient Appraisal, Care Planning and Evaluation (PACE) system and extend it to all health care facilities both institutional and noninstitutional.

PREVENTIVE HEALTH CARE

The nation's health care system has grown in response to acute needs of the sick. Manpower in the health field is oriented to illness. Major expenditures at all levels of public and private interest are made to support the provision of acute care. Health insurance plans tend to cover costs only after a well-defined illness. The individual often finds himself at the risk of various illnesses most often because of his or her own behavior. Industrialization and urbanization frequently create unhealthy and unsafe living and working conditions for those who for economic reasons are attracted to the major cities. The rural population is also threatened by an increased exposure to toxic materials and by risk of injury in increasing numbers of new machinery. Similarly, the demands and expectations of our social system create a stressful environment.

Prevention is clearly identified as the number one priority for a future health-care system that would be basic to national health insurance. Although much is known about the cause of diseases, the scientific and technological capacity to prevent major diseases is limited because of lack of knowledge and in most cases lack of approaches to change individuals' behavior and attitudes.[21]

Public health programs have not been able to keep pace with the risks created by the newer technologies and altered life styles in the United States. For example, hypertension can now be alleviated by continual medication, using antihypertensive drugs. But, how can individuals be motivated to take these drugs for the rest of their lives, particularly when no overt symptoms are evident to the individual? Likewise, cancer of the lung is a preventable disease in most cases, with cigarette smoking identified as a leading cause. Yet the number of individuals who smoke, particularly women, is on the increase. At present, and at today's level of scientific knowledge, technologies for the prevention of most cases of heart disease, cancer, and stroke are lacking. Nurse researchers can contribute greatly by undertaking studies to influence individuals and institutions to change to more healthful behavior.

The ever-increasing American expenditures on health care could be controlled by giving greater attention to the prevention of the major chronic and disabling diseases.

Health education activities have often followed the same disease orientation approach. Information is dispensed through public media, community meetings, and in publications of many agencies and special interest groups, on the impact of disease on various human biological systems. In recent years, patient education programs have been developed to provide specific information to patients afflicted with a specific disease.

Community health education programs operated by public health agencies, for example, often have no relationship to school health education programs. Patient education is sometimes disregarded by community health educators but quite often is considered to be the only health education of importance by disease-oriented health service providers.

Rural Health Services for the Long-Term Care Patient/Resident

There is an inability to provide the full range of preventive health service to migrants and seasonal farmworkers and their families which include the elderly and disabled. The success of these and rural programs is too often contingent upon the ability of nonphysician providers to generate income from third party reimbursement.

In the field of rural health, nonphysician providers are trained with federal funds and utilized, and yet Medicare, which is federally administered, needs to recognize such personnel as eligible for reimbursement as does Medicaid.

Population Research

The rapid increase in world population demands attention in this area. Modern contraceptive techniques have significant limitations. "Improvement in methods of fertility control can be one of the most welcome and important contributions of the biological sciences to the betterment of life for all people." (DHEW, Public Health Service, Biomedical Research Panel).[22] Greatly needed is high quality and imaginative research of an interdisciplinary nature. The nurse having ready access to the patient and the trust of that patient engendered by her profession is in an enviable position to conduct significant research in this area.

Genetics of Human Diseases

Recent advances in the understanding of genetic mechanisms are contributing to a scientific base of knowledge. The prevention of psychoses, diabetes, high blood pressure, coronary heart disease, and cancer can be more readily achieved if one can understand the degree to which genetic factors underlie susceptibility to these diseases.

Neurobiology

The challenge in this area is to find ways to understand the human organism, how the brain and nervous system develop, how they function in health and disease, how thought occurs, how memory is stored, how we reason, how we are motivated. Interdisciplinary research would be very appropriate in this area.

Nutrition

Research is needed to determine how healthful food consumption practices can be fostered. All health personnel need to integrate sound nutritional health care practices into their daily activities.

Child Health

Much research needs to be undertaken to decrease the incidence and severity of disabling conditions. Amniocentesis has proven to be an effective procedure in which inborn genetic defects such as Down's syndrome and metabolic diseases can be detected. Amniocentesis needs to be made more generally available to pregnant women over 35. In addition, research needs to be undertaken to develop simple laboratory tests to screen for environmental mutagens leading to genetic diseases.

Increased emphasis on preventive health care in childhood could prove successful in reducing the likelihood of chronic heart disease in later life. Williams and Wynder state that atherosclerosis, which kills 900,000 people each year, is a basically pediatric problem, and we should "place a high priority on modifying current lifestyles—particularly lowering the consumption of saturated fats and cholesterol in the diet, encouraging nonsmoking, maintaining ideal body weight and keeping physically fit."[23] Research is needed to identify the major intervention goals to bring about needed change. The concept of a "health passport" beginning with infancy is a concept meriting exploration.

Teenage Pregnancies

Teenage pregnancies represent one of the leading causes contributing to infant mortality and birth defects. Nurse researchers could contribute greatly in this area by undertaking contraceptive and social science research, exploring ways to prevent unplanned pregnancies, and by developing a systems approach to strengthen comprehensive health, education, and social services.

Immunization

Many children (close to 50 per cent) remain unimmunized, two-thirds of them are in families with income above the poverty line. Research efforts here also have to be directed to parents to find ways of changing behavioral patterns.

Mental Health

The number of children in mental health institutions has more than doubled between 1955 and 1973. Most psychosocial disability can be prevented. Social and behavioral research is needed to learn how to deal with the mother/infant relationship.

Health Care Systems Research

Equity of access to health care services of a high quality necessitates that research be undertaken to develop health care delivery systems that provide a full range of health services; ability to serve a population defined by geography and enrollment; a built-in capability that assures that the system has a corporate identity; a unit record system that is a family-linked system; capability of providing 24-hour accessible services; and transportation and linkage with an emergency health services system.[24]

A health care system having these characteristics will require major changes in what we now consider appropriate facilities in which health services are to be provided. Major structural reforms of traditional patterns of providing health services are needed. Most health services need to be extended into the community through Health Maintenance Organizations (HMOs), neighborhood health centers, home health agencies, day care centers, and so forth. The National Health Planning and Resources Development Act of 1974 (P.L. 93–641) represents milestone legislation in which nurses everywhere must take an active role in shaping health care delivery systems and identifying our specific roles in providing needed health services.

Health Care Training

Research needs to be undertaken to determine if the American health economy will support a growing array of health specialists needed to function in a variety of health care delivery systems. How should they be educated? The growth of health and medical manpower has risen to 4.7 million, about 7 per cent of the total U.S. work force. Serious attention needs to be given to this area.[25]

There are major areas that impact on new roles in nursing that need to evolve if we are to meet the health needs of Americans and develop necessary strategies to meet these needs.

First, what has happened to the population over the past decade? The annual death rate has declined in recent years but there remain variations in segments of the population, such as males versus females, whites versus nonwhites.

Inpatient facilities have increased to approximately 7,000 hospitals and 28,000 long-term care facilities. The number of acute care beds has risen to 850,000 and 228,000 are unoccupied. More than 4.5 million men and women in 200 occupations are employed in the delivery of health services. Expenditures for illness and injury have risen to over $200 billion, $80 billion of which represents direct costs for personal health care services. Hospital costs per admission have risen from $127 in 1950 to over $500 in 1979 with a predicted increase to $1,000 by the time gasoline gets to be $1 a gallon. Who provides for the health dollar? Third-party payers now cover 90 per cent of the total expenditures for hospitalization. Public funds cover one-third of the total for persons under 65, and two-thirds of the total expenditures of those over 65. In spite of this, recipients of Medicare pay more out-of-the-pocket expenses for health services now than they did before the advent of Medicare (Title XVIII) in 1966. There are obvious problems of distribution, provision, utilization, and unparalleled rising costs of providing health services. As some form of national health insurance evolves, never before in the history of American nursing does a greater challenge confront us in nursing.

As we view the impact of new roles in nursing, can we in all good conscience believe that health is a *right* of every American? A "right" is more than just an interest that an individual might have or a state of being that an individual might prefer. A "right" refers to entitlements— not those things that would be nice for people to have but rather those things they are *entitled* to have. The term "right" is often confused with the concept of equality and this is particularly true when we speak of rights to health care and equality in respect to health care. The right to health care for every American is an idealistic goal, but equality of health care in terms of access, provision of services, and costs may not be attainable. Therefore, nurses need to look at new roles in nursing and develop strategies that are based on an optimum level of health services to be provided rather than upon a maximum level. For example, more than 10 million Americans could benefit immediately from renal dialysis. Yet neither the persons nor the facilities are available to provide these needed services. Another example is the need to activate a national program of home health services to provide for services for one-third of long-term care patients who do not belong in institutions such as nursing homes. There is now no national community network to provide the needed back-up services. A realistic fact is that 50 per cent of the visiting nurses' associations have only two or fewer nurses on their staffs.

If health care is a right of every American we must recognize that medical care with its emphasis upon "curing" rather than "caring" represents only a very small if not marginal contribution of health care services. It has been stated that 80 per cent of illness is functional and can be effectively treated by any talented healer who displays warmth, interest, and compassion. Another 10 per cent of illness is wholly incurable and only in the remaining 10 per cent does scientific medicine—at considerable cost—have any value at all. Our dilemma is that not only are 228,000 beds unoccupied, but also that our present costly institutional facilities are designed predominantly to meet the requirements of the 10 per cent of individuals who can benefit from scientific medicine. Recognizing the many dilemmas with which we are faced we would like to address the four points mentioned initially.

The Recipient of Services

The client, that is, the patient, the resident, or individual recipient of health services, is a part of a delivery system of health. Such a health care delivery system must:

- Provide a full range of medical and health services;
- Have the capability of serving a population defined by geography and enrollment;
- Provide a unit record system that is a family-oriented system;
- Provide an organization and a system of accountability;
- Have the capability of providing 24-hour accessible services; and
- Provide transportation and linkage with an emergency health services system.

Several models for health care delivery are presented in a recent American Academy of Nursing publication.[26]

An integral part of the health care delivery system is *primary* care which is unavailable to many people today. Primary care is a continuous source of care to which an individual or family *first* must turn for help in each episode of illness. Primary care must also ". . . educate clients to preventive measures and offer them regularly, whether these are immunization of a child, antepartal care, or alcohol and drug prevention." Doris Schwartz describes six stages of primary care:[27]

- 1st stage: Purely preventive—the preservation of existing health both physical and mental.
- 2nd stage: Also preventive but addressed particularly to those individuals at special risk for a variety of reasons, e.g., genetic (sickle cell anemia), poverty, lack of motivation.
- 3rd stage: Early detection of existing problems both physical and mental.
- 4th stage: Manifest illness: the acute stage to which the present health system directs its greatest effort.
- 5th stage: Rehabilitation needs to be activated from the time the individual is identified as a patient.
- 6th stage: Those persons for whom care or some degree of rehabilitation is not possible. Primary care is also concerned with monitoring to alleviate unnecessary suffering and prevent crippling complications, according to Virginia Henderson, "letting the chronically ill person die as he would want to die if he had the strength and the will and the knowledge to control the circumstances for himself."

Providers of Services

The roles of nurses already are undergoing many changes. Also, licensed nurse practitioners will increase substantially, as they become more independent in their practice. The Billings, Montana, ruling* concerning the firing of physician assistants for practicing nursing without a license is a significant legal decision, supporting the right of only *licensed* nurses to function as independent nurse practitioners and practice nursing. New types of nurses will appear in addition to those now highly specialized in acute care—the family nurse practitioner who can deal with major health problems, particularly those that are preventable (e.g., smoking, alcoholism, drug addiction, stress problems, child abuse, mental illness). Multiple health care delivery systems will require nurses to assume leadership roles in administering these systems, e.g., HMOs, ambulatory clinics, planning for health services, and delivery of health services. We are moving steadily toward securing a direct reimbursement mechanism that will cover payment for nursing services provided in community settings and homes.

Research in nursing practice will be key to identifying strategies to cope with health problems and outcome measures to assess the services provided. Some of the problems basic to nursing that must be addressed are:

* State of Montana, Office of the Attorney General, State Capitol, Helena, Montana, August 28, 1975, Volume 36, Opinion No. 18.

1. Paucity of nurses prepared and functioning as nurse researchers.
2. Lack of financial support for nursing research.
3. Lack of incorporation of research findings into practice.
4. Lack of integration of researcher role into the employment situation.
5. Dearth of good clinical studies.
6. Need for instruments and criterion measures to evaluate effects of nursing care.

Educating Providers of Health Care Services

Many changes in the systems of nursing education are required if the strategies outlined previously are to be achieved, and if health care services are to be related to those who need these services. Primary health care practitioners and gerontological nurse practitioners are top priorities. Both undergraduate and graduate nursing programs need to be redesigned to prepare these individuals. Preparation in leadership and decision-making skills is paramount. We no longer can afford the proliferation of nursing schools. Educational efforts, due to limited economic resources, will have to be accountable to society and the demands of the consumer. Hospital-based programs will decrease. Baccalaureate and higher degree programs will undergo major changes in order to adapt to the demands of health care delivery systems. Clinical practice will shift drastically to community health settings and long-term care facilities. The shift of the base of employment away from acute care settings to community-based settings will occur. Numerous surgical procedures will be carried out on an outpatient basis requiring the increased skills of the surgical nurse practitioner.

PROBLEMS IN CONDUCTING RESEARCH IN NURSING

In every field of research there are obstacles that tend to block research progress. These problems are not unique to nursing research, but they must be overcome if progress is to be made. Some of the major problems are summarized by the authors in the following paragraphs.

Political and Social Pressures

The public's continuing dissatisfaction with nursing care, the increasing costs of nursing services, the continued shortages, are problems to be faced. The nation's health needs are changing, and the nursing profession has not kept pace with these changes. Knowledge needed to evaluate nursing practice must become ". . . truly scientific, embracing all values relevant to formal organizations."[28] Improvement of patient care through nursing practice involves more than making a novel change such as constructing a circular unit or employing electronic gadgets. Likewise all the money in the world will not achieve worthwhile research results unless there are prepared researchers with freedom to undertake the research.

Supply

The shortage of prepared professional nursing personnel is acute, drastically reducing the number of nurses who might pursue a career of research in nursing. Some of this is due to the increased demand for nursing services and some to the poor distribution and utilization of nursing services. There is a reduced percentage of high school graduates entering nursing due in part to an increasing percentage who pursue college careers and who prepare themselves for other professions. Other problems are: A continued high rate of drop-outs during the educational program; wide fluctuations in availability of nurses in different parts of the country; low economic status as compared with other professions; and an old-fashioned public image of nursing that continues to picture the nurse functioning in an era of simple medical care practices.

Communications

There is a widening gap between the faculties of nursing schools and nurse practitioners. In situations where this exists the discovery of new knowledge in the laboratory and its application to the care of patients can be halted. There must be a close working relationship between the faculty and nurse practitioners if discoveries of the laboratory are to be transmitted to the bedside. Some new knowledge does reach the nurse practitioner, but application of new research findings cannot be achieved without authoritative support from both nursing education and nursing service.

Models to Emulate

It has only been recently that nursing has been able to identify the nurse researcher and/or nurse scientist as models to emulate. The nurse teacher-investigator functions within a circumscribed environment where her satisfaction stems from her academic colleagues and students. The nurse practitioner, on the other hand, must seek her satisfaction from patient care. The motivation of both groups is different. This must be recognized as a factor in recruiting nurses into research. More needs to be known about the effect of the nursing school upon the student in influencing her career choice in research.

Education and Training

What is the responsibility of the school of nursing for preparing nurse researchers? The school has a major responsibility to impart broad concepts and methods of approach and to assist the student in developing habits of thought and basic attitudes. The nursing school can help immeasurably in providing a student with a sound basis for her career choice. Likewise the school, using a scientific approach to the practice of nursing and fully utilizing a problem-solving approach in teaching and clinical practice, can help the student to form sound habits of scientific inquiry. Education and training in many schools of nursing are outmoded. Nurse educators need to modernize pedagogic methods and utilize many more teaching aids, such as closed-circuit television and teaching machines. A scientific approach to clinical teaching can be a challenging opportunity for the budding researcher and needs to be incorporated in basic core material. Postgraduate education can serve as an important link between the nursing school and the nurse practitioner. The nurse scientist finds her roots in a core of basic knowledge and skills in the biological as well as the behavioral, physical, and social sciences. It is the mission of the school of nursing to see that these foundations are initially established. (As indicated previously, this might be done by offering a minor or second major in one of the sciences).

If the nursing profession is to achieve a pool of nurse scholars and researchers that would compose one per cent of the active professional nursing population, the following barriers must be overcome:

Prepare nurse faculties in centers for nursing research
Improve methods for reaching nurses with research potential and interests
Identify and nurture creative talent and scientific ability
Research into the content of curriculums to find ways of preparing nurse researchers

Defining the Research Problem

Two-thirds of the research grant applications that are submitted to the U.S. Public Health Service that are disapproved are done so by the reviewers because of the lack of a clear statement of the research problem.

Some progress has been made in defining criteria for patient selection and comparison,[29] but it is difficult to define the nonmedical or environmental situations influencing recovery or disease progression. There are many unknowns in nursing, such as the components of patient care, the amount of nursing care necessary, and valid criteria of nursing practice (tools for measurement are not available). There is also a discrepancy between nursing care needed and nursing care received. The dearth of clinical specialists in nursing further aggravates the problem, as these are the persons most likely to pose the research questions in nursing practice that need to be answered.

Access to Study Populations

Nurses must have access to study populations where nursing experimentation is applicable. Finding suitable study populations is extremely difficult, as this involves the willingness of individuals or families to be studied, the cooperation of professional workers in the field, the willingness of patients to participate in experimental research, and many other problems.[30] Many subjects may be poorly educated or have different values from the researcher or the person who designed the research.

Methodological Problems

Once the research question has been clearly defined, there are numerous methodological problems that must be faced in designing the research. Selecting a sample of study subjects from the target population is one of these. Scientific sampling requires random selection, which may be difficult to achieve among human subjects. In explanatory experiments, random assignment of subjects to the experimental and control groups and the use of a placebo and the double blind techniques are methods of research controls that are difficult to apply in many conceivable nursing studies.

Another methodological problem is the lack of valid and reliable measuring instruments for gathering data in nursing research. Many studies now depend on subjective observations of patients' behavior. Unless the skill and training of the observers are at a high level, such observations can be crude and inconclusive.

Cost

Patient care research is costly. Longitudinal studies of population groups are badly needed but are costly and difficult to finance over long periods of time. Stable financing of research projects is not easy, particularly where funds are dependent upon demonstration of annual progress. This in turn presents problems in recruiting prepared research personnel who are solely dependent upon research grant funds.

Interdisciplinary Research

Almost all future research in nursing will be interdisciplinary, for there are facts, concepts, and theories from the physical, biological, and social sciences that have relevance for nursing. Those with research skills cannot be isolated from their own discipline.[31] Dual appointments with the nursing department and the appropriate discipline (e.g., department of sociology) are essential if the research investigator is to thrive. There is beginning to appear the nurse clinician-scholar and/or nurse scientist who will be able to converse directly and cogently with specialists in the other sciences. Nursing must not make the mistake of isolating them from teaching and contacts with undergraduate students. "Interdisciplinary research has difficulties of its own. Not only is there the problem of needing an effective research team composed of diverse personalities, but there are problems of language, communication, understanding, and mutual confidence and respect among various members of the team from different disciplines."[32]

Conceptualization of Research

In nursing there are lacking conceptual models and theories for research. A few attempts have been made in this direction, as has been indicated previously. The conceptual basis for research can help the investigator select appropriate variables that can be measured and will serve as indicators of the processes postulated.

DISCOVERY OF NEW KNOWLEDGE AND ITS APPLICATION

More than 1,000 studies have been completed since 1950 that have specific relevance for nursing.[33,34] There is an urgency to prepare a critique of these studies and to replicate those which have findings that are applicable. The gap between what is known through research and what is applied is broadening.[35] It will take time to identify significant concepts and theories that will represent breakthroughs for nursing education or practice.

Application of research findings can be speeded up by stimulating regional and national conferences where clinical papers can be presented and challenged. The now completed American Nurses' Association's clinical sessions are an example of a pioneering endeavor to achieve this aim.

Another important endeavor was a workshop conducted by the American Nurses' Foundation to stimulate the utilization of research findings in the improvement of nursing care of the aging.[36] Findings of research studies, and reports of informed groups relevant to the care of the aged, were presented in general sessions of the workshop. Emphasis was placed upon relevant and recent findings concerning the scientific bases of aging and the care of the aged. Participants at the workshop were given an opportunity to give direct patient care and to apply their newly learned knowledge. Such workshops should be stimulated throughout the country.

Continued participation by researchers in contributing the critique column of *Nursing Research* is one way in which critical thinking can be stimulated and significant research findings identified. Investigators also have the obligation of contributing summaries of their ongoing research to the Science Information Exchange and to the Health Information Foundation. It is only through continued effort on the part of all those concerned with research in nursing that significant findings can be brought to light and communicated.

References

1. Editorial, "Directions Apparent in Nursing Research." *Nursing Res.,* **8:** 187–188, fall 1959.

2. Rozella Schlotfeldt, "Summaries of Workshop Group Discussions, Conferences and Workshop on Research in Nursing." Cleveland, Ohio, September 14–17, 1958, American Nurses' Foundation, Inc.

3. *Ibid.,* p. 4.

4. Dale R. Lindsay and Ernest M. Allen, "Medical Research: Past Support, Future Directions." *Science,* **134:**2017–2024, December 22, 1961.

5. Charles D. Flagle, "Operational Research in the Health Services," *Research Methodology and Potential in Community Health and Preventive Medicine. Ann. New York Acad. Sc.,* **107:**752, May 22, 1963.

6. *Ibid.*

7. W. C. Meierhenny (ed.), "Learning Theory and AV Utilization." *AV Communication Review,* **9:** No. 5, September–October 1961, Supplement 4.

8. Rena E. Boyle, "Critical Issues in Collegiate Nursing Education." Report of the Conference of the Council of Member Agencies of the Department of Baccalaureate and Higher Degree Programs. Kansas City, Kansas, National League for Nursing, November 8–10, 1961.

9. Martha E. Rogers, "Some Comments on the Theoretical Basis of Nursing Practice." *Nursing Sc.,* **1:**11, April–May 1963.

10. Faye G. Abdellah *et al., Patient-Centered Approaches to Nursing.* New York, Macmillan Publishing Co., Inc., 1960, p. 12.

11. Martha E. Rogers, *loc. sit.*

12. Faye G. Abdellah, *op. cit.,* p. 27.

13. Mildred Konlande, "Nursing Care Based Upon Selected Concepts from Biological Sciences." Report of the Conference of the Council of Member Agencies of the Department of Baccalaureate and Higher Degree Programs, Kansas City, Kansas, National League for Nursing, Department of Baccalaureate and Higher Degree Programs, November 8–10, 1961, pp. 39–40.

14. Rhoda Bowen, "Nursing Care Based Upon Selected Concepts from Physics." Report of the Conference of the Council of Member Agencies of the Department of Baccalaureate and Higher Degree Programs, Kansas City, Kansas, National League for Nursing, Department of Baccalaureate and Higher Degree Programs, November 8–10, 1961, pp. 41–44.

14a. Faye G. Abdellah, *op. cit.*

15. William A. Glaser, "Hospital Organization—A Comparison of American and Foreign Systems." Paper presented at the Advanced Institute of American College Administrators, The Roosevelt Hospital, New York, April 4, 1963, unpublished.

16. William A. Glaser, "American and Foreign Hospitals—Some Sociological Comparisons," Eliot Freidsen (ed.), *The Hospital.* New York, The Free Press of Glencoe, 1963.

17. Ruth Freeman *et al.,* "Patient Care Research: Report of a Symposium." *Am. J. Pub. Health,* **56:**965–969, June 1963.

18. *Ibid.,* p. 966.

19. *Ibid.,* pp. 966–968.

20. American Academy of Nursing, "Long-Term Care in Perspective: Past, Present, and Future Directions for Nursing." (ANA Publ. G-120) Kansas City, Mo., The Academy, 1976.

21. U.S. Public Health Service, *Forward Plan for Health*, FY 1978–82. [DHEW Publ. No. (OS) 76–50046] Washington, D.C., Government Printing Office, 1976.

22. U.S. Public Health Service, *Report of the President's Biomedical Research Panel.* [DHEW Publ. No. (OS) 76–501] Washington, D.C., Government Printing Office, 1976 Appendix A.

23. C. E. Williams and E. L. Wynder, "A Blind Spot In Preventive Medicine." *JAMA,* **236:**2196–2197, November 8, 1976.

24. Faye G. Abdellah, "Models for Health Care Systems." Kansas City, Mo., The Association, ANA Publ. G-119:1–13, 1975.

25. E. E. Flook and P. J. Sanazaro, Jr., *Health Services Research and R&D in Perspective.* Ann Arbor, Mich., Health Administration Press, 1973.

26. Faye G. Abdellah, "Models for Health Care Systems," *op. cit.*

27. Doris Schwartz, "One Suggestion for a Primary Health System for the Nation," in *Models for Health Care Delivery: Now and for the Future.* Kansas City, Mo., American Academy of Nursing, 1975, pp. 20–26.

28. Andrew C. Fleck, "Evaluation Research Programs in Public Health Practice," *Research Methodology and Potential in Community Health and Preventive Medicine. Ann. New York Acad. Sc.,* **107:**717–724, May 22, 1963.

29. U.S. Department of Health, Education, and Welfare, *Elements of Progressive Patient Care.* Public Health Service, Division of Hospital and Medical Facilities, U.S. Public Health Service Publication No. 930–C–1, September 1962, p. 10.

30. William R. Willard, "The Present Status and Future Development of Community Health Research—A Critique: From the Viewpoint of Educational Institutions," *Research Methodology and Potential in Community Health and Preventive Medicine. Ann. New York Acad. Sc.,* **107:**771, May 22, 1963.

31. John S. Millis, remarks made by Dr. John S. Millis, President, Western Reserve University, at the National Conference on Nursing Research, Cleveland, Ohio, September 15, 1958, American Nurses' Foundation, Inc.

32. William R. Willard, *op. cit.,* p. 775.

33. U.S. Public Health Service, *Research in Nursing 1955–1968.* Division of Nursing, Research Grants Branch, PHS Publication No. 1356, 1969.

34. Virginia A. Henderson, *Nursing Studies Index,* Volume 4, 1957–1959. Philadelphia, J. B. Lippincott Co., 1964.

35. Calvin W. Taylor *et al.,* "Bridging the Gap." *Nat. Ed. A. J.,* **51:**23–25, January 1962.

36. Alice M. Forman and M. Irene Brown, "The Utilization of Research Findings in the Improvement of Nursing Care of the Aging." Report of a Workshop Project for Staff Nurses of Upper New England. New York, American Nurses' Foundation, Inc., April 1963.

Suggestions for Further Reading

1. Rozella M. Schlotfeldt, "Cooperative Nursing Investigations: A Role for Everyone." *Nursing Res.* **23:**452–456, November–December 1974.

2. "Health and Society." *The Milbank Memorial Fund Quarterly,* **52:**225–346, Summer 1974.

3. Marjorie V. Batey (ed.). *Communicating Nursing Research. Nursing Research in the Bicentennial Year,* Vol. 9. Boulder, Colorado, Western Interstate Commission for Higher Education, April 1977.

4. National Commission for the Protection of Human Subjects of Biomedical and Behavioral Research. *Special Study. Implications of Advances in Biomedical and Behavioral Research,* Washington, D.C., DHEW Publication No. (OS) 78–0015, September 30, 1978.

5. DHEW, PHS. *National Conference on Health Promotion Programs in Occupational Settings. The Proceedings.* Washington, D.C., DHEW Publication, Office of Health Information and Health Promotion, January 17–19, 1979.

GLOSSARY AND BRIEF DEFINITIONS
OF SELECTED RESEARCH TERMS

algorithm: A name that is sometimes used for iterative solution procedures. It is a common name for solution procedures used in obtaining an optimal integer linear programing model. The algorithm requires that all new variables must also be integers. These algorithms have been inefficient for most problems, requiring a prohibitive amount of electronic computer time even to solve small problems involving only a few constants and a few variables.[1]

analysis of covariance: A statistical procedure for adjusting the data to equalize the groups studied in terms of important extraneous variables (covariables) *after* the independent variable has been applied to the subjects and measurements have been made of the dependent variable. Combines the two techniques of analysis of variance and regression analysis.

analysis of variance: A statistical test of significance of the results of a study in which the effects on the dependent variable of more than two alternatives of an independent variable (or more than one independent variable) are being tested simultaneously. In testing multiple independent variables this procedure can provide valuable information on the effects of not only each independent variable, but also of combinations of these variables. In the test of significance the F-test is employed. Analysis of variance is the analytical method for treating data obtained from such experimental designs as the latin square and the factorial.

associative relationships: A change in the dependent variable is related to a change in the independent variable, but we cannot with certainty say that the effect on the dependent variable was directly caused by the independent variable.

assumption: A statement whose correctness or validity is taken for granted.

balancing: A procedure for equating the subjects in the experimental and control groups of an experiment in terms of important organismic variables by matching the groups as a whole in terms of these variables rather than by matching the individuals composing the groups, as in pairing.

Bayesian statistics: An approach to statistical inference that employs Bayes' probability theorem. Since prior knowledge is used in testing the significance of the results of a study, Bayesian inference is considered to be a subjective approach to statistical inference.

bimodal: A frequency distribution in which the values of the measurements that have been made for a group of study subjects form two peaks (modes).

binary: Composed of two elements or parts—e.g., binary logarithm or binary number system. As compared with the decimal system, the binary number system is composed of only zero and 1. This system is used in electronic computers and in information theory.

calibration: The marking off of the intervals that make up the scale of a measuring instrument.

case study: A detailed, factual, largely narrative description and analysis of individuals, institutions, communities, whole societies, incidents, situations, inanimate objects, plants or animals.

causation: The process whereby a given event or phenomenon, called the cause, invariably precedes a certain other event, called the effect.

cause and effect: The cause of a certain effect is some appropriate factor that is invariably related to the effect.

central limit theorem: "A statistical theorem stating that the *sampling distribution* of a mean approaches the normal distribution as the number of random samples becomes very large, even if the values that comprise the sample means and the population from which the random samples are drawn do not form a normal distribution."[2]

central tendency, measure of: "Any of various statistical measures used to obtain a single number that is considered the most representative value of a series of data. Commonly referred to as an *average,* this number is the central point in the frequency distribution of a single variable about which the other values are distributed. The center of the distribution may vary according to the particular measure of central tendency used—the mean, median, or mode."[3]

chi-square test: A nonparametric statistical test of significance based on the chi-square distribution. It can be used to analyze the significance of differences among groups that are being compared in terms of qualitative variables. The data, called frequency distributions, consist of counts of the number of study subjects in each group found to possess each of the scale values of the variables measured. The test is performed by calculating theoretical frequencies for each scale value (i.e., for each cell of the table into which the frequencies are tabulated), subtracting the theoretical from the actual frequencies, squaring the differences, dividing by the theoretical frequency, and then summing up all the quotients. This sum is the computed value of chi-square for the sample data. The larger the computed value of chi-square, for specified-size samples, the smaller is the probability that the differences in the frequency distributions being compared are due to random sampling.

class interval: "An arbitrary, convenient subdivision of a quantitative *variable.* The total *range* of the variable is divided into class intervals, preferably equal in size. Both continuous and discrete variables are so divided to facilitate analysis."[4]

cluster: A subgroup of variables each of which is more closely correlated with other members of the subgroup than with the other variables in the larger group.

cluster analysis: A technique for determining clusters. It is analogous to the technique of factor analysis.

cluster sampling: See **sampling.**

coefficient of correlation: A summary measure called r that varies between -1 and $+1$. Its value is a measure of the degree of relationship between the variables studied. The closer the computed value of r is to $+1$ or -1, the higher is the degree of relationship among the variables studied.

cohort: A set of study subjects who are grouped together according to certain characteristics and observed longitudinally. In explanatory studies these characteristics would be the independent variables. Cohort studies are essentially repeated cross-sectional studies that involve the same subjects.

comparative experiments: Explanatory experiments in which the effects produced by the application of alternative values of the independent variable to different groups of study subjects are compared in terms of some criterion measure to find out which alternative produces the most desirable effect.

conceptual framework: A theoretical approach to the study of problems that are scientifically based which emphasizes the selection, arrangement, and clarification of its concepts. A conceptual framework states functional relationships between events and is not limited to statistical relationships.

conceptualization: The ordering of data by means of concepts (general meanings, ideas, properties)—i.e., the appropriate concepts that will put a group of facts into a rational or useful order.

concomitant variation: Whenever two phenomena vary together in a consistent and persistent manner either the variations represent a direct causal connection between the two phenomena, or else both are being affected by some common causal factor.

confidence interval: A measure of the precision with which a sample statistic (summary measure) estimates the parameter of the population from which the sample was randomly selected. Determined from the standard error of the statistic, the confidence interval provides a range within which we estimate that the true value of the population parameter lies at a stated level of probability (confidence coefficient). Thus, for example, the 95 per cent confidence interval—the value of the sample statistic ± 2 standard errors—tells us that the probability that the interval embraces the true parameter value is nineteen to one.

consensual validation: The determination that something is real by the fact of agreement between the perceiving of several persons.

constellation: Any inclusive and organized grouping of phenomena.

construct: "A concept devised to aid in scientific analysis and generalization. A construct is generally inferred indirectly from observable phenomena. It is an abstraction from reality, selecting and focusing on certain aspects of reality and ignoring others. It is a *heuristic assumption* designed to guide and suggest fruitful areas of investigation; it is not intended as a direct description of concrete phenomena."[5]

continuum: Describes the scale for a variable in which within the interval between any two values it is always possible to have a third value.

control: Any operation that is designed to test or limit any of the conceivable sources of error and distortion in knowledge. In research, experimental control refers to the manipulation or modification of the conditions under which the observations are to be made. Statistical control involves the treatment of the data to remove the effects of extraneous factors.

control group: Subjects who are as closely as possible equivalent to an experimental group and exposed to all the conditions of the investigation except the experimental (treatment, stimulus) variable.

correlation: "1. The interrelationship of two (or more) quantitative variables so that an increase in the magnitude of one of the variables is associated with an increase or decrease in the magnitude of the other. Thus when two variables are highly correlated it is possible to predict with reasonable accuracy the magnitude of the other. The term 'correlation' usually is not used to refer to the association of two qualitative variables or of a quantitative variable and a qualitative variable. 2. Occasionally the term 'correlation' is used to refer to the interrelationship of any two (or more) variables whether quantitative or qualitative."[6]

counseling: "The process of using interviews, psychological tests, guidance, and other techniques to help an individual solve his personal problems and plan his future realistically."[7]

covariance, analysis of: "The extension of the basic technique of the analysis of *variance* to the situation in which there are two or more quantitative variables. The *covariance* of the quantitative variables is measured for each of the categories of the qualitative variable, and the resulting measures are compared to see if they differ significantly. The categories of the qualitative variable (or variables) may be referred to as separate samples, and thus it may be said that the covariances of two or more quantitative variables in two or more samples are compared to see if there is a statistically significant difference between the samples."[8]

criterion measure: A measure of the dependent variable that serves to indicate the effects of the independent variable upon the subjects being studied.

criterion measures (evaluation of):
   meaningfulness: Pragmatic test of the measure as a whole. Does the measure have any practical, real-life meaning and application?
   reliability: The consistency or precision of the measure. A measure is considered reliable if it is consistently reproducible.
   sensitivity: Ability of the measure to detect fine differences among the subjects being studied.
   validity: Does the measure actually measure what it is supposed to measure? Also referred to as relevance.

cross-sectional design: A type of research design in which data from a specific point in time are collected and analyzed, as in a descriptive survey.

cybernetics: The scientific study of messages and of regulatory or control mechanisms whether found in machines, persons, social groups, or institutions (e.g., communication theory, information theory). Originated by Norbert Wiener.

decision-making research: A study conducted for the purpose of selecting a course of action from several alternative courses of action that could be taken.

deduction: A process of reasoning that starts with given premises and attempts to derive valid conclusions. Reasoning from the general to the particular.

demography: "The study of population size, composition, and distribution, and the patterns of change therein. The narrowest conception of demography views it as the study of vital statistics (the study of birth and death rates and related statistics). However, as vital statistics are analyzed and interpreted, demography develops into social demography or population studies. In the broadest view population composition and distribution include not only such variables as fertility, mortality, age and sex, but also marriage, divorce, family size, race, education, illiteracy, unemployment, distribution of wealth, occupational distribution, crime rates, density of population, migration, etc."[9]

demonstration: The aim of a demonstration is to show how a particular research finding can be applied to a specific situation. A demonstration differs from research in that it does not seek answers to questions nor does it require a tight research design.

double-blind: A control technique in an experiment in which neither the investigator nor the study subject knows which subject receives the placebo and which the actual treatment. It is employed to provide additional assurance that the experimental and control groups are identical in every way except in terms of the independent variable that is being tested.

ecology: The study of organisms in reference to their physical environment—i.e., the ways in which humans adapt to an environment and the resulting geographic distribution. An attempt to determine which parts of the physical and social environment (for a specific period) are transformed into goals, barriers, boundaries, and other psychological factors that constitute an individual's *life space*.

effect: An event or phenomenon that follows another phenomenon; a result as manifested in an effect (dependent) variable.

empirical: Based on factual investigation, experience, or observation.

empirical law: A law based on facts or observations and expressing in general form the relationships between two or more sets of data.

empirical test: "A test of a hypothesis in which the investigator observes the phenomena in question (either under experimental or 'natural' conditions) to determine whether the hypothesis is supported or contradicted by these observations. Ideally, the investigator should be as interested in disproving as in verifying the hypothesis, and should consider all other possible explanations for the observed events. Moreover, the scientific validity of any set of observations depends upon their confirmation by other qualified observers. Any other qualified investigator following the specified procedure should reach the same conclusion about a hypothesis as the original investigator."[10]

empiricism (scientific): A philosophical movement in which the instruments of all sciences are the experience of the scientist himself.

epistemology: Philosophical study of the origin, nature, and limits of knowledge.

equal-appearing intervals method: A method of scaling variables developed by L. Thurstone that is an adaptation of the logical principles of the equal sense differences method to the task of scaling judgments of any kind, such as attitudes and opinions.

error, alpha: "The rejection of a true null hypothesis. Since null hypotheses are accepted or rejected on the basis of statistical probability, the possibility exists that a true null hypothesis may be erroneously rejected. Generally speaking, in the use of statistical probability to accept and reject null hypotheses, the risk of rejecting a true null hypothesis increases as the risk of accepting a false null hypothesis decreases. The level of significance used indicates the probability of making an alpha error, a higher level indicating a greater chance of this type of error. Alpha error is sometimes referred to as type I error."[11]

error, beta: "The retaining of a false null hypothesis. Since null hypotheses are accepted or rejected on the basis of tests of statistical probability, the possibility exists that a false null hypothesis may be accepted. The degree of danger of accepting a false null hypothesis depends upon the level of significance used in testing the hypothesis: the lower the level of significance used, the greater the probability of making a beta error. Beta error is sometimes referred to as type II error."[12]

errors in research: In addition to sampling error, the following are the three major sources of error in research:

observer error: These may be random or systematic. The latter can result from inadequate training or psychological biases of the observer.

processing error: A type of error resulting from faulty data processing such as the errors in translation of open-ended responses, arithmetical mistakes.

response error: May also be random or systematic (bias) and arise where there is no observer to check the accuracy or completeness of responses.

experiment: An arrangement of conditions under which the phenomenon to be observed shall take place. In explanatory experiments the aim is to determine for that phenomenon the causal influences of these conditions.

experimental design: The step-by-step plan of an experiment, including the determination of the conceptual basis for the research, the selection of study subjects, the specification of instruments for data collection, and the determination of the analysis and interpretation of the findings. Experimental designs set forth the conduct of the research under highly controlled conditions. In explanatory experiments subjects are randomly assigned to the alternative groups being studied.

experimental group: Subjects who are exposed to the experimental (treatment, stimulus) variable and whose reactions will reflect the *effect,* if any, of that variable.

explanatory research: The purpose of this type of research is to seek answers to questions concerned with "Why does something happen?" "What would happen if . . .?" Explanatory research is essentially concerned with studying the relationship among two or more variables. Explanatory research can be employed to discover causal relationships, to establish predictive relationships, or to evaluate a method, program, or procedure.

exploratory study: "A preliminary study the major purpose of which is to become familiar with a phenomenon that is to be investigated, so that the major study to follow may be designed with greater understanding and precision. The exploratory study (which may use any of a variety of techniques, usually with a small sample) permits the investigator to define his research problem and formulate his hypotheses more accurately. It also enables him to choose the most suitable techniques for his research and to decide on the questions most in need of emphasis and detailed investigation, and it may alert him to potential difficulties, sensitivities, and areas of resistance."[13]

extrapolation: ". . . any process of estimating values of a function beyond the range of available data . . . the process of extending a norm line beyond the limits of actually obtained data, in order to permit interpretation of extreme scores. The extension may be done mathematically by fitting a curve to the obtained data or, as is more common, by less rigorous methods, usually graphic. Considerable judgment on the test maker's part enters into any extrapolation process, which means that extrapolated norm values are likely to be to some extent arbitrary."[14]

fact: An event, a phenomenon; something that has actually happened.

factor: In psychological research, a factor is considered to be any one of several conditions that together may be the cause of an event or phenomenon.

factor analysis: A statistical technique for interpreting scores and correlations among scores from a number of tests. It attempts to find functionally unitary traits in two or more correlated variables.

factorial design: This design tests the simultaneous effects of several independent variables on a dependent variable. The design may also involve multiple alternatives for each of the independent variables.

field surveys: The gathering of statistical data from the study subjects in their natural habitat. Data are collected either directly as in an interview or indirectly as in a mailed questionnaire.

frequency distribution: A grouping of data collected in a study that indicates the number of study subjects possessing the different values of the scale of the variable measured.

F-test: A test of the significance of differences in the values of summary measures, based on the F distribution. It is employed in such statistical procedures as the analysis of variance. The F-test, which is the ratio of:

$$\frac{\text{variance among groups}}{\text{variance within groups}}$$

provides the relative frequency (5 times out of 100, 1 time out of 100, etc.) of obtaining by randomization a value as large as that computed by the ratio. The higher the value of the F ratio, for specified-size samples, the greater is the probability that the summary measures being compared are significantly different from each other rather than their differences being attributable to random sampling. A parametric test.

generalization: Application of a general concept or idea to a relatively new object or situation.

general linear hypothesis: The statistical model underlying many hypotheses tested in explanatory research, such as comparative experiments. It expresses the statistical relationship between independent and dependent variables. In its most elementary form it can be stated as: $Y = a + (b)X$ in which Y, the dependent variable, is a function of X, the independent variable.

Hawthorne effect: A term used to describe the way people who are put in a specialized research setting tend to respond psychologically to the conditions of the study—i.e., to the novelty of the situation or to the fact of having been treated in a special way. It was first described in the classic experiments at the Hawthorne plant of the Western Electric Company in Chicago during the late 1920's and early 1930's. The psychological reaction to the study conditions can be mistaken for the effect of the explanatory independent variable manipulated by the experimenter and can lead to spurious inferences.

historical method: A study of persons by tracing the events in their life history.

hypothesis(es): Statement(s) of the expected relationship(s) among the phenomena being studied; tentative explanation of a complex set of data not yet proved; a tentative deduction; usually the first step in problem solving.

induction: A process of reasoning that starts with facts about specific situations and attempts to establish general propositions. Reasoning from the particular to the general.

inference: A judgment based on other information rather than on direct observation. Statistical inference is the process by which one is able to make generalizations from the data. The process consists of conducting an experiment in such a way that it is possible to replicate the exact experiment in other situations or groups. Statistical methods make it possible to determine to what extent the new averages, measures of variation, and relationships differ from those obtained by prior experiments.

interviewing: A process by which the observer gathers data by verbal questioning of the study subjects to elicit data on the variables being studied.

investigation: The systematic examination of phenomena to describe or explain them.

Kolmogorov-Smirnov D test: "A nonparametric statistical test designed to measure whether the difference between two frequency distributions probably is significant or is merely due to chance. The two frequency distributions being compared may be the distributions of two independent samples or the comparison may be between the distribution of one sample and a theoretical distribution. In the Kolmogorov-Smirnov test the cumulative percentages of the two distributions in each category or *class interval* are compared."[15]

Kuder-Richardson formula: ". . . provides estimates of the reliability of a single test from a single administration. The information ordinarily required is the number of items in the test, the standard deviation of the test scores, and the difficulty of each item in the test, or the average difficulty of all items as reflected in the mean test score. Because of this convenience and their statistical soundness, the Kuder-Richardson formulas are now widely used in the estimation of test reliability."[16]

latin-square design: A type of experimental design involving multiple comparisons that was developed to make efficient use of the study subjects. In this design the number of times each alternative of the independent variable is replicated is equal to the number of different comparison groups.

level of significance: States the risk of rejecting the null hypothesis and accepting the alternative hypothesis when in fact the null hypothesis is true.

Likert scale: "A summated attitude scale consisting of a series of items (attitude statements) each of which is rated by the respondent to indicate his degree of agreement or disagreement. Typically each statement has five possible responses: strongly agree, agree, uncertain, disagree, strongly disagree."[17]

Mann-Whitney U test: "A nonparametric statistical test based on rank order. When data from two samples are in the form of ranks, or relative position in terms of magnitude, this test may be used to determine whether one sample has significantly higher ranks than the other sample. On this basis the test indicates whether the two samples probably are drawn from different populations or from the same population with the observed differences due merely to chance. The Mann-Whitney U test is generally regarded as one of the most powerful nonparametric tests available for determining differences in central tendency in a series of data. It provides a nonparametric alternative for the parametric *t* test."[18]

measure of central tendency: A summary measure of the values of the measurements of a particular variable that represents the most typical, common, central, or average value for all the subjects studied. The three most frequently employed measures of central tendency are the mean, median, and mode. In a normal distribution of measurement values the mean, median, and mode are identical in value.

  mean: The sum of all the values in the distribution divided by the number of values.

median: When the values of the measurements are arranged in order of magnitude the median is the value that is larger than half of the values and smaller than the other half. It is the middle value of a distribution—the fiftieth percentile.

mode: The most common value in a distribution of measurements.

measure of variation: A summary measure of the dispersion of the values of the measurements of a particular variable among the study subjects. Common measures of variation are: range, standard deviation, and variance.

range: The lowest and the highest values in the set of measurements. Sometimes considered as the difference between the lowest and highest values.

standard deviation: The most widely used measure of variation. It is computed as follows: the difference between the value of each individual measurement and the mean is determined and each deviation is squared. The sum of all the squared deviations is divided by the number of measurements, and the square root of this quotient is obtained.

variance: The square of the standard deviation.

MEDLARS: Medical Literature Analysis and Retrieval System is a computer-based bibliographic system making possible the publication of an index to the published medical and related literature and the retrieval of specialized bibliographic information on both recurring and demand bases.

method of agreement: If the circumstances that lead up to the occurrence of a given event, *B*, have during every occurrence of the event only one factor in common. *A*, then *A* is probably the cause of *B*.

method of difference: If two or more sets of circumstances are different in respect to only one factor, *A*, and if a given event, *B* occurs only when *A* is present, then *A* is likely to be the cause of *B*.

method of residues: When the factors that are known to cause a part of some phenomenon are isolated, the remaining part of the phenomenon is the effect of the residual factors.

model, conceptual: A diagrammatic representation of a postulate or concept. A model in research is a symbolic or physical visualization of a theory, law, or other abstract construct. It is an analogy of the actual phenomenon expressed in a format that is more readily grasped and understood than the abstract conceptual scheme it is used to describe. Models can either be physical or symbolic. Physical models include life-like physical representations, abstract physical representations, and schematic and other diagrams. Symbolic models include mathematical and statistical models in which letters of the alphabet are used to represent the various elements included in the model, while specially devised symbols are used to indicate the mathematical operations designated by the model. Mathematical models are an exact quantitative formulation of the relationship among the factors they include. A statistical model states the quantitative relationship among the factors in probabilistic terms.

Neyman-Pearson approach to statistical inference: This approach uses traditional tests of significance in which all elements of the research design—the null hypothesis, the alternative hypotheses, and the level of significance—are established in advance of the actual data collection and kept fixed during the course of the study. An objective approach to significance testing as compared to the personalistic approach of Bayesian inference.

normal curve: A bell-shaped curve that indicates that the majority of the values of the measurements of a variable for a group of study subjects cluster together and possess about the same scale value while fewer and fewer subjects possess the more extreme values—those away from the values held by the majority of subjects. Also called the guassion curve after its discoverer, the German mathematician, Karl F. Gauss. The properties of the normal curve are very valuable in statistical analysis of data. In a normal curve:

± 1 standard deviations from the mean =   68 per cent of all the values.
± 2 standard deviations from the mean =   95 per cent of all the values.
± 3 standard deviations from the mean = 100 per cent of all the values.

norms: A set of scores on a test derived from a representative group of respondents. Norms are used as standards for evaluating the scores obtained by users of the test.

null hypothesis: When we are studying the differences between experimental and control groups, or in any research in which we are comparing summary measures determined from samples, we usually wish to test some hypothesis about the nature of the true difference between the populations represented by the samples. Most commonly, the statistical analysis is directed toward testing the *null hypothesis,* which states that the obtained differences in the values of the summary measures between the groups being compared could have occurred by chance alone, because of having sampled, and there really is no difference between the groups. This means that if we repeated our experiment many times and calculated the differences in the values of the criterion measures between the experimental and the control groups for each experiment, the average difference would be zero. (We add the positive differences together and subtract the negative differences, and divide by the number of differences we have measured.)

If our statistical analysis (called the statistical test of significance) leads us to the conclusion that the observed differences in our samples could have arisen by chance *only* a small percentage of times in the absence of true differences between the populations represented by our samples, we reject the null hypothesis, that is, we conclude that there probably is a genuine difference between the two populations. In the social sciences, it is more or less conventional to reject the null hypothesis when the statistical analysis indicates that the observed difference would not occur by chance alone more often than 5 times out of 100 repeated experiments (called the .05 level of significance).

In addition to the null hypothesis every explanatory study also includes *alternative hypotheses.* These may express the expectation of the researcher—that there *is* a genuine difference between the groups he is studying. If on the basis of the study findings we reject the null hypothesis, we have thus accepted the alternative hypothesis. Conversely, when we accept the null hypothesis, we reject the alternative hypothesis.

nursing: It is a service to individuals and to families, therefore to society. It is based upon an art and science which mold the attitudes. intellectual competencies, and technical skills of the individual nurse into the desire and ability to help people, sick or well, cope with their health needs.

nursing diagnosis: Determination of the nature and extent of nursing problems presented by individual patients receiving nursing care and their families.

nursing research: A systematic, detailed attempt to discover or confirm the facts that relate to a specific problem or problems in the field of nursing. It has as its goal the provision of scientific knowledge in nursing. Research in nursing is primarily interdisciplinary.

nursing science: A body of scientific knowledge from the physical, biological, and social sciences that is uniquely nursing.

observers: Research personnel who collect the data.

nonparticipant observer: Serves as the recorder of the data, but is not one of the study subjects.

participant observer: Collects the required data while taking part in the activity being studied.

operational definition: A series of words that clearly designate performable and observable acts or operations that can be verified by others.

optimum allocation: A technical procedure to determine the best possible allocation of the sampling units into strata. Can tell the researcher what is the most efficient size sample for each stratum.

pairing: A method of matching the individual members of the experimental and control samples with respect to relevant organismic covariables. Helps to equate the groups more closely than what can be achieved by randomization alone.

panel design: A technique in which a selected sample of subjects is interviewed, usually about the same variable (e.g., income), recurrently over an extended period of time to study the change that has taken place.

parameters: Summary measures, such as means and standard deviations, that are computed from data obtained from all the sampling units in the target population.

percentage: A type of summary measure known as a rate. A rate expresses the relative frequency of occurrence of the particular scale value for which it is computed among the subjects studied. (See page 290 for definitions and types of rates commonly used in the health field.)

percentile (P): "A point (score) in a distribution below which falls the percent of cases indicated by the given percentile. Thus the 15th percentile denotes the score or point below which 15 per cent of the scores fall. 'Percentile' has nothing to do with the per cent of correct answers an examinee has on a test."[19]

phenomenon: That which is open to observation; an event; a fact.

pilot study: A study carried out before a research design is completely formulated to assist in (a) the formulation of the problem, or (b) the development of hypotheses, or (c) the establishment of priorities for further research. Also called an exploratory study.

placebo (Latin—"I will please."): Term used in clinical trials of drugs to describe an inert capsule tablet or injection given to members of the control group that is disguised to serve as an imitation of the drug actually being tested among the experimental subjects. It is used to control psychological bias by matching the experimental and control groups in terms of equivalent exposure to the *process* of drug administration.

poisson distribution: A binomial distribution where the probability of occurrence of a defined event is extremely small.

prediction: A statement about an event not yet observed detailing what will be found when it is observed.

premise: A proposition stated or assumed as leading to a conclusion. Something taken for granted.

pretest: This test takes place *after* the research design has been formulated (a) to develop the procedures for applying the research instruments, or (b) to test the wording of questions, or (c) to insure, as far as practical, that the specific questions or observations are relevant and precise.

product-moment method: A technique used to compute the coefficient of correlation (r) for quantitative variables. It is the ratio of two standard deviations. The numerator of the ratio is the standard deviation of the values of the dependent variable *calculated* from the regression equation, and the denominator is the standard deviation of the *actual* values of the dependent variable that were obtained from the sample.

projective techniques: A method for collecting data in which the subjects are asked to respond to nonstructured or ambiguous stimuli—an ambiguity that the investigator may make no attempt to conceal. Examples of projective techniques are the Rorschach test, the thematic apperception test, and the word association test.

prospective design: A type of research design in which the collection of data proceeds forward in time. It includes such studies as an experiment in which the study begins with alternative groups of study subjects who are exposed to the independent variable and then followed up over a period of time and compared in terms of some criterion measure. Prospective designs are also used in nonexperimental research.

A cohort study is a type of prospective nonexperimental study in which the same group of subjects—e.g., all graduates from a school of nursing in 1965—are followed up over a period of years, and data are routinely gathered from them on variables of interest to the researcher.

Q-sort: A technique originally developed to explore the personality of individuals. Provides a method for deriving an ordinal scale for measuring certain kinds of variables. A sorting process is employed in which the rater is given a collection of items to sort into a number of piles to determine the rater's own attitudes toward the object being rated (e.g., satisfaction with nursing care). It is a *forced choice* method of scaling a variable in that the number of items that can be sorted into any one pile is predetermined. In the Q-sort the number of items that can be placed in each pile follows the pattern of the normal curve.

random sample: "A sample of the members of a population drawn in such a way that every member of the population has an equal chance of being included —that is, drawn in a way that precludes the operation of bias or selection. The purpose in using a sample thus free of bias is, of course, that the sample be fairly 'representative' of the total population, so that sample findings may be generalized to the population. A great advantage of random samples is that formulas are available for estimating the expected variation of the sample statistics from their true values in the total population; in other words, we know how precise an estimate of the population value is given by a random sample of any given size."[20]

random start: In systematic sampling, as in sampling from names on a list, the first name is chosen randomly from among the first n names, and after that every nth name is selected for the sample.

randomization: A technique in experimental research to equalize the composition of the various groups under study so that they are identical in respect to all pertinent organismic variables. Subjects are allocated to the different study groups according to the laws of chance. The procedure of randomization is known as random assignment or allocation.

regression analysis: In studies of independent and dependent variables that are both measurable in terms of quantitative scales, if a sufficiently large number of measurements were obtained, it would be possible to fit an equation, called a regression equation, to the data which would express the relationship between the variables. The test of significance between the variables is an evaluation of the slope of the line that is fitted to the data, called the regression coefficient.

reliability: A criterion for assessing the quality of data. Data are reliable if they are consistent, accurate, and precise. Another term for reliability is precision.

replication: The subdividing of an experiment into a number of parts—the replicas—each of which contains all the essential elements with which the experiment is concerned. The term is also applied to a repetition of the identical study design among a different set of study subjects.

research: An activity whose purpose is to find a valid answer to some question that has been raised. The answers provide new knowledge to the world at large. It is a purposeful activity.

applied research: To obtain new facts and/or identify relationships among facts that are intended to be used in a real-life situation. Specifically, applied research is intended to solve a problem, make a decision, or develop or evaluate a program, procedure, process, or product.

basic or pure research: To establish fundamental theories, facts and/or statements of relationships among facts in some area of knowledge that are *not* intended for immediate use in some real-life situation. The aim of basic research is to advance scientific knowledge and to facilitate further research in the area of knowledge.

descriptive research: The research is primarily concerned with obtaining accurate and meaningful descriptions of the phenomena under study. "Absolute" research is sometimes used as a designation of a descriptive study.

developmental research: The aim of this research is to develop a new procedure, program, or product.

evaluative research: A program, method, procedure, or product is tested to assess the quality, applicability, feasibility, desirability, or worth in terms of some meaningful criterion measure.

experimental and nonexperimental research: In experimental research all elements of the research are under control of the investigator, and it is often conducted in a specialized research setting: laboratory, experimental unit, or research center. This type of research is prospective. In nonexperimental research all elements of the research are not under direct control of the investigator, and it is conducted in a natural setting such as a school, a public health agency, a hospital, or a patient's home. This type of research is frequently retrospective.

explanatory research: The aim of this type of research is to test a hypothesis about a relationship between an independent variable (causal, treatment, stimulus variable) and a dependent variable (effect, response, or criterion variable). The independent variable is manipulated by the researcher.

methodological research: To develop methods, tools, products, or procedures for conducting further research or for use in practice; to develop theories and models.

research design: Plan of the research that is developed prior to the actual launching of the study. It is part of a number of steps beginning with the formulation of the problem and ending with a report of the findings of the study.

Sometimes referred to as a research proposal or research protocol. Research designs may be experimental or nonexperimental, prospective or retrospective, longitudinal or cross-sectional.

research personnel:

principal investigator: One designated as assuming major responsibility for the administration of the research. The individual who originated the study, developed the initial research plan, and is responsible for the scientific merit of the research.

project director: An individual who is designated to work under the direction of the principal investigator and is responsible for the technical aspects of the research, such as data collection. Some studies designate only a project director, in which case the individual carries out the functions of both the principal investigator and the project director.

research associate or assistant: A junior investigator who works under the direction of the project director.

research problem: The motivation for undertaking a study that consists of a definition of concepts and terms narrowed down from a broadly stated question into one more restricted in scope and related to research findings that have been obtained by others.

retrospective design: In nonexperimental explanatory studies it is the type of design in which the dependent variable is observed first and the data are traced back and related to possible relevant independent variables that are hypothesized as being associated with the dependent variable. Nonexperimental descriptive studies can also be retrospective in that the data collected refer back to a prior point in time.

role analysis: A sociological technique based on the concept of a role as a patterned sequence of learned actions or deeds performed by a person in an interaction situation.

Rorschach test: A projective test utilizing 10 cards printed with inkblots to which the subject responds. The test is diagnostic of personality as a whole.

sampling: The process of selecting a fraction of the sampling units of a target population for inclusion in a study.

cluster sampling (multistage): Used in large-scale descriptive studies involving target populations with geographically dispersed sampling units. The cluster, or primary sampling unit, might represent a hospital or a block within a neighborhood. The elementary sampling unit on which measurements are desired might be the patients in the hospital or the residents of the block. Commonly used in epidemiological studies.

convenience sampling: Subjects are selected because they happen to be available for participation in the study at a certain time.

probability sampling: A method whereby each sampling unit in the target population has a known—greater than zero—probability of being selected in the sample. Neither the sampler nor the sampling unit has any conscious influence over the inclusion in the sample of a specific sampling unit, since the sampling units are selected by chance. Also known as random and scientific sampling. Distinguished from purposive sampling (convenience, quota, and purposive sampling) where the sampling units are deliberately selected according to certain criteria.

purposive sampling: A sample in which the sampling units are deliberately (nonrandomly) selected according to certain criteria that are known to be important and are considered to be representative of the target population. Purposive sampling is also known as judgment sampling.

quota sampling: Similar to a convenience sample, but in which the use of controls prevents overloading the sample with subjects having certain characteristics. The controls are established by determining the distribution of the sampling units according to those variables deemed to be important.

sequential sampling: The sampling units are taken into the study sequentially and the number to be included in the study is not fixed in advance. Useful in testing the effects of drugs on patients.

simple random sampling: Each sampling unit has an equal probability of being selected for the sample.

stratified random sample: The target population is subdivided into homogeneous subpopulations. Then, a random sample or a systematic sample is selected from each subpopulation.

systematic sampling: After a random start, every *n*th unit (name on a list, patient in a bed, house on block) is selected in the order in which the units are arranged.

sampling error (standard error): A measure of the extent to which the sample findings are different from what they would be if all the sampling units in the target population had been studied. For summary measures like the mean and percentage, the sampling error is the ratio of the variation (standard deviation) of the values of the measurements among the sampling units in the target population to the square root of the number of sampling units in the sample. This formula is modified according to the type of sampling design used. Measures of sampling error are also known as standard errors.

sampling units: The individual discrete members of a target population. Sampling units can consist of human beings, animals, plants, or inanimate objects.

scale: A device for determining the magnitude or quantity of the variable being measured possessed by the study subjects to whom it is applied (quantitative variables) or for determining the appropriate discrete class or category of the variable to which the study subject belongs (qualitative variables).

graphic rating scale: A scale in which the variable is qualitatively scaled along a continuum from one extreme to the other. A rater makes a direct rating on the scale.

Guttman-type scale: A scale in which the different items composing the scale have a cumulative property so that a person who responds a certain way to, say, the third item on a scale is almost certain to have responded the same way to the preceding two items.

interval scale: A quantitative scale in which the distance between the points is equal, so we can justifiably break the intervals down into finer subdivisions that will provide us with more refined distinctions among the study subjects we are measuring. An interval scale has no zero point (e.g., scale for body temperature) in contrast to a ratio scale (weight scale), which does.

Likert-type scale: An ordinal-type scale in which the variable is evaluated by a series of statements that when responded to by study subjects, according to, say, degree of favorableness or unfavorableness toward each statement, can provide a criterion measure of the variable.

nominal scale: A qualitative scale consisting of a number of discrete, mutually exclusive and exhaustive categories of a variable, each possessing a distinctive attribute in terms of the variable (e.g., sex: female-male; types of illnesses).

ordinal scale: A qualitative scale in which the different categories included in the scale are related in terms of a graded order (e.g., excellent, very good, average, poor).

qualitative scale: A type of scale in which the subject is observed, and on the basis of the definition of the variable the subject is placed into one of its categories. The numerical data yielded by such a scale are called frequency data and show the number of subjects who are classified into each of the discrete categories of the scale. Sometimes called enumeration scales. Nominal and ordinal scales are examples of qualitative scales.

ratio scale: A quantitative scale possessing a true zero point. A scale with an absolute zero point—the total absence of the variable—makes it possible to determine not only how much greater one measurement is from another as in an interval scale, but also how many times greater it is (e.g., a scale for the variable "time").

Thurstone-type scale: An ordinal scale useful in studying attitude-type variables in which an attempt is made to establish the quantitative distance between the categories included in the scale. Also known as the method of "equal-appearing intervals." A battery of statements, each with its own scale value, is presented to the rater, and he checks those statements which most closely represent his own position. An overall scale value is assigned on the basis of the average value of the items checked by the respondent.

science: A systematic method of describing and controlling the material world.

Science Information Exchange (S.I.E.): A clearinghouse for information on current scientific research actually in progress, originally maintained by the Smithsonian Institution, Washington, D.C., and transferred to National Technical Information Service (NTIS).

score: A quantitative value assigned to a scale, test, or other type of data-gathering instrument to indicate the degree to which the respondent possesses the variable being measured.

serendipity: A situation in which a secondary discovery is more significant than the original objective of the research.

spurious correlation: This is said to occur when a direct cause and effect relationship is inferred between two variables when no such relationship actually exists. Instead, both variables are dependent upon a third variable that has not been controlled in the study.

statistical significance: To test whether two or more groups being compared in terms of a summary measure—a mean, a standard deviation, a percentage, or, nonparametrically, in terms of their rank order on a qualitative scale—could be considered to have come from the same target population or not (i.e., that they are essentially two independent samples from the same population).

statistics: Summary measures, such as percentages, means, medians, percentiles, and standard deviations, that are computed from measurements obtained from a sample of the total population. Estimates of population parameters.

stochastic process: A series of events for which the estimate of the probability of a certain outcome approaches the true probability as the number of events increases.

subjects in research: The persons or things from whom data are collected. Study subjects can be human beings, animals, plants, cells, or inanimate objects.

survey: Nonexperimental research conducted in a natural setting in which there is less control over the study subjects and the setting than in an experiment.

target population: The total membership of a defined set of subjects from which a sample of the study subjects is selected. Projection of data obtained in a study proceeds from the sample to the target population.

test of statistical significance: A statistical technique to test whether the summary measures being compared, after allowing for a sampling error, could be independent estimates of the same population parameter. If so, they can be considered as identical, and any differences among them can be attributed to sampling error.

nonparametric tests of statistical significance: Tests of significance, sometimes called order statistics. Many of these tests treat data in terms of ordinal rankings or comparisons, as in rank correlation and the sign test techniques as well as in the other nonparametric methods such as the runs tests, median test, and Mann-Whitney U test. Nonparametric tests, also known as distribution-free tests of statistical significance, make no assumptions about the nature of the distribution of the values of the measurements in the target population from which the sampling units were selected and require only that the sampling units be selected randomly and the measurements be independent.

parametric tests of statistical significance: Tests of parameters such as the mean and standard deviation that are based on random sampling distributions as the normal curve, the t distribution, and the F distribution. Parametric tests require that certain assumptions be met concerning the distribution of the values of the measurements in the target population from which the sampling units were selected. Parametric tests are useful in testing variables having quantitative scales, interval or ratio. Parametric tests are more sensitive than nonparametric tests.

power of a test of statistical significance: The probability of rejecting the null hypothesis when it is actually false. It is a measure of the sensitivity of the test —the extent to which it isolates real differences among the groups that were studied.

Type I error in a test of statistical significance: This error is incurred in a test of statistical significance when we reject the null hypothesis and accept the alternative hypothesis when in fact the null hypothesis is true. The level of significance selected in the test of significance (e.g., .05) is the risk of committing this error.

Type II error in a test of statistical significance: This error is incurred in a test of statistical significance when we accept the null hypothesis and reject the alternative hypothesis when the alternative hypothesis is actually true. Reducing the risk of Type I error increases the risk of committing a Type II error.

thermatic apperception test (T.A.T.): A projective test in which a person is asked to tell a story suggested by a series of pictures.

theory: Summarizes existing knowledge, provides an explanation for observed facts and relationships, and predicts the occurrence of as yet unobserved events and relationships on the basis of explanatory principles, embodied in the theory. Scientific theory is composed of definitions, postulates, and deductions.

t-test: A parametric statistical test for small samples based on students *t* distribution. It can be used to test the significance of the difference in the values of summary measures for two samples. Significance is assessed by determining whether this difference exceeds the amount that could be attributed to random sampling. If it does not, the two sample summary measures can be considered to be independent estimates of the same population parameter and the two samples as having been randomly drawn from the same population. In a test of the differences between two sample means, the t-test is in the form of the following ratio (under the null hypothesis the difference in population means is considered to be zero):

$$\frac{\text{Difference in sample means minus difference in population means}}{\text{Standard error of the difference in sample means}}$$

When the number of sampling units is large, the test is known as the T-test and is based on the normal rather than the t distribution.

two-tailed test: "A *statistical test* used to test a hypothesis when the direction of the difference between samples or relationship between variables is not predicted in the hypothesis. That is, the null hypothesis merely states that there will not be significant difference between the samples, or relationship between the variables, and the alternative hypothesis does not specify which sample will be further in a given direction (score higher, be more favorable, etc.) if there is a difference, or if there is a relationship between the variables whether it will be positive or negative. The term 'two-tailed' refers to the fact that there is a *region of rejection* of the null hypothesis at both ends (or tails) of the *sampling distribution*.[21]

validity: A criterion for evaluating the quality of data. Data are valid if they actually measure what they are supposed to measure. Another term for validity is relevance.

value: The individual's evaluation of the positive, neutral, or negative character of an object, someone's behavior, or a situation.

variable: The characteristic, property, trait, or attribute of the person or thing observed in a study. Variables must have a scale of measurement possessing at least two mutually exclusive values and must give rise to statistical data.

   dependent variable: The variable that is observed to determine the effect of the manipulation of the independent variable. It can be called the criterion, effect, or response variable.

   environmental variable: Relates to the many factors in the setting in which the individual is studied that can impinge on the individual (e.g., economic, anthropological, sociological, and physical factors).

   extraneous variable: The variable(s) that are not of primary interest to the researcher but are present in large numbers in any study involving human beings. They include organismic and environmental variables. They may be controlled or uncontrolled.

   independent variable: The variable that is changed or manipulated by the researcher. It may be called the experimental, treatment, causal, or stimulus variable.

   organismic variable: Deals with all the many personal characteristics of human beings as individuals—physiological, psychological, and demographic.

weighted scoring: ". . . the number of points awarded for the correct response is not the same for all items in the test. In some cases, weighted scoring involves the award of different numbers of points for the choice of different responses to the same item."[22]

Yule's coefficient of association: A technique to estimate the coefficient of correlation for qualitative variables, each having two categories. $A = \dfrac{ad - bc}{ad + bc}$ where a, b, c, d are the four cells in a 2×2 table: $\begin{array}{c|c} a & b \\ \hline c & d \end{array}$,

References

1. S. Hillier Frederick, and Jerald Lieberman, *Introduction to Operations Research*. Holden-Day, Inc., San Francisco, 1967, p. 555.
2. George Theodorsen and Achilles Theodorson, *Modern Dictionary of Sociology*. Apollo Editions, Thomas T. Crowell Company, 1969, p. 41.
3. *Ibid.*, p. 42.
4. *Ibid.*, pp. 50–51.
5. *Ibid.*, p. 74.
6. *Ibid.*, p. 80.
7. *Ibid.*, p. 85.
8. *Ibid.*, pp. 85–86.
9. *Ibid.*, p. 108.
10. *Ibid.*, p. 130.
11. *Ibid.*, p. 133.
12. *Ibid.*, p. 133.
13. *Ibid.*, p. 142.
14. Test Department, *Test Service Notebook, N. 13*. Tarrytown, N.Y., Harcourt, Brace, and World, Inc., (No. Date), p. 2.
15. Theodorson, *op. cit.*, pp. 221–22.
16. Ebel Robert, "Appendix Glossary of Terms Used in Educational Measurement," in *Measuring Education Achievement*. Englewood Cliffs, N.J., Prentice-Hall, 1965, p. 454.
17. Theodorson, *op. cit.*, p. 232.
18. *Ibid.*, pp. 241–42.
19. Test Department, *op. cit.*, p. 4.
20. *Ibid.*, p. 5.
21. Theodorson, *op. cit.*, p. 444.
22. Ebel, *op. cit.*, p. 468.

BIBLIOGRAPHY

Selected Research References

1. Abdellah, F. G., *Overview of Nursing Research, 1955–1968*. National Center for Health Services Research and Development, Rockville, Md., 1971. Also see by the same author "Overview of Nursing Research, 1955–1968." *Nurs. Res.,* **19:**6–17, January–February 1970; **19:**157–62, March–April 1970; **19:**239–52, May–June, 1970; and "U.S. Public Health Service's Contribution to Nursing Research—Past, Present, Future." *Nurs. Res.,* **26:**244–49, July–August 1977.

2. Abdellah, F. G., "The Nature of Nursing Science. Conference on the Nature of Science in Nursing." *Nurs. Res.,* **18:**390–93, September–October 1969.

3. Abdellah, F. G., and Levine, E., *Appraising the Clinical Resources in Small Hospitals*. U.S. Public Health Service Monograph No. 24. Government Printing Office, Washington, D.C., 1954.

4. Abdellah, F. G., "Criterion Measures in Nursing." *Nurs. Res.,* **10:**21–26, winter 1961.

5. Abdellah, F. G., and Levine, E., "Developing a Measure of Patient and Personnel Satisfaction with Nursing Care." *Nurs. Res.,* **5:**100–108, February 1957.

6. Abdellah, F. G., and Levine, E., *Effect of Nurse Staffing on Satisfactions with Nursing Care*. Hospital Monograph Series No. 4. American Hospital Association, Chicago, 1958.

7. Abdellah, F. G., and Levine, E., *Patients and Personnel Speak* (rev. ed.). U.S. Public Health Service Publication No. 527. Government Printing Office, Washington, D.C., 1964.

8. Abdellah, F. G., Beland, I., Martin, A., and Matheney, R., *Patient-Centered Approaches to Nursing*. Macmillan Publishing Co., Inc., New York, 1960.

9. Abdellah, F. G., and Levine, E., "Work Sampling Applied to the Study of Nursing Personnel." *Nurs. Res.,* **3:**11–16, June 1954.

10. Ackoff, R. L., *The Design of Social Research*. University of Chicago Press, Chicago, 1953.

11. Aday, L. A., *The Utilization of Health Services: Indices and Correlates*. DHEW Publication No. (HSM) 73–3003. National Center for Health Services Research and Development, Hyattsville, Md., 1973.

12. Altman, S. H., *Present and Future Supply of Registered Nurses.* DHEW Publication No. (NIH) 73–134. U.S. Government Printing Office, Washington, D.C., 1972.

13. American Nurses' Association, *Facts About Nursing, 78–79.* The Association, Kansas City, Mo., 1979.

14. American Nurses' Association, "The Improvement of Nursing Practice." American Nurses' Association, New York, 1961.

15. American Nurses' Foundation, "Research-Pathway to Future Progress in Nursing Care." *Nurs. Res.,* **9:**4–7, winter 1960.

16. Anderson, E. T., et al., *The Development and Implementation of a Curriculum Model for Community Nurse Practitioners.* U.S. Government Printing Office, Washington, D.C., 1977.

17. Anscombe, F. J., "Sequential Medical Trials." *J. Am. Statistical A.,* **58:** 365–83, June 1963.

18. Applied Management Sciences, *Review of Health Manpower Population Requirements Standards.* DHEW Publication No. (HRA) 77–22. Health Resources Administration, Hyattsville, Md., 1976.

19. Applied Management Sciences, *The Area Resource File.* DHEW Publication No. (HRA) 78–69. Health Resources Administration, Hyattsville, Md., 1978.

20. Armitage, P., *Sequential Medical Trials.* John Wiley & Sons, Inc., New York, 1975.

21. Army Air Forces's Aviation Psychology, Program Research Reports, *Psychological Research in the Theatres of War, Report No. 17* (ed., W. M. Lepley). U.S. Government Printing Office, Washington, D.C., 1947.

22. Arnstein, M. G. (ed.), *International Conference on the Planning of Nursing Studies.* International Council of Nurses, Florence Nightingale Foundation, London, 1956.

23. Ashby, W. R., *An Introduction to Cybernetics.* John Wiley & Sons, Inc., New York, 1958.

24. Aspen Systems Corporation, *Selected Bibliographic References on Methodologies for Community Health Status Assessment.* DHEW Publication No. (HRA) 77–14550. Health Resources Administration, Hyattsville, Md., 1976.

25. Aydelotte, M. K., *Nurse Staffing Methodology: A Review and Critique of Selected Literature.* DHEW Publication No. (NIH) 73–433. U.S. Government Printing Office, Washington, D.C., 1973.

26. Aydelotte, M. K., and Tener, M. E., *An Investigation of the Relation Between Nursing Activity and Patient Welfare.* State University of Iowa, Iowa City, 1960.

27. Bacon, Francis, "Advancement of Learning," in *Great Books of the Western World.* Encyclopaedia Britannica, Inc., Chicago, 1952.

28. Bailey, J. T., "The Critical Incident Technique in Identifying Behavioral Criteria of Professional Nursing Effectiveness." *Nurs. Res.,* **5:**52–64. 1956.

29. Bales, R. F., *et al., Interaction Process Analysis.* Addison-Wesley Publishing Co., Inc., Cambridge, Mass., 1950.

30. Barber, T. X., *Pitfalls in Human Research: Ten Pivotal Points.* Pergamon Press, Inc., New York, 1976.

31. Barzun, J., and Graff, H. P., *The Modern Researcher,* 3rd. ed. Harcourt Brace Jovanovich, Inc., New York, 1977.

32. Batey, M. V. (ed.), *Communicating Nursing Research: Vol. 4: Is the Gap Being Bridged?* Western Interstate Commission for Higher Education, Boulder, Col., July 1971.

33. Batey, M. V. (ed.), *Communicating Nursing Research: Vol. 7: Critical Issues in Access to Data.* Western Interstate Commission for Higher Education, Boulder, Col., January 1975.

34. Batey, M. V. (ed.), *Communicating Nursing Research: Vol. 8: Nursing Research Priorities: Choice or Chance.* Western Interstate Commission for Higher Education, Boulder, Col., March 1977.

35. Batey, M. V. (ed.), *Communicating Nursing Research, Vol. 9: Nursing Research in the Bicentennial Year.* Western Interstate Commission for Higher Education, Boulder, Col., April 1977.

36. Batey, M. V. (ed.), *Communicating Nursing Research, Vol. 10: Optimizing Environments for Health: Nursing's Unique Perspective.* Western Interstate Commission for Higher Education, Boulder, Col., September 1977.

37. Battistella, R. M., and Weil, T. P., *Health Care Organization. Bibliography and Guidebook.* Association of University Programs in Hospital Administration, Washington, D.C., 1971.

38. Bennis, W. G., *et al.,* "Reference Group and Loyalties in the Outpatient Department." *Admin. Sci. Qt.,* **2:**481–500, March 1958.

39. Bennis, W. G., *et al., The Role of the Nurse in the Outpatient Department.* American Nurses' Foundation, Inc., New York, 1961.

40. Bergan, T., and Hirsch, G., *A National Model of Nurse Supply, Demand, and Distribution: Summary Report.* Western Interstate Commission on Higher Education, Boulder, Col., 1976.

41. Bermosk, L. S., and Mordam, M. J., *Interviewing in Nursing.* Macmillan Publishing Co., Inc., New York, 1973.

42. Berthold, J. S., Curran, M. A., and Barhyte, D. Y., *Educational Technology and the Teaching-Learning Process: A Selected Bibliography.* Division of Nursing, Bethesda, Md., 1970.

43. Beshers, J. M., "Models and Theory Construction." *Am. Sociol. Rev.,* **22:** 32–38, February 1957.

44. Beveridge, W. I. B., *The Art of Scientific Investigation* (rev. ed.). W. W. Norton and Co., New York, 1957.

45. Bircher, A. U., "On the Development and Classification of Diagnoses." *Nurs. Forum,* **14:**10–29, winter 1975.

46. Blalock, H. M., Jr., *Theory Construction.* Prentice-Hall, Englewood Cliffs, New Jer., 1970.

47. Blalock, H. M., Jr. (ed.), *Causal Methods in the Social Sciences.* Aldine Publishing Co., Chicago, 1971.

48. Blankenship, A., *Consumer and Opinion Research.* Harper and Row, New York, 1949.

49. Bloch, D., "Some Crucial Terms in Nursing: What Do They Really Mean?" *Nurs. Outlook,* **22:**689–94, November 1974.

50. Blumberg, M., and Drew, J. A., "Methods for Assessing Nursing Care Quality." *Hospitals, J.A.H.A.,* **37:**72–80, November 1, 1963.

51. Borger, R., and Cioffi, F., *Explanation in the Behavioral Sciences.* The University Press, Cambridge, 1970.

52. Boyle, R., *A Study of Student Nurse Perception of Patient Attitudes.* U.S. Public Health Service Publication No. 769. Government Printing Office, Washington, D.C., 1960.

53. Braithwaite, R. B., *Scientific Explanation: A Study of the Functions of Theory, Probability and Law in Science.* Cambridge University, Cambridge, England, 1953.

54. Brink, P. J., and Wood, M. J., *Basic Steps in Planning Nursing Research: From Question to Proposal.* Duxbury Press, North Scituate, Mass., 1978.

55. Brook, R. H., *Quality of Care Assessment: A Comparison of Five Methods of Peer Review.* DHEW Publication No. (HRA) 74–3100. National Center for Health Services Research and Development, Hyattsville, Md., 1973.

56. Bross, I. D. J., *Design for Decision.* Macmillan Publishing Co., Inc., New York, 1953.

57. Brown, E. L., *Newer Dimensions of Patient Care—Part I.* Russell Sage Foundation, New York, 1961.

58. Brown, E. L., *Newer Dimensions of Patient Care—Part II: Improving Staff Motivation and Competence in the General Hospital.* Russell Sage Foundation, New York, 1962.

59. Brown, M. (ed.), *Readings in Gerontology.* C. V. Mosby Co., St. Louis, 1978.

60. Brown, R., *Explanation in Social Science.* Aldine Publishing Co., Chicago, 1963.

61. Buckley, W. (ed.), *Modern Systems Research for the Behavioral Scientist.* Aldine Publishing Co., Chicago, 1968.

62. Bunge, H. L., "Research Is Every Professional Nurse's Business." *Am. J. Nurs.,* **58:**816–19, 1958.

63. Burling, T., Lentz, E. M., and Wilson, R. N., *The Give and Take in Hospitals.* G. P. Putnam's Sons, New York, 1956.

64. Bush, G. P., and Hattery, L. H., *Scientific Research, Its Administration and Organization.* American University Press, Washington, D.C., 1950.

65. Cambridge Research Institute, *Trends Affecting the U.S. Health Care System,* DHEW Publication No. (HRA) 76–14503. U.S. Government Printing Office, Washington, D.C., 1975.

66. Campbell, C., *Nursing Diagnosis and Intervention in Nursing Practice.* John Wiley & Sons, Inc., New York, 1978.

67. Campbell, D. T., "Factors Relevant to the Validity of Experiments in Social Settings." *Psychol. Bull.,* **54:**297–312, 1957.

68. Campbell, N., "Measurement," in *The World of Mathematics,* J. R. Newman (ed.). Simon and Schuster, New York, 1956, Vol. 3, pp. 1797–1813.

69. Cannon, W. B., "The Role of Chance in Discovery." *Scientific Monthly,* **51:**204–209, 1940.

70. Cannon, W. B., *The Wisdom of the Body,* 2nd ed., rev. W. W. Norton and Co., New York, 1939.

71. Cartwright, D., and Zander, A. (eds.), *Group Dynamics: Research and Theory*. Harper and Row, New York, 1968.

72. Chapin, F. S., *Experimental Designs in Sociological Research*. Greenwood Press, Inc., Westport, Conn., 1974.

73. Chew, V., *Experimental Designs in Industry*. John Wiley & Sons, Inc., New York, 1958.

74. Churchman, C. W., *The Systems Approach*. Dell Publishing Co., New York, 1968.

75. Clearinghouse on Health Indexes, *Cumulated Annotations, 1976*. DHEW Publication No (PHS) 78–1225. National Center for Health Statistics, Hyattsville, Md., 1978.

76. Coch, L., and French, J. R. P., Jr., "Overcoming Resistance to Change," in D. Cartwright and A. Zander (eds.), *Group Dynamics: Research and Theory*, 2nd ed. Harper and Row, New York, 1953, pp. 257–79.

77. Cochran, W. G., and Cox, G. M., *Experimental Designs*, 2nd ed. John Wiley & Sons, Inc., New York, 1957.

78. Cochran, W. G., "Matching in Analytical Studies." *Am. J. Pub. Health,* **43:**684–91, June 1953.

79. Cochran, W. G., "Research Techniques in the Study of Human Beings." *Milbank Mem. Fund Qt.,* **33:**121–36, April 1955.

80. Cochran, W. G., *Sampling Techniques*. John Wiley & Sons, Inc., New York, 1977.

81. Cohen, J., and Cohen, P., *Applied Multiple Regression/Correlation Analysis for the Behavioral Sciences*. John Wiley & Sons, Inc., New York, 1975.

82. Cohen, M. R., and Nagel, E. *An Introduction to Logic and Scientific Method*. Harcourt, Brace and Co., New York, 1934.

83. Colton, T., *Statistics in Medicine*. Little, Brown and Co., Boston, 1974.

84. Commission on Human Resources, National Research Council, *Personnel Needs and Training for Biomedical and Behavioral Research,* Vols. I and II. National Academy of Sciences, Washington, D.C., 1977.

85. Conant, J. B., *On Understanding Science*. The New American Library of World Literature, New York, 1951.

86. Cronbach, L., *Essentials of Psychological Testing*, 3rd ed. Harper and Row, New York, 1970.

87. Dampier, Sir W. C., *A History of Science*. 4th ed. rev. Macmillan Publishing Co., Inc., New York, 1949.

88. Dawes, R. M., *Fundamentals of Attitude Measurement*. John Wiley & Sons, Inc., New York, 1972.

89. DeGeyndt, W., and Ross, K. B., *Evaluation of Health Programs: An Annotated Bibliography*. Systems Development Project, Minneapolis, 1968.

90. DeGroot, A. D., *Methodology: Foundations of Inference and Research in the Behavioral Sciences*. Mouton and Co., The Hague, 1969.

91. DHEW/Public Health Service, *National Conference on Health Promotion Programs in Occupational Settings: The Proceedings*. DHEW Publication, Office of Health Information and Health Promotion, Washington, D.C., January 17–19, 1979.

92. Division of Manpower Intelligence, *An Annotated Bibliography of Basic*

Documents Related to Health Manpower Programs. DHEW Publication No. (HRA) 75–7. U.S. Government Printing Office, Washington, D.C., 1974.

93. Division of Nursing, *Effectiveness and Efficiency of Nursing Programs.* DHEW Publication No. (HRA) 74–23. Health Resources Administration, Hyattsville, Md., 1973.

94. Division of Nursing, *First Report to the Congress, February 1, 1977. Nurse Training Act of 1975.* Report of the Secretary of Health, Education, and Welfare on the Supply and Distribution of and Requirements for Nurses as Required by Section 951, Nurse Training Act of 1975. Title IX, Public Law 94–63. DHEW Publication No. (HRA) 78–38. U.S. Government Printing Office, Washington, D.C., 1978.

95. Division of Nursing, *Source Book: Nursing Personnel.* DHEW Publication No. (HRA) 75–43. U.S. Government Printing Office, Washington, D.C., 1974.

96. Division of Nursing, *Survey of Registered Nurses Employed in Physicians' Offices.* DHEW Publication No. (HRA) 75–50. U.S. Government Printing Office, Washington, D.C., 1975.

97. Donabedian, A., "Some Issues in Evaluating the Quality of Nursing Care." *Am. J. Pub. Health,* **59:**1833–36, October 1969.

98. Downs. F. S., and Newman, M. A., *A Source Book of Nursing Research.* F. A. Davis, Philadelphia, 1973.

99. Doyle, T., *et al., The Impact of Health System Changes on the Nation's Requirements for Registered Nurses.* DHEW Publication No. (HRA) 78–9. U.S. Government Printing Office, Washington, D.C., 1978.

100. Dubin, R., *Theory Building.* Free Press, New York, 1968.

101. Dunn, H. L., "The Biological Basis for High-Level Wellness." Council for High-Level Wellness, Washington, D.C., October 1959.

102. Dunn, H. L., "Points of Attack for Raising the Levels of Wellness." *J. Nat. Med. A.,* **49:**225–55, 1957.

103. Eddington, E. S., *Statistical Inference: The Distribution-Free Approach.* McGraw-Hill Book Co., New York, 1969.

104. Edwards, A. L., *Experimental Design in Psychological Research,* 4th ed. Holt, Rinehart and Winston, New York, 1972.

105. Edwards, A. L., *Statistical Analysis,* 4th ed. Holt, Rinehart and Winston, New York, 1974.

106. Edwards, W. M., and Flynn, F., *Gerontology: A Core List of Significant Works.* Institute of Gerontology, The University of Michigan–Wayne State University, Ann Arbor, Mich., 1978.

107. Elliott, J. E., and Kearns, J. (eds.), *Analysis and Planning for Improved Distribution of Nursing Personnel and Services: Final Report.* DHEW Publication No. (HRA) 79–16, Government Printing Office, Washington, D.C., 1979.

108. English, H. B., and English, A. C., *A Comprehensive Dictionary of Psychological and Psychoanalytical Terms.* Longmans, Green and Co., New York, 1958.

109. Ericksen, G. L., *Scientific Inquiry in the Behavioral Sciences.* Scott, Foresman and Co., Glenview, Ill., 1970.

110. Federer, W. T., *Experimental Designs: Theory and Application*. Macmillan Publishing Co., Inc., New York, 1955.

111. Feibleman, J. K., "The Nature of the Hypothesis." *Nurs. Forum*, **1:**46–60, winter 1961–1962.

112. Festinger, L., and Katz, D. (eds.), *Research Methods in the Behavioral Sciences*. The Dryden Press, New York, 1953.

113. Fidler, N. D., "The Need for Research in Nursing." *Can. Nurse*, **55:**224–26, March 1969.

114. Finney, D. J., *Experimental Design and Its Statistical Basis*. University of Chicago Press, Chicago, 1974.

115. Fisher, R. A., *The Design of Experiments*, 2nd ed. Oliver and Boyd, London, 1935. (See also 1974 edition with G. T. Prance).

116. Flagle, C. D., "How to Allocate Progressive Patient Care Beds," in L. E. Weeks and J. R. Griffith (eds.), *Progressive Patient Care: An Anthology*. The University of Michigan, Ann Arbor, 1964, pp. 47–57.

117. Flagle, C. D., "Operational Research in the Health Services," in *Research Methodology and Potential in Community Health and Preventive Medicine. Ann. N.Y. Acad. Sci.*, **107:**748–59, May 23, 1963.

118. Flanagan, J. C., "Critical Requirements: A New Approach to Employee Evaluation." *Personnel Psychology*, **2:**419–25, winter 1949.

119. Flanagan, J. C., *Principles and Procedures in Evaluating Performance*. American Management Association, New York, 1952.

120. Flanagan, J. C., *The Critical Incident Technique in the Study of Individuals*. American Council on Education, Washington, D.C., 1952.

121. Fleck, A. C., "Evaluation Research Programs in Public Health Practice," in *Research Methodology and Potential in Community Health and Preventive Medicine, Ann. N.Y. Acad. Sci.*, **107:**717–24, May 22, 1963.

122. Flook, E. E., and Sanazaro, P. J., (eds.), *Health Services Research and R&D in Perspective*. Health Administration Press, The University of Michigan, Ann Arbor, 1973.

123. Foerst, H. V., *et al.*, *Planning for Nursing Needs and Resources*. DHEW Publication No. (NIH) 72–87. U.S. Government Printing Office, Washington, D.C., 1972.

124. Fortin, F., and Kerouac, S., "Validation of Questionnaires on Physical Function." *Nurs. Res.*, **26:**128–35, March–April 1977.

125. Freeman, R., *et al.*, "Patient Care Research: Report of a Symposium." *Am. J. Pub. Health*, **56:**965–69, June 1963.

126. French, D., *An Approach to Measuring Results in Social Work*. Columbia University Press, New York, 1952.

127. French, J. R. P., Jr., "Experiments in Field Settings," in L. Festinger and D. Katz, *Research Methods in the Behavioral Sciences*. The Dryden Press, New York, 1953, pp. 98–135.

128. Gebbie, K. M. (ed.), *Summary of the Second National Conference on Classification of Nursing Diagnoses*. National Group for the Classification of Nursing Diagnoses, St. Louis, 1976.

129. George, F. L., and Kuehn, R. P., *Patterns of Patient Care*. Macmillan Publishing Co., Inc., New York, 1955.

130. Georgopoulos, B. S. (ed.), *Organization Research on Health Institutions.* Institute for Social Research, The University of Michigan, Ann Arbor, 1972.

131. Georgopoulos, B. S., and Mann, F. C., *The Community General Hospital.* Macmillan Publishing Co., Inc., New York, 1962.

132. Georgopoulos, B. S., and Tannenbaum, A. S., "A Study of Organizational Effectiveness." *Am. Sociol. Rev.,* **22:**534–40, October 1957.

133. Gingras, P. (ed.), *National Conferences.* DHEW Publication No. (HRA) 77–3. U.S. Government Printing Office, Washington, D.C., 1977.

134. Giovannetti, P., *Patient Classification Systems and Their Uses: A Description and Analysis.* DHEW Publication No. (HRA) 78–22, National Technical Information Service, Springfield, Va., 1978.

135. Glock, C. Y., (ed.), *Survey Research in the Social Sciences.* Russell Sage Foundation, New York, 1967.

136. Goldfarb, M., "Methodological Approaches for Determining Health Manpower Planning Models." *Medical Care Rev.,* **32:**1–27, June 1975.

137. Goldstein, P., *How to Do an Experiment.* Harcourt, Brace and Co., New York, 1957.

138. Gomberg, W., *The Validity of Time Study Techniques.* Science Research Associates, Chicago, 1948.

139. Good, C. V., and Scates, D. E. *Methods of Research.* Appleton-Century-Crofts, Inc., New York, 1954.

140. Goode, W. J., "A Theory of Role Strain." *Am. Sociol. Rev.,* **25:**483–96, August 1960.

141. Goode, W. J., and Hatt, E., *Methods in Social Research.* McGraw-Hill, New York, 1952.

142. Gordon, M., *A First Course in Statistics.* Macmillan Publishing Co., Inc., New York, 1978.

143. Gortner, S. R., and Nahm, H., "An Overview of Nursing Research in the United States." *Nurs. Res.,* **26:**10–33, January–February 1977.

144. Gray, R., and Sauer, K., *Nursing Resources and Requirements: A Guide for State Level Planning.* Western Interstate Commission on Higher Education, Boulder, Col., 1978.

145. Greenberg, B. G., "The Philosophy and Methods of Research," in *Report on Nursing Research Conference,* H. H. Werley (ed.). Walter Reed Army Institute of Research, Washington, D.C., 1962, pp. 1–100.

146. Greenberg, B. G., "The Use of Analysis of Covariance and Balancing in Analytical Surveys." *Am. J. Pub. Health,* **43:**692–99, June 1953.

147. Gross, N. C., Mason, W. S., and McEachern, A. W.. *Explorations in Role Analysis: Studies of the School Superintendency Roles.* John Wiley & Sons, Inc., New York, 1958.

148. Guthrie, E. R., "Psychological Facts and Psychological Theory." *Psychol. Bull.,* **43:**1, January 1946.

149. Guttentag, M., and Struening, E. L., *Handbook of Evaluation Research.* Sage Publications, Inc., Beverly Hills, Calif., 1975.

150. Guttman L., "A Basis for Scaling Qualitative Data." *Am. Sociol. Rev.,* 9: 139–50, April 1944.

151. Habenstein, R. A., and Christ, E. A., *Professionalizer, Traditionalizer, and Utilizer*. University of Missouri Press, Columbia, 1955.

152. Habenstein, R. W. (ed.), *Pathways to Data*. Aldine Publishing Co., New York, 1970.

153. Hadley, B. J. (ed.), *Methods for Studying Nurse Staffing in a Patient Unit*. DHEW Publication No. (HRA) 78–3, U.S. Government Printing Office, Washington, D.C., 1978.

154. Hagen, E., and Wolff, L., *Nursing Leadership Behavior in General Hospitals*. Teachers College, Columbia University, New York, 1961.

155. Hagood, M. J., and Price, D. O., *Statistics for Sociologists* (rev. ed.). Holt, Rinehart and Winston, New York, 1952.

156. Haldeman, J. C., and Abdellah, F. G., "Concepts of Progressive Patient Care." *Hospitals, J.A.H.A.*, **33:**38–42, 142, 144, 41–46, May 16 and June 1, 1959.

157. Hammond, K. R., and Householder, J. E., *Introduction to the Statistical Method*. Alfred A. Knopf, New York, 1962.

158. Hanchett, E. S., *The Problem Oriented System: A Literature Review*. DHEW Publication No. (HRA) 78–6. Health Resources Administration, Hyattsville, Md., 1977.

159. Hansen, M. H., Hurwitz, W. N., and Madow, W. G., *Sample Survey Methods and Theory*. 2 vols. John Wiley & Sons, Inc., New York, 1953.

160. Hasselmeyer, E. G., *Behavior Patterns of Premature Infants*. U.S. Public Health Service Publication No. 840. Government Printing Office, Washington, D.C., 1961.

161. Hardy, M. E., "Theories: Components, Development, Evaluation." *Nurs. Res.*, **23:**100–107, March–April 1974.

162. Hardy, M. E., *Theoretical Foundations for Nursing*. MSS Information Corp., New York, 1973.

163. Harris, M. I., "Theory Building in Nursing." *Image*, **4:**6–10, 1971.

164. Haussmann, R. K. D., and Hegyvary, S. T., *Monitoring Quality of Nursing Care, Part III: Professional Review for Nursing: An Empirical Investigation*. DHEW Publication No. (HRA) 77–70. Health Resources Administration, Hyattsville, Md., 1977.

165. Haussmann, R. K. D., Hegyvary, S. T., and Newman, J. F., *Monitoring Quality of Nursing Care, Part II: Assessment and Study of Correlates*. DHEW Publication No. (HRA) 76–7. Health Resources Administration, Hyattsville, Md., 1976.

166. Hawley, P. R., "Evaluation of the Quality of Patient Care." *Am. J. Pub. Health*, **45:**1533–37, December 1955.

167. Health Resources Administration, *Conditions for Change in the Health Care System*. DHEW Publication No. (HRA) 78–642, U.S. Government Printing Office, Washington, D.C., 1978.

168. Henderson, V., "An Overview of Nursing Research." *Nurs. Res.*, **6:**61–71, October 1957.

169. Henderson, V., *Nursing Studies Index*, Vol. IV, 1957–1959. J. B. Lippincott Co., Philadelphia, 1963. See also Vol. III, 1950–1956 (1966); Vol. II, 1930–1949 (1970); and Vol. I, 1900–1929 (1972).

170. Henderson, V., "Research in Nursing Practice—When?" *Nurs. Res.,* **4:**99, February 1956.

171. Henderson, V., *The Basic Principles of Nursing Care.* Cornwell Press, Ltd., London, 1958.

172. Herzog, E., "Research, Demonstrations and Common-Sense." *Child Welfare, J. Child Welfare League of America,* **41:**243–48, June 1962.

173. Herzog, E., *Some Guidelines for Evaluative Research.* Childrens Bureau Publication No. 375. U.S. Department of Health, Education and Welfare, Washington, D.C., 1959.

174. Heslin, P., "Evaluating Clinical Performance." *Nurs. Outlook,* **11:**344–45, May 1963.

175. Hess, I., Riedel, D. C., and Fitzpatrick, T. B., *Probability Sampling of Hospitals and Patients,* 2nd ed. Bureau of Hospital Administration, Research Series No. 1, University of Michigan, Ann Arbor, 1975.

176. Hiestand, D., and Ostow, M., *Health Manpower Information for Policy Guidance.* Ballinger Publishing Co., Cambridge, Mass., 1976.

177. Hilbert, H., and Hildebrand, E. M., "Studies in Nursing: Notes and Observations." *Nurs. Outlook,* **10:**44–46, January 1962.

178. Hildebrand, D. K., Laing, J. D., and Rosenthal, H., *Prediction Analysis of Cross Classifications.* John Wiley & Sons, Inc., New York, 1977.

179. Hill, A. B., *Principles of Medical Statistics,* 4th ed. rev. Oxford University Press, New York, 1971.

180. Hillway, T., *Introduction to Research.* Houghton Mifflin Co., Boston, 1964.

181. Hollander, M., and Wolfe, D. A., *Nonparametric Statistical Methods.* Wiley-Interscience, New York, 1973.

182. Hopkins, C. E., *et al., Outcomes Conference I–II: Methodology of Identifying, Measuring and Evaluating Outcomes of Health Service Programs, Systems and Sub-systems.* National Technical Information Service, Springfield, Va., 1970. (Report No. HSRD 70–39.)

183. Horn, B. J., and Swain, M. A., *Criterion Measures of Nursing Care Quality.* DHEW Publication No. (PHS) 78–3187. National Center for Health Services Research, Hyattsville, Md., 1978.

184. Howland, D., "A Hospital System Model." *Nurs. Res.,* **12:**232–36, fall 1963.

185. Howland, D., "Approaches to the Systems Problem." *Nurs. Res.,* **12:** 172–74, summer 1963.

186. Howland, D., "Engineering in Interdisciplinary Research." *J. Engineering Ed.,* **52:**664–70. June 1962.

187. Howland, D., and McDowell, W. E., "The Measurement of Patient Care: A Conceptual Framework." *Nurs. Res.,* **13:**4–7, winter 1964.

188. Hughes, E. C., Hughes, H. M., and Deutscher, I., *Twenty-Thousand Nurses Tell Their Story.* J. B. Lippincott Co., Philadelphia, 1958.

189. Hyde, A., "The American Nurses' Foundation's Contributions to Research in Nursing." *Nurs. Res.,* **26:**225–27, May–June 1977.

190. Hyman, H. H., *Interviewing in Social Research.* University of Chicago Press, Chicago, 1954.

191. Hyman, H. H., *Survey Design and Analysis*. The Free Press of Glencoe, New York, 1955.

192. Institute of Medicine, *A Manpower Policy for Primary Health Care*. National Academy of Sciences, Washington, D.C., 1978.

193. Jackson, J. M., "The Effect of Changing the Leadership of Small Groups." *Human Relations,* **6:**25–44, 1953.

194. Jacox, A., and Prescott, P., "Determining a Study's Relevance for Clinical Practice." *Am. J. Nurs.,* **78:**1882–89, November 1978.

195. Jelinek, R. C., and Dennis, L. C., *A Review and Evaluation of Nursing Productivity*. DHEW Publication No. (HRA) 77–15. U.S. Government Printing Office, Washington, D. C., 1976.

196. Jelinek, R. C., Haussman, R. K. D., Hegyvary, S. T., and Newman, J. F., Jr., *A Methodology for Monitoring Quality of Nursing Care*. DHEW Publication No. (HRA) 76–25. U.S. Government Printing Office, Washington, D.C., 1975.

197. Jessen, R. J., *Statistical Survey Techniques*. John Wiley & Sons, Inc., New York, 1978.

198. John, A. L., *A Study of the Psychiatric Nurse*. Livingstone, Edinburgh, 1961.

199. Johns, E., and Pfefferkorn, B., *An Activity Analysis of Nursing*. Committee on the Grading of Nursing Schools, New York, 1934.

200. Johnson, D. E., "The Nature of a Science of Nursing." *Nurs. Outlook,* **7:**291–94, May 1959.

201. Johnson, D. E., "A Philosophy of Nursing." *Nurs. Outlook,* **7:**198–200, April 1959.

202. Johnson, D. E., "The Significance of Nursing Care." *Am. J. Nurs.,* **61:** 63–66, November 1961.

203. Johnson, W. L., "Longitudinal Study of Family Adjustments to Myocardial Infarction." *Nurs. Res.,* **12:**242–47, fall 1963.

204. Johnson, W. L., "Research Programs of the National League for Nursing." *Nurs. Res.,* **26:**172–76, May–June, 1977.

205. Johod, G., *Information Storage and Retrieval Systems for Individual Researchers*. Wiley-Interscience, New York, 1970.

206. Jones, D. C., *et al., Trends in Registered Nurse Supply*. DHEW Publication No. (HRA) 76–15. U.S. Government Printing Office, Washington, D.C., 1976.

207. Jones, P. E., and Jakob, D. F., *An Investigation of the Definition of Nursing Diagnoses*. University of Toronto, Toronto, 1977.

208. Jones, P. S., "An Adaptation Model for Nursing Practice." *Am. J. Nurs.,* **78:**1900–1906, November 1978.

209. Kahn, R. L., and Cannell, C. F., *The Dynamics of Interviewing*. John Wiley & Sons, Inc., 1957.

210. Kalisch, P. A., and Kalisch, B. J., *Nursing Involvement in the Health Planning Process*. DHEW Publication No. (HRA) 78–25. (HRP-0500201.) National Technical Information Service, Springfield, Va., 1977.

211. Kalisch, P. A., and Kalisch, B. J., *The Advance of American Nursing*. Little Brown and Co., Boston, 1978.

212. Kant, I., "The Critique of Pure Reason," in *Great Books of the Western World,* Vol. 42. Encyclopaedia Britannica, Inc., Chicago, 1952.

213. Katz, D., "Field Studies," in L. Festinger and D. Katz (eds.), *Research Methods in the Behavioral Sciences.* The Dryden Press, Inc., New York, 1 953, pp. 56–97.

214. Kaufmann, F., *Methodology of Research in the Social Sciences.* Oxford University Press, New York, 1944.

215. Kempthorne, O., *The Design and Analysis of Experiments.* Robert E. Krieger Publishing Co., New York, 1973.

216. Kendall, P. L., "Methodological Appendix," in R. K. Merton, G. G. Reader, and P. L. Kendall (eds.), *The Student Physician.* Harvard University Press, Cambridge, Mass., 1957.

217. Kendall, M. G., and Buckland, W. R., *A Dictionary of Statistical Terms,* 3rd ed. Longman Group Ltd., London, 1976.

218. Ketefian, S., (ed.). *Translation of Theory into Nursing Practice and Education.* Division of Nursing, School of Education, Health, Nursing and Arts Professions. New York University, New York, 1975.

219. Kidd, C. V., *American Universities and Federal Research.* Belknap Press of Harvard University Press, Cambridge, Mass., 1959.

220. Kidd, C. V., "The Effect of Research Emphasis on Research Itself." *Res. and Med. Ed.,* **37:**95–100, December 1962.

221. Kish, L., "Some Statistical Problems in Research Design." *Am. Sociol. Rev.,* **24:**328–38, June 1959.

222. Klein, M. W., Malone, M. F., Bennis, W. G., and Berkowitz, N. H., "Problems of Measuring Patient Care in an Out-Patient Department." *J. Health and Human Behavior,* **2:**138–44, 1961.

223. Knapp, R. G., *Basic Statistics for Nurses.* John Wiley & Sons, Inc., New York, 1978.

224. Knopf, L., *From Student to Registered Nurse: A Report of the Nurse Career-Pattern Study.* DHEW Publication No. 72–130. U.S. Government Printing Office, Washington, D.C., 1972.

225. Knopf, L., *Registered Nurses One and Five Years After Graduation.* National League for Nursing, New York, 1975.

226. Kodadek, S. (ed.), *Inventory of Innovations in Nursing.* DHEW Publication No. (HRA) 77–2. U.S. Government Printing Office, Washington, D.C., 1976.

227. Kraft, C. H., and Elder, C. V., *Introduction to Statistics.* Macmillan Publishing Co., Inc., New York, 1968.

228. Kruskal, W. H., and Tanur, J. M., *International Encyclopedia of Statistics.* The Free Press, New York, 1978.

229. Lazarsfeld, P. F., *et al., The People's Choice.* Columbia University Press, New York, 1948.

230. Lazarsfeld, P. F., "The Sociology of Empirical Social Research." *Am. Sociol. Rev.,* **27:**757–67, December 1962.

231. Lazarsfeld, P. F., and Rosenberg, M., *The Language of Social Research.* The Free Press of Glencoe, New York, 1955.

232. Lentz, E. M., and Michaels, R. W., "Comparisons Between Medical and Surgical Nurses." *Nurs. Res.,* **8:**192–97, fall 1959.

233. Leone, L. P., "Research in Nursing and Nursing Education," in L. E. Heidgerken (ed.), *The Improvement of Nursing Through Research*. Catholic University of America Press, Washington, D.C., 1959, pp. 17–28.

234. Levine, E.,"Experimental Design in Nursing Research." *Nurs. Res.*, **9**:203–12, fall 1960.

235. Levine, E., "The A.B.C.'s of Statistics." *Am. J. Nurs.*, **59**:71–75, January 1959.

236. Levine, E., "What Do We Know About Nurse Practitioners." *Am. J. Nurs.*, **77**:1799–1803, November 1977.

237. Levine, E. (ed.), *Research on Nurse Staffing in Hospitals: Report of the Conference*. DHEW Publication No. (NIH) 73–434. U.S. Government Printing Office, Washington, D.C., 1973.

238. Levine, E., and Wright, S., "New Ways to Measure Personnel Turnover." *Hospitals, J.A.H.A.*, **31**:38–42, August 1, 1957.

239. Levine, H. D., and Phillip, P. J., *Factors Affecting Staffing Levels and Patterns of Nursing Personnel*. DHEW Publication No. (HRA) 75–6. U.S. Government Printing Office, Washington, D.C., 1975.

240. Levinson, D. J., "Role, Personality and Social Structure in the Organization Setting." *J. Abnorm. Psychol.*, **58**:170–80, 1959.

241. Lewin, K., *Field Theory in Social Science-Selected Theoretical Papers*. Harper and Row, New York, 1951.

242. Li, C. C., *Path Analysis*. Boxwood Press, Pacific Grove, Calif., 1975.

243. Likert, R., *New Patterns of Management*. McGraw-Hill, New York, 1961.

244. Lindsay, D. R., and Allen, E. M., "Medical Research: Past Support, Future Directions." *Science*, **134**:2017–24, December 22, 1961.

245. Lindzey, G. (ed.), *Handbook of Social Psychology*, 5 vols. Addison-Wesley, Cambridge, Mass., 1968.

246. Little, A. D., Inc., *Computer-Based Patient Monitoring Systems*. DHEW Publication No. (HRA) 76–3143. National Center for Health Services Research, Hyattsville, Md., 1976.

247. Little, D. E., and Carnevali, D. L., *Nursing Care Planning*. J. B. Lippincott Co., Philadelphia, 1969.

248. Lum, J., and Leonhard G. (eds.), *Report of the Panel of Expert Consultants*. Western Interstate Commission for Higher Education, Boulder, Col., 1978.

249. Lundberg, G. A., *Social Research: A Study in Methods of Gathering Data*, rev. ed. Greenwood Press, Inc., Westport, Conn., 1968.

250. Macgregor, F. C., *Social Science in Nursing*. Russell Sage Foundation, New York, 1960.

251. Madge, J. H., *The Tools of Social Science*. Longmans, Green and Co., New York, 1953.

252. Mainland, D., *Elementary Medical Statistics*. W. B. Saunders Co., Philadelphia, 1963.

253. Mainland, D., "The Clinical Trial—Some Difficulties and Suggestions." *J. Chron. Dis.*, **11**:484–96, May 1960.

254. Malone, M. F., "Research as Viewed by Researcher and Practitioner." *Nurs. Forum*, **1**:39–55, spring 1962.

255. Manaser, J. C., and Werner, A. M., *Instruments for the Study of Nurse-Patient Interaction.* Macmillan Publishing Co., Inc., New York, 1964.

256. Maranell, G. M., *Scaling: A Source Book for Behavioral Scientists.* Aldine Publishing Co., Chicago, 1974.

257. Marascuilo, L. A., *Statistical Methods for Behavioral Science Research.* McGraw-Hill Book Co., New York, 1971.

258. Matarazzo, J. D., Saslow, G., and Matarazzo, R. G. "The Interaction Chronograph as an Instrument for Objective Measurement of Interaction Patterns During Interviews." *J. Psychol.,* **41:**347–67, 1956.

259. Matek, S. J., *Accountability: Its Meaning and Its Relevance to the Health Care Field.* DHEW Publication No. (HRA) 77–72. (HRP–0500101.) National Technical Information Service, Springfield, Va., 1977.

260. Mathews, B. P., "Measurement of Psychological Aspects of the Nurse-Patient Relationship." *Nurs. Res.,* **11:**154–62, summer 1962.

261. Mayers, M. G., *A Systematic Approach to the Nursing Care Plan.* Appleton-Century-Crofts, New York, 1972.

262. McGinnis, R., "Randomization and Inference in Sociological Research." *Am. Sociol. Rev.,* **23:**408–14, August 1958.

263. McNerney, W. J., *et al., Hospital and Medical Economics.* Hospital Research and Educational Trust, Chicago, 1962.

264. Mechanic, D., "Approaches to Controlling the Costs of Medical Care: Short-Range and Long-Range Alternatives." *New Engl. J. Med.,* **298:**249–54, Feb. 2, 1978.

265. Mechanic, D., and Volkart, E. H., "Stress Illness, Behavior, and the Sick Role." *Am. Sociol. Rev.,* **26:**51–58, 1961.

266. Medicus Systems Corporation, *Effects of Nursing Education on Nursing Performance.* Prepared under contract No. HRA 231–77–0121 with Division of Nursing, HRA. Hyattsville, Md., 1979.

267. Merton, R. K., Reader, G. G., and Kendall, P. L. (eds.), *The Student Physician.* Harvard University Press, Cambridge, Mass., 1957.

268. Merton, R. K., Broom, L., and Cottrell, L. S. (eds.), *Sociology Today.* Basic Books, Inc., New York, 1959.

269. Merton R. K., Fiske, M., and Kendall, P. L., *The Focused Interview.* Bureau of Applied Social Research, Columbia University, New York, 1952.

270. Meyer, B., and Heidgerken, L. E., *Research in Nursing.* J. B. Lippincott Co., Philadelphia, 1962.

271. Meyer, G. R., *Tenderness and Technique: Nursing Values in Transition.* Institute of Industrial Relations, University of California, Los Angeles, 1960.

272. Millman, M. L. (ed.), *Nursing Personnel and the Changing Health Care System.* Ballinger Publishing Co., Cambridge, Mass., 1978.

273. Mills, J. S., *A System of Logic,* 8th ed. Harper and Row, New York, 1874.

274. Mosteller, F., Rourke, R. E. K., and Thomas, G. B., Jr., *Probability with Statistical Applications.* Addison-Wesley Publishing Co., Inc., Reading, Mass, 1974.

275. Mosteller, F., and Tukey, J. W., *Data Analysis and Regression.* Addison-Wesley Publishing Co., Reading, Mass., 1977.

276. Mullane, M. K., "A Self-Appraisal Guide for Hospital Nursing Services." Detroit and Tri-County League for Nursing, Detroit, 1959.

277. Nash, P. M., *Evaluation of Employment Opportunities for Newly Licensed Nurses.* DHEW Publication No. (HRA) 75–12, U.S. Government Printing Office, Washington, D.C., 1975.

278. Nathan, R. A., Associates, Inc., *Methodological Approaches for Determining Health Manpower Supply and Requirements. Vol. 1. Analytical Perspective. Vol. 2. Practical Planning Manual.* DHEW Publication No. (HRA) 76–14511 and DHEW Publication No. (HRA) 76–14512. National Technical Information Service, Springfield, Va., 1976.

279. National Center for Health Services Research, *Criterion Measures of Nursing Care Quality.* NCHSR Research Summary Series, DHEW Publication No. (PHS) 78–3187, Washington, D.C., August 1978.

280. National Center for Health Services Research, *Recent Studies in Health Services Research.* DHEW Publication No. (HRA) 77–3162. National Center for Health Services Research, Hyattsville, Md., 1977.

281. National Center for Health Statistics, *Health United States, 1978.* DHEW Publication No. (PHS) 78–1232. U.S. Government Printing Office, Washington, D.C., 1979.

282. National Commission for Manpower Policy, *Employment Impacts of Health Policy Developments.* Special Report No. 11. The Commission, Washington, D.C. October 1976.

283. National League for Nursing, "The National League for Nursing—Its Role in Nursing Research." *Nurs. Res.,* **9:**190–95, fall 1960.

284. National League for Nursing, *Selected Management Information Systems for Public Health/Community Health Agencies.* National League for Nursing, New York, 1978.

285. National League for Nursing, *Nursing Data Book.* National League for Nursing, New York, 1978.

286. National League of Nursing Education, *A Study of Nursing Service in One Children's and Twenty-one General Hospitals.* National League of Nursing Education, New York, 1948.

287. National League of Nursing Education, *A Study of Pediatric Nursing.* National League of Nursing Education, New York, 1947.

288. Naval Research Advisory Committee, *Basic Research in the Navy,* Vol. 1 of a Report to the Secretary of the Navy on Basic Research in the Navy, Department of Navy, Washington, D.C., June 1, 1959.

289. New, P. K., *et al., Report: Nursing Research Conference.* Community Studies, Inc., Kansas City, Mo., 1957.

290. Newcomb, T. M., "An Approach to the Study of Communicative Acts," in P. Hare, E. F. Borgatta, and R. F. Bales (eds.), *Small Groups.* Alfred A. Knopf, New York, 1955, pp. 149–63.

291. Newcomb, T. M., "Role Behavior in the Study of Individual Personality and of Groups." *J. Personality,* **18:**273–89, 1950.

292. Newman, J. R., *What Is Science?* Washington Square Press, New York, 1961.

293. Nite, G., and Willis, F., *The Coronary Patient: Hospital Care and Rehabilitation.* Macmillan Publishing Co., Inc., New York, 1964.

294. Notter, L., and Spector, A. F., *Nursing Research in the South: A Survey.* Southern Regional Education Board, Atlanta, 1974.

295. Nuffield Provincial Hospitals Trust, *Problems and Progress in Medical Care.* Oxford University Press, London, 1964.

296. Office of Federal Statistical Policy and Standards, *Social Indicators, 1976.* U.S. Government Printing Office, Washington, D.C., 1977.

297. O'Malley, M., and Kossack, C. F., "A Statistical Study of Factors Influencing the Quality of Patient Care in Hospitals." *Am. J. Pub. Health,* **40:** 1428–36, November 1950.

298. O'Neil, W. M., *Fact and Theory.* Sydney University Press, Sydney, Australia, 1969.

299. Orlando, I. J., *The Dynamic Nurse-Patient Relationship.* G. P. Putnam's Sons, New York, 1961.

300. Parten, M. B., *Surveys, Polls, and Samples.* Harper and Row, New York, 1950.

301. Patrick, C., "Scientific Thought." *J. Psychol.,* **5:**55–83, 1938.

302. Payne, S. L., *The Art of Asking Questions.* Princeton University Press, Princeton, New Jer., 1951.

303. Peak, Helen, "Problems of Objective Observations," in L. Festinger and D. Katz (eds.), *Research Methods in the Behavioral Sciences.* The Dryden Press, Inc., New York, 1953, pp. 243–99.

304. Peatman, J. G., *Descriptive and Sampling Statistics.* Harper and Row, New York, 1947.

305. Peirce, C. S. S., *Values in a Universe of Chance.* Doubleday and Co., New York, 1958.

306. Peplau, H. E., *Interpersonal Relations in Nursing.* G. P. Putnam's Sons, New York, 1952.

307. Phillips, D. S., *Basic Statistics for Health Science Students.* W. H. Freeman and Co., San Francisco, 1978.

308. Phillips, J. S., and Thompson, R. F., *Statistics for Nurses: The Evaluation of Quantitative Information.* Macmillan Publishing Co., Inc., New York, 1967.

309. Phillips, T. P. (ed.), *The Doctorally Prepared Nurse. Report of Two Conferences on the Demand for and Education of Nurses with Doctoral Degrees.* DHEW Publication No. (HRA) 76–18. U.S. Government Printing Office, Washington, D.C., 1976.

310. Polit, D., and Hungler, B., *Nursing Research: Principles and Methods.* J. B. Lippincott Co., Philadelphia, 1978.

311. Reiter, F., and Kakosh, M. E., *Quality of Nursing Care.* A Report of a Field Study to Establish Criteria, 1950–1954, Institute of Research and Studies in Nursing Education, Division of Nursing Education, Teachers College, Columbia University, New York, 1963.

312. Riehl, J. P., and Roy, Sister C., *Conceptual Models for Nursing Practice.* Appleton-Century-Crofts, New York, 1974.

313. Roberts, D. E., and Freeman, R. B. (eds.), *Redesigning Nursing Education for Public Health: Report of the Conference, May 23–25, 1973.* DHEW Publication No. (HRA) 75–75, Health Resources Administration, Hyattsville, Md., 1975.

314. Rogers, M. E., "Some Comments on the Theoretical Basis of Nursing Practice." *Nurs. Sci.,* **1:**11–13, 60–61, April–May 1963.

315. Rogers, M. E., *An Introduction to the Theoretical Basis of Nursing.* F. A. Davis Co., Philadelphia, 1970.

316. Ruesch, J., and Kees, W., *Nonverbal Communication: Notes on the Visual Perception of Human Relations.* University of California Press, Berkeley, 1956.

317. Runkel, P. J., and McGrath, J. E., *Research on Human Behavior: A Systematic Guide to Method.* Holt, Rinehart and Winston, Inc., New York, 1972.

318. Rutman, L., *Evaluation Research Methods: A Basic Guide.* Sage Publications, Beverly Hills, 1977.

319. Safford, B. J., and Schlotfeldt, R. M., "Nursing Service Staffing and Quality of Nursing Care." *Nurs. Res.,* **9:**149–54, summer 1960.

320. Schlotfeldt, R. M., "Reflections on Nursing Research." *Am. J. Nurs.,* **60:**492–94, April 1960.

321. Schlotfeldt, R. M., "Summaries of Workshop Group Discussions, Conferences and Workshops on Research in Nursing, Cleveland, Ohio," Sept. 14–17, American Nurses' Foundation, Inc., New York, 1958.

322. Schlotfeldt, R. M., "The Significance of Empirical Research for Nursing." *Nurs. Res.,* **20:**140–42, March–April 1971.

323. Schwartz, D., Henley, B., and Zeitz, L., *The Elderly Ambulatory Patient: Nursing and Psychosocial Needs.* Macmillan Publishing Co., Inc., New York, 1964.

324. Schwirian, P. M., *Prediction of Successful Nursing Performance, Part I and Part II.* DHEW Publication No. (HRA) 77–27. U.S. Government Printing Office, Washington, D.C., 1977.

325. See, E. M., "The American Nurses' Association and Research in Nursing." *Nurs. Res.,* **26:**165–71, May–June 1977.

326. Seeman, M., and Evans, J. W., "Stratification and Hospital Care: II. The Objective Criteria of Performance." *Am. Sociol. Rev.,* **26:**193–204, 1961.

327. Segall, M., and Sauer, K., "Nurse Staffing in the Context of Institutional and State-Level Planning." *Nurs. Admin. Q.,* **2:**39–50, fall 1977.

328. Selltiz, C., Jahoda, M., Deutsch, M., and Cook, S. W., *Research Methods in Social Relations,* 3rd ed. Holt, Rinehart and Winston, New York, 1976.

329. Selvin, H. C., "A Critique of Tests of Significance in Survey Research." *Am. Sociol. Rev.,* **22:**519–27, October 1957.

330. Selye, H., *From Dream to Discovery: On Being a Scientist.* Arno, New York, 1975.

331. Sheps, M. C., "Approaches to the Quality of Hospital Care." *Pub. Health Rep.,* **70:**877–86, September 1955.

332. Shuman, L. S., Speas, R. D., Jr., and Young, J. P., *Operations Research in Health Care: A Critical Analysis.* The Johns Hopkins University Press, Baltimore, 1975.

333. Sidman, M., *Tactics of Scientific Research.* Basic Books, Inc., New York, 1960.

334. Simmons, L. W., and Henderson, V., *Nursing Research: A Survey and Assessment.* Appleton-Century-Crofts, Inc., New York, 1964.

335. Simon, J. R., "Nurses' Ratings of Patient Welfare as Criterion Measures in the Health Sciences." *Occupational Psychology,* **35:**10–22, 1961.

336. Sloan, F. A., *Equalizing Access to Nursing Services: The Geographic Dimension.* DHEW Publication No. (HRA) 78–51, U.S. Government Printing Office, Washington, D.C., 1978.

337. Slonim, M. J., "Sampling in a Nutshell." *J. Am. Statistical A.,* **52:**146–61, June 1957.

338. Smith, D. M., "Myth and Method in Nursing Practice." *Am. J. Nurs.,* **64:**68–72, February 1964.

339. Solon, J. A., Sheps, C. G., Lee, S. S., and Barbano, J. P., "Patterns of Medical Care: Validity of Interview Information on Use of Hospital Clinics." *J. Health Hum. Behav.,* **3:**21–30, Spring, 1962.

340. Som, R. K., *A Manual of Sampling Techniques.* Crane, Russak and Co., Inc., New York, 1973.

341. Somers, A. R., *Health Care in Transition: Directions for the Future.* Hospital Research and Educational Trust, Chicago, 1971.

342. Spiegelman, M., *Introduction to Demography.* Harvard University Press, Cambridge, Mass., 1968.

343. Stanford, E. D., and Kinsella, C. R., *Assessment of Nursing Services: Report of the Conference, June 1974.* DHEW Publication No. (HRA) 75–40. Health Resources Administration, Bethesda, Md., 1975.

344. Stephan, F. F., "History of the Uses of Modern Sampling Procedures." *J. Am. Statistical A.,* **43:**12–39, March 1948.

345. Stephenson, W., *The Study of Behavior: Q-Technique and Its Methodology.* The University of Chicago, Chicago, 1953.

346. Stewart, I. M., "Possibilities of Standardization in Nursing Techniques." *Mod. Hosp.,* **12:**541, June 1919.

347. Stodgill, R., *et al., Methods in the Study of Administrative Leadership.* Ohio Studies in Personnel Research, Monograph No. 80. Bureau of Business Research, Ohio State University, Columbus, Ohio, 1955.

348. Stumpf, J. C., "Communication Abilities of Veterans Administration Nurses." Doctoral Dissertation, University of Utah, Salt Lake City, 1961.

349. Sudman, S., *Applied Sampling.* Academic Press, New York, 1976.

350. Sultz, H. A., Zielezny, M., and Kinyon, L., *Longitudinal Study of Nurse Practitioners—Phase I.* DHEW Publication No. (HRA) 76–43. U.S. Government Printing Office, Washington, D.C., 1976.

351. Surgeon General's Consultant Group on Nursing, *Toward Quality in Nursing: Needs and Goals.* Government Printing Office, Washington, D.C., February 1963.

352. Swanson, G. E., Newcomb, T. M., Hartley, E. L. (eds.), *et al., Readings in Social Psychology.* Holt, Rinehart and Winston, New York, 1952.

353. System Sciences, Inc., *The Physician Extender Reimbursement Study,* Social Security Administration, Washington, D.C., 1978.

354. Tai, S. W., *Social Science Statistics: Its Elements and Applications.* Goodyear Publishing Co., Santa Monica, Calif., 1978.

355. Taton, R. (translated by A. J. Pomerans); *Reason and Chance in Scientific Discovery.* Hutchinson Co., Ltd., London, 1957.

356. Taylor, C. W., *et al.,* "Bridging the Gap Between Basic Research and Educational Practice." *Nat. Ed. A. J.,* **51:**23–25, January 1962.

357. Taylor, S. F., *A Short History of Science and Scientific Thought.* W. W. Norton and Co., New York, 1949.

358. Taylor, S. P., "Bibliography on Nursing Research, 1950–1974." *Nurs. Res.,* **24:**207–25, May–June 1975.

359. Theobold, D. W., *An Introduction to the Philosophy of Science.* Methuen and Co., London, 1968.

360. Tippett, L. H. C., *Random Sampling Numbers.* Cambridge University Press, Cambridge, London, 1927.

361. Travers, R. M. W., *An Introduction to Educational Research,* 3rd ed. Macmillan Publishing Co., Inc., New York, 1969.

362. Tryon, R. C., "Communality of a Variable: Formulation by Cluster Analysis." *Psychometrika,* **22:**241–60, 1957.

363. Tudor, G. E., "A Socio-psychiatric Nursing Approach to Intervention in a Problem of Mutual Withdrawal on a Mental Hospital Ward." *Psychiatry,* **15:**193, 1952.

364. Turk, H., and Ingles, T., *Clinic Nursing: Explorations in Role Innovations.* F. A. Davis Co., Philadelphia, 1963.

365. Underwood, B. J., *Psychological Research.* Appleton-Century-Crofts, Inc., New York, 1957.

366. United States Public Health Service, *Research in Nursing 1969–1972.* DHEW Publication No. (NIH) 73–489. Division of Nursing, Bethesda, Md., 1973. See also *Research in Nursing 1955–1968.* PHS Publication No. 1356. Division of Nursing, Bethesda, Md., 1970.

367. U.S. Public Health Service, Division of Hospital and Medical Facilities, *Elements of Progressive Patient Care.* U.S. Public Health Service Publication No. 930-C-1. Government Printing Office, Washington, D.C., 1962.

368. Van Den Berg, J. H., *Medical Ethics and Medical Power.* W. W. Norton and Co., New York, 1978.

369. Verhonick, P. J., *Descriptive Study Methods in Nursing.* Scientific Publication No. 219. Pan American Health Organization, Washington, D.C., 1971.

370. Veterans Administration, Department of Medicine and Surgery, "Report of the Committee on Measurement of the Quality of Medical Care." Washington, D.C., 1959.

371. Vreeland, E. M., "Nursing Research Programs of the Public Health Service." *Nurs. Res.,* **13:**148–58, spring 1964.

372. Vreeland, E. M., "The Nursing Research Grant and Fellowship Program in the Public Health Service." *Am. J. Nurs.,* **58:**1700–1702, December 1958.

373. Wallis, W. A., and Roberts, H. V., *Statistics: A New Approach.* The Free Press of Glencoe, New York, 1956.

374. Wardwell, W. I., and Bahnson, C. B., "Problems Encountered in Behavioral Science Research in Epidemiological Studies." *Am. J. Pub. Health,* **54:**972–81, June 1964.

375. Watt, J., "Nursing and Research in the Biological Sciences." *Nurs. Res.,* **6:**57–60, October 1957.

376. Weatherall, M., *Scientific Method*. The English Universities Press, Ltd., London, 1968.

377. Webb, S., and Webb, B., *Methods of Social Study*. Longmans, Green and Co., London, 1932.

378. Weeks, L. E., and Griffith, J. R. (eds.), *Progressive Patient Care: An Anthology*. University of Michigan Press, Ann Arbor, 1964.

379. Weisberg, H. F., and Bowen, B. D., *An Introduction to Survey Research and Data Analysis*. W. H. Freeman and Co., San Francisco, 1977.

380. Werley, H., "Promoting the Research Dimension in the Practice of Nursing Through the Establishment and Development of a Department of Nursing in an Institute of Research." *Military Med.*, **127:**219–31, March 1962.

381. Wessen, A., "Hospital Ideology and Communication Between Ward Personnel," in E. G. Jaco (ed.), *Patients, Physicians, and Illness*. Free Press of Glencoe, New York, 1958, pp. 448–68.

382. Wexler, D., *et al.*, "Sensory Deprivation: A Technique for Studying Psychiatric Aspects of Stress." *Arch. Neurol. Psychiat.*, **79:**225–33, 1958.

383. White, C. M., *Sources of Information in the Social Sciences*. American Library Association, Chicago, 1973.

384. Whiting, J. F., "Needs, Values, Perceptions, and the Nurse-Patient Relationship." *J. Clin. Psychol.*, **15:**146–50, 1959.

385. Whiting, J. F., *The Nurse-Patient Relationship and the Healing Process*. Pittsburgh Veterans Administration Hospital, Pittsburgh, 1958.

386. Wiener, N., *Cybernetics*. John Wiley & Sons, Inc., New York, 1957.

387. Wilcox, J., "Observer Factors in the Measurement of Blood Pressure." *Nurs. Res.*, **10:**4–17, winter 1961.

388. Willard, W. R., "The Present Status and Future Development of Community Health Research—A Critique: From the Viewpoint of Educational Institutions." *Ann. N.Y. Acad. Sci.*, **107:**776, May 22, 1963.

389. Williams, M. E., "The Patient Profile." *Nurs. Res.*, **9:**122–24, summer 1960.

390. Williamson, H. M., *et al.*, "Use of the EPPS for Identifying Personal Role Attributes Desirable in Nursing." *J. Health Hum. Behav.*, **4:**266–75, winter 1963.

391. Wilson, E. B., *An Introduction to Scientific Research*. McGraw-Hill, New York, 1952.

392. Wold, H., "Causal Inference from Observational Data." *J. Royal Statistical Society* (series A, Part 1), **119:**28–61, January 1956.

393. Wooden, H. E., "The Hospital's Purpose Is the Patient, But ——." *Mod. Hosp.*, **92:**90–96, January 1959.

394. Wooldridge, P. J., Leonard, R. C., and Skipper, J. K., Jr., *Methods of Clinical Experimentation to Improve Patient Care*. C. V. Mosby Co., St. Louis, 1978.

395. Wright, B., and Evitts, M. S., "Direct Factor Analysis in Sociometry." *Sociometry*, **24:**82–98, March 1961.

396. Wright, M. G., *The Improvement of Patient Care. A Study at Harper Hospital*. G. P. Putnam's Sons, New York, 1954.

397. Wright, S., "Turnover and Job Satisfaction." *Hospitals, J.A.H.A.*, **31**:47–52, October 1, 1957.

398. Young, P. V., *Scientific Social Surveys and Research*, 4th ed. Prentice-Hall, Englewood Cliffs, New Jer., 1966.

399. Yura, H., Ozimek, D., and Walsh, M. B., *Nursing Leadership: Theory and Process*. Appleton-Century-Crofts, New York, 1976.

400. Yura, H., and Walsh, M. B., *The Nursing Process: Assessing, Planning, Implementing, Evaluating,* 2nd ed. Appleton-Century-Crofts, New York, 1973.

INDEX FOR THE BIBLIOGRAPHY

INDEX TO AUTHORS
CITED IN REFERENCES

SUBJECT INDEX